Health Benefits of Fermented Foods and Beverages

Health Benefits of Fermented Foods and Beverages

EDITED BY
JYOTI PRAKASH TAMANG

CRC Press
Taylor & Francis Group
Boca Raton London New York

CRC Press is an imprint of the
Taylor & Francis Group, an **informa** business

CRC Press
Taylor & Francis Group
6000 Broken Sound Parkway NW, Suite 300
Boca Raton, FL 33487-2742

Printed on acid-free paper
Version Date: 20150204

International Standard Book Number-13: 978-1-4665-8809-7 (Hardback)

Visit the Taylor & Francis Web site at
http://www.taylorandfrancis.com

and the CRC Press Web site at
http://www.crcpress.com

Contents

Preface

Fermented foods contribute an important part of the diet of industrialized countries, and an equally essential role in nutrition in developing countries. More than 5000 varieties of common and uncommon fermented foods and alcoholic beverages are consumed in the world. About 80% of global fermented foods are naturally fermented by both cultivable and uncultivable microorganisms. The application of molecular and modern identification tools through culture-dependent and culture-independent techniques including next-generation sequence techniques has thrown new light on the diversity of a number of previously unknown and uncultivable microorganisms in naturally fermented foods. Ethnic food fermentations represent a precious cultural heritage in most regions, and harbor a huge genetic potential of valuable but hitherto undiscovered strains.

The sustainable use of microorganisms in food fermentation is based on an interrelationship between indigenous knowledge of food fermentation, modern expertise and information, a basic understanding of the microbial background of fermentation and of good hygienic practices (GHP), some experience of handling microbial cultures, and conservation of microbial strains. The diversity of functional microorganisms in fermented foods and beverages consists of bacteria, yeasts, and fungi. Microorganisms establish relevant substrates for survival and produce bioactive compounds that enrich the human diet, thereby benefiting the health of mankind. Ethnic fermented foods of the world are considered to be a means to preserve microbial diversity *ex situ*; they are custodians of microbial diversity and play a key role in the storage and supply of authentic reference material for research and development.

The most remarkable aspects of fermented foods are their biological functions that enhance several health benefits to consumers due to the functional microorganisms associated with them. Functional properties of fermented foods are acidification, bio-preservation, bio-transformation of bland substrates, bio-enrichment of nutritional value, bio-degradation of undesirable compounds, probiotic properties, bio-production of peptides, enzymes, antimicrobial properties, protective cultures, production of isoflavones, saponin and polyglutamic acid, and antioxidant activity. The health-promoting benefits of fermented foods and beverages are prevention of cardiovascular disease, cancer, hepatic disease, gastrointestinal disorders and inflammatory bowel disease; protection from hypertension, thrombosis, osteoporosis, allergic reactions, diabetes, from spoilage and toxic pathogens and synthesis of nutrient and bioavailability; reduction of obesity; increased immunity; alleviation of lactose intolerance; antiaging effects; and therapeutic values/medicinal values. Today, some ethnic fermented foods and alcoholic beverages are commercialized and marketed globally as health foods, functional foods, therapeutic foods, nutraceuticals, or health foods/drinks. Increased understanding of the viability of probiotic bacteria, interactions between gut microbiota, diet, and the host will open up new possibilities of producing new ingredients for nutritionally optimized foods that promote consumer health through microbial activities in the gut. Introduction of new fermented food products containing friendly/good bacteria will emerge such as cereals, energy bars, cheese, juices, disease-specific medical foods and infant foods. However, 90% of health-benefiting naturally fermented foods and alcoholic beverages in the world are still produced at home by traditional methods.

This book has 21 chapters covering the health benefits of fermented foods of the world. There is a separate chapter on microorganisms in fermented foods and beverages of the world. We attempted to update and collate information and research carried out on various aspects of health-promoting benefits of fermented foods and beverages. We are grateful to all contributing authors who accepted our invitation to contribute to this book. Some of them are well recognized scientists and researchers with vast experience in the field of fermented foods and beverages. We are happy to bring them all together on the same platform to bring out this book. Our thanks to Nagendra Shah of Hong Kong, Toshirou Nagai of Japan, Dong-Hwa Shin, Han Eung-Soo and Hyun Ju Kim of Korea, Raha Abdul Rahim of Malaysia, Anil Anal of Thailand, Yearul Kabir of Bangladesh, Baltasar Mayo of Spain, Mary Astuti of Indonesia, Ramesh Chandan of the United States, Rintu Banerjee, Rabindra Malik, Rekha Singhal, Prakash Halami, Anu Appaiah, Usha Rani, Kumaraswamy Jeyaram, Santa Ram Joshi, Binaya Nayak, Namrata Thapa, G. Balakrish Nair, Neerja Hajela and Sarath Gopalan—all from different parts of India. We are also grateful to the Taylor & Francis Group, CRC Press for publishing out this comprehensive book and we hope it will be read by researchers, students, teachers, nutritionists, dieticians, food entrepreneurs, agriculturalists, government policy makers, ethnologists, sociologists, and people in the electronic media who are interested in the health benefits of fermented foods and beverages. Although there are hundreds of research articles, review papers, and limited books on fermented foods and beverages, this book *Health Benefits of Fermented Foods and Beverages* is the first of this kind, a compilation of various aspects of functionality and health benefits of fermented foods and beverages of the world.

I dedicate this book to the creators of the indigenous knowledge of traditional food fermentation technologies for putting together both an ocean of knowledge and the basis for research to study indepth molecular nutrition and bioactive compounds in fermented foods and beverages.

Jyoti Prakash Tamang
Gangtok, India

Editor

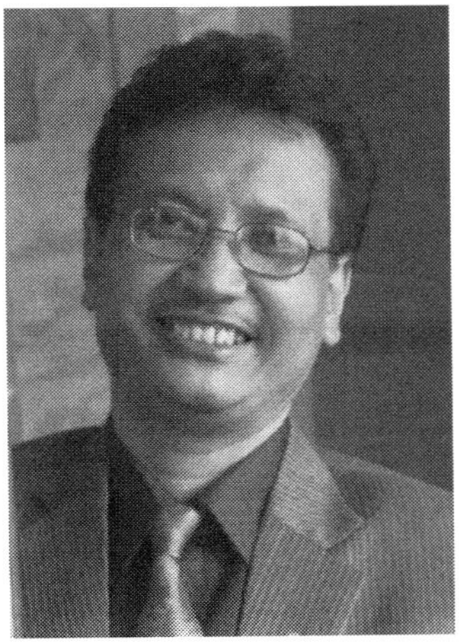

Professor Jyoti Prakash Tamang has been one of the authorities on global fermented foods and beverages for the last 27 years. He earned a PhD in microbiology from North Bengal University (1992), did postdoctoral research work at the National Food Research Institute, Tsukuba, Japan (1995), and at the Institute of Hygiene and Toxicology, Germany (2002). He was awarded the National Bioscience Award of the Department of Biotechnology by the Government of India in 2005, and the Gourmand Best Cookbook Award in Paris in 2010. He is a fellow of the National Academy of Agricultural Sciences (2012), the Indian Academy of Microbiological Sciences (2010), and the Biotech Research Society of India (2006). He has published more than 120 research papers, and authored several books including *Himalayan Fermented Foods: Microbiology, Nutrition, and Ethnic Values,* and *Fermented Foods and Beverages of the World,* both published by CRC Press, Taylor & Francis Group, USA in 2010. He has one patent, and has mentored several PhD students. He is a member of several prestigious national and international academic groups including the International Yeast Commission and the Asian Federation of Lactic Acid Bacteria, among others. Dr. Tamang is a professor in the Department of Microbiology and also dean of the School of Life Sciences of Sikkim University, a national university in Sikkim. He has served as the first registrar of Sikkim University appointed by the president of India.

Contributors

Sunita Adak
Microbial Biotechnology and Downstream Processing Laboratory
Agricultural and Food Engineering Department
Indian Institute of Technology
Kharagpur, West Bengal, India

Saeed Akhter
Department of Food Science and Technology
Bahauddin Zakariya University
Multan, Pakistan

Leocadio Alonso
Departamento de Microbiología y Bioquímica
Instituto de Productos Lácteos de Asturias (IPLA-CSIC)
Villaviciosa, Asturias, Spain

Anil Kumar Anal
Food Engineering and Bioprocess Technology
Asian Institute of Technology
Pathumthani, Thailand

Anu Appaiah K. A.
Food Microbiology
CSIR-Central Food Technological Research Institute
Mysore, Karnataka, India

Mary Astuti
Universitas Gadjah Mada
Yogyakarta, Indonesia

Lionel In Lian Aun
Department of Biotechnology
UCSI University
Kuala Lumpur, Malaysia

Rintu Banerjee
Microbial Biotechnology and Downstream Processing Laboratory
Agricultural and Food Engineering Department
Indian Institute of Technology
Kharagpur, West Bengal, India

Moumita Bishai
Microbial Biotechnology and Downstream Processing Laboratory
Agricultural and Food Engineering Department
Indian Institute of Technology
Kharagpur, West Bengal, India

Koel Biswas
Department of Biotechnology and Bioinformatics
North-Eastern Hill University
Shillong, Meghalaya, India

Soo-Wan Chae
Clinical Trial Center for Functional Foods
Division of Pharmacology
Chonbuk National University Medical School
Jeonju, South Korea

Ramesh C. Chandan
Global Technologies, Inc.
Minneapolis, Minnesota

Rajen Chettri
Department of Microbiology
School of Life Sciences
Sikkim University (Central University)
Gangtok, Sikkim, India

Hak-Jong Choi
World Institute of Kimchi
Gwangju, South Korea

Son Chu-Ky
School of Biotechnology and Food Technology
Hanoi University of Science and Technology
Hanoi, Vietnam

Shweta Deshaware
Food Engineering and Technology Department
Institute of Chemical Technology
Mumbai, Maharashtra, India

Sheenam Garg
Dairy Microbiology Division
National Dairy Research Institute
Karnal, Haryana, India

Sarath Gopalan
Pushpawati Singhania Research Institute
New Delhi, India

Neerja Hajela
Yakult India Microbiota and Probiotic Science Foundation
New Delhi, India

Prakash M. Halami
Department of Food Microbiology
CSIR-Central Food Technological Research Institute
Mysore, Karnataka, India

Eung Soo Han
World Institute of Kimchi
Gwangju, South Korea

Ashfaque Hossain
Department of Microbiology
College of Medicine
University of Hail
Hail, Saudi Arabia

Swati B. Jadhav
Food Engineering and Technology Department
Institute of Chemical Technology
Mumbai, Maharashtra, India

Kumaraswamy Jeyaram
Microbial Resources Division
Institute of Bioresources and Sustainable Development (IBSD)
Imphal, Manipur, India

Santa Ram Joshi
Microbiology Laboratory
Department of Biotechnology & Bioinformatics
North-Eastern Hill University
Shillong, Meghalaya, India

Su-Jin Jung
Clinical Trial Center for Functional Foods
Division of Pharmacology
Chonbuk National University Medical School
Jeonju, Republic of Korea

Yearul Kabir
Department of Biochemistry and Molecular Biology
University of Dhaka
Dhaka, Bangladesh

Hyun Ju Kim
World Institute of Kimchi
Gwangju, Republic of Korea

Sanath Kumar H.
Post Harvest Technology Department
Central Institute of Fisheries Education (CIFE)
Mumbai, Maharashtra, India

Adelene Song Ai Lian
Department of Cell and Molecular Biology
Universiti Putra Malaysia
Selangor, Malaysia

Foo Hooi Ling
Department of Bioproccess Technology
Universiti Putra Malaysia
Selangor, Malaysia

R. K. Malik
Dairy Microbiology Division
National Dairy Research Institute
Karnal, Haryana, India

Baltasar Mayo
Departamento de Microbiología y Bioquímica
Instituto de Productos Lácteos de Asturias (IPLA-CSIC)
Villaviciosa, Asturias, Spain

Toshirou Nagai
Genetic Resources Center
National Institute of Agrobiological Sciences
Tsukuba, Ibaraki, Japan

G. Balakrish Nair
Translational Health Science and Technology Institute
Gurgaon, Haryana, India

Binaya Bhusan Nayak
Post Harvest Technology Department
Central Institute of Fisheries Education (CIFE)
Mumbai, Maharashtra, India

Raha Abdul Rahim
Department of Cell and Molecular Biology
Universiti Putra Malaysia
Selangor, Malaysia

Amit Kumar Rai
Regional Center of Institute of Bioresources and Sustainable Development (RCIBSD)
Tadong, Sikkim, India

Arun Rai
Department of Botany
Sikkim Government College
Tadong, Sikkim, India

Usha Rani M.
Food Microbiology
CSIR-Central Food Technological Research Institute
Mysore, Karnataka, India

Samira Sarter
CIRAD UMR Qualisud
Hanoi, Vietnam

and

CIRAD, UMR Qualisud
Montpellier, France

Nagendra P. Shah
School of Biological Sciences
The University of Hong Kong
Pokfulam, Hong Kong

Dong-Hwa Shin
Shindonghwa Food Research Institute
Jeonju, South Korea

Rekha S. Singhal
Food Engineering and Technology Department
Institute of Chemical Technology
Mumbai, Maharashtra, India

Buddhiman Tamang
Department of Microbiology
School of Life Sciences
Sikkim University (Central University)
Gangtok, Sikkim, India

Jyoti Prakash Tamang
Department of Microbiology
School of Life Sciences
Sikkim University (Central University)
Gangtok, Sikkim, India

Namrata Thapa
Department of Zoology
School of Life Sciences
Sikkim University (Central University)
Gangtok, Sikkim, India

Lakshmishri Upadrasta
Microbial Biotechnology and Downstream Processing Laboratory
Agricultural and Food Engineering Department
Indian Institute of Technology
Kharagpur, West Bengal, India

S. V. N. Vijayendra
Department of Food Microbiology
CSIR-Central Food Technological Research Institute
Mysore, Karnataka, India

Chapter 1

Microorganisms in Fermented Foods and Beverages

Jyoti Prakash Tamang, Namrata Thapa, Buddhiman Tamang, Arun Rai, and Rajen Chettri

Contents

1.1 Introduction

Traditionally boiled rice is the staple diet with ethnic fermented and nonfermented legume products, vegetables, pickles, fish and meat on the side in the Far East, South and North Asia and the Indian subcontinent excluding western and northern India. In the west and north of India, wheat/barley-based breads/loaves is the staple diet together with milk and fermented milk products, meat and fermented meats. This diet is also followed in West Asia, Europe, North America and in Australia and New Zealand. Sorghum/maize porridges are the main diet with ethnic fermented and nonfermented sorghum/maize/millet, cassava, wild legume seeds, meat and milk products in Africa and South America (Tamang 2012a). Fermented foods are popular throughout the world and in some regions make a significant contribution to the diet of millions of individuals. The fermented food products supply protein, minerals, and other nutrients that add variety and nutritional fortification to otherwise starchy, bland diets.

Fermentation was traditionally a process which enabled the preservation of perishable food and has been used for centuries (www.eolss.net/sample-chapters/c06/e6-34-09-09.pdf; Hansen 2004). The term fermentation comes from the Latin word *fermentum* (to ferment). Throughout the world there are many different types of fermented foods, in which a range of different substrates are metabolized by a variety of microorganisms to yield products with unique and appealing characteristics. Fermented foods and alcoholic beverages are produced from raw materials or substrates of plant or animal origins mostly by natural fermentation or in the case of a few products by black-slopping or the addition of a traditionally prepared starter culture(s) containing functional microorganisms which modify the substrates biochemically and organoleptically into edible products that are socially acceptable to consumers (Tamang 2010b).

1.1.1 History of Fermented Foods

Methods for fermentation of vegetables might have developed in Asia (Pederson 1979), or in the Mediterranean (Hulse 2004), or in Europe (Tamang and Samuel 2010). Methods for pickling vegetables were well established during the Song dynasty in China (960–1279 AD), and have remained more or less the same to the present day (Tamang and Samuel 2010). *Suau cai*, the ethnic fermented mixed vegetable product of China, was one of the main meals for workers during the construction of the Great Wall of China in 300 BC (Pederson 1979). The history of *kimchi*, a fermented vegetable product of Korea, was traced back to 3–4 AD (Chang 1975). The traditional preparation of *kimchi* was mentioned in someKorean historical documents recorded during 1759–1829 AD (Cheigh 2002). *Sauerkraut* or *sauerkohl* meaning sour cabbage in German was documented in the seventeenth century (Pederson and Albury 1969). Olives were preserved or fermented with various methods in Roman times during 50–150 AD (Sealey and Tyers 1989). The oral history of the origin of some common Himalayan fermented vegetables such as *gundruk*, ethnic fermented leafy vegetables and *sinki*, ethnic fermented radish tap roots were documented by Tamang (2010a).

Bread-making is one of the oldest food processing practices in the food history of human beings. There are ample archaeological remains of tools and installations which were used to make bread in ancient Egypt (Samuel 2002), and descriptions of baking in Roman texts and tombs are available (Curtis 2001). About 250 bakeries were reported to have operated in ancient Rome around 100 BC (Pederson 1979). *Dosa*, the ethnic fermented pancake made from rice and black gram in South India was first noted in the Tamil Sangam literature in India about the sixth century AD (Srinivasa 1930). The traditional preparation of *idli,* an ethnic fermented rice-black gram food of India and Sri Lanka, eaten at breakfast, has been described by the poet Chavundaraya of South India in 1025 AD (Iyengar 1950). *Dhokla*, a fermented mixture of wheat and Bengal gram of western India was first mentioned in 1066 AD (Prajapati and Nair 2003). *Jalebi*, the fermented cereal-based pretzel-like product of India and Pakistan has been known since 1450 AD and is probably of Arabic or Persian origin (Gode 1943).

Soybean was probably introduced to India from China through the Himalayas several centuries ago and some believe that soybeans were also brought via Myanmar by traders from Indonesia (Shurtleff and Aoyagi 2010). *Kinema,* a fermented sticky soybean food of India, Nepal and Bhutan might have originated in east Nepal around 600 BC to 100 AD during the Kirat dynasty (Tamang 2010a). The word *kinema* was derived from the word *kinamba* of the Limboo language of the Kirat race, *ki* means fermented and *namba* means flavor (Tamang 2001). A hypothetical triangle "*natto*-triangle" was initially proposed by Nakao (1972) and was based on the distribution of plasmids (Hara et al. 1986, 1995) and the 16s RNA sequencing (Tamang et al. 2002) of the *Bacillus* species from common nonsalted sticky fermented soybean foods of Asia. An imaginary triangle known as "*Kinema-Natto-Thua nao* triangle" (KNT-triangle) was proposed by Tamang (2010a). Within the KNT-triangle in Asia only *Bacillus*-fermented soybean foods are prepared and consumed starting from Japan (*natto*), touching the Korean peninsula (*chungkokjang*), South China (*douchi*), North Thailand (*thua-nao*), Myanmar (*pepok*), Cambodia and Laos (*sieng*), southern Bhutan, the Darjeeling hills and Sikkim in India, and eastern Nepal (*kinema*), and the North East Indian states of Meghalaya (*tungrymbai*), Manipur (*hawaijar*), Mizoram (*bekang*), Nagaland (*aakhone*), and Arunachal Pradesh (*peruyaan*). The proposed "KNT triangle" does not include nonsticky and nonbacilli fermented soybean products such as *tempeh, miso, sufu, shoyu,* and so on.

Asian fermented soybean foods might have originated from *douchi* or *tau-shi*, during the Han dynasty in southern China around 206 BC (Bo 1984a,b, Zhang and Liu 2000). *Natto,* a fermented sticky soybean, was introduced to Japan from China by Buddhist priests during the Nara period around 710–794 AD (Itoh et al. 1996, Kiuchi 2001). Production of *shoyu* and *miso* in China was recorded around 1000 BC with the transfer of knowledge of production of *shoyu* and *miso* to Japan in around 600 AD (Yokotsuka 1985). *Tempeh,* the mold-fermented soybean food of Indonesia was originally introduced by ethnic Chinese traders in the early seventeenth century and the earliest record of the word tempeh appeared in the Serat Centini manuscript around 1815 AD (Astuli 1999).

The oldest sacred books of the Hindus, the *Rig Veda* and the *Upanishads* mentioned the origin of *dahi,* one of the oldest yoghurt-like fermented milk products of India during 6000–4000 BC (Yegna Narayan Aiyar 1953). Some milk products of Sudan and Egypt consumed in modern Africa such as *rob* (made from cow/goat/sheep milk), *gariss* (from camel milk), *biruni* (cow/camel milk) of Sudan, and *mish* (cow/camel milk) were mentioned by medieval Arab travelers (Odunfa 1988, Dirar 1993). The ancient Turkish people in Asia who lived as nomads were the first to make yoghurt, called "yoghurut" (Rasic and Kurmann 1978). The Babylonian records refer to cheese in 2000 BC (Davis 1964). The importance of cheese in the food habits of people in Greece (1500 BC) and Rome (750 BC) has been well documented (Scott 1986).

The Mekong basin of south-west China, Laos and northern and north-west Thailand were the most probable place of origin of fermented fish products in Asia (Ishige 1993, Ruddle 1993). Consumption of sausage by the ancient Babylonians was recorded around 1500 BC (Pederson 1979). The name *salami* is believed to have originated from the city of Salamis located on the east cost of Cyprus, which was destroyed in 449 BC (Lücke 1985).

1.1.2 History of Alcoholic Drinks

Fermented beverages appeared in 5000 BC in Babylon, 3150 BC in Ancient Egypt, 2000 BC in Mexico and 1500 BC in Sudan (www.eolss.net/sample-chapters/c06/e6-34-09-09.pdf). The earliest evidence of the grape in Egypt is seeds in jars imported from the Levant, dating to about 3150 BC indicating that wine was possibly produced in Egypt itself by 3000 BC (Murray 2000). Archaeological findings and chemical analyses of residues recovered from the Neolithic (6th millennium BC) Hajji Firuz Tepe, and the Early Bronze Age (4th millennium BC) Godin Tepe, both in western Iran, is commonly reported to represent the earliest evidence of wine making (Renfrew 1999, Wilson 1999).

Early Mesopotamian beer was based on barley malt, that is, sprouted and dried grain (Curtis 2001). Analysis of ancient beer residues using scanning electron microscopy was more focused on archaeological evidence (Samuel 1996, 2000). The whole starch remaining in the unheated malt would have broken down more slowly and the source of fermentation is uncertain (Samuel 2000). Archaeobotanical evidence from northern Germany and Scandinavia shows that hops and sweet gale (*Myrica gale*) became important beer flavorings in early medieval times (ninth to tenth century AD) (Behre 1984).

Pulque, one of the ancient alcoholic beverages of South America, which is fermented from *agave* juice and now is the national drink of Mexico was inherited from the Aztecs (Goncalves de Lima 1975). Another ancient alcoholic drink of the Andes Indians living in the lower altitude regions of South America is *chicha*, prepared from maize through human saliva which serves as the source of amylase for conversion of starch into fermentation sugars (Escobar 1977).

During the *Vedic* period of Indian history (2500–200 BC), based originally around the Indus River system, alcoholic drink *soma rus* was common and was worshipped as the liquid god *Soma* because of its medicinal attributes (Bose 1922, Sarma 1939). Drinking of alcohol in India has been mentioned in the *Ramayana* during 300–75 BC (Prakash 1961). The malting process as well as wine fermentation is rarely used in traditional fermentation processes in Asia, instead, amylolytic mixed starters prepared from the growth of molds and yeasts on raw or cooked cereals are more commonly used (Tamang 2010c). The use of traditionally prepared amylolytic mixed starters, common to the Himalayas and South East Asia, might have its origins during the time of Euchok, the daughter of the legendary king of Woo of China, known as the goddess of rice-wine in Chinese culture in 4000 BC (Lee 1984). The first documentation of *chu*, the mixed amylolytic starter of China (use for production of fermented beverages and alcoholic drinks), was found in the Shu-Ching document written during the Chou dynasty (1121–256 BC) (Haard et al. 1999). The use of *chu* for fermentation of rice-based alcoholic beverages and drinks was recorded in the beginning of the Three Nations' Periods in Korea during first century BC to second century AD (Lee 1995). The word *ragi*, an amylolytic starter of Indonesia, was first noted on an ancient inscription called the Kembang Arum near Yogyakarta in Java around 903 AD (Astuli 1999). *Kodo ko jaanr*, the ethnic fermented finger millet alcoholic beverage of the Himalayas was mentioned in the history of Nepal during the Kirat dynasty in 625 BC to 100 AD (Adhikari and Ghimirey 2000). The Newar community of Nepal used to ferment alcoholic beverages from rice during the Malla dynasty in 880 AD (Khatri 1987). There are brief descriptions of the fermented millet beverages of the Darjeeling hills and Sikkim in India in historical documents (Hooker 1854, Risley 1928, Gorer 1938).

1.2 Protocol for Studying Fermented Foods

Protocols for studies of ethnic fermented foods and alcoholic beverages primarily focus on the following parameters (Tamang 2014):

1. Documentation of the indigenous knowledge of the local people of traditional preparation, culinary practices, mode of consumption, ethnical values, therapeutic uses, socio-economy, market survey of marginal producers of fermented foods/alcoholic beverages using standard format; photography.
2. Sensory character(s) of a fermented food or alcoholic beverage by a researcher: taste, texture, aroma/flavor, and appearance.
3. Calculation of per capita consumption and annual production of ethnic fermented foods and alcoholic beverages of the particular region/village.
4. Determination of pH, temperature of the product *in situ*.
5. Collection of samples aseptically in pre-sterile containers.
6. Microbiology of fermented foods: determination of microbial loads of microorganisms (bacteria, yeasts, molds) and pathogenic contaminants (colony forming unit per gram or liter of sample), isolation of cultivable microorganisms.
7. Identification of isolates: phenotypic (morphological, physiological, and biochemical tests) and molecular identifications, assigning the proper identification of functional microorganisms following the standard norm of ICBN for microorganisms and well-authenticated taxonomical keys.

8. Isolation of uncultured microorganisms directly from food samples, and identification by culture-independent molecular techniques.
9. Preservation of identified strains of microorganisms in 15% glycerol at 80°C, or lyophilized, and deposited at authorized culture collection centers.
10. Experiments on fermentation dynamics or microbial changes during *in situ* fermentation to understand the role of functional or nonfunctional microorganism(s) using culture-independent techniques during natural fermentation.
11. Determination of the proximate composition and nutritional values of the products.
12. Determination of functional properties: probiotics, antioxidants, antimicrobial activities, tyrosinase inhibition, cell proliferation and MMP-2 inhibition activities, degradation of antinutritive compounds, bioactive compounds, unsaturated fatty acids, including omega 3-fatty acids, isoflavones and saponins, total phenolic compounds, total anthocyanin, saponin, and so on.
13. Studies on food safety: occurrence of pathogenic and spoilage microorganisms, toxin production, shelf-life of the products.
14. Optimization of a traditional process using a starter culture(s), consisting either of a pure culture or of a consortium of identified native microorganism(s) with desirable functional properties.
15. Organoleptic evaluation and consumer preference trials of the product prepared on laboratory scale.

1.3 Microorganisms

Microorganisms determine the characteristics of fermented food, for example, acidity, flavor and texture, as well as the health benefits that go beyond simple nutrition (Vogel et al. 2011). Microorganisms may be present as the indigenous microbiota of the food or as a result of the intentional addition of microorganisms as starter cultures in an industrial food fermentation process (Stevens and Nabors 2009). Also, microbial cultures can be used to produce several compounds (enzymes, flavors, fragrances, etc.) either specifically for application as food additives or *in situ* as a part of food fermentation processes (Longo and Sanromán 2006).

With an estimated 5000 varieties of fermented foods and beverages, worldwide, only a small fraction of these artisanal products have been subjected to scientific studies so far (Tamang 2010b). In many of these foods, the biological and microbiological bases of the fermentation processes are poorly understood. What little information is available often deals with the identification and perhaps preliminary characterization of the primary microbiota in the finished product. This in turn will necessitate a more thorough understanding of the microorganisms involved, in terms of the types and their specific activities, so that the fermentation process can be made more reliable and predictable.

With the discovery of microorganisms, it became possible to understand and manage food fermentation. Methods for isolating and purifying microbial cultures became available in the nineteenth century. Sterilization or pasteurization of the raw materials prior to inoculation with well-defined cultures allowed the fermentation processes to be managed with little variation. The use of defined cultures became the industrial standard in breweries by the nineteenth century. During the twentieth century, the wine, dairy, and meat industries also shifted production procedures toward the use of well-characterized and defined starter cultures. In the beginning, starter cultures were isolates from earlier fermentations that were maintained and propagated at the site of production. The application of microbiology and process technology resulted in large improvements in the quality of the fermented food products. The quality improvements have been so great that today all significant production of fermented food is industrial. The small amount of "home fermentation" conducted in the form of baking, home brewing and private cheese making usually rely on commercially available yeast and bacterial cultures. The maintenance of the microorganisms differs between the different food industries in the sense that some fermentation industries, such as breweries and vinegar producers maintain their own stains and inocula. In the dairy industry, as well as in the meat industry and bakeries, cultures are usually obtained from suppliers dedicated to the production of high-quality food ingredients (Mogensen et al. 2002, Hansen 2004).

Fermentation can basically be performed either by natural or spontaneous fermentation, by back-slopping or by the addition of starter cultures. By spontaneous fermentation, the raw material and its initial treatment will encourage the growth of an indigenous microbiota. In most spontaneous fermentation, a microbial succession takes place: quite often lactic acid bacteria (LAB) will initially dominate followed by various species of yeasts. Molds only grow aerobically, limiting their occurrence in certain types of fermented products. LAB produce lactic acid and other antimicrobial substances that inhibit the growth of harmful bacteria along with reducing the sugar content, thereby prolonging the shelf life of the product. Yeasts mostly produce aroma components and alcohols. When molds are involved in fermentation, they generally contribute by producing both intra- and extracellular proteolytic and lipolytic enzymes that highly influence the flavor and texture of the product (Tamang and Fleet 2009).

In back-slopping, a part of a precious batch of a fermented product is used to inoculate the new batch. This procedure produces a higher initial number of beneficial microorganisms than that found in the raw material and ensures a faster and more reliable fermentation than that which occurs in spontaneous fermentation. Examples of back-slopping are home-made fermentation of milk, vegetables, and cereals (Josephsen and Jespersen 2004).

Novel insights into the metabolism of LAB offer perspectives for the application of a new generation of starter cultures. Functional starter cultures are starters that possess at least one inherent functional property. These can contribute to food safety and/or offer one or more organoleptic, technological, nutritional, or health advantage. The implementation of carefully selected strains as starter cultures or co-cultures in fermentation processes can help to achieve *in situ* expression of the desired property, maintaining a perfectly natural and healthy product. A functional LAB starter culture is able to produce antimicrobial substances, sugar polymers, sweeteners, aromatic compounds, useful enzymes, or nutraceuticals, while-the so-called probiotic strains, mainly LAB, exhibit health-promoting properties. Such functionalities also lead to a wider application area and higher flexibility of starter cultures (Leroy and De Vuyst 2004). Nowadays, there are many commercial suppliers of starter cultures worldwide, such as Alce and CSL (Italy), ASCRS (Australia), Chr. Hansen and Danisco (Denmark), CSK and DSM (the Netherlands), Degussa and Gewürzmüller (Germany), Lallemand (Canada), NZDRI (New Zealand), Quest International (UK), Rhodia (France), and so on. All companies can easily be found on the Internet/World wide Web (Hansen 2002, 2004).

Fermented foods are the hubs of consortia of microbiota and mycobiota (functional, nonfunctional, and pathogenic contaminants), which may be present as natural indigenous microbiota in uncooked plant or animal substrates, utensils, containers, earthen pots, or environments (Hesseltine 1983, Tamang 1998), or as a result of the intentional addition of the microorganisms as starter cultures in an industrial food fermentation process (Stevens and Nabors 2009). Functional microorganisms transform the chemical constituents of raw materials of plant/animal sources during fermentation thereby enhancing the nutritional value of the products, enriching them with improved flavor and texture, prolonging their shelf live, and fortifying them with health-promoting bio-active compounds (Farhad et al. 2010). Species of lactic acid bacteria and *Bacillus*, and amylolytic and alcohol-producing yeasts and filamentous molds are the major microbiota in the fermented foods and alcoholic beverages of Asia, whereas LAB or a combination of bacteria (LAB, non-LAB, micrococci)-yeast mixtures and filamentous molds are more prominent in Africa. Filamentous molds and bacilli are rare in the fermented foods and beverages of Africa, Europe, Australia, and America (Tamang 1998), although fermented legume products, based on *Bacillus* fermentation, are common in West Africa (Oguntoyinbo et al. 2007).

1.3.1 Isolation by Culture-Dependent and Culture-Independent Methods

The classical phenotypic identification methods are totally based on culture-dependent techniques for only cultivable microorganisms in culture media, ignoring several unknown uncultivable microorganisms that may have major or minor functional roles in the production of fermented foods. Direct DNA extraction from samples of fermented foods commonly referred to as culture-independent methods are nowadays commonly used in food microbiology to profile both cultivable and uncultivable microbial populations from fermented foods (Cocolin and Ercolini 2008). Culture independent techniques first appeared in food microbiology at the end of the 1990s and since then they have been applied extensively. These methods do not rely on cultivation and target nucleic acids (DNA and RNA) to identify and follow the changes that occur in the main populations present in a specific ecosystem (Cocolin et al. 2013). The most popular culture-independent technique being used in the isolation of microorganisms from fermented foods is a PCR-DGGE analysis to profile bacterial populations (Cocolin et al. 2011, Tamang 2014) and yeast populations in fermented foods (Cocolin et al. 2002, Jianzhonga et al. 2009). Culture-dependent and culture-independent methods are contradictory to each other (Alegría et al. 2011), but for microbial taxonomy both methods are equally important and complementary. Both cultivable and uncultivable microorganisms from any fermented food and beverage may be identified using culture-dependent and -independent methods to document a complete profile of native functional and nonfunctional microorganisms, and to study both inter- and intra-species diversity within a particular genus or among genera (Ramos et al. 2010, Yan et al. 2013, Tamang 2014). Greppi et al. (2013a) first reported the combination of both culture-dependent and independent methods to reveal predominant yeast species and biotypes in the traditional fermented maize foods of Benin. The DGGE analysis on the DNA directly extracted from fermented maize products demonstrated the presence of *Dekkera bruxellensis* and *Debaryomyces hansenii*, not detected by the culture-based approach (Greppi et al. 2013b).

1.3.2 Identification: Phenotypic and Biochemical

Phenotypic characteristics include colony appearance, cell morphology, Gram staining, growth at different temperatures (8–65°C), pH (3.9–9.6), and salt tolerance (4.0%–18%). Biochemical tests are based on the metabolic activities of microorganisms such as carbon and nitrogen sources, energy sources, sugar fermentation, secondary metabolite formation, and enzyme production (Tamang 2014). A few ready-to-use commercial identification kits are commonly used such as API 50CH (bioMérieux, France) for rapid sugar fermentation tests, and the Biolog Microbial Identification System, for identification of different groups of bacteria and yeasts.

1.3.3 Identification: Genotypic or Molecular

Molecular identification is emerging as an accurate and reliable identification tool, and is widely used in identification of both culture-dependent and culture-independent microorganisms from fermented foods. Owing to a variety of tools that provide advanced molecular differentiation of microorganisms, microbial populations can be quantified and new microbial species isolated and identified (Giraffa and Carminati 2008). Some common molecular tools used in identification of microorganisms isolated from fermented foods are species-specific PCR, qPCR, rep-PCR, AFLP, RAPD, DGGE, TGGE, ARDRA, mtDNA-RFLP, mCOLD-PCR, MLSA, and MLST.

Species-specific PCR primers are used to identify a particular species of the genus (Tamang et al. 2005); this technique is widely applied in the identification of LAB isolated from fermented foods (Robert et al. 2009). The application of real-time quantitative PCR (qPCR) with specific primers provides the specific detection and quantification of LAB species in fermented foods (Park et al. 2009). The repetitive extragenic palindromic sequence-based PCR (rep-PCR) technique permits typing at a subspecies level and reveals significant genotypic differences between strains of the same bacterial species from fermented foods (Tamang et al. 2008). Amplified fragment-length polymorphism (AFLP) is a technique based on the selective amplification and separation of genomic restriction fragments, and its applicability is for the identification of various LAB strains in fermented foods (Tanigawa and Watanabe 2011). Random amplification of polymorphic DNA (RAPD) is commonly used for discrimination of LAB strains from fermented foods (Schillinger et al. 2003, Chao et al. 2008). The amplified ribosomal DNA restriction analysis (ARDRA) technique using restriction enzymes is also useful in identification of uncultivable microorganisms from fermented foods (Jeyaram et al. 2010). The mt DNA-RFLP technique showed discriminating power similar to microsatellite typing and interdelta analysis (Schuller et al. 2007) and is considered as a useful genetic marker for *Saccharomyces cerevisiae* in amylolytic starters (Jeyaram et al. 2011). Techniques of denaturing gradient gel electrophoresis (DGGE) and temperature gradient gel electrophoresis (TGGE) have been developed to profile microbial communities directly from fermented foods, and are based on sequence-specific distinctions of 16S rDNA or 26S rDNA amplicons produced by PCR (Ongol and Asano 2009, Alegría et al. 2011). A modified CO-amplification at lower denaturation temperature PCR (mCOLD-PCR) method has been developed to detect low-abundant microorganisms using a double-strand RNA probe to inhibit the amplification of the sequence of a major microorganism in wine fermentation (Takahashi et al. 2014). Multilocus sequence analysis (MLSA) using housekeeping genes as molecular markers alternative to the 16S rRNA genes, has been proposed for LAB species identification from fermented foods (Naser et al. 2005, de Bruyne et al. 2007, 2008, 2010). Multilocus sequence typing (MLST) has also been used for discriminating LAB strains from fermented foods (Diancourt et al. 2007, Picozzi et al. 2010, Tanigawa and Watanabe 2011).

Effective tools of next-generation sequencing (NGS) such as phylobiomics, metagenomics, and metatranscriptomics are required for the documentation of cultures in traditional fermented products, for sensory quality and safety improvements, in some cases for starter culture design for commercialization and potentially for supporting sustainable food systems (van Hijum et al. 2013). A proteomics identification method using matrix-assisted laser desorption ionizing-time of flight mass spectrometry (MALDI-TOF MS) is used to identify the species of *Bacillus* in the fermented foods of Africa (Savadogo et al. 2011), *Lactobacillus* strains isolated from fermented foods (Dušková et al. 2012, Sato et al. 2012), sub-speciation of *Lactococcus* (*Lc.*) *lactis* (Tanigawa et al. 2010), LAB from traditional fermented vegetables of Vietnam (Nguyen et al. 2013b), probiotics from yoghurt (Angelakis et al. 2011), and *Tetragenococcus halophilus* and *Tetra. muriaticus* from fermented foods

(Kuda et al. 2014). The application of NGS such as metagenomic approaches using massively parallel pyrosequencing of tagged 16S rRNA gene amplicons provide detailed information on microbial communities associated with *kimchi* (Jung et al. 2011, Park et al. 2012), *nukadoko*, a fermented rice bran mash used for pickling vegetables in Japan (Sakamoto et al. 2011), *narezushi*, a fermented salted fish with cooked rice in Japan (Kiyohara et al. 2012), and *ben-saalga*, a traditional gruel of pearl millet in Burkina Faso (Humblot and Guyot 2009). The 16S rRNA gene sequence-based pyrosequencing method enables a detailed, comprehensive and high-throughput analysis of microbial ecology (Sakamoto et al. 2011), and this method has been applied to various traditional fermented foods (Oki et al. 2014). Compared to the pyrosequencing analysis, the DGGE method only revealed some of the major bacterial species such as *Bacillus thermoamylovorans* and *B. licheniformis* in *chungkokjang* (the sticky fermented soybean food of Korea) and could not detect a large number of predominant or diverse rare bacterial species identified in the pyrosequencing analysis. Also the regional differences of the bacterial community were more clearly represented in the pyrosequencing method than in the DGGE analysis (Nam et al. 2011).

Metabolomics, also called metabonomics or metabolic profiling, deals with the simultaneous determination and quantitative analysis of intracellular metabolites or low-molecular-mass molecules and can be used as a tool for the comprehensive understanding of fermented and functional foods with LAB (Mozzi et al. 2013). The application of species-independent functional gene microarray for identification of LAB in fermented foods has been developed (Weckx et al. 2009). Up-to-date analytical methods have also been applied in the identification and discrimination of some microbial species/strains from fermented foods such as length heterogeneity PCR (LH-PCR), high-throughput sequencing (HTS), BOX-PCR (Zhu et al. 2014), and so on.

1.4 Main Types of Microorganisms in Global Food Fermentation

Main types (with genera) of microorganisms associated with global fermented foods and beverages are grouped as follows (Bernardeau et al. 2006, Tamang and Fleet 2009, Tamang 2010a,b,c, Bourdichon et al. 2012, Alexandraki et al. 2013):

- Bacteria: *Acetobacter, Arthrobacter, Bacillus, Bifidobacterium, Brachybacterium, Brevibacterium, Carnobacterium, Corynebacterium, Enterobacter, Enterococcus, Gluconacetobacter, Hafnia, Halomonas, Klebsiella, Kocuria, Lactobacillus, Lactococcus, Leuconostoc, Macrococcus, Microbacterium, Micrococcus, Oenococcus, Pediococcus, Propionibacterium, Staphylococcus, Streptococcus, Streptomyces, Tetragenococcus, Weisella, Zymomonas.*
- Fungi: *Actinomucor, Aspergillus, Fusarium, Lecanicillium, Mucor, Neurospora, Penicillium, Rhizopus, Scopulariopsis, Sperendonema.*
- Yeasts: *Candida, Cyberlindnera, Cystofilobasidium, Debaryomyces, Dekkera, Hanseniaspora, Kazachstania, Galactomyces, Geotrichum, Guehomuces, Kluyveromyces, Lachancea, Metschnikowia, Pichia, Saccharomyces, Schizosaccharomyces, Schwanniomyces, Starmerella, Torulaspora, Trigonopsis, Wickerhamomyces, Yarrowia, Zygosaccharomyces, Zygotorulaspora.*

1.4.1 Bacteria

Bacteria are the most dominant microorganisms in both naturally fermented foods or foods fermented by the use of starter cultures. Among the bacteria, lactic acid bacteria are commonly associated with acidic fermented foods, while non-LAB bacteria such as *Bacillus*, micrococcaceae, *Bifidobacterium, Brachybacterium, Brevibacterium,* and *Propionibacterium* etc., are also involved in food fermentation, frequently as minor or secondary groups.

1.4.1.1 Lactic Acid Bacteria

Lactic acid bacteria are Gram-positive, catalase-negative bacteria that produce large amounts of lactic acid. The bacterial groups that make up the LAB are among the most familiar to humans, because of their association with the human environment, and with a wide range of naturally fermented dairy products, grain crops, vegetables, and so on. The LAB comprise a large bacterial group consisting of about 380 species in 40 genera of 6 families, belonging phylogenetically to the order *Lactobacillales* within the phylum *Firmicutes* (Stiles and Holzapfel 1997). Common genera of the LAB isolated from various fermented foods of the world are *Alkalibacterium, Carnobacterium, Enterococcus, Lactococcus, Lactobacillus, Leuconostoc, Oenococcus, Pediococcus, Streptococcus, Tetragenococcus, Vagococcus*, and *Weissella* (Carr et al. 2002, Salminen et al. 2004, MetaMicrobe.com/Lactic Acid Bacteria 2013).

1.4.1.2 Non-Lactic Acid Bacteria

Bacillus is reported from the alkaline-fermented foods of Asia and Africa (Parkouda et al. 2009). Species of *Bacillus* present in fermented foods mostly soybean-based foods are *B. amyloliquefaciens, B. circulans, B. coagulans, B. firmus, B. licheniformis, B. megaterium, B. pumilus, B. subtilis, B. subtilis* variety *natto* and *B. thuringiensis* (Kiers et al. 2000, Kubo et al. 2011), while strains of *B. cereus* have been isolated from the fermentation of *Prosopis africana* seeds for the production of *okpehe* in Nigeria (Oguntoyinbo et al. 2007). Some strains of *B. subtilis* produce λ-polyglutamic acid (PGA) which is an amino acid polymer commonly present in Asian fermented soybean foods giving the characteristic sticky texture to the product (Urushibata et al. 2002, Meerak et al. 2007, Nishito et al. 2010).

Species of *Bifidobacterium, Brachybacterium, Brevibacterium,* and *Propionibacterium* have been isolated from cheese and other fermented milks (Bourdichon et al. 2012). Several species of *Kocuria, Micrococcus,* and *Staphylococcus* have been reported from fermented milk products, fermented sausages and meat and fish products (Wu et al. 2000, Martín et al. 2006, Coton et al. 2010). *Enterobacter cloacae, Klebsiella pneumoniae, K. pneumoniae* subsp. *ozaenae, Haloanaerobium, Halobacterium, Halococcus, Propionibacterium, Pseudomonas*, and so on, are also present in many fermented foods (Tamang 2010b). Species of *Arthrobacter* and *Hafnia* are involved in meat fermentation (Bourdichon et al. 2012).

1.4.2 Yeasts

The role of yeasts in food fermentation is to ferment sugar, produce secondary metabolites, inhibit growth of mycotoxin-producing molds and display several enzymatic activities such as lipolytic, proteolytic, pectinolytic, glycosidasic and urease activities (Aidoo et al. 2006, Romano et al. 2006). Genera of yeasts reported from fermented foods, alcoholic beverages and nonfood mixed amylolytic starters are *Brettanomyces, Candida, Cryptococcus, Debaryomyces, Dekkera, Galactomyces, Geotrichum, Hansenula, Hanseniaspora, Hyphopichia, Issatchenkia, Kazachstania, Kluyveromyces, Metschnikowia, Pichia, Rhodotorula, Rhodosporidium, Saccharomyces,*

Saccharomycodes, Saccharomycopsis, Schizosaccharomyces, Sporobolomyces, Torulaspora, Torulopsis, Trichosporon, Yarrowia, and *Zygosaccharomyces* (Watanabe et al. 2008, Tamang and Fleet 2009, Kurtzman et al. 2011, Lv et al. 2013).

1.4.3 Fungi

The major roles of fungi, mostly filamentous molds, in fermented foods and alcoholic beverages are the production of intra- and extracellular proteolytic and lipolytic enzymes that highly influence the flavor and texture of the product, and also the degradation of antinutritive factors improving bioavailability of minerals (Josephsen and Jespersen 2004, Aidoo and Nout 2010). Species of *Actinomucor, Amylomyces, Aspergillus, Monascus, Mucor, Neurospora, Penicillium, Rhizopus*, and *Ustilago* are reported from many fermented foods, Asian nonfood amylolytic starters and alcoholic beverages (Hesseltine 1991, Nout and Aidoo 2002).

1.4.4 Pathogenic Contaminants

About 80% of fermented foods are produced by natural fermentation and may contain functional, nonfunctional, and pathogenic microorganisms during initial fermentation. Pathogenic bacteria commonly reported for fermented foods are *Escherichia coli, Listeria monocytogenes, Yersinia enterocolitica, Bacillus cereus, Clostridium botulinum*, and so on (Lindqvist and Lindblad 2009, Rossi et al. 2011).

1.4.5 Gut Microflora

The human gastrointestinal tract (GIT) houses over 10^{14} microbial cells with over 1000 diverse bacterial types, mostly in the colon (Lepage et al. 2012, Purchiaroni et al. 2013). Colonization of the gut is initiated before birth following ingestion of microbe-containing amniotic fluid by the fetus (Mshvildadze and Neu 2010, Aagaard et al. 2014). The majority of bacteria in the adult gut are nonsporing anaerobes, the most numerically predominant of which include species of *Bacteroides, Bifidobacterium, Eubacterium, Clostridium, Lactobacillus, Fusobacterium*, and various Gram-positive cocci and bacteria that are present in lower numbers include *Enterococcus* spp., Enterobacteriaceae, methanogens, and dissimilatory sulfate-reducing bacteria (Wallace et al. 2011). Microorganisms colonize different parts of GIT and bacterial population density varies along the GIT (Romano-Keeler et al. 2014). The GIT is one of the most complex ecosystems of microorganisms ranging from bacteria (mostly LAB), archaea (e.g., methanogens), and eukarea (fungi, helminthes, and protozoa) as well as viruses (Mitsuoka 1992, Holzapfel et al. 1997, Norman et al. 2014). In healthy adults, 80% of the identified fecal microbiota belong to four dominant phyla: the Gram-negative *Bacteroides* and *Proteobacteria* and the Gram-positive *Actinobacteria* and *Firmicutes* which include at least 17 families, corresponding to no less than 1250 different species of bacteria (Schuijt et al. 2013). The composition and distribution of gut microbiota (Purchiaroni et al. 2013) are as follows: in the stomach (*Lb. reuteri, Lb. delbrueckii, Lb. gastricus, Lb. antri*), in the small intestine (*Lb. reuteri, Lb. bulgaricus, Lb. acidophilus, Enterococcus avium, Ent. dispar, Ent. durans, Ent. faecalis, Ent. faecium, Ent. flavescens, Ent. gallinarum, Ent. hirae, Ent. mundtii, Ent. raffinosus*), and in the large intestine (*Ent. faecalis, Bacteroides, Bifidobacterium, Eubacterium, Peptococcurs, Clostridium, Lactobacillus*).

1.5 Types of Fermented Foods

The major groups of substrates-based fermented foods are as follows:

1. Fermented milk foods
2. Fermented cereal foods
3. Fermented vegetable foods
4. Fermented soybean and non-soybean foods
5. Fermented meat products
6. Fermented fish products
7. Fermented root/tuber products
8. Fermented beverages and Asian amylolytic starters
9. Miscellaneous fermented products (fermented tea, cocoa, vinegar, *nata, pidan*, etc.)

1.5.1 Fermented Milks

Fermented milks (Table 1.1) are classified into two major groups based on the presence of dominant microorganisms: (i) lactic fermentations which are dominated by species of LAB, and consist of the thermophilic type (e.g., yogurt, Bulgarian buttermilk), probiotic type (acidophilus milk, yakult, bifidus milk), and the mesophilic type (e.g., natural fermented milk, cultured milk, cultured cream, cultured buttermilk); and (ii) fungal-lactic fermentations where LAB and yeasts species cooperate to generate the final product and consist of alcoholic milks (e.g., *kefir, koumiss*, acidophilus-yeast milk), and moldy milks (e.g., *viili*) (Mayo et al. 2010). Starter cultures in milk fermentation are of two types depending on the principal function, primary cultures to participate in the acidification, and secondary cultures for flavor, aroma, and maturing activities (Topisirovic et al. 2006). The main species involved as primary cultures in milk fermentation are *Lactococcus lactis* subsp. *cremoris, Lc. lactis* subsp. *lactis, Lactobacillus delbrueckii* subsp. *delbrueckii, Lb. delbrueckii* subsp. *lactis, Lb. helveticus, Leuconostoc* spp., and *Streptococcus thermophilus* (Parente and Cogan 2004). Secondary cultures used in cheese making are *Brevibacterium linens, Propionibacterium freudenreichii, Debaryomyces hansenii, Geotrichum candidum, Penicillium camemberti*, and *P. roqueforti* for the development of flavor and texture during the ripening of cheese (Coppola et al. 2006, Quigley et al. 2011). Besides primary and secondary cultures, some nonstarter lactic acid bacteria (NSLAB) microbiota are usually present in high numbers which include *Enterococcus durans, Ent. faecium, Lb. casei, Lb. plantarum, Lb. salivarius*, and *Staphylococcus* spp. (Briggiler-Marcó et al. 2007). Yogurt is a widely consumed highly nutritious fermented milk as a coagulated milk product resulting from the fermentation of milk by *Strep. thermophilus* and *Lb. delbrueckii* subsp. *bulgaricus* (formerly *Lb. bulgaricus*) (Tamime and Robinson 2007). *Lb. acidophilus, Lb. casei, Lb. rhamnosus, Lb. gasseri, Lb. johnsonii*, and *Bifidobacterium* spp., are among the most common adjunct cultures in yogurt fermentation (Guarner et al. 2005). Fermented milk products that are manufactured using starter cultures containing yeasts include acidophilus-yeast milk, *kefir, koumiss*, and *viili* (de Ramesh et al. 2006). *Lb. acidophilus, Lb. amylovorus, Lb. crispatus, Lb. gallinarum, Lb. gasseri*, and *Lb. johnsonii* are reported from acidophilus milk (Berger et al. 2007).

Natural fermented milks are one of the oldest methods of milk fermentation using raw or boiled milk to ferment spontaneously or by using the back-slopping method (Robinson and Tamime 2006). In back-slopping, a part of a precious batch of a fermented product is used to inoculate the new batch

Table 1.1 Some Common and Uncommon Ethnic Fermented Milk Products of the World

Product	*Substrate*	*Sensory Property and Nature*	*Microorganisms*	*Country*	*References*
Acidophilus milk	Cow milk	Acidic, sour, drink	Species of *Lactobacillus*, *Lactococcus*	Russia, East Europe, Greece, Turkey, North America, Scandinavia	Mayo et al. (2010)
Airag	Mare or camel milk	Acidic, sour, mild alcoholic, drink	*Lb. helveticus*, *Lb. kefiranofaciens*, *Bifidobacterium mongoliense*, *Kluyveromyces marxianus*	Mongolia	Watanabe et al. (2008, 2009b)
Ayib	Goat milk		*Canida* sp., *Saccharomyces* sp., *Lactobacillus* sp., *Leuconostoc* sp.	East and Central Africa	Odunfa and Oyewole (1997)
Biruni	Cow/camel milk	Acidic, semi-liquid, drink	LAB	Sudan	Jung (2012)
Butter	Animal milk	Soft paste, butter	LAB	Worldwide	Mayo et al. (2010)
Buttermilk		Acid fermented butter milk	*Lb. bulgaricus*	Bulgaria	Mayo et al. (2010)
Cheese	Animal milk	Soft or hard, solid; side dish, salad	*Lc. lactis* subsp. *cremoris*, *Lc. lactis* subsp. *lactis*, *Lb. delbrueckii* subsp. *delbrueckii*, *Lb. delbrueckii* subsp. *lactis*, *Lb. helveticus*, *Lb. casei*, *Lb. plantarum*, *Lb. salivarius*, *Leuconostoc* spp., *Strep. thermophilus*, *Ent. durans*, *Ent. faecium*, and *Staphylococcus* spp., *Brevibacterium linens*, *Propionibacterium freudenreichii*, *Debaryomyces hansenii*, *Geotrichum candidum*, *Penicillium camemberti*, *P. roqueforti*.	Worldwide	Parente and Cogan (2004), Quigley et al. (2011)

Chhu	Yak/cow milk	Cheese like product, curry, soup	*Lb. farciminis, Lb. brevis, Lb. alimentarius, Lb. salivarius, Lact. lactis, Saccharomycopsis* sp., *Candida* sp.	India, Nepal, Bhutan, China (Tibet)	Dewan. and Tamang (2006)
Chhurpi (hard)	Yak/cow milk	Chewable milk, masticator	*Lb. farciminis, Lb. casei, Lb. biofermentans, W. confusus*	India, Nepal, Bhutan, China (Tibet)	Tamang (2010a)
Chhurpi (soft)	Yak/cow milk	Cheese-like product, soup, curry, pickle	*Lb. farciminis, Lb. paracasei, Lb. biofermentans, Lb.plantarum, Lb. curvatus, Lb. fermentum, Lb. alimentarius, Lb. kefir, Lb. hilgardii, W. confusus, Ent. faecium, Leuc. mesenteroides*	India, Nepal, Bhutan, China (Tibet)	Tamang et al. (2000)
Dahi	Cow/buffalo milk, starter culture	Curd, savory	*Lb. bifermentans, Lb. alimentarius, Lb. paracasei, Lact. lactis, Strep. cremoris, Strep. lactis, Strep. thermophilus, Lb.bulgaricus, Lb. acidophilus, Lb. helveticus, Lb. cremoris, Ped. pentosaceous, P. acidilactici, W. cibara, W. paramesenteroides, Lb. fermentum, Lb. delbrueckii* subsp. *indicus, Saccharomycopsis* sp., *Candida* sp.	India, Nepal, Sri Lanka, Bangladesh, Pakistan	Harun-ur-Rashid et al. (2007), Patil et al. (2010)
Ergo	Milk	Acid fermented butter milk	*Lactobacillus* sp., *Lactococcus* sp.	Ethiopia	Steinkraus (1996)
Filmjölk	Cow milk	Less-sour than yoghurt, yoghurt-like	*Lc. lactis* and *Leuc. mesenteroides*	Sweden	Kosikowski and Mistry (1997)
Gariss	Camel milk	Acidic, liquid, refreshing beverage	LAB	Sudan	Akabanda et al. (2013)
Gheu/ghee	Cow milk	Soft, oily mass, solid, butter	*Lc. lactis* subsp. *lactis, Lc. lactis* subsp. *cremoris*	India, Nepal, Bhutan, Bangladesh, Pakistan	Tamang (2010a)

(Continued)

Table 1.1 (*Continued*) Some Common and Uncommon Ethnic Fermented Milk Products of the World

Product	*Substrate*	*Sensory Property and Nature*	*Microorganisms*	*Country*	*References*
Kefir	Goat, sheep, cow	Alcoholic fermented milk, effervescent milk	*Tor. holmii, Tor. delbruechii, Lb. brevis, Lb. caucasicus,Strep. thermophilus, Lb. bulgaricus, Lb. plantarum, Lb. casei, Lb. brevis*	Russia	Bernardeau et al. (2006)
Kesong Puti, Keso, Kesiyo	Carabao's (buffalo) milk or cow carabao's milk, salt, Abomasal extracts coagulant, starter	White cheese, soft cheese	*Lb. helveticus, Lact. lactis, Lb. rhamnosus, Leuc. mesenteroides, Lb. acidophilus, Lb. plantarum, Lb. brevis, Lb. curvatus*	Philippines	Kisworo (2003)
Kishk	Milk, wheat	Fermented milk wheat mix, drink	*Lb. plantarum, Lb. brevis, Lb. bulgaricus, Lb. casei, Strep. thermophilus*	Egypt	Bernardeau et al. (2006)
Kurut	Yak milk	Naturally fermented milk, drink	LAB	China	Sun et al. (2010)
Kushuk	Milk, wheat	Fermented milk wheat mix, drink	*Lb. plantarum, Lb. brevis*	Iraq	Bernardeau et al. (2006)
Koumiss	Milk	Acid fermented milk, drink	*Lb. bulgaricus, Torula* sp., *Lb. salivarius, Lb. buchneri, Lb. heveticus, Lb. plantarum, Lb. acidophilus*	Russia	Hao et al. (2010)
Laban rayeb	Milk	Acid fermented milk, yoghurt-like	*Lb. casei, Lb. plantarum, Lb. brevis, Lact. lactis, Sacch. kefir, Leuconostoc* sp.	Egypt	Bernardeau et al. (2006)

Laban zeer	Milk	Acid fermented milk	*Lb. casei, Lb. plantarum, Lb. brevis, Lc. lactis, Lc. lactis*	Egypt	Bernardeau et al. (2006)
Lassi	Cow milk	Acidic, buttermilk, refreshing beverage	*Lb. Acidophilus, Strep. thermophilus*	India, Nepal, Bhutan, Bangladesh, Pakistan	Patidar and Prajapati (1998)
Långfil	Cow milk	Elastic texture, sour, yoghurt-like	LAB	Sweden	Tamime (2005)
Leben/Lben	Cow milk	Sour milk	*Candida* sp., *Saccharomyces* sp., *Lactobacillus* sp., *Leuconostoc* sp.,	North, East Central Africa	Odunfa and Oyewole (1997)
Liban-argeel	Sheep, goat, cow, buffalo milk	Acid fermented milk	LAB	Iraq	Bernardeau et al. (2006)
Maa	Yak milk	Mild-acidic, viscous, butter	LAB, yeasts	China (Tibet), India, Bhutan	Tamang (2010a)
Maziwa lala	Milk	Yoghurt-like	*Strep. lactis, Strep. thermophilus*	Kenya	Olasupo et al. (2010)
Mohi	Cow milk	Acidic, buttermilk, refreshing beverage	*Lb. alimentarius, Lc. lactis* subsp. *lactis, Lc. lactis* subsp. *cremoris; Saccharomycopsis* spp. and *Candida* spp.	Nepal, India, Bhutan	Dewan and Tamang (2007)
Mish	Cow/camel milk	Acidic, semi-liquid, refreshing beverage	LAB	Sudan, Egypt	Bernardeau et al. (2006)
Misti dahi (mishti doi, lal dahi, payodhi)	Buffalo/cow milk	Mild-acidic, thick-gel, sweetened curd, savory	*Strep. salivarius* subsp. *thermophilus, Lb. acidophilus, Lb. delbrueckii* subsp. *bulgaricus, Lc. lactis* subsp. *lactis, Sacch. cerevisiae.*	India, Bangladesh	Ghosh and Rajorhia (1990), Gupta et al. (2000)

(Continued)

Table 1.1 (*Continued*) Some Common and Uncommon Ethnic Fermented Milk Products of the World

Product	*Substrate*	*Sensory Property and Nature*	*Microorganisms*	*Country*	*References*
Nunu	Raw cow milk	Naturally fermented milk	*Lb. fermentum, Lb. plantarum, Lb. helveticus, Leuc. mesenteroides, Ent. faecium, Ent. italicus, Weissella confuse; Candida parapsilosis, C. rugosa, C. tropicalis, Galactomyces geotrichum, Pichia kudriavzevii, Sacch. cerevisiae*	Ghana	Akabanda et al. (2013)
Paneer	Buffalo or cow milk	Whey, soft, cheese-like product, fried snacks, curry	LAB	India, Nepal, Pakistan, Bangladesh, Middle East	Tamang (2012b)
Phrung	Yak milk	Mild-acidic, hard-mass like *chhurpi*, masticator	Unknown	India, China (Tibet)	Tamang (2010a)
Philu	Cow or yak milk, bamboo vessels	Cream like product, curry	*Lb. paracasei, Lb. bifermentans, Ent. faecium*	India, Nepal, Tibet (China)	Dewan and Tamang (2007)
Pheuja or suja	Tea-yak butter, salt	Salty with buttery flavor, liquid, Refreshing tea	Unknown	India, China (Tibet), Bhutan, Nepal	Tamang (2010a)
Rob	Cow, goat, sheep milk	Mild-acidic, savory	LAB	Sudan	Akabanda et al. (2013)
Shrikhand	Cow, buffalo milk	Acidic, concentrated sweetened viscous, savory	*Lc. lactis* subsp. *lactis, Lc. lactis* subsp. *diacetylactis, Lc. lactis* subsp. *cremoris, Strep. thermophilus, Lb. delbruecki* subsp. *Bulgaricus*	India	Aneja et al. (2002)

Somar	Yak or cow milk	Buttermilk	*Lb. paracasei, Lact. Lactis*	India, Nepal	Dewan and Tamang. (2007)
Sour milk kerbah	Milk	Acid fermented milk	*Lact. lactis, Sacch. kefir, Lb. casei, Lb. brevis, Lb. plantarum*	Egypt	Mayo et al. (2010)
Sua chua	Dried skim milk, starter, sugar	Acid fermented milk	*Lb. bulgaricus, Strep. thermophilus*	Vietnam	Alexandraki et al. (2013)
Shyow	Yak milk	Acidic, thick-gel viscous, curd-like, savory	LAB, yeasts	China (Tibet), Bhutan, India	Tamang (2010a)
Tarag	Cow, yak, goat milk	Acidic, sour, drink	*Lb. delbrueckii* subsp. *bulgaricus, Lb. helveticus, Strep. thermophilus, Sacch. cerevisiae, Issatchenkia orientalis, Kazachstania unispora*	Mongolia	Watanabe et al. (2008)
Viili	Cow milk	Thick and sticky, sweet taste, breakfast	*Lc. lactis* subsp. *lactis, Lc. lactis* subsp. *cremoris, Lc. lactis* subsp. *lactis* biovar. *Diacetylactis, Leuc. mesenteroides* subps. *cremoris, G. candidum, K. marxianus, P. fermentans*	Finland	Kahala et al. (2008)
Wara	Milk	Sweet taste, beverage	*Lc. lactis, Lactobacillus* sp.	West Africa	Olasupo et al. (2010)
Yoghurt	Animal milk	Acidic, thick-gel viscous, curd-like product, savory	*Strep. thermophilus, Lb. delbrueckii* subsp. *bulgaricus, Lb. acidophilus, Lb. casei, Lb. rhamnosus, Lb. gasseri, Lb. johnsonii, Bifidobacterium* spp.	Europe, Australia, America	Tamime and Robinson (2007)

(Josephsen and Jespersen 2004). Examples of naturally fermented milks are *dahi, lassi, misti dahi, srikhand, chhu, chhurpi, mohi, philu, shoyu, somar* (cow/buffalo/yak milk) of India, Nepal, Pakistan, Bhutan, and Bangladesh (Harun-ur-Rashid et al. 2007, Sarkar 2008, Patil et al. 2010, Tamang 2010a, Tamang et al. 2012), *kurut* of China (Sun et al. 2010), *aaruul, airag, byasulag, chigee, eezgii, tarag,* and *khoormog* of Mongolia (Watanabe et al. 2008, Takeda et al. 2011, Oki et al. 2014), *ergo* of Ethiopia, *kad, lben, laban, rayeb, zabady, zeer* of Morocco and Northern African and Middle East countries, *rob* (from camel milk), *biruni* (cow/camel milk), *mish* (cow/camel milk) of Sudan, *amasi* (*hodzeko, mukaka wakakora*) of Zimbabwe, *nunu* (from raw cow milk) of Ghana (Akabanda et al. 2013), *filmjölk* and *långfil* of Sweden (Mayo et al. 2010), *koumiss* or *kumis* or *kumys* or *kymys* of the Caucasian area (Wu et al. 2009).

Lc. lactis subsp. *cremoris,* and *Lc. lactis* subsp. *lactis* are found among the dominant microbiota along with other mesophilic lactobacilli (*Lb. casei/Lb. paracasei, Lb. fermentum, Lb. helveticus, Lb. plantarum,* and/or *Lb. acidophilus*), *Ent. faecium,* and species of *Leuconostoc* and *Pediococcus* in naturally fermented milks (Tamang et al. 2000, Mathara et al. 2004, Patrignani et al. 2006, Dewan and Tamang 2006, 2007, Yu et al. 2011, Akabanda et al. 2013). Yeasts present in naturally fermented milks are *Candida lusitaniae, C. parapsilosis, C. rugosa, C. tropicalis, Kluyveromyces* (*Kl.*) *marxianus, Sacch. cerevisiae, Galactomyces geotrichum, Pichia kudriavzevii,* and others (Gadaga et al. 2000, Dewan and Tamang 2006, Akabanda et al. 2013). *Koumiss* or *kumis* or *kumys* or *kymys* is a natural fermented dairy product of the Caucasian area. *Lb. casei, Lb. coryniformis, Lb. curvatus, Lb. helveticus, Lb. kefiranofaciens, Lb. kefiri, Lb. paracasei, Lb. plantarum, Lb. fermentum,* and *Leuc. mesenteroides* (Ying et al. 2004, Watanabe et al. 2008, Wu et al. 2009), *Lb. acidophilus, Lb. fermentum,* and *Lb. kefiranofaciens* (dominant LAB), *E. faecalis, Lc. lactis, Lb. buchneri, Lb. jensenii, Lb. kefiri, Lb. kitasatonis, Lb. paracasei, Leuc. mesenteroides,* and *Strep. thermophilus* (Hao et al. 2010), yeasts *Sacch. cerevisiae, Issatchenkia orientalis, Kazachstania unispora, Kl. marxianus, Pichia mandshurica* (Watanabe et al. 2008) were isolated from *koumiss.*

1.5.2 Fermented Cereal Foods

The well-documented fermented cereal foods of the world (Table 1.2) are sourdough of Europe, America, and Australia (de Vuyst et al. 2009), *selroti* of India and Nepal (Yonzan and Tamang 2009), *idli* of India and Sri Lanka (Sridevi et al. 2010), *dosa* of India and Sri Lanka (Soni et al. 1986), *mawè* and *gowé* of Benin (Vieira-Dalodé et al. 2007), *ben-saalga* of Burkino Faso and Ghana (Humblot and Guyot 2009), *kisra* of Sudan (Hamad et al. 1997), *kenkey* of Ghana (Oguntoyinbo et al. 2011), *togwa* of Tanzania (Mugula et al. 2003), *ting* of Botswana (Sekwati-Monang and Gänzle 2011), *ogi* and *kunu-zaki* of Nigeria (Oguntoyinbo et al. 2011), and *tarhana* of Turkey, Cyprus and Greece (Sengun et al. 2009). Cereal fermentation is characterized by a complex microbial ecosystem, mainly represented by the species of LAB and yeasts (Corsetti and Settanni 2007), whose fermentation confers to the resulting bread its characteristic features such as palatability and high sensory quality (Blandino et al. 2003). The species of *Enterococcus, Lactococcus, Lactobacillus, Leuconostoc, Pediococcus, Streptococcus,* and *Weissella* are commonly associated with cereal fermentation (Guyot 2010). A native strain of *Sacch. cerevisiae* is the principal yeast of most bread fermentations (Hammes et al. 2005). Other non-*Saccharomyces* yeasts are also significant in many cereal fermentations which include *Candida, Debaryomyces, Hansenula, Pichia, Trichosporon, Yarrowia* (Foschino et al. 2004, Veinocchi et al. 2006). *Lb. plantarum, Lb. panis, Lb. sanfrancisensis, Lb. pontis, Lb. brevis, Lb. curvatus, Lb. sakei, Lb. alimentarius, Lb. fructivorans, Lb. paralimentarius, Lb. pentosus, Lb. spicheri, Lb. crispatus, Lb. delbrueckii, Lb. fermentum, Lb. reuteri, Lb. acidophilus, Lc. lactis, Leuc. mesenteroides, Ped. pentosaceus, W. confuse.* The yeasts

Table 1.2 Some Common and Uncommon Ethnic Fermented Cereal Foods of the World

Product	*Raw Material/ Substrate*	*Sensory Property and Nature*	*Microorganisms*	*Country*	*References*
Abreh	Sorghum	Solid state and submerged	*Lb. plantarum*	Sudan	Odunfa and Oyewole (1997)
Aliha	Maize, sorghum	Nonalcoholic beverage	LAB	Ghana, Togo, Benin	Odunfa and Oyewole (1997)
Ambali	Millet, rice	Acidic, pan cake Shallow-fried, staple	LAB	India	Tamang (2010a)
Ang-kak	Red rice	Colorant	*Monascus purpureus*	China, Taiwan, Thailand, Phillipines	Steinkraus (1996)
Banku	Maize and cassava	Staple food	*Lactobacillus* sp., yeasts	Ghana	Campbell-Platt (1987)
Bahtura	Wheat flour	Deep-fried bread	LAB, yeasts	India	Campbell-Platt (1987)
Boza	Cereals	Sour refreshing liquid	*Lactobacillus* sp., *Lactococcus* sp., *Pediococcus* sp., *Leuconostoc* sp., *Sacch. cerevisiae*	Bulgaria, Balkan	Blandino et al. (2003)
Burukutu	Sorghum and cassava	Creamy, liquid, drink	*Sacch. cerevisiae*, *Sacch. chavelieri*, *Leuc. mesenteroides*, *Candida* sp., *Acetobacter* sp.	Nigeria	Odunfa and Oyewole (1997), Kolawole et al. (2013)
Busa	Maize, sorghum, millet	Submerged	*Sacch. cerevisiae*, *Schizosacchromyces pombe*, *Lb. plantarum* ,*Lb. helveticus*, *Lb. salivarius*, *Lb. casei*, *Lb. brevis*, *Lb. buchneri*, *Leuc. mesenteroides*, *Ped. damnosus*	East Africa, Kenya	Odunfa and Oyewole (1997), Blandino et al. (2003)

(*Continued*)

Table 1.2 (*Continued*) Some Common and Uncommon Ethnic Fermented Cereal Foods of the World

Product	*Raw Material/ Substrate*	*Sensory Property and Nature*	*Microorganisms*	*Country*	*References*
Ben-saalga	Pearl millet	Weaning food	*Lactobacillus* sp., *Pediococcus* sp., *Leuconostoc* sp., *Weissela* sp., yeasts	Burkina Faso, Ghana	Tou et al. (2007)
Chilra	Wheat, barley, buckwheat	Staple	LAB, *Sacch. cerevisiae*	India	Thakur et al. (2004)
Dégué	Millet	Condiment	*Lb. gasseri, Lb. fermentum, Lb. brevis, Lb. casei, Enterococcus* sp.	Burkina Faso	Abriouel et al. (2006)
Dosa	Rice and black gram	Thin, crisp pancake, Shallow-fried, staple	*Leuc. mesenteroides, Ent. faecalis, Tor. candida, Trichosporon pullulans*	India, Sri Lanka, Malaysia, Singapore	Soni et al. (1986)
Enjera/Injera	Tef flour, wheat	Acidic, sourdough, leavened, pancake-like bread, staple	*Lb. pontis, Lb. plantarum, Leuc. mesenteroides, Ped. cerevisiae, Sacch. cerevisiae, Cand. glabrata*	Ethiopia	Olasupo et al. (2010)
Gowé	Maize	Intermediate product used to prepare beverages, porridges	*Lb. fermentum, Lb. reuteri, Lb. brevis, Lb. confusus, Lb. curvatus, Lb. buchneri, Lb. salivarius, Lact. lactis, Ped. pentosaceus, Ped. acidilactici, Leuc. mesenteroides; Candida tropicalis, C. krusei, Kluyveromyces marxianus*	Benin	Vieira-Dalodé et al. (2007), Greppi et al. (2013a)
Hakua	Rice	Strong off-flavor, therapeutic uses	Unknown	Nepal, India	Tamang (2005)
Hopper	Rice, coconut water	Steak-baked, pancake, staple	*Sacch. cerevisiae*, LAB	Sri Lanka	Steinkraus (1996)
Hussuwa	Sorghum	Cooked dough	*Lb. fermentum, Ped. acidilactici, Ped. pentosaceus*, Yeasts	Sudan	Yousif et al. (2010)

Huitlacoche or 'maize mushroom'	cobs of pre-harvest maize	Large fruiting body edible, condiment	*Ustilago maydis*	Mexico	Alexandraki et al. (2013)
Hulumur	Sorghum, rice, millet	Nonalcoholic drink	*Leuc. mesenteroides, Lb. Plantarum, Lactobacillus* sp.	Sudan, Turkey	Campbell-Platt (1987)
Idli	Rice, blackgram dhal or other dehusked pulses	Mild-acidic, soft, moist, spongy pudding; staple, breakfast	*Leuc. mesenteroides, Lb. delbrueckii, Lb. fermenti, Lb. coryniformis, Ped. acidilactis, Ped. cerevisae, Streptococcus* sp., *Ent. faecalis, Lact. lactis, B. amyloliquefaciens, Cand. cacaoi, Cand. fragicola, Cand. glabrata, Cand. kefyr, Cand. pseudotropicalis, Cand. sake, Cand. tropicalis, Deb. hansenii, Deb. tamarii, Issatchenkia terricola, Rhiz. graminis, Sacch. cerevisiae, Tor. candida, Tor. holmii*	India, Sri Lanka, Malaysia, Singapore	Steinkraus et al. (1967), Sridevi et al. (2010)
Jalebi	Wheat flour	Crispy sweet, donut-like, deep-fried, snacks	*Sacch. Bayanus, Lb. fermentum, Lb. buchneri, Lact. lactis, Ent. faecalis, Sacch. cerevisiae*	India, Nepal, Pakistan	FAO (1999)
Kenkey	Maize	Acidic, solid, steamed dumpling, staple	*Lb. plantarum, Lb. brevis, Ent. cloacae, Acinetobacter* sp., *Sacch. cerevisiae, Cand. mycoderma*	Ghana	Odunfa and Oyewole (1997), Oguntoyinbo et al. (2011)
Khanom-jeen	Rice	Noodle, staple	*Lactobacillus* sp., *Streptococcus* sp., *Rhizopus* sp., *Mucor* sp.	Thailand	Blandino et al. (2003)
Khamak (Kao-mak)	Glutinous rice, *Look-pang* (starter)	Dessert	*Rhizopus* sp., *Mucor* sp., *Penicillum* sp., *Aspergillus* sp., *Endomycopsis* sp., *Hansenula* sp., *Saccharomyces* sp.	Thailand	Alexandraki et al. (2013)

(Continued)

Table 1.2 (*Continued*) Some Common and Uncommon Ethnic Fermented Cereal Foods of the World

Product	*Raw Material/ Substrate*	*Sensory Property and Nature*	*Microorganisms*	*Country*	*References*
Kichudok	Rice	Steamed cake, side dish	*Leuc. mesenteroides, Ent. faecalis, Saccharomyces* sp.	Korea	Von Mollendorff (2008)
Kunu-zaki	Maize, sorghum, millet	Mild-acidic, viscous, porridge, staple	*Lb. plantarum, Lb. pantheris, Lb. vaccinostercus, Corynebacterium* sp., *Aerobacter* sp., *Cand. mycoderma, Sacch. cerevisiae, Rhodotorula* sp., *Cephalosporium* sp., *Fusarium* sp., *Aspergillus* sp., *Penicillium* sp.	Nigeria	Oguntoyinbo et al. (2011)
Kisra	Sorghum	Thin pancake bread, staple	*Ped. pentosaceus, Lb. confusus, Lb. brevis, Lactobacillus* sp., *Erwinia ananas, Klebsiella pneumoniae, Ent. cloacae, Cand. intermedia, Deb. hansenii, Aspergillus* sp., *Penicillium* sp., *Fusarium* sp., *Rhizopus* sp.	Sudan	Mohammed et al. (1991), Hamad et al. (1997)
Kishk	Wheat, milk	Refreshing beverage	*Lb. plantarum, Lb. brevis, Lb. casei, B. subtilis*, Yeasts	Egypt	Blandino et al. (2003)
Koko	Maize	Porridge	*Ent. clocae, Acinetobacter* sp., *Lb. plantarum, Lb. brevis, Sacch. cerevisiae, Cand. mycoderma*	Ghana	Blandino et al. (2003)
Kunu-zaki	Maize (white and yellow), red sorghum	Mild, sour liquid/ porridge, staple	*W. confusa, Strep. lutetiensis, Strep. gallolyticus* subsp. *macedonicus,*	West Africa, Nigeria	Olasupo et al. (2010)
Lao-chao	Rice	Paste, soft, juicy, glurinous desert	*Rhiz. oryzae, Rhiz. Chinensis, Chlamydomucor oryzae, Sacchromycopsis* sp.	China	Blandino et al. (2003)

Maheu	Maize, sorghum, millet	Refreshing beverage	*Lb. delbrueckii*	South Africa	Steinkraus (2004)
Mahewu	Maize	Refreshing beverage	*Lb. delbruchi, Lact. lactis*	South Africa	Blandino et al. (2003)
Mawè	Maize	Intermediate product used to prepare beverages, porridges	*Lb. fermentum, Lb. reuteri, Lb. brevis, Lb. confusus, Lb. curvatus, Lb. buchneri, Lb. salivarius, Lact. lactis, Ped. pentosaceus, Ped. acidilactici, Leuc. mesenteroides; Candida glabrata, Sacch. cerevisiae, Kluyveromyces marxianus, Clavispora lusitaniae*	Benin, Togo	Hounhouigan et al. (1993), Greppi et al. (2013a,b)
Masvusvu	Maize	Refreshing beverage	LAB	Zimbabwe	Alexandraki et al. (2013)
Marchu	Wheat flour	Baked bread	Unknown	India, Pakistan	Tamang (2010a)
Mbege	Maize, sorghum, millet	Submerged	*Sacch. cerevisiae, Schizosaccharomyces pombe, Lb. plantarum, Leuc. mesenteroides*	Tanzania	Odunfa and Oyewole (1997)
Me	Rice	Acidic, sour, condiment	LAB	Vietnam	Alexandraki et al. (2013)
Minchin	Wheat gluten	Solid, condiment	*Paceilomyces* sp., *Aspergilus* sp., *Cladosporium* sp., *Fusarium* sp., *Syncephalastum* sp., *Penicillium* sp., *Trichothecium* sp.	China	Blandino et al. (2003)
Mungbean starch	Mungbean	Fermented noodle	*Leuc. mesenteroides*	Thailand	Alexandraki et al. (2013)

(*Continued*)

Table 1.2 (*Continued*) Some Common and Uncommon Ethnic Fermented Cereal Foods of the World

Product	*Raw Material/ Substrate*	*Sensory Property and Nature*	*Microorganisms*	*Country*	*References*
Naan	Wheat flour	Leaved bread, baked	*Sacch. cerevisiae*, LAB	India, Pakistan, Afghanistan	Batra (1986)
Ogi	Maize, sorghum, millet	Mild-acidic, viscous, porridge, staple	*Lb. plantarum, Lb. pantheris, Lb. vaccinostercus, Corynebacterium* sp., *Aerobacter* sp., *Candida krusei, Clavispora lusitaniae, Sacch. cerevisiae, Rhodotorula* sp., *Cephalosporium* sp., *Fusarium* sp., *Aspergillus* sp., *Penicillium* sp.	Nigeria	Odunfa and Oyewole (1997), Greppi et al. (2013a)
Perkarnaya	Rye	Acidic, aerated bread	Yeasts, LAB	Russia	Alexandraki et al. (2013)
Pito	Maize, sorghum, millet	Submerged	*Geotrichum candidum, Lactobacillus* sp., *Candida* sp.	West Africa	Odunfa and Oyewole (1997)
Poto poto (Gruel)	Maize	Slurry	*Lb. gasseri, Lb. plantarum/ paraplantarum, Lb. acidophilus, Lb. delbrueckii, Lb. reuteri, Lb. casei, Bacillus* sp., *Enterococcus* sp., yeasts	Congo	Abriouel et al. (2006)
Pozol	Maize	Mild-acidic, thick viscous, porridge, staple	*Lactobacillus* sp., *Leuconostoc* sp., *Candida* sp., *Enterobacteriaceae, B. cereus, Paracolobactrum aerogenoides, Agrobacterium azotophilum, Alkaligenes pozolis, E. coli* var. *napolitana, Pseudomonas mexicana, Kleb. pneumoniae, Saccharomyces* sp., molds	Mexico	FAO (1998)
Pumpernickel	Rye	Acidic, full-grain, aerated bread; long shelf-life	Yeasts, LAB, as for rye sourdough	Switzerland, Germany	Alexandraki et al. (2013)

Puto	Rice	Steamed cake, breakfast	*Leuc. mesenteroides, Ent. faecalis, Ped. cerevisiae,* yeasts	Philippines	Steinkraus (1996)
Rabadi	Buffalo or cow milk and cereals, pulses	Mild-acidic, thick slurry-like product	*Ped. acidilactici, Bacillus* sp., *Micrococcus* sp.; Yeasts	India, Pakistan	Ramakrishnan (1979), Gupta et al. (1992)
Sourdough bread	Rye	Sandwich, bread	*Lb. pontis* and *Lb. panis, Lb. amylovorus, Lb. acidophilus, Lb. crispatus, Lb. delbrueckii, Lb. fermentum, Lb. reuteri, Sacch. cerevisiae, Issatchenkia orientalis*	Germany, Northern Europe	Iacumin et al. (2009)
San Francisco	(Rye), mainly wheat	Mild-acidic, leavened bread	*Lb. sanfrancisensis, Lb. alimentarius, Lb. brevis, Lb. fructivorans, Lb. paralimentarius, Lb. pentosus, Lb. plantarum, Lb. pontis, Lb. spicheri, Leuc. mesenteroides, W. confusa*	USA	Gänzle et al. (1998)
Seera	Wheat grains	Dried, sweet dish	Unknown	India, Pakistan	Thakur et al. (2004)
Selroti	Rice-wheat flour-milk	Pretzel-like, deep-fried bread, staple	*Leuc. mesenteroides, Ent. faecium, Ped. pentosaceus* and *Lb. curvatus, Sacch. cerevisiae, Sacch. kluyveri, Deb. hansenii, P. burtonii, Zygosaccharomyces rouxii*	India, Nepal, Bhutan	Yonzan and Tamang (2010, 2013)
Siddu	Wheat flour, opium seeds, walnut	Steamed bread, oval-shaped, staple	*Sacch. cerevisiae, Cand. valida*	India	Thakur et al. (2004)
Sourdough bread	Rye, wheat	Mild-acidic, leavened bread	*Lb. sanfranciscensis, Lb. alimentarius, Lb. buchneri, Lb. casei, Lb. delbrueckii, Lb. fructivorans, Lb. plantarum, Lb. reuteri, Lb. johnsonii, Cand. humili, Issatchenkia orientalis*	America, Europe, Australia	de Vuyst et al. (2009)

(*Continued*)

Table 1.2 (*Continued*) Some Common and Uncommon Ethnic Fermented Cereal Foods of the World

Product	*Raw Material/ Substrate*	*Sensory Property and Nature*	*Microorganisms*	*Country*	*References*
Tapai Pulut	Glutinous rice, *Ragi*		*Chlamydomucor* sp., *Endomycopsis* sp., *Hansenula* sp.	Malaysia	Steinkraus (1996)
Tape Ketan	Glutinous rice, *Ragi*		*Thizopus* sp., *Chlamydomucor* sp., *Candida* sp., *Endomycopsis* sp., *Saccharomyces* sp.	Indonesia	Steinkraus (1996)
Tepache	Maize, pineapple, apple or orange		*B. subtilis*, *B. graveolus* and the yeasts, *Tor. insconspicna*, *Sacch. cerevisiae* and *Cand. queretana*	Mexico	FAO (1998)
Ting	Sorghum	Sour taste	LAB	Botswana	Sekwati-Monang and Gänzle (2011)
Togwa	Cassava, maize, sorghum, millet	Fermented gruel or beverage	*Lb. brevis*, *Lb. cellobiosus*, *Lb. fermentum*, *Lb. plantarum and Ped. pentosaceus*, *Candida pelliculosa*, *C. tropicalis*, *Issatchenkia orientalis*, *Sacch. cerevisiae*	Tanzania	Mugula et al. (2003)
Tarhana	Sheep milk, wheat	Mild-acidic, sweet-sour, soup or biscuit	*Lb. bulgaricus*, *Strep. thermophilus*, yeasts	Cyprus, Greece, Turkey	Karagozlu et al. (2008)
Taotjo	Wheat, rice, soybeans	Semi-solid food, condiment	*Asp. oryzae*	East Indies	Blandino et al. (2003)
Uji	Maize, sorghum, millet, cassava flour	Acidic, sour, porridge, staple	*Leuc. mesenteroides*, *Lb. plantarum*	Kenya, Uganda, Tanzania	Odunfa and Oyewole (1997)

Sacch. cerevisiae, Sacch. exiguus, Candida humilis, C. milleri, Issatchenkia orientalis were isolated from sourdough (Iacumin et al. 2009, Weckx et al. 2010). Gluten-free sourdough was prepared from buckwheat and/or teff flours using *Ped. pentosaceus, Leuc. holzapfelii, Lb. gallinarum, Lb. vaginalis, Lb. sakei, Lb. graminis, W. cibaria* (Moroni et al. 2011).

1.5.3 Fermented Vegetable Products

People eat plants, both domesticated and wild, preparing them according to a variety of recipes. Perishable and seasonal leafy vegetables, radish, cucumbers including young edible tender bamboo shoots are traditionally fermented into edible products using the indigenous knowledge of biopreservation. Mostly species of *Lactobacillus* and *Pediococcus,* followed by *Leuconostoc, Weisella, Tetragenococcus,* and *Lactococcus* (Watanabe et al. 2009a, Savadogo et al. 2011) have been isolated from various fermented vegetable foods of the world (Table 1.3). Species of LAB present in Korean *kimchi* are *Lc. lactis, Lb. brevis, Lb. curvatus, Lb. plantarum, Lb. sakei* subsp. *sakei, Luec. citreum, Leuc. gasicomitatum, Leuc. gelidum, Leuc. kimchii, Leuc. mesenteroides* subsp. *mesenteroides, Ped. pentosaceus, Weissella confusa, W. kimchii,* and *W. koreensis* (Shin et al. 2008, Nam et al. 2009, Park et al. 2010, Jung et al. 2011). A few species of non-LAB and yeasts were also reported from *kimchi* which included species of *Halococcus, Haloterrigena, Candida, Kluyveromyces, Lodderomyces, Natrialba, Natronococcus, Pichia, Saccharomyces, Sporisorium,* and *Trichosporon* (Chang et al. 2008). The species of LAB reported from *sauerkraut* are *Lc. lactis* subsp. *lactis, Lb. brevis, Lb. curvatus Lb. plantarum, Lb. sakei, Leuc. fallax, Leuc. mesenteroides* and *Ped. pentosaceus* (Johanningsmeier et al. 2007, Plengvidhya et al. 2007). *Lb. brevis, Lb. casei, Lb. casei* subsp. *pseudoplantarum, Lb. fermentum, Lb. plantarum, Leuc. fallax, Ped. pentosaceus* constitute the native lactic flora in the Himalayan fermented vegetables such as *gundruk, sinki, goyang, khalpi, inziangsang* (Karki et al. 1983, Tamang et al. 2005, Tamang and Tamang 2007, 2010). *Lb. brevis, Lb. lactis, Lb. fermentum, Lb. pentosus, Lb. plantarum, Leuc. mesenteroides* and *Ped. pentosaceus* are the functional LAB in *pao cai* or *suan cai,* the naturally fermented vegetable products of China and Taiwan (Yan et al. 2008, Huang et al. 2009). A complex microbial community in the brines of fermented olives based on a culture-independent study consisted of LAB (*Lb. pentosus/Lb. plantarum, Lb. paracollinoides, Lb. vaccinostercus/Lb. suebicus* and *Pediococcus* sp.), both cultivable and uncultivable non-lactics (*Gordonia* sp./*Pseudomonas* sp., *Halorubrum orientalis, Halosarcina pallid, Sphingomonas* sp./*Sphingobium* sp./*Sphingopyxis* sp., *Thalassomonas agarivorans*) and yeasts (*Candida* cf. *apicola, Pichia* sp., *Pic. manshurica/Pic. galeiformis, Sacch. cerevisiae*) (Abriouel et al. 2011).

Sunki is an ethnic nonsalted and fermented vegetable product of Japan prepared from the leaves and stems of the red turnip (Wacher et al. 2010). *Lb. plantarum, Lb. brevis, Lb. buchneri, Lb. kisonensis, Lb. otakiensis, Lb. rapi, Lb. sunkii,E. faecalis, B. coagulans,* and *P. pentosaceus* have been isolated from *sunki* (Endo et al. 2008, Watanabe et al. 2009a). *Fu-tsai* and *suan-tsai* are the ethnic fermented mustard products of Taiwan prepared by the Hakka tribes eaten as soup, fried with shredded meat, or stewed with meat (Chao et al. 2009). *Ped. pentosaceus* and *Tetragenococcus halophilus* (Chen et al. 2006), *Lb. farciminis, Leuc. mesenteroides, Leuc. pseudomesenteroides, W. cibaria,* and *W. paramesenteroides* (Chao et al. 2009), *Lb. futsaii* (Chao et al. 2012) are isolated from *fu-tsai* and *suan-tsai.*

Ent. durans,Lb. brevis, Lb. coryniformis, Lb. curvatus, Lb. delbrueckii, Lb. plantarum, Lb. xylosus, Leuc. citreum, Leuc. fallax, Leuc. lactis, Leuc. mesenteroides, Ped. pentosaceus, Tetra. halophilus were reported from Indian fermented bamboo shoots (Tamang and Sarkar 1996, Tamang et al. 2008, Tamang and Tamang 2009, Tamang et al. 2012, Sonar and Halami 2014). Species of *B. cereus, B. pumilus, B. subtilis* and *Pseudomonas fluorescens* along with LAB were also isolated

Table 1.3 Some Common and Uncommon Ethnic Fermented Vegetable Products of the World

Product	*Substrate/Raw Materials*	*Sensory Property and Nature*	*Microorganisms*	*Country*	*References*
Anishi	Taro leaves	Acidic, wet	LAB	India	Tamang (2010a)
Bastanga	Bamboo shoot	Acidic, soft	LAB	India	Tamang (2010a)
Burong mustala	Mustard	Acidic, wet	*Lb. brevis, Ped. cerevisiae*	Philippines	Rhee et al. (2011)
Cucumbers (pickles)	Cucumbers	Acidic, wet, pickle	*Leuc. mesenteroides, Ped. cerevisiae, Ped. acidilactici, Lb. plantarum, Lb. brevis*	Europe, USA, Canada	Vaughn (1985)
Dha muoi	Mustard and beet (*dha muoi*), eggplant (*ca muoi*)	Acidic, wet	*Lb. fermentum, Lb. pentosus, Lb. plantarum, Ped. pentosaceus, Lb. brevis, Lb. paracasei, Lb. pantheris, Ped. acidilactici*	Vietnam	Nguyen et al. (2013b)
Dakguadong	Mustard leaf	Salad	*Lb. plantarum*	Thailand	Rhee et al. (2011)
Ekung	Bamboo shoot	Acidic, sour, soft, curry	*Lb. plantarum, Lb. brevis, Lb. casei, Tor. halophilus*	India	Tamang and Tamang (2009)
Eup	Bamboo shoot	Acidic, sour, dry, curry	*Lb. plantarum, Lb. fermentum, Lb. brevis, Lb. curvatus, Ped. pentosaceus, Leuc. mesenteroides, Leuc. fallax, Leuc. lactis, Leuc. citreum, Ent. durans*	India	Tamang and Tamang (2009)
Fu-tsai	Mustard	Acidic, sour	*Ent. faecalis, Lb. alimentarius, Lb. brevis, Lb. coryniformis, Lb. farciminis, Lb. plantarum, Lb. versmoldensis, Leuc. citreum, Leuc. mesenteroides, Leuc. pseudomesenteroides, Ped. pentosaceus, W. cibaria, W. paramesenteroides*	Taiwan	Chao et al. (2009, 2012)

Goyang	Wild vegetable	Acidic, sour, wet, soup	*Lb. plantarum, L. brevis, Lact. lactis, Ent. faecium, Ped. pentosaceus, Candida* sp.	India, Nepal	Tamang and Tamang (2007)
Gundruk	Leafy vegetable	Acidic, sour, dry, soup, side-dish	*Lb. fermentum, Lb. plantarum, Lb. casei, Lb. casei* subsp. *pseudoplantarum, Ped. pentosaceus ,*	India, Nepal, Bhutan	Karki et al. (1983), Tamang et al. (2005)
Hirring	Bamboo shoot tips	Acidic, sour, wet, pickle	*Lb. brevis, Lb. plantarum, Lb. curvatus, Ped. pentosaceus, Leuc. mesenteroides, Leuc. fallax, Leuc. lactis, Leuc. citreum, Ent. durans, Lact. lactis*	India	Tamang and Tamang (2009)
Hom-dong	Red onion	Fermented red onion	*Leuc. mesenteroides, Ped. cerevisiae, Lb. plantarum, Lb. fermentum, Lb. buchneri*	Thailand	Phithakpol et al. (1995)
Hum-choy	Gai-choy	Chinese sauerkraut	*Pediococcus* sp., *Streptococcus* sp.,	China	Phithakpol et al. (1995)
Inziang-sang	Mustard leaves	Acidic, sour, dry, soup	*Lb. plantarum, Lb. brevis, Ped. acidilactici*	India	Tamang et al. (2005)
Jeruk	Fruits and vegetables	Acidic, wet	LAB	Malaysia	Merican (1996)
Jiang-sun	Bamboo shoot, salt, sugar, *douchi* (fermented soybeans)	Fermented bamboo, side dish	*Lb. plantarum, Ent. faecium, Lc. lactis* subsp. *lactis*	Taiwan	Chen et al. (2010)
Khalpi	Cucumber	Acidic, sour, wet, pickle	*Lb. brevis, Lb. plantarum, Ped. pentosaceus, Ped. Acidilactici, Leuc. Fallax*	India, Nepal	Tamang et al. (2005), Tamang and Tamang (2010)

(Continued)

Table 1.3 (*Continued*) Some Common and Uncommon Ethnic Fermented Vegetable Products of the World

Product	*Substrate/Raw Materials*	*Sensory Property and Nature*	*Microorganisms*	*Country*	*References*
Kimchi (beachoo)	Cabbage, green onion, hot pepper, ginger	Acidic, mild-sour, wet, side-dish	*Leuc. mesenteroides, Leuc. citreum, Leuc. gasicomitatum, Leuc. kimchii, Leuc. inhae, W. koreensis, W. cibaria, Lb. plantarum, Lb. sakei, Lb. delbrueckii, Lb. buchneri, Lb. brevis, Lb. fermentum, Ped. acidilactici, Ped. pentosaceus*	Korea	Nam et al. (2009), Jung (2012)
Kimchi (Dongchimi)	Radish, salt, water	Acidic, mild-sour, wet, soup, side-dish	*Leuc. mesenteroides, Lb. plantarum, Lb. brevis, Ped. cerevisiae*	Korea	Nam et al. (2009), Jung (2012)
Kimchi (Kakdugi)	Radish, salt, garlic, green onion, hot pepper, ginger	Acidic, mild-sour, wet, side-dish	*Leuc. mesenteroides, , Lb. plantarum, Lb. brevis, Ped. cerevisiae*	Korea	Nam et al. (2009), Jung (2012)
Lung-siej	Bamboo shoot	Sour-acidic, soft	*Lb. brevis, Lb. plantarum, Lb. curvatus, Ped. pentosaceus, Leuc. mesenteroides, Leuc. fallax, Leuc. lactis, Leuc. citreum, Ent. durans*	India	Tamang (2010a)
Naw-mai-dong	Bamboo shoots	Acidic, wet	*Leuc. mesenteroides, Ped. cerevisiae, Lb. plantarum, Lb. brevis, Lb. fermentum, Lb. buchneri*	Thailand	Phithakpol et al. (1995)
Mesu	Bamboo shoot	Acidic, sour, wet	*Lb. plantarum, Lb. brevis, Lb. curvatus, Leu, citreum, Ped. pentosaceus*	India, Nepal, Bhutan	Tamang and Sarkar (1996), Tamang et al. (2008)
Oiji	Cucumber, salt, water	Fermented cucumber	*Leuc. mesenteroides, Lb. brevis, Lb. plantarum, Ped. cerevisiae*	Korea	Alexandraki et al. (2013)

Olives (fermented)	Olive	Acidic, wet, Salad, side dish	*Leuc. mesenteroides, Ped. pentosaceus; Lb. plantarum Lb. pentosus/Lb. plantarum, Lb. paracollinoides, Lb. vaccinostercus/ Lb. suebicus* and *Pediococcus* sp. non-lactics (*Gordonia* sp./*Pseudomonas* sp., *Halorubrum orientalis, Halosarcina pallid, Sphingomonas* sp./ *Sphingobium* sp./*Sphingopyxis* sp., *Thalassomonas agarivorans*) and yeasts (*Candida* cf. *apicola, Pichia* sp., *Pic. manshurica/Pic. galeiformis, Sacch. cerevisiae*)	USA, Spain, Portugal, Peru, Chile	Abriouel et al. (2011)
Pak-gard-dong	Leafy vegetable, salt, boiled rice	Acidic, wet, side dish	*Lb. plantarum, Lb. brevis, Ped. cerevisiae*	Thailand	Phithakpol et al. (1995)
Pak-sian-dong	Leaves of *Gynandropis pentaphylla*	Acidic, wet, side dish	*Leuc. mesenteroides, Ped. cerevisiae, Lb. plantarum, Lb. germentum, Lb. buchneri*	Thailand	Phithakpol et al. (1995)
Poi	Taro corms	Acidic, semi-solid	LAB, yeasts	Hawaii	Alexandraki et al. (2013)
Pao cai	Cabbage	Sweet and sour rather than spicy, breakfast	*Lb. pentosus, Lb. plantarum, Lb. brevis, Lb. lactis, Lb. fermentum, and Leuc. mesenteroides*, and *Ped. pentosaceus*	China	Yan et al. (2008)
Sauerkraut	Cabbage	Acidic, sour, wet, salad, side dish	*Leuc. mesenteroides, Ped. pentosaceus; Lb. brevis, Lb. plantarum, Lb. sakei*	Europe, USA, Canada, Australia	Johanningsmeier et al. (2007)

(*Continued*)

Table 1.3 (*Continued*) Some Common and Uncommon Ethnic Fermented Vegetable Products of the World

Product	*Substrate/Raw Materials*	*Sensory Property and Nature*	*Microorganisms*	*Country*	*References*
Sayur asin	Mustard leaves, cabbage, salt, coconut	Acidic, sour, wet, salad	*Leuc. mesenteroides, Lb. plantarum, Lb. brevis, Lb. confuses, Ped. pentosaceus*	Indonesia	Puspito and Fleet (1985)
Sinnamani	Radish	Acidic, sour, wet	LAB	Nepal	Tamang (2010a)
Soibum	Bamboo shoot	Acidic, sour, soft, curry	*Lb. plantarum, Lb. brevis, Lb. coryniformis, Lb. delbrueckii, Leuc. fallax, Leuc. Lact. lactis, Leuc. mesenteroides, Ent. durans, Strep. lactis, B. subtilis, B. lichniformis, B. coagulans, B. cereus, B. pumilus Pseudomonas fluorescens, Saccharomyces* sp., *Torulopsis* sp.	India	Jeyaram et al. (2009), Tamang et al. (2012)
Soidon	Bamboo shoot tips	Acidic, sour, soft, curry	*Lb. brevis, Leuc. fallax, Lact. lactis*	India	Tamang et al. (2008)
Soijim	Bamboo shoot	Acidic,liquid, condiment	*Lb. brevis, Lb. plantarum, Lb. curvatus, Ped. pentosaceus, Leuc. mesenteroides, Leuc. fallax, Leuc. lactis, Leuc. citreum, Ent. durans*	India	Tamang et al. (2008)
Sinki	Radish tap-root	Acidic, sour, dry, soup, pickle	*Lb. plantarum, Lb. brevis, Lb. casei, Leuc. fallax*	India, Nepal, Bhutan	Tamang and Sarkar (1993), Tamang et al. (2005)
Suan-cai	Vegetables	Acidic, sour, wet	*Ped. pentosaceus, Tetragenococcus halophilus*	China	Chen et al. (2006)

Suan-tsai	Mustard	Acidic, sour, dry	*Ent. faecalis, Lb. alimentarius, Lb. brevis, Lb. coryniformis, Lb. farciminis, Lb. plantarum, Lb. versmoldensis, Leuc. citreum, Leuc. mesenteroides, Leuc. pseudomesenteroides, Ped. pentosaceus, W. cibaria, W. paramesenteroides*	Taiwan	Chao et al. (2009)
Sunki	Turnip	Acidic, sour, wet	*Lb. plantarum, Lb. fermentum, Lb. delbrueckii, Lb. parabuchneri, Lb. kisonensis, Lb. otakiensis, Lb. rapi, Lb. sunkii*	Japan	Endo et al. (2008), Watanabe et al. (2009a)
Takuanzuke	Japanese radish, salt, sugar, *Shochu*	Pickle radish	*Lb. plantarum, Lb. brevis, Leuc. mesenteroides, Streptococcus* sp., *Pediococcus* sp., yeasts	Japan	Alexandraki et al. (2013)
Takanazuke	Broad leaved mustard, red pepper, salt, turmeric	Vegetable pickle Takuanzuke	*Ped. halophilus, Lb. plantarum, Lb. brevis*	Japan	Alexandraki et al. (2013)
Tuaithur	Bamboo shoot	Solid, wet, sour, curry	*Lb. plantarum, Lb. brevis, Ped. pentosaceou, Lc. lactis, Bacillus circulans, B. firmus, B. sphaericus, B. subtilis*	India	Chakrabarty et al. (2014)
Tuairoi	Bamboo shoot	Solid, dry, sour, curry	*Lb. plantarum, Ent. faecium, Ped. pentosaceous, Leuc. mesenteroides, B. laterosporus, B. circulans, B. stearothermophilus, B. firmus, B. cereus*	India	Chakrabarty et al. (2014)
Yan-Jiang	Ginger	Pickle	LAB	Taiwan	Chang et al. (2011)

from the fermented bamboo shoots of India (Jeyaram et al. 2010). *Jiang-sun* is a traditional fermented bamboo shoot food in Taiwan (Chen et al. 2010).

1.5.4 Fermented Legumes

Among the fermented legumes (Table 1.4), most of the products are of soybean origin. Two types of fermented soybean foods are produced: soybeans which are naturally fermented by *Bacillus* spp. (mostly *B. subtilis*) with characteristic stickiness, and soybeans which are fermented by filamentous molds (mostly *Aspergillus, Mucor, Rhizopus*). The *Bacillus*-fermented sticky soybean foods of Asia are *natto* of Japan (Kubo et al. 2011), *chungkokjang* of Korea (Shin et al. 2012), *kinema* of India, Nepal, and Bhutan (Tamang 2001), *aakhune, bekang, hawaijar, peruyaan*, and *tungrymbai* of India (Tamang et al. 2009), *thua nao* of Thailand (Dajanta et al. 2011), *pepok* of Myanmar (Tamang 2010b) and *sieng* of Cambodia and Laos (Tamang 2010b). Mold-fermented soybean products are *miso* and *shoyu* of Japan (Sugawara 2010), *tempeh* of Indonesia (Nout and Kiers 2005), *douchi* of China (Zhang et al. 2007), *sufu* of China (Han et al. 2001), *doenjang* of Korea (Kim et al. 2009). Among the common non-soybean fermented legumes of the world are *bikalga, dawadawa, iru, soumbala, ugba* of Africa (Parkouda et al. 2009, Ouoba et al. 2010), *dhokla, papad*, and *wari* of India (Nagai and Tamang 2010), *ontjom* of Indonesia (Nagai and Tamang 2010), and *maseura* of India and Nepal (Chettri and Tamang 2008).

The species of *Bacillus* isolated from *kinema* include *B. cereus, B. circulans, B. licheniformis, B. sphaericus, B. subtilis*, and *B. thuringiensis* (Sarkar et al. 1994, 2002, Tamang 2003), however, *B. subtilis* is the dominant functional bacterium in *kinema* (Sarkar and Tamang 1994, Tamang and Nikkuni 1996). *Ent. faecium* is also present in *kinema* (Sarkar et al. 1994). Based on molecular identification tools using ARDRA, ITS-PCR, and RAPD-PCR techniques, the species of *Bacillus* were isolated from *tungrymbai (*or *turangbai)* and *bekang*, naturally fermented soybean foods of the states of Meghalaya and Mizoram in North East India and were identified as *B. subtilis, B. pumilus, B. licheniformis, B. cereus, B. coagulans, B. circulans, B. brevis*, and *Lysinibacillus fusiformis* (Chettri 2013). *B. subtilis, B. licheniformis, B. cereus, Staphylococcus aureus, Staph. sciuri, Alkaligenes* spp., *Providencia rettgeri* were isolated from *hawaijar* of the state of Manipur in India (Jeyaram et al. 2008a).

Species of *Bacillus* isolated from naturally fermented *chungkokjang* are *B. amyloliquefaciens B. licheniformis*, and *B. subtilis* (Tamang et al. 2002, Choi et al. 2007, Kwon et al. 2009), *B. subtilis* subsp. *chungkokjang* (Park et al. 2005), *B. megaterium* (Shon et al. 2007). *Ent. faecium* is also present in *chungkukjang* (Yoon et al. 2008). Nam et al. (2012) analyzed 12,697 bacterial pyrosequences in *chungkukjang* and found that almost all the bacteria were members of the phylum *Firmicutes* (>95%), with only a small portion belonging to *Proteobacteria* (<5%). In various samples, specific unclassified *Bacillus* species and LAB existed as the dominant microbes of *chungkukjang* (Nam et al. 2012).

Japanese *natto* is the only *Bacillus*-fermented soybean food which is now produced by commercial mono-culture starter *B. natto*, first isolated from naturally fermented *natto* by Sawamura (1906). *B. natto* differs from *B. subtilis* on account of biotin requirement, production of polyglutamate, possession of 5.7-kb and 60-kb plasmids (Hara et al. 1983, Nagai et al. 1997), and insertion sequences (Nagai et al. 2000, Kimura and Itoh 2007). *Thua nao*, an ethnic fermented nonsalty sun-dried wafer-type soybean food of Thailand, is used as a seasoning. *B. subtilis* is a functional bacterium in *thua nao* (Chunhachart et al. 2006, Inatsu et al. 2006).

Rhizopus microsporus is a functional mold for fermentation of *tempeh* with varieties *Rhi. microsporus, Rhi. oligosporus, Rhi. rhizopodiformis, Rhi. tuberosus*, and *Rhi. chinensis*

Table 1.4 Some Common and Uncommon Ethnic Fermented Legume (Soybeans and Non-Soybean) Products of the World

Product	*Substrate/Raw Material*	*Sensory Features and Nature*	*Microorganisms*	*Country*	*References*
Aakhone	Soybean	Alkaline, sticky, paste	*B. subtilis, Proteus mirabilis*	India	Singh et al. (2014)
Bekang	Soybean	Alkaline, sticky, Paste, curry	*B. subtilis, B. pumilus, B. licheniformis, B. sphaericus, B. brevis, B. coagulans, B. circulans, B. amyloliquefaciens, Ent. faecium, Ent. durans, Ent. hirae, Ent. Raffinossus, Ent. cecorum, Proteus mirabilis Sacch. cerevisiae, Debaryomyces hansenii, Pic. burtonii.*	India	Chettri (2013), Singh et al. (2014)
Bhallae	Black gram	Mild acidic, side dish	*B. subtilis, Candida curvata, C. famata, C. membraneafaciens, C. variovaarai, Cryptococcus humicoius, Deb. hansenii, Geotrichum candidum, Hansenula anomala, H. polymorpha, Kl. marxianus, Lb. fermentum, Leuc. mesenteroides, Ped. membranaefaciens, Rhiz. marina, Sacch. cerevisiae, Ent. faecalis, Trichosporon beigelii, Trichosporon pullulans, Wingea robertsii*	India	Rani and Soni (2007)
Bikalga	Roselle (*Hibiscus sabdariffa*)	Condiment	*B. subtilis, B. licheniformis, B. megaterium, B. pumilus*	Burkina Faso	Ouoba et al. (2007a,b)
Ce-lew	Soybean, corn flour, rice flour, salt	Soya sauce	*Ped. halopholus, Bacillus* sp., *Asp. oryzae, Asp. flavus*	Thailand	Alexandraki et al. (2013)
Chee-fan	Soybean whey curd	Cheese-like, solid	*Mucor* sp., *Asp. glaucus*	China	Blandino et al. (2003)

(*Continued*)

Table 1.4 (*Continued*) Some Common and Uncommon Ethnic Fermented Legume (Soybeans and Non-Soybean) Products of the World

Product	*Substrate/Raw Material*	*Sensory Features and Nature*	*Microorganisms*	*Country*	*References*
Chungkokjang (or *jeonkukjang, cheonggukjang*	Soybean	Alkaline, sticky, soup	*B. subtilis, B. amyloliquefaciens, B. licheniformis, B. cereus, Pantoea agglomerans, Pantoega ananatis, Enterococcus* sp., *Pseudomonas* sp., *Rhodococcus* sp.	Korea	Hong et al. (2012), Shin et al. (2012)
Dage	Coconut press cake, *Ragi*	Solid, side dish	*Rhizopus* sp.,	Indonesia	Alexandraki et al. (2013)
Douchi	Soybean	Alkaline, paste	*B. amyloliquefaciens, B. subtilis, Asp. oryzae*	China, Taiwan	Wang et al. (2006), Zhang et al. (2007)
Dawadawa	Locust bean	Alkaline, sticky	*B. pumilus, B. licheniformis, B. subtilis, B. firmus, B. atrophaeus, B. amyloliquefaciens, B. mojavensis, Lysininbacillus sphaericus.*	Ghana, Nigeria	Amoa-Awua et al. (2006), Meerak et al. (2008)
Dhokla	Bengal gram	Mild acidic, spongy, Steamed, snack	*Leuc. mesenteroides, Lb. fermenti, Ent. faecalis, Tor. candida, Tor. pullulans*	India	Blandino et al. (2003)
Doenjang	Soybean	Alkaline, paste	*B. subtilis, B. licheniformis, B. pumilis, Mu. plumbeus, Asp. oryzae, Deb. hansenii, Leuc. mesenteroides, Tor. halophilus, Ent. faecium, Lactobacillus* sp.	Korea	Kim et al. (2009), Shin et al. (2012)
Dosa	Rice, blackgram dhal (*Phaselus mango*)	Fermented fan cake	*Leuc. mesenteroides, Lb. delbrueckii, Lb. fermenti, Ent. faecalis, B. amyloliquefaciens, Cand. boidini, Cand. glabrata, Cand. sake, Deb. hansenii, Hansenula polymorpha, Issatchenkia terricola, Rhiz. graminis*	India, Sri Lanka	Soni et al. (1986)

Furu	Soybean curd	Mild acidic	*B. pumilus, B. megaterium, B. stearothermophilus, B. firmus, Staph. hominis*	China	Sumino et al. (2003)
Gochujang	Soybean, red pepper	Hot-flavored seasoning	*B. velegensis, B. amyloliquefacious, B. subtilis, B. liqueformis,* spcecis of *Oceanobacillus, Zygosaccharomyses, Candida lactis, Zygorouxii, Aspergillus, Penicillium, Rhizopus*	Korea	Nam et al. (2012), Kim et al. (2013).
Hawaijar	Soybean	Alkaline, sticky	*B. subtilis, B. licheniformis, B. amyloliquefaciens, B. cereus, Staph. aureus, Staph. sciuri, Alkaligenes* sp., *Providencia rettgers, Proteus mirabilis*	India	Jeyaram et al. (2008a), Singh et al. (2014)
Hishiho-Miso	Soybean, barley or wheat, salt, vegetables, Mizuame, sugar, shoyu	Sweetend Miso	*Asp. oryzae, Ped. halophilus, Sacch. Rouxii, Streptococcus* sp.	Japan	Sugawara (2010)
Iru	Locust bean	Alkaline, sticky	*B. subtilis, B. pumilus, B. licheniformis, B. megaterium, B. fumus, B. atrophaeus, B. amyloliquefaciens, B. mojavensis, Lysininbacillus sphaericus, Staph. saprophyticus*	Nigeria, Benin	Odunfa and Oyewole (1997), Meerak et al. (2008)
Kanjang	Soybean, meju, salt, water	Soya sauce	*Asp. oryzae, B. subtilis, B. pumillus, B. citreus, Sarcina mazima, Sacch. Rouxii*	Korea	Shin et al. (2012)
Kawal	Leaves of legume (*Cassia* sp.)	Alkaline, strong flavored, dried balls	*B. subilis, propionibacterium* sp., *Lb. plantarum, Staph. sciuri,* Yeasts	Sudan	Dirar et al. (2006)
Kecap	Soybean, wheat	Liquid	*Rhiz. oligosporus, Rhiz. oryzae, Asp. oryzae, Ped. halophilus, Staphylococcus* sp., *Candida* sp., *Debaromyces* sp., *Sterigmatomyces* sp.	Indonesia	Alexandraki et al. (2013)

(Continued)

Table 1.4 (*Continued*) Some Common and Uncommon Ethnic Fermented Legume (Soybeans and Non-Soybean) Products of the World

Product	*Substrate/Raw Material*	*Sensory Features and Nature*	*Microorganisms*	*Country*	*References*
Ketjap	Soybean (black)	Syrup	*Asp. oryzae, Asp. flavus, Rhiz. oligosporus, Rhiz. arrhizus*	Indonesia	Alexandraki et al. (2013)
Kinda	Locust bean	Alkaline, sticky	*B. pumilus, B. licheniformis, B. subtilis, B. atrophaeus, B. amyloliquefaciens, B. mojavensis, Lysininbacillus sphaericus.*	Sierra Leone	Meerak et al. (2008)
Kinema	Soybean	Alkaline, sticky	*B. subtilis, B. licheniformis, B. cereus, B. circulans, B. thuringiensis, B. sphaericus, Ent. faecium, Cand. parapsilosis, Geotrichum candidum*	India, Nepal, Bhutan	Sarkar et al. (1994), Tamang (2003)
Khaman	Bengal gram	Mild acidic, spongy	*Leuc. mesenteroides, Lb. fermentum, Lact. lactis, Ped. acidilactici, Bacillus* sp.	India	Ramakrishnan (1979)
Koikuchi Shoyu	Defatted soybean flake, wheat, brine, tane-koji	Soy sauce	*Aspergillus sojae, Asp. oryzae, Sacch. rouxii, Tor. versatilis, Tor. echellsii, Ped. halophilus, Sacch. halomembransis, Ent. faecalis, Bacillus* sp.	Japan	Sugawara (2010)
Maseura	Black gram	Dry, ball-like, brittle, condiment	*B. subtilis, B. mycoides, B. pumilus, B. laterosporus, Ped. acidilactici, Ped. pentosaceous, Ent. durans, Lb. fermentum, Lb. salivarius, Sacch. cerevisiae, Pic. burtonii, Cand. castellii*	Nepal, India	Chettri and Tamang (2008)
Meitauza	Soybean	Liquid	*B. subtilis, Asp. oryzae, Rhiz. oligosporus, Mu. meitauza, Actinomucor elegans*	China, Taiwan	Zhu et al. (2008)

Meju	Soybean	Alkaline, paste	*Asp. flavus, Asp. fumigatus, Asp. niger, Asp. oryzae, Asp. retricus, Asp. spinosa, Asp. terreus, Asp. Wentii, Botrytis cineara Mu. adundans, Mu. circinelloides, Mu. griseocyanus, Mu. hiemalis, Mu. jasseni, Mu. Racemosus, Pen. citrinum, Pen. griseopurpureum, Pen. griesotula, Pen. kaupscinskii, Pen. lanosum, Pen. thomii, Pen. turalense, Rhi. chinensis, Rhi. nigricans, Rhi. oryzae, Rhi. Sotronifer; Candida edax, Can. incommenis, Can. utilis Hansenula anomala, Han. capsulata, Han. Holstii, Rhodotorula flava, Rho. glutinis, Sacch. exiguus, Sacch. cerevisiae, Sacch. kluyveri , Zygosaccharomyces japonicus, Zyg. rouxii; Bacillus citreus, B. circulans, B. licheniformis, B. megaterium, B. mesentricus, B. subtilis, B. pumilis, Lactobacillus* sp., *Ped. acidilactici*	Korea	Choi et al. (1995)
Miso	Soybean	Alkaline, paste	*Ped. acidilactici, Leuc. paramesenteroides, Micrococcus halobius, Zygosaccharomyces rouxii, Asp. oryzae*	Japan	Asahara et al. (2006)
Miso (Hishiho)	Soybean, barley or wheat, salt, vegetables, Mizuame (dextrose syrup), sugar, *shoyu*	Sweet miso	*Asp. oryzae, Ped. halophilus, Sacch. rouxii, Streptococcus* sp.	Japan	Sugawara (2010)

(*Continued*)

Table 1.4 (*Continued*) Some Common and Uncommon Ethnic Fermented Legume (Soybeans and Non-Soybean) Products of the World

Product	*Substrate/Raw Material*	*Sensory Features and Nature*	*Microorganisms*	*Country*	*References*
Miso (Kome Ama)	Rice, soybean, salt, *tane-koji*	Sweet rice miso	*Asp. oryzae, Streptococcus* sp., *Pediococcus* sp., *Sacch. rouxii*	Japan	Sugawara (2010)
Miso (Kome Kara)	Rice, soybean, salt, *tane-koji*, salt	Salt rice miso	*Asp. oryzae, Sacch. rouxii, Ped. halophilus, Tor. versalis, Tor. echellsii, Bacillus* sp.	Japan	Sugawara (2010)
Miso (Mame)	Cereal, soybean, salt		*Asp. oryzae, Asp. sojae, Ent. faecalis, Tor. versatilis, Bacillus* sp.	Japan	Sugawara (2010)
Miso (Mugi)	Barley, soybean, salt, *koji*	Barley Miso	*Asp. oryzae, Sacch. rouxii, Ped. halophilus, Ent. faecalis, Tor. versatilis, Tor. echellsii, Bacillus* sp.	Japan	Sugawara (2010)
Moromi	Soybean		*Aspergillus* sp., *Sacch. rouxii*	Japan	FAO (1998, 1999)
Natto	Soybean	Alkaline, sticky	*B. subtilis (natto)*	Japan	Nagai and Tamang (2010)
Oncom Hitam (Black *Oncom*) And *Oncom Merah* (Orange *Oncom*	Peanut press cake, tapioca, soybean curd starter	Fermented peanut press cake, roasted or fried	*Neurospora intermedia, N. crassa, N. sitophila* (from red *oncom*), *Rhi. oligosporus* (from black *oncom)*	Indonesia	Ho (1986)
Ogiri/Ogili	Melon seeds, castor oil seeds, pumpkin bean, sesame		*B. subtilis, B. pumilus, B. licheniformis, B. megaterium, B. rimus, Pediococcus* sp., *Staph. saprophyticus, Lb. plantarum*	West, East and Central Africa	Odunfa and Oyewole (1997)

Okpehe	Seeds from *Prosopis africana*	Alkaline, sticky	*B. subtilis, B. amyloliquefaciens, B. cereus, B. licheniformis*	Nigeria	Oguntoyinbo et al. (2010)
Owoh	Cotton seed		*B. subtilis, B. pumilus, B. licheniformis, Staph. saprophyticus*	West Africa	Odunfa and Oyewole (1997)
Papad	Black gram	Circular wafers	*Cand. krusei, Deb. hansenii, Lb. fermentum, Leuc. mesenteroides, P. membranaefaciens, Sacch. cerevisiae, Ent. faecalis, Trichosporon beigelii*	India, Nepal	Rani and Soni (2007)
Pepok	Soybean	Alkaline, sticky	*Bacillus* sp.	Myanmar	Nagai and Tamang (2010)
Peruyaan	Soybean	Alkaline, sticky	*B. subtilis, B. amyloliquefaciens, Vagococcus lutrae, Ped. acidilactici, Ent. faecalis*	India	Singh et al. (2014)
Sieng	Soybean	Alkaline, sticky	*Bacillus* sp.	Cambodia, Laos	Nagai and Tamang (2010)
Soumbala	Locust bean	Alkaline, sticky	*B. pumilus, B. atrophaeus, B. amyloliquefaciens, B. mojavensis, Lysininbacillus sphaericus. B. subtilis, B. thuringiensis, B. licheniformis, B. cereus, B. badius, B. firmus, B. megaterium, B. mycoides, B. sphaericus, Peanibacillus alvei, Peanibacillus larvae, Brevibacillus laterosporus*	Burkina Faso	Ouoba et al. (2003a,b, 2004)
Soy sauce	Soybean	Alkaline, liquid	*Asp. oryzae, Asp. niger, Sacch. rouxii, Ped. acidilactis, Ped. cerevisae, Ped. halophilus, Lb. delbrueckii*	Worldwide	Sugawara (2010)
Shoyu	Soybean	Alkaline, liquid, Seasoning	*Asp. oryzae* or *Asp. sojae, Z. Rouxii, C. versatilis*	Japan, Korea, China	Sugawara (2010)

(Continued)

Table 1.4 (*Continued*) Some Common and Uncommon Ethnic Fermented Legume (Soybeans and Non-Soybean) Products of the World

Product	*Substrate/Raw Material*	*Sensory Features and Nature*	*Microorganisms*	*Country*	*References*
Sufu	Soybean curd	Mild-acidic, soft	*Actinomucor elenans, Mu. silvatixus, Mu. corticolus, Mu. hiemalis, Mu. praini, Mu. racemosus, Mu. subtilissimus, Rhiz. chinensis*	China, Taiwan	Han et al. (2001)
Tamari Shoyu	Defatted soybean, salt, water, wheat	Soybean rich Shoyu	*Asp. sojae, Asp. oryzae, Sacch. rouxii, Tor. versaltilis, Tor. echellsii, Ped. halophilus, Ent. faecalis, Bacillus* sp.	Japan	Alexandraki et al. (2013)
Tauco	Soybean	Alkaline, paste, use as flavoring agent	*Rhiz. oryzae, Rhiz. ologosporus, Asp. oryzae, Lb. delbrueckii, Zygosaccharomyces soyae*	Indonesia	Winarno et al. (1973)
Tao-si	Soybean, salt, rice bran, wheat flour	Fermented soybean curd	*Asp. oryzae*	Philippines	Blandino et al. (2003)
Tempe	Soybean	Alkaline, solid, fried cake, breakfast	*Asp. niger, Rhiz. oligosporus, Rhiz. arrhizus, Rhiz. oryzae, Rhiz. stolonifer, Citrobacter freundii, Enterobacter cloacae, K. pneumoniae, K. pneumoniae* subsp. *ozaenae, Pseudomas fluorescens* as vitamin B_{12}-producing bacteria, *Lb. fermentum, Lb. lactis, Lb. plantarum, Lb. reuteri*	Indonesia (Origin), the Netherlands, Japan, USA	Nout and Kiers (2005), Jennessen et al. (2008)
Tempe Benguk	Velvet bean seeds, *Ragi* Tempe	Alkaline, solid, fried cake, breakfast	*Rhizopus* sp., *Rhiz. oligosporus, Rhiz. arrhizus*	Indonesia	Nagai and Tamang (2010)

Tempe Gembus	Solid residue of soybean curd, tapioca, *Ragi* tempe	Alkaline, solid, fried cake, breakfast	*Rhizopus* sp. *Rhiz. oryzae*, *Rhiz. oligosporus*	Indonesia	Alexandraki et al. (2013)
Tempe Kecipir	Winged bean seed, *Ragi*, old Tempe	Alkaline, solid, fried cake, breakfast	*Rhiz. oryzae*, *Rhiz. arrhizus*, *Rhiz. oligosporus*, *Rhiz. achlamydosporus*	Indonesia	Alexandraki et al. (2013)
Tempe Kedelai	Soybean, tapioca flour, maize, young papaya, cassava, coconut press cake, starter	Alkaline, solid, fried cake, breakfast	*Rhizopus* sp., *Rhiz. oryzae*, *Rhiz. oligosporus*	Indonesia	Alexandraki et al. (2013)
Tempe Koro Pedang	Jack bean seed (*Canavalia ensiformis*), *ragi*, old *tempe*	Alkaline, solid, fried cake, breakfast	*Rhiz. oryzae*, *Rhiz. arrhizus*, *Rhiz. achlamydosporus*	Indonesia	Alexandraki et al. (2013)
Tempe Lamtoro	Wied Tamarind (*Leucaena Leucocephala*)	Alkaline, solid, fried cake, breakfast	*Rhizopus* sp., *Rhiz. oryzae*	Indonesia	Alexandraki et al. (2013)
Thua nao	Soybean	Alkaline, paste, dry, side dish	*B. subtilis*, *B. pumilus*, *Lactobacillus* sp.	Thailand	Chunhachart et al. (2006)

(Continued)

Table 1.4 (*Continued*) Some Common and Uncommon Ethnic Fermented Legume (Soybeans and Non-Soybean) Products of the World

Product	*Substrate/Raw Material*	*Sensory Features and Nature*	*Microorganisms*	*Country*	*References*
Tofu (stinky tofu)	Soybean	Alkaline, liquid	*Bacillus* sp., *Ent. hermanniensis, Lb. agilis, Lb. brevis, Lb. buchneri, Lb. crispatus, Lb. curvatus, Lb. delbrueckii, Lb. farciminis, Lb. fermentum, Lb. pantheris, Lb. salivarius, Lb. vaccinostercus, Lc. lactis, Lactococcus* sp., *Leuc. camosum, Leuc. citreum, Leuc. fallax, Leuc. lactis, Leuc. mesenteroides, Leuc. pseudomesenteroides, Ped. acidilactici, Strep. bovis, Strep. macedonicus, W. cibaria, W. confusa, W. paramesenteroides, W. soli*	China, Japan	Chao et al. (2008)
Toyo	Soybean, salt, brown sugar, wheat starter	Cowpea sauce	*Asp. oryzae, Hansenula anomala, Hansenula subpelliculosa, Lb. delbrueckii*	Philippines	Alexandraki et al. (2013)
Tungrymbai/ turangbai	Soybean	Alkaline, sticky, curry, soup	*B. subtilis, B. pumilus, B. licheniformis, B. amyloliquefaciens, Lb. brevis, Ent. faecium, Ent. durans, Ent. hirae, Ent. Raffinossus, Ent. cecorum, Vagococcus carniphilus Sacch. cerevisiae, Debaryomyces hansenii, Pic. burtonii,*	India	Chettri (2013), Singh et al. (2014)

Tuong	Rice, maize, salt	Staple	*Asp. oryzae, Sacch. rouxii, Ped. halophilus*	Vietnam	Alexandraki et al. (2013)
Ugba	African oil bean (*Pentaclethra macrophylla*)	Alkaline, flat, glossy, brown in color	*B. subtilis, B. pumilus, B. licheniformis, Staph. saprophyticus*	Nigeria	Odunfa and Oyewole (1997)
Uri	Locust bean	Alkaline, sticky, condiment, soup	*Bacillus* spp.	West Africa	Alexandraki et al. (2013)
Usukuchi Shoyu	Soybean, wheat, Tane-Koji, Amasake	Soy sauce, seasoning	*Asp. oryzae, Sacch. rouxii,* tor. *versatilis, Tor. echellsii, Ped. halophilus, Sacch. halomembransis, Ent. faecalis, Bacillus* sp.	Japan	Alexandraki et al. (2013)
Vadai	Black gram	Paste, side dish	*Pediococcus* sp., *Streptococcus* sp., *Leuconostoc* sp.	India	Blandino et al. (2003)
Wari	Black gram	Ball-like, brittle, side dish	*B. subtilis, Cand. curvata, Cand. famata, Cand. krusei, Cand. parapsilosis, Cand. vartiovaarai, Cryptococcus humicolus, Deb. hansenii, Deb. tamarii, Geotrichum candidum, Hansenula anomala, Kl. marxianus, Sacch. cerevisiae, Rhiz. lactosa, Ent. faecalis, Wingea robetsii, Trichosporon beigelii*	India	Rani and Soni (2007)

(Nout and Kiers 2005, Jennessen et al. 2008). *Citrobacter freundii, Enterobacter cloacae, Kl. pneumoniae, Kl. pneumoniae* subsp. *ozaenae, Pseudomonas fluorescens* as vitamin B_{12}-producing bacteria, and LAB—*Lb. fermentum, Lb. lactis, Lb. plantarum, Lb. reuteri* are important microorganisms in naturally fermented *tempeh* (Denter and Bisping 1994, Feng et al. 2005). Four types of *douchi* are produced in China: *Mucor*-fermented *douchi, Aspergillus*-fermented *douchi, Rhizopus*-fermented *douchi,* and *Bacillus*-fermented *douchi* (Zhang et al. 2007). *Aspergillus awamori, Asp. kawachii, Asp. oryzae, Asp. Shirousamii,* and *Asp. sojae* have been widely used as the starter in preparation of *koji* in Japan for production of *miso* and *shoyu* (Kitamoto 2002, Matsushita et al. 2009). *B. subtilis, B. licheniformis, Ent. faecium, Leuc. mesenteroides, Tetra. halophilus,* and *Asp. oryzae, Debaryomyces hansenii,* and *Mucor plumbeus* were isolated from *doenjang* (Kim et al. 2009). Using next-generation sequencing, Nam et al. (2011) have analysed the microbial community of traditional Korean soybean pastes, and derived 17,675 bacterial sequences from nine local and two commercial brands of *doenjang* samples.

Bikalga, dawadawa, iru, mbodi, ntoba and *soumbala* are the ethnic nonsalted fermented locust bean (*Parkia biglobosa*) foods of Africa. Microorganisms involved are *B. amyloliquefaciens, B. lichenifornis, B. megaterium, B. pumilus, B. subtilis, Enterococcus avium, Ent. casseliflavus, Ent. faecalis, Ent. faecium, Ent. hirae, Lb. plantarum, Micrococcus* spp., *Ped. acidilactici, Ped. pentosaceus, Staphylococcus* (*Staph.*) *hominis, Staph. saprophyticus, Staph. xylosus,, Weissella cibaria,* and *W. confusa* (Amoa-Awua et al. 2006, Azokpota et al. 2006, Meerak et al. 2008, Ouoba et al. 2010). Although *B. subtilis* has been reported as the dominant bacterium involved in the fermentation, other *Bacillus* spp. such as *B. amyloliquefaciens, B. cereus,* and *B. licheniformis* have also been detected, for example, in *okpehe* produced in Nigeria from *Prosopis africana* (legume) seeds, thus suggesting the inter-species diversity in these kinds of products (Oguntoyinbo et al. 2010). A study by Ouoba et al. (2008) reflects the interspecies diversity characterizing this fermentation, comprising *B. subtilis* as the predominant organism followed by *B. licheniformis,* while strains of *B. cereus, B. pumilus, B. badius, Brevibacillus bortelensis, B. sphaericus,* and *B. fusiformis* were also detected. A number of studies have been undertaken to develop starter cultures for the fermentation of indigenous legumes, such as the seeds of *Prosopis africana* (Oguntoyinbo et al. 2007), and of the African locust bean (*Parkia biglobosa*) (Ouoba et al. 2003a,b, 2004, 2005, 2007a,b).

1.5.5 Fermented Root Crop and Tuber Products

Cassava (*Manihot esculenta*) root is traditionally fermented into staple foods such as *gari* of Nigeria, *fufu* of Togo, Burkina Faso, Benin, Nigeria and Ghana, *agbelima* of Ghana, *chikawgue* of Zaire, *kivunde* of Tanzania, and *kocho* of Ethiopia (Table 1.5). *Gari* making involves several stages including fermentation, dextrinization, partial gelatinization, and tetrogradation (Abimbola 2007). In initial stage of fermentation of cassava is dominated by *Corynebacterium manihot* (Oyewole et al. 2004). *Lb. acidophilus, Lb. casei, Lb. fermentum, Lb. pentosus, Lb. plantarum* are present in *gari* (Oguntoyinbo and Dodd 2010). *Lb. plantarum, Leuconostoc* sp., and *Streptococcus* spp. play a major role in detoxification of the cyanogenic glucosides during *gari* fermentation (Ngaba and Lee 1979). *Geotrichum candidum* is the dominant yeast responsible for the characteristic taste and aroma of *gari* (Okafor and Ejiofor 1990).

Cassava root is also traditionally fermented into a sweet dessert such as *tapé* in Indonesia (Ardhana and Fleet 1989). A mixed culture of *Streptococcus, Rhizopus,* and *Saccharomycopsis* produces the aroma in the *tapé,* whereas *Sm. fibuligera* produces α-amylase and *Rhizopus* sp. produces glucoamylase (Suprianto et al. 1989). *Simal tarul ko jaanr* is a mild-alcoholic food beverage prepared from cassava root in Nepal and India (Tamang et al. 1996).

Table 1.5 Some Ethnic Fermented Root Crop Products of the World

Product	*Substrate/ Raw Materials*	*Sensory Property and Nature*	*Microorganisms*	*Country*	*References*
Chikwangue	Cassava	Solid state, staple	Species of *Corynebacterium, Bacillus, Lactobacillus, Micrococcus, Pseudomonas, Acinetobacter, Moraxella*	Central Africa, Zaire	Odunfa and Oyewole (1997)
Cingwada	Cassava	Solid state	Species of *Corynebacterium, Bacillus., Lactobacillus, Micrococcus*	East and Central Africa	Odunfa and Oyewole (1997)
Dage	Coconut press cake, *ragi*		*Rhizopus* sp.	Indonesia	Alexandraki et al. (2013)
Fufu	Cassava	Submerged, staple	*Bacillus* sp., *Lb. plantarum, Leuc. mesenteroides, Lb. cellobiosus, Lb. brevis; Lb. coprophilus, Lact. lactis; Leuc. lactis, Lb. bulgaricus, Klebsiella* sp., *Leuconostoc* sp., *Corynebacterium* sp., *Candida* sp.	West Africa	Odunfa and Oyewole (1997)
Iape Ketela	Cassava, *ragi*		Species of *Rhizopus, Chlamydomucor, Candida, Saccharomyces, Endomycopsis*	Indonesia	Alexandraki et al. (2013)
Gari	Cassava	Solid state, staple	*Corynebacterium mannihot, Geotrichum* sp., *Lb. plantarium, Lb. buchnerri, Leuconostoc* sp., *Streptococcus* sp.	West and Central Africa	Oyewole et al. (2004)
Lafun/ Konkonte	Cassava	Submerged, staple	*Bacillus* sp., *Klebsiella* sp., *Candida* sp., *Aspergillus* sp., *Leuc. mesenteroides, Corynebacterium manihot, Lb. plantarum, Micrococcus luteus, Geotrichum candidum*	West Africa	Odunfa and Oyewole (1997)

(*Continued*)

Table 1.5 (*Continued*) Some Ethnic Fermented Root Crop Products of the World

Product	*Substrate/ Raw Materials*	*Sensory Property and Nature*	*Microorganisms*	*Country*	*References*
Peujeum	Cassava roots	Acidic, solid, eaten after baking	Yeasts, mold	Indonesia	Alexandraki et al. (2013)
Simal tarul to jaanr	Cassava	Sweet, mild-alcoholic food, staple	*Mu. circinelloides, Rhi. Chinensis,- Pichia anomala, Sacch. cerevisiae, Candida glabrata, Saccharomycopsis fibuligera, Ped. pentosaceus, Lb. bifermentans*	India and Nepal	Tamang (2005)
Tapé	Cassava	Sweet dessert	*Streptococcus* sp., *Rhizopus* sp., *Saccharomycopsis fibuligera*	Indonesia	Suprianto et al. (1989)
Tapai Ubi	Cassava, Ragi	Sweet dessert	*Saccharomycopsis fibuligera, Amylomyces rouxii, Mu. circinelloides, Mu. javanicus, Hansenula* spp., *Rhi. arrhizus, Rhi. oryzae, Rhi. chinensis*	Malaysia	Merican and Yeoh (1989)

1.5.6 Fermented Fruit Products

Some fermented fruit pickles are *atchara* (green unripe papaya), *burong mangga* (green unripe mango), *burong prutas* (local fruits) of the Philippines, *achar* of India and Nepal, and so on (Table 1.6). *Ca muoi* is a fermented fruit of Vietnam, and *tempoyak* is a fermented durian fruit of Malaysia. *Sacch. cerevisiae, Schizosaccharomyces pombe, Lb. plantarum*, and *Leuc. mesenteroides* were isolated from *palm wine/emu*, a fermented palm fruit of West Africa (Odunfa and Oyewole 1997). *Lb. plantarum* strains were isolated from Thai fermented fruits (Tanganurat et al. 2009).

1.5.7 Fermented Meat Products

Traditionally preserved and fermented meat products (Table 1.7) of many countries are the *salami* of Europe (Toldra 2007), *alheira* of Portugal (Albano et al. 2009), *androlla* of Spain (Garcia-Fontan et al. 2007), *nham* of Thailand (Chokesajjawatee et al. 2009), *kargyong, satchu*, and *suka ko masu* of India and Nepal (Rai et al. 2009, 2010), *arjia, chartayshya* and *jamma* of India (Oki et al. 2011), and *nem chua* of Vietnam (Khanh et al. 2011, Nguyen et al. 2011). The major microorganisms involved in meat fermentation are a species of LAB and coagulase-negative cocii, however, yeasts and enterococci are also present in some meat products (Rantsiou and Cocolin 2006). Identification based on the culture-independent approach using the DGGE-method has revealed *Lb. curvatus* and *Lb. sakei* as the main species of LAB involved in the transformation process, accompanied by coagulase-negative cocci *Staphy. xylosus* during meat fermentation and ripening (Cocolin et al. 2011). *Lb. curvatus, Lb. paraplantarum, Lb. plantarum, Lb. sakei, Lb. brevis, Lb. carnis, Lb. casei, Lb. curvatus, Lb. divergens, Lb. sanfransiscensis, Leuc. carnosum, Leuc. gelidium, Leuc. pseudomesenteroides, Leuc. citreum, Leuc. mesenteroides, Ped. acidilactici, Ped. pentosaceus, W. cibaria, W. viridescens, B. lentus, B. licheniformis, B. mycoides, B. subtilis, B. thuringiensis, E. cecorum, E. durans, E. faecalis, E. faecium, E. hirae* are the dominant LAB in fermented meats (Albano et al. 2009, Rai et al. 2010, Cocolin et al. 2011, Oki et al. 2011, Nguyen et al. 2013a); and also coagulase-negative staphylococci, micrococci, Enterobacteriaceae in fermented meats (Marty et al. 2011). The species of yeasts present in Spanish fermented sausages are *C. intermedia/curvata, C. parapsilosis, C. zeylanoides, Citeromyces matritensis, Trichosporon ovoides*, and *Yarrowia lipolytica* (Encinas et al. 2000).

1.5.8 Fermented, Dried and Smoked Fish Products

Preservation of fish through fermentation, sun drying, smoking and salting is traditionally performed by people living in coastal regions, or near lakes and rivers, and such preserved/fermented fish products are consumed as seasoning, condiments, curry and on the side (Salampessy et al. 2010). Some ethnic fermented fish products of the world (Table 1.8) are *hentak, ngari*, and *tungtap* of India (Thapa et al. 2004), and *bordia, karati*, and *lashim* of India (Thapa et al. 2007), *jeotgal* or *jeot* or *saeu-jeot* of Korea (Guan et al. 2011, Jung et al. 2013), *plaa-som* of Thailand (Saithong et al. 2010), *shiokara* of Japan (Fujii et al. 1999), *patis* of the Philippines (Steinkraus 1996), *surströmming* of Sweden (Kobayashi et al. 2000a), and sun-dried or smoked fish products such as *gnuchi, sidra, sukuti* of India, Nepal, and Bhutan (Thapa et al. 2006), *Ent. faecalis, Lb. plantarum, Lb. reuteri, Strep. salivarius*, species of *Bacillus, Micrococcus, Pediococcus* and yeasts including species of *Candida* and *Saccharomyces* are reported from fermented fish products of Thailand (Saithong et al. 2010, Hwanhlem et al. 2011). *Micrococcus* and *Staphylococcus* are dominant bacterial genera during ripening of *shiokara* (Wu et al. 2000). *Haloanaerobium praevalens* has been

Table 1.6 Some Ethnic Fermented Fruit Products of the World

Product	*Substrate/Raw Materials*	*Sensory Property and Nature*	*Microorganisms*	*Country*	*References*
Achar/ chatney	Fruits, vegetables, oil, salt	Acidic, hot and sour, pickle	LAB	India, Nepal, Pakistan, Bangladesh	Tamang (2010b)
Atchara	Green unripe papaya, onion, red pepper, garlic, ginger, salt	Unripe papaya pickle	*Leuc. mesenteroides, Lb. brevis, Lb. plantarum, Strep. faecalis, Ped. cerevisiae*	Philippines	Alexandraki et al. (2013)
Burong Mangga	Green unripe mango, salt	Pickled green mango		Philippines	Alexandraki et al. (2013)
Burong Prutas	Fruits, salt, sugar	Picked fruits	*Lb. brevis, Lb. plantarum, Leuc. mesenteroides*	Philippines	Alexandraki et al. (2013)
Chuk	Fruits	Sour, dark-brown paste, therapeutic uses	unknown	Nepal, India	Tamang (2005)
Ogiri	Melon seeds	Alkaline, condiment	LAB, *Bacillus* spp.	Nigeria	Tamang (2010b)
Owoh	Cotton seeds	Alkaline, condiment	LAB, *Bacillus*	Nigeria	Tamang (2010b)
Tempoyak	Durian fruit	Fermented durian fruit	Yeast, *Bacillus* sp., *Acetobacter* sp., *Lactobacilus* sp.	Malaysia	Merican (1996)

Table 1.7 Some Common and Uncommon Ethnic Fermented Meat Products of the World

Product	*Substrate/Raw Materials*	*Sensory Property and Nature*	*Microorganisms*	*Country*	*References*
Alheira	Pork or beef, bread chopped fat, spices, salt	Dry/ semi-dry, sausage	LAB, staphylococci, micrococci, yeast	Portugal	Albano et al. (2009)
Androlla	Ground lean pork	Dry, sausage	LAB, micrococci, yeast	Spain	Garcia-Fontan et al. (2007)
Arjia	Large intestine of chevon	Sausage, curry	*Ent. faecalis, Ent. faecium, Ent. hirae, Leuc. citreum, Leuc. mesenteroides, Ped. pentosaceus, Weissella cibaria*	India, Nepal	Oki et al. (2011)
Bacon	Cured pork, beef	Dry, semi-dry, staple	LAB, yeast, micrococci	Germany, Belgium, Spain	Tanaka et al. (1980)
Chartayshya	Chevon	Dried, smoked meat, curry	*Ent. faecalis, Ent. faecium, Ent. hirae, Leuc. citreum, Leuc. mesenteroides, Ped. pentosaceus, Weissella cibaria*	India	Oki et al. (2012)
Chorizo	Pork, coarse chopped, spices, salt	Dry	*Lb. sake, Lb. curvatus, Lb. plantarum*	Spain	Garcia-Varona et al. (2000)
Chilu	Yak, beef, sheep fat	Hard, oily, edible oil	LAB	India, China (Tibet), Bhutan	Tamang et al. (2009)
Ham	Cured pork	Semi-dry, breakfast	LAB, yeasts, micrococci	Spain, Italy	Simoncini et al. (2007)
Honoheigrain	Pig/boar meat	Rough, hard, dried meat; curry	*Lb. brevis, Lb. plantarum, Leuc. mesenteroides, E. faecium, B. cereus, B. pumilus, B. firmus, B. circulans, B. stearothermophilus, Micrococcus, Staphylococcus; Debaryomyces hansenii, Sacch. cerevisae*	India	Chakrabarty et al. (2014)

(Continued)

Table 1.7 (*Continued*) Some Common and Uncommon Ethnic Fermented Meat Products of the World

Product	*Substrate/Raw Materials*	*Sensory Property and Nature*	*Microorganisms*	*Country*	*References*
Kargyong	Yak, beef, pork, crushed garlic, ginger, salt	Sausage like meat product, curry	*Lb. sakei, Lb. divergens, Lb. carnis, Lb. sanfrancensis, Lb. curvatus, Leuc. mesenteroides, Ent. faecium, B. subtilis, B. mycoides, B. thuringiensis, Staph. aureus, Micrococcus* sp., *Deb. hansenii, Pic. anomala*	India	Rai et al. (2010)
Kheuri	Yak, beef	Chopped intestine of yak, curry	LAB	India, China (Tibet), Bhutan	Tamang et al. (2009)
Jerky	Beef	Dry, semi-dry, side dish	LAB, yeast, molds, micrococci	South America	Delong (1992)
Longanisa	Pork lean, pork backfat, ground pork, salt, sugar, soysauce, vinegar, anisado wine, potassium nitrate		LAB	Philippines	Alexandraki et al. (2013)
Mortadello	Pork	Unsmoked chopped meat, sausage	LAB, micrococci	Italy, France, USA	
Nham (Musom)	Pork meat, pork skin, salt, rice, garlic	Fermented pork	*Ped. cerevisiae, Lb. plantarum, Lb. brevis*	Thailand	Chokesajjawatee et al. (2009)

Nem-chua	Pork, salt, cooked rice	Fermented sausage	*Lb. pentosus, Lb. plantarum, Lb. brevis, Lb. paracasei, Lb. fermentum, Lb. acidipiscis, Lb. farciminis, Lb. rossiae, Lb. fuchuensis, Lb. namurensis, Lc. lactis, Leuc. citreum, Leuc. fallax, Ped. acidilactici, Ped. pentosaceus, Ped. stilesii, Weissella cibaria, W. paramesenteroides.*	Vietnam	Nguyen et al. (2011)
Pastirma	Chopped beef lean meat with lamb fat, not smoked, heavily seasoned	Dry/semi-dry, sausage	*Lb. plantarum, Lb. sake, Pediococcus, Micrococcus, Staph. xylosus, Staph. carnosus*	Turkey, Iraq	Aksu et al. (2005)
Peperoni	Pork, beef	Dried meat, smoked, sausage	LAB, micrococci	Europe, America, Australia	Adams (2010)
Salami	Pork	Sausage	LAB, micrococci	Europe	Adams (2010)
Sai-krok-prieo	Pork, rice	Sausage	LAB	Thailand	Phithakpol et al. (1995)
Soppressata	Chopped lean pork meat, NaCl and spices	Dry/ semi-dry, sausage	LAB, yeast, staphylococci, micrococci, enterobacteriaceae	Italy	Parente et al. (1994)
Salchichon	Pork or beef meat, fat, NaCl, spices	Dry, sausage	LAB, Yeast, micrococcaceae, enterobacteriaceae, molds	Spain	Fernandez-Lopez et al. (2008)
Salsiccia	Chopped pork meat, spices, NaCl	Dry/ semi-dry, sausage	LAB, yeast, enterobacteriaceae staphylococci, micrococci	Italy	Parente et al. (2001a,b)
Sucuk	Chopped meat, pork or beef, curing salts and various spices	Dry, sausage	LAB, micrococci, staphylococci, enterobacteriaceae	Turkey	Genccelep et al. (2008)

(Continued)

Table 1.7 (*Continued*) Some Common and Uncommon Ethnic Fermented Meat Products of the World

Product	*Substrate/Raw Materials*	*Sensory Property and Nature*	*Microorganisms*	*Country*	*References*
Sai-krok-prieo	Pork, rice, garlic, salt	Fermented sausage	*Lb. plantarum, Lb. salivarius, Ped. pentosacuns*	Thailand	Adams (2010)
Satchu	Beef, yak, port, tumeric powder, edible oil, butter, salt	Ethnic dried meat, curry	*Ped. pentosaceuous, Lb. casei, Lb. carnis, Ent. faecium, B. subtilis, B. mycoides, B. lentus, Staph. aureus, Micrococcus* sp., *Deb. hansenii, Pic. anomala*	India	Tamang et al. (2012)
Suka ko masu	Goat, buffalo meat, tumeric powder, mustard oil, salt	Dried or smoked meat, curry	*Lb. carnis, Ent. faecium, Lb. plantarum, B. subtilis, B. mycoides, B. thuringiensis, Staph. aureus, Micrococcus* sp., *Debaromyces hansenii, Pic. burtonii*	India	Rai et al. (2010)
Sukula	Buffalo	Dried, smoked, curry	LAB	Nepal	Tamang (2010a)
Tocino	Pork, salt, sugar, potassium nitrate	Fermented cured pork	*Ped. cerevisiae, Lb. brevis, Leuc. mesenteroides*	Philippines	Alexandraki et al. (2013)

Table 1.8 Some Common and Uncommon Ethnic Fermented Fish Products of the World

Product	*Substrate/Raw Materials*	*Sensory Property and Nature*	*Microorganisms*	*Country*	*References*
Ayaiba	Fish	Smoked fish, pickle, curry	unknown	India	Tamang (2010a)
Bagoong Alamang (Bagoong Isda, Bagoong)	Fish/shrimp, salt	Fish/shrimp paste, condiment	*Bacillus* sp., *Pediococcus* sp.	Philippines	Alexandraki et al. (2013)
Balao-balao (Burong Hipon Tagbilao)	Shrimp, rice, salt.	Fermented rice shrimp, condiment	*Leuc. mesenteroides, Ped. cerevisiae, Lb. plantarum, Lb. brevis, Ent. faecalis*	Philippines	Alexandraki et al. (2013)
Balao-balao (Burong Hipon Tagbieao)	Shrimp, rice, salt	Fermented fish-rice, condiment	*Leuc. mesenteroides, Ped. cerevisiae*	Philippines	Arroyo et al. (1978)
Belacan (Blacan)	Shrimp, salt	Shrimp paste, condiment	*Bacillus, Pediococcus, Lactobacillus, Micrococcus, Sarcina, Clostridium, Brevibacterium, Flavobacterium, Corynebacteria*	Malaysia	Salampessy et al. (2010)
Bagoong	Fish	Fish paste; condiment	*Bacillus* sp., *Micrococcus* sp., *Moraxella* sp.	Philippines	Mabesa and Babaan (1993)
Bagoong alamang	Shrimp	Shrimp paste; condiment	LAB	Philippines	Mabesa and Babaan (1993)
Bakasang	Fish, shrimp	Fish or shrimp paste, condiment	*Pseudomonas, Enterobacter, Moraxella, Micrococcus, Streptococcus, Lactobacillus, Pseudomonas, Moraxella, Staphylococcus, Pediococcus* spp.	Indonesia	Ijong and Ohta (1996)

(Continued)

Table 1.8 (*Continued*) Some Common and Uncommon Ethnic Fermented Fish Products of the World

Product	*Substrate/Raw Materials*	*Sensory Property and Nature*	*Microorganisms*	*Country*	*References*
Burong Bangus	Milkfish, rice, salt, vinegar	Fermented milkfish, sauce	*Leuc. mesenteroides, Lb. plantarum, W. confusus*	Philippines	Alexandraki et al. (2013)
Burong Isda	Fish, rice, salt	Fermented fish, sauce	*Leuc. mesenteroides, Ped. cerevisiae, Lb. plantarum, Strep. faecalis, Micrococcus* sp.	Philippines	Sakai et al. (1983a,b)
Budu	Marine fishes, salt, sugar	Fish sauce	*Ped. halophilus, Staph. aureus, Staph. epidermidis, B. subtilis, B. laterosporus, Proteus* sp., *Micrococcus* sp., *Sarcina* sp., *Corynebacterium* sp.	Thailand, Malaysia	Merican (1977), Phithakpol et al. (1995)
Gnuchi	Fish (*Schizothorax richardsonii*), salt, tumeric powder	Eat as curry	*Lb. plantarum, Lact. lactis, Leuc. mesenteroides, Ent. faecium, Ent. faecalis, Ped. pentosaceus, Cand. chiropterorum, Cand. bombicola, Saccharomycopsis* sp.	India	Tamang et al. (2012)
Gulbi	Shell-fish	Salted and dried, side dish	*Bacillus licheniformis, Staphylococcus* sp., *Aspergillus* sp., *Candida* sp.	Korea	Kim et al. (1993)
Hákarl	Shark flesh	Fermented, side dish	LAB	Iceland	Alexandraki et al. (2013)
Hentak	Finger sized fish (*Esomus danricus*)	Condiment	*Lact. lactis, Lb. plantarum, Lb. fructosus, Lb. amylophilus, Lb. coryniformis, Ent. faecium, B. subtilis, B. pumilus, Micrococcus* sp., *Candida* sp., *Saccharomycopsis* sp.	India	Thapa et al. (2004)

Hoi-malaeng pu-dong	Mussel (*Mytilus smaragdinus*), salt	Fermented mussel	*Ped. halophilus, Staph. aureus, Staph. epidermidis*	Thailand	Phithakpol et al. (1995)
Ika-Shiokara	Squid, salt	Fermented squid	*Micrococcus* sp., *Staphylococcus* sp., *Debaryomyces* sp.	Japan	Alexandraki et al. (2013)
Jaadi	Fish, salt	Salted fish, curry, condiment	LAB	Sri Lanka	Alexandraki et al. (2013)
Jeot kal	Fish	High-salt fermented, staple	LAB	Korea	Guan et al. (2011)
Kapi	Small fish	Paste, condiment	Micrococci, LAB	Thailand	Phithakpol (1993)
Karati, Bordia, Lashim	Fish (*Gudushia chapra, Pseudeutropius atherinoides, Cirrhinus reba*), salt	Dried, salted, side dish	*Lact. lactis, Leuc. mesenteroides, Lb. plantarum, B. subtilis, B. pumilus, Candida* sp.	India	Thapa et al. (2007)
Kung-chom	Shrimp, salt, sweetened rice	Fermented fish-rice	*Ped. cerevisiae*	Thailand	Phithakpol (1993)
Kung chom	Shrimp (*Macrobrachum lanchesteri*), salt, garlic, rice	Fermented shrimp	*Ped. halophilus, Staph. aureus, Staph. epidermidis*	Thailand	Phithakpol (1993)
Kusaya	Horse mackerel, salt	Fermented dried fish	*Corynebacterium kusaya, Spirillum* sp., *C. bifermentans, Penicillium* sp.	Japan	Alexandraki et al. (2013)
Mehiawah	Marine fish	Fermented paste; side-dish		Middle-East	Al-Jedah et al. (1999)

(*Continued*)

Table 1.8 (*Continued*) Some Common and Uncommon Ethnic Fermented Fish Products of the World

Product	*Substrate/Raw Materials*	*Sensory Property and Nature*	*Microorganisms*	*Country*	*References*
Myulchijeot	Small sardine, salt	Fermented small sardine	*Ped. cerevisiae, Staphylococcus* sp., *Bacillus* sp., *Micrococcus* sp.	Korea	Alexandraki et al. (2013)
Narezushi	Sea water fish, cooked millet, salt	Fermented fish-rice	*Leuc. mesenteroides, Lb. plantarum*	Japan	Alexandraki et al. (2013)
Nam pla (Nampla-dee, Nampla-sod)	*Solephorus* sp. *Ristelliger* sp. *Cirrhinus* sp., water, brackish water, marine fish, salt	Fish sauce	*Micrococcus* sp., *Pediococcus* sp., *Staphylococcus* sp., *Streptococcus* sp., *Sarcina* sp., *Bacillus* sp., *Lactobacillus* sp., *Corynebacterium* sp., *Pseudomonas* sp., *Halococcus* sp., *Halobacterium* sp.	Thailand	Saisithi (1987), Wongkhalaung (2004)
Ngari	Fish (puntius sophore), salt	Fermented fish	*Lact. lactis, Lb. plantarum, Ent. faecium, Lb. fructosus, Lb. amylophilus, Lb. coryniformis, B. subtilis, B. pumilus, Micrococcus* sp., *Candida* sp., *Saccharomycopsis* sp.	India	Thapa et al. (2004)
Nga pi	Fish	Fermented paste, condiment	LAB	Myanmar	Tyn (1993)
Ngan pyaye	Fish	Fish sauce, condiment	LAB	Myanmar	Tyn (1993)
Nuoc mam	Marine fish	Fish sauce, condiment	*Bacillus* sp., *Pseudomonas* sp., *Micrococcus* sp., *Staphylococcus* sp., *Halococcus* sp., *Halobacterium salinarium, H. cutirubrum*	Vietnam	Lopetcharat et al. (2001)

Patis	*Stolephorus* sp., *Clupea* sp., *Decapterus* sp., *Leionathus* sp., fish, salt, food color-optional	Fish sauce	*Ped. halophilus, Micrococcus* sp., *Halobacterium* sp., *Halococcus* sp., *Bacillus* sp.	Philippines, Indonesia	Baens-Arega (1977)
Pla-ra	Fresh water fish, salt, roasted rice	Fermented fish-rice	*Pediococcus* sp.	Thailand	Phithakpol (1993)
Pla-chao (Pla-Khaomak)	Fresh water fish, salt, Khaomak	Thai sweetened fish	*Ped. cerevisiae, Staphyloccous* sp., *Bacillus* sp., *Micrococcus* sp.	Thailand	Phithakpol et al. (1995)
Pla-chom (Pla-khoa-kour)	Fresh water or marine anchovy, boiled rice, salt, garlic, roasted rice flour	Fermented fish, Thai anchovy	*Ped. cerevisiae, Lb. brevis, Bacillus* sp.	Thailand	Phithakpol et al. (1995)
Pekasam	Freshwater fish-rice	Fermented fish, side dish	LAB	Malaysia	Karim (1993)
Pindang	Fish	Dried, salted, side dish	LAB	Indonesia	Putro (1993
Pla-paeng-daeng	Marine fish, red molds rice (*Ang-kak*), salt	Red fermented fish	*Pediococcus* sp., *Ped. halophilus, Staph. aureus, Staph. epidermidis,*	Thailand	Phithakpol et al. (1995)
Pla ra (Pla-dag, Pla-ha, Ra)	Fresh water fish, brackish water fish, marine fish	Fermented fish	*Ped. cerevisiae, Lb. brevis, Staphylococcus* sp., *Bacillus* sp.	Thailand	Phithakpol et al. (1995)

(*Continued*)

Table 1.8 (*Continued*) Some Common and Uncommon Ethnic Fermented Fish Products of the World

Product	*Substrate/Raw Materials*	*Sensory Property and Nature*	*Microorganisms*	*Country*	*References*
Pla-som (Pla-khao-sug)	Marine fish, salt, boiled rice, garlic	Fermented fish	*Ped. cerevisiae, Lb. brevis, Staphylococcus* sp., *Bacillus* sp.	Thailand	Saithong et al. (2010)
Saeoo Jeot (Jeotkal)	Shrimp (*Acetes chinensis*), salt	Fermented shrimp	*Halobacterium* sp., *Pediococcus* sp.	Korea	Guan et al. (2011)
Som-fug (Som-dog, Pla-fu, Pla-muig, Fug-som)	Fresh fish, boiled rice, salt, garlic	Thai fermented fish, condiment	*Ped. cerevisiae, Lb. brevis, Staphylococcus* sp., *Bacillus* sp.	Thailand	Phithakpol et al. (1995)
Shottsuru	Anchovy, opossum shrimp, salt	Fish sauce, condiment	*Halobacterium* sp., *Aerococcus viridians (Ped. homari)*, halotolerant and halophilic yeasts	Japan	Itoh et al. (1993)
Sidra	Fish (*Punitus sarana*)	Dried fish, curry	*Lact. lactis, Lb. plantarum, Leuc. mesenteroides, Ent. faecium, Ent. facalis, Ped. pentosaceus, W. confusus, Cand. chiropterorum, Cand. bombicola, Saccharomycopsis* sp.	India	Thapa et al. (2006)
Sikhae	Sea water fish, cooked millet, salt	Fermented fish-rice, sauce	*Leuc. mesenteroides, Lb. plantarum*	Korea	Lee (1993)
Shiokara	Squid	Fermented; side-dish	LAB	Japan	Fujii et al. (1999)

Suka ko maacha	River fish (*Schizothorax richardsoni*), salt, turmeric powder	Smoked, dried, curry	*Lact. lactis, Lb. plantarum, Leuc. mesenteroides, Ent. faecium, Ent. faecalis, Ped. pentosaceus, Cand. chiropterorum, Cand. bombicola, Saccharomycopsis* sp.	India	Thapa et al. (2006)
Sukuti	Fish (*Harpodon nehereus*)	Pickle, soup, and curry	*Lact. lactis, Lb. plantarum, Leuc. mesenteroides, Ent. faecium, Ent. faecalis, Ped. pentosaceus, Cand. chiropterorum, Cand. bombicola, Saccharomycopsis* sp.	India	Thapa et al. (2006)
Surströmming	Fish	Fermented herrings	*Haloanaerobium praevalens*	Sweden	Kobayashi et al. (2000a)
Tai-pla	Fresh water fish, brackish water fish, marine fishes, salt	Fermented fish, condiment	*Pediococcus* sp., *Ped. halophilus, Staph. aureus, Staph. epidermidis*	Thailand	Phithakpol et al. (1995)
Trassi	Shrimps/fish	Fermented paste; side-dish	LAB, micrococci	Indonesia	Van Veen (1965)
Tungtap	Fish	Fermented fish, paste, pickle	*Lc. lactis* subsp. *cremoris, Lc. plantarum, Ent. faecium, Lb. fructosus, Lb. amylophilus, Lb. corynifomis* subsp. *Torquens, Lb. plantarum, B. subtilis, B. pumilus, Micrococcus*, yeasts-species of *Candida, Saccharomycopsis.*	India	Thapa et al. (2004)
Yu lu	Small fish like sardine or anchovies	Fish sauce	LAB, micrococci	China	Jiang et al. (2007)

reported from *surströmming*, the fermented herrings of Sweden and *Haloanaerobium fermentans*, *Tetra. muriaticus* and *Tetra. halophilus* from the Japanese puffer fish ovaries (Kobayashi et al. 2000b,c). *B. subtilis*, *B. pumilus*, *E. faecalis*, *E. faecium*, *Lc. lactis* subsp. *cremoris*, *Lc. lactis* subsp. *lactis*, *Lc. plantarum*, *Lb. amylophilus*, *Lb. fructosus*, *Lb. confusus*, *Lb.corynifomis* subsp. *torquens*, *Lb. plantarum*, *Leuc. mesenteroides*, *P. pentosaceus*, *Micrococcus*; yeasts—*Candida bombicola*, *C. chiropterorum*, and *Saccharomycopsis* spp. were isolated from Indian fermented and sun-dried fish products (Thapa et al. 2004, 2006, 2007).

1.5.9 Vinegar

Vinegar (Table 1.9) is one of the most popular condiments in the world and is prepared from any sugar containing substrates and hydrolyzed starchy materials by acetic acid fermentation. *Acetobacter aceti* subsp. *aceti*, *A. oryzae*, *A. pasteurianus*, *A. polyxygenes*, *A. xylinum*, *A. malorum*, *A. pomorum* are the dominant bacteria for vinegar fermentation (Haruta et al. 2006, Bourdichon et al. 2012). Yeast species in vinegar fermentation are *Candida lactis-condensi*, *C. stellata*, *Hanseniaspora valbyensis*, *H. osmophila*, *Saccharomycodes ludwigii*, *Sac. cerevisiae*, *Zygosaccharomyces bailii*, *Z. bisporus*, *Z. lentus*, *Z. mellis*, *Z. pseudorouxii*, and *Z. rouxii* (Solieri and Giudici 2008).

1.5.10 Ethnic Fermented Tea

Tea, the second most popular beverage in the world after water, originated in China and two common species of tea are *Camellia sinensis* var. *sinensis* and *Camellia sinensis* var. *assamica* (Schillinger et al. 2010). Though normal black tea is drunk everywhere, however, some ethnic Asian communities have special fermented tea such as *miang* of Thailand, *puer* tea and *fuzhuan brick* of China, and *kombucha*. Fermented tea (Table 1.10) is *puer tea*, *kombucha*, and *fuzuan* brick tea of China (Mo et al. 2008), and *miang* of Thailand (Tanasupawat et al. 2007).

Aspergillus niger is the predominant fungus in *puer tea*; *Blastobotrys adeninivorans*, *A. glaucus*, species of *Penicillium*, *Rhizopus* and *Saccharomyces*, and the bacterial species *Actinoplanes* and *Streptomyces* were also isolated from *puer tea* (Jeng et al. 2007, Abe et al. 2008). *Brettanomyces bruxellensis*, *Candida stellata*, *Rhodotorula mucilaginosa*, *Saccharomyces* spp., *Schizosaccharomyces pombe*, *Torulaspora delbrueckii*, *Zygosaccharomyces bailii*, *Z. bisporus*, *Z. kombuchaensis*, and *Z. microellipsoides* were isolated from *kombucha* (Kurtzuman et al. 2001, Teoh et al. 2004). The major bacterial genera present in *kombucha* were *Gluconacetobacter* (>85%), *Acetobacter* (<2%), *Lactobacillus* (up to 30%), and the yeast populations were found to be dominated by *Zygosaccharomyces* (>95%) (Marsh et al. 2014). *Lb. thailandensis*, *Lb. camelliae*, *Lb. plantarum*, *Lb. pentosus*, *Lb. vaccinostercus*, *Lb. pantheris*, *Lb. fermentum*, *Lb. suebicus*, *Ped. siamensis*, *E. casseliflavus*, and *E. camelliae* are involved in the fermentation of *miang* production (Sukontasing et al. 2007, Tanasupawat et al. 2007). Species of *Aspergillus*, *Penicillium* and *Eurotium* are major fungi for fermentation of *fuzhuan brick* tea (Mo et al. 2008).

1.5.11 Bacterial Cellulose

Nata or bacterial cellulose (Table 1.10) produced by *Acetobacter xylinum* is a candied delicacy of the Philippines (Kozaki 1976, Jagannath et al. 2010, Adams 2014). Two types of *nata* are well known: *nata de piña*, produced from the juice from pineapple trimmings, and *nata de coco*, produced from coconut water or coconut skim milk. Species identification using 16S rDNA sequencing revealed that the two strains belong to two different species of

Table 1.9 Some Common and Uncommon Vinegar Products of the World

Product	*Substrate*	*Sensory Property and Nature*	*Microorganisms*	*Country*	*References*
Cuka Aren	Sap from flower stalk of Aren	Vinegar, seasoning	*Acetobacter* sp.	Indonesia	Alexandraki et al. (2013)
Cuka Nipah	Sap from inflorescence stalk of Nipa fruiticans	Vinegar, seasoning	*Acetobacter* sp.	Malaysia	Alexandraki et al. (2013)
Sirca	Gur of molasses or grains	Vinegar, seasoning	*Sacch. cerevisiae, Acetobacter* sp.	Pakistan	Alexandraki et al. (2013)
Sirka	Fruit juices or sugar cane juices	Vinegar, seasoning	*Acetobacter* sp.	Bangladesh	Alexandraki et al. (2013)
Suka	Coconut water or fruits or sugar or palm sap or rice washings	Vinegar, seasoning	*Lb. fermentum, Lb. plantarum, Lb. panis, Lb. pontis, W. cibaria, Acetobacter pomoum, Actobacter ghanensis, Acetobacter orientalis, Acetobacter pasteurianus*	Philippines	Dalmacio et al. (2011)
Vinegar	Sugar containing substrates	Acetic acid flavored, liquid, condiment, seasoning	*Acetobacter aceti* subsp. *aceti, A. oryzae, A. pasteurianus, A. polyxygenes, A. xylinum, A. malorum, A. pomorum; Candida lactis-condensi, C. stellata, Hanseniaspora valbyensis, H. osmophila, Saccharomycodes ludwigii, Sacch. cerevisiae, Zygosaccharomyces bailii, Z. bisporus, Z. lentus, Z. mellis, Z. pseudorouxii, Z. rouxii*	Worldwide	Solieri and Giudici (2008), Sengum and Karabiyikli (2011)

Table 1.10 Some Miscellaneous Fermented Products of the World

Fermented Products	*Substrate/Raw Materials*	*Sensory Property and Nature*	*Microorganisms*	*Country*	*References*
Fermented Tea					
Fuzhuan brick	Tea	Fermented tea, drink	*Aspergillus, Penicillium, Eurotium*	China	Mo et al. (2008)
Kombucha or Tea fungus	Tea liquor	Flavored, drink	*Acetobacter xylinum, Zygosaccharomyces kombuchaensis, Z. bailii, Z. bisporus, Z. microellipsoides, Brettanomyces, Saccharomyces, Schizosaccharomyces pombe, Torulaspora delbrueckii, Rhodotorula mucilaginosa, Candida stellata, Brettanomyces bruxellensis*	China (Tibet), India	Schillinger et al. (2010)
Miang	Tea	Fermented tea, flavored, drink	*Lb. thailandensis, Lb. camelliae, Lb. plantarum, Lb. pentosus, Lb. vaccinostercus, Lb. pantheris, Lb. fermentum, Lb. suebicus, Pediococcus siamensis, E. casseliflavus* and *E. camelliae*	Thailand	Tanasupawat et al. (2007)
Puer	Tea	Fermented tea, brownish red, and a fragrance produced, drink	*Asp. glaucus*, species of *Penicillium*, and *Rhizopus, Blastobotrys adeninivorans*, and *Saccharomyces Actinoplanes, Streptomyces*	China	Jeng et al. (2007), Abe et al. (2008)
Bacterial Cellulose					
Nata de coco	Coconut water or coconut skim milk	Thick white or cream-colored, candied, ice cream, fruit salads	*Acetobacter* xylinus and A. hansenii	Philippines	Bernardo et al. (1998)

Nata de piña	Juice from pineapple	Insoluble gelatinous film of polysaccharides, ice cream, fruit salads	*Acetobacter* xylinus and A. hansenii	Philippines	Bernardo et al. (1998)
Chocolate					
Cacao	Cacao beans in pods of tree *Theobroma cocao*	Chocolate, confectionery	*Lb. fermentum, Acetobacter pasteurianus, A. senegalensis, Lb. ghanensis, Lb. plantarum, Lb. cacaonum, Lb. fabifermentans, Weissella fabaria, W. ghanensi, Fructobacillus pseudoficulneus, Tatumella ptyseos, Tatumella citrea, Bacillus coagulans; Hanseniaspora uvarum, H. quilliermundii, Issatchenkia orientalis (Candida krusei), Pichia membranifaciens, Sacch. cerevisiae, Kluyveromyces* sp.	Worldwide	Papalexandratou et al. (2011)
Coffee					
Coffee	Coffee	Flavored coffee, refreshing drink	*Ent. cloacae, Klebsiella oxytoca, Hafnia alvei, Lactobacillus, Leuconostoc, Weissella* spp.	Worldwide	Holzapfel and Müller (2007), Schillinger et al. (2008)
Fermented egg					
Pidan	Duck egg	Alkaline, side dish	*B. cereus, B. macerans, Staphylococcus cohnii, Staph. epidermidis, Staph. haemolyticus, Staph. warneri*	China	Wang and Fung (1996)

Acetobacter: A. xylinus and *A. hansenii* and may be a new subspecies under these species designation (Bernardo et al. 1998). Bacterial cellulose, a microbial polysaccharide, has significant potential as a food ingredient in view of its high purity, *in situ* change of flavor and color, and its ability to form various shapes and textures (Shi et al. 2014).

1.5.12 Cocoa/Chocolates

Chocolate (Table 1.10) is also a fermented product obtained from cocoa beans which require fermentation as one of the first stages. *Lb. fermentum* and *Acetobacter pasteurianus* were the predominating bacterial species during cocoa fermentation (Lefeber et al. 2010, Papalexandratou et al. 2011). Diverse LAB species appear to be typically associated with the fermentation of cocoa beans in Ghana, and, in fact, a number of new species have been described in recent years, for example, *Lb. ghanensis* (Nielsen et al. 2007), *Weissella ghanensis* (de Bruyne et al. 2008), *Lb. cacaonum, Lb. fabifermentans* (de Bruyne et al. 2009) and *Weissella fabaria* (de Bruyne et al. 2010). *Fructobacillus pseudoficulneus, Lb. plantarum*, and *Acetobacter senegalensis* were among the prevailing species during the initial phase of cocoa fermentation, and *Tatumella ptyseos* and *Tatumella citrea* were the prevailing enterobacterial species in the beginning of the fermentation (Papalexandratou et al. 2011). *Bacillus coagulans* are also recovered in vinegar (Bourdichon et al. 2012). Yeasts involved during spontaneous cocoa fermentation are *Hanseniaspora uvarum, H. quilliermundii, Issatchenkia orientalis* (*Candida krusei*), *Pichia membranifaciens, Sacch. cerevisiae,* and the *Kluyveromyces* species for flavor development (Ardhana and Fleet 1989).

1.5.13 Coffee Cherries

Coffee cherries are harvested from *Coffea arabica* trees and are processed by either wet or dry methods to remove the pulp and mucilaginous materials that surround the seeds (Silva et al. 2008). Species of yeasts and bacteria grow throughout these processes, producing pectinolytic, hemicellulolytic, and other enzymes that facilitate pulp and mucilage degradation (Masoud et al. 2004). *Ent. cloacae, Klebsiella oxytoca,* and *Hafnia alvei* have been isolated from coffee berries of Ethiopia (Holzapfel and Müller 2007), while LAB represented by *Lactobacillus, Leuconostoc,* and *Weissella* spp. seem to be typically associated with desirable fermentations of the coffee cherry (Schillinger et al. 2008).

1.5.14 Fermented Eggs

Pidan (Table 1.10), consumed by the Chinese, are preserved eggs prepared from alkali-treated fresh duck eggs, which have a strong smell of hydrogen sulfide and ammonia (Ganasen and Bejakul 2010). The main alkaline chemical reagent used for making *pidan* is sodium hydroxide, which is produced by the reaction of sodium carbonate, water, and calcium oxide of pickle or coating mud. *B. cereus, B. macerans, Staphy. cohnii, Staph. epidermidis, Staph. haemolyticus,* and *Staph. warneri* are predominant in *pidan* (Wang and Fung 1996).

1.6 Types of Fermented Beverages

1.6.1 Amylolytic Mixed Starters

The production of amylolytic starters (Table 1.11) are a unique traditional technology of preservation of the essential consortia of microorganisms (filamentous molds, amylolytic and

Table 1.11 Some Ethnic Amylolytic Starter Cultures of Asia

Product	*Substrate*	*Sensory Property and Nature*	*Microorganisms*	*Country*	*References*
Balan	Wheat	Dry, ball-like starter	Molds, yeasts	India	Tamang (2010a)
Bakhar	Rice-herbs	Dry, ball-like starter	Yeasts	India	Tamang (2010a)
Budod	Rice, starter	Basi production	*Mu. circinelloides, Mu. grisecyanus, Rhi. cohnii, Sacch. cerevisiae, Saccharomycopsis fibuligera*	Philippines	Kozaki and Uchimura (1990)
Binubudan (Binuburan, Purad)	Milled rice + Budod	Basi production	*Debarymyces hansenni, Cand. parapsilosis, Trichosporon fennicum*	Philippines	Tanimura et al. (1978)
Binokhok	Roast rice	Starter	Unknown	Philippines	Alexandraki et al. (2013)
Chiu-yueh	Rice, wild herbs	Gray-white, dry ball to preparae *lao-chao*	Species of *Rhizopus, Amylomyces, Torulopsis, Hansenula*	China, Taiwan, Singapore	Wei and Jong (1983)
Chou or chu or shi or qu	Rice, wheat, sorghum or barley flour	Dry, ball, cake or brick shaped	Species of Aspergillus, Candida, Weissella, Staphylococcus	China	Yan et al. (2013)
Chuzo	Rice, wild herbs	Dry, ball-like starter	Molds, yeasts, LAB	Mongolia	Alexandraki et al. (2013)
Dabai	Rice, wild herbs	Dry, ball-like starter	Molds, yeasts, LAB	India	Sha et al. (2012)

(Continued)

Table 1.11 (*Continued*) Some Ethnic Amylolytic Starter Cultures of Asia

Product	*Substrate*	*Sensory Property and Nature*	*Microorganisms*	*Country*	*References*
Hamei	Rice	Starter to make *atingbai*	*Mucor* sp., *Rhizopus* sp., *Sacch. cerevisiae*, *Pic. anomala*	India	Jeyaram et al. (2008b)
Hong qu (*hóng qu*)	Rice	Starter to make Chinese wine	*Saccharomycopsis fibuligera*, *Sacch. cerevisiae*, *Pichia*, *Candida*, *Cryptococcus*, *Rhodotorula*, *Sporobolomyces*, *Rhodosporidium*	China	Lv et al. (2013)
Humao	Rice, barks of wild plants	Dry, flat, cake-like starter for *Judima* production	*Ped. Pentosaceous*, *B. polymyxa*, *B. licheniformis*, *B. stearothermophilus*, *D. hansenii*, *Sacch. cerevisiae*, *Rhizopus*, *Mucor*	India	Chakrabarty et al. (2014)
Jui paing	Rice, wild herbs	Dry, ball-like starter to preparae *tapai*	Molds, yeasts, LAB	Malaysia	Alexandraki et al. (2013)
Ipoh/Siye	Rice, wild herbs	Dry, mixed starter	Molds, yeasts, LAB	India	Tamang (2010a)
Koji	Rice, wheat	Dry, black-yellow colored, mold-culture to produce *saké*, *miso*, *shoyu*	*Asp. awamori*, *Asp. kawachii*, *Asp. oryzae*, *Asp. shirousamii*, *Asp. Sojae*, yeasts	Japan	Lee et al. (2007), Suganuma et al. (2007)
Khekhrii	Germinated rice	Dry starter to make *Zutho*	Yeasts, LAB	India	Tamang (2010a)
Loogpang	Rice flour, powder of Kha root, spices	Starter, cake	*Rhizopus* sp., *Mucor* sp., *Chlamydomucor* sp., *Penicillum* sp., *Aspergillus* sp., *Asp. niger*, *Asp. flavus*, *Endomycopsis* sp., *Hansenula* sp., *Saccharomyces* sp.	Thailand	Tamang (2012b)

Marcha	Glutinous rice, roots, wild herbs, ginger, red dry chili	Starter	*Mu. circinelloides, Mu. hiemalis, Rhiz. chinensis, Rhiz. stolonifer, Saccharomycopsis fibuligera, Saccharomycopsis capsularis, Pichia anomala, Pichia burtonii, Sacch. cerevisiae, Sacch. bayanus, Cand. glabrata, Ped. pentosaceus, Lb. bifermentans, Lb. brevis*	India	Tsuyoshi et al. (2005)
Mana	Wheat, herbs	Dry, granulated starter to produce alcoholic drinks	*Asp. oryzae, Rhizopus* spp.	Nepal	Nikkuni et al. (1996)
Manapu	Rice-wheat, herbs	Dry, mixed starter to produce *poko*	Molds, yeasts	Nepal	Shrestha et al. (2002)
Men	Rice, wild herbs, spices	Dry, ball-like starter to produce *Ruou*	*Rhi. oryzae, Rhi. microsporus, Absidia corymbifera, Amylomyces rouxii, Saccharomycopsis fibuligera, Sacch. cerevisiae, Issatchenkia* sp., *Pic. anomala, Pic. ranongensis, Candida tropicalis, Clavispora lusitaniae, Xeromyces bisporus, Botryobasidium subcoronatum; Ped. pentosaceus, Lb. plantarum, Lb. brevis, Weissella confusa, W. paramesenteroides, Bacillus subtilis, B. circulans, B. amyloliquefaciens, B. sporothermodurans, Acetobacter orientalis, A. pasteurianus, Burkholderia ubonensis, Ralstonia solanacearum, Pelomonas puraquae*	Vietnam	Dung et al. (2006), Thanh et al. (2008)
Meju	Soybean	Fermented soybean starter	*Asp. oryzae, B. subtilis*	Korea	Alexandraki et al. (2013)

(*Continued*)

Table 1.11 (*Continued*) Some Ethnic Amylolytic Starter Cultures of Asia

Product	*Substrate*	*Sensory Property and Nature*	*Microorganisms*	*Country*	*References*
Nuruk (Kokja)	Wheat	Starter to produce *Takju, sojo, yakju*	*Asp. oryzae, Candida* sp., *Asp. niger, Rhizopus* sp., *Penicillum* sp., *Mucor* sp., *Hansenula anomala, Leuc. mesenteroides, B. subtilis*	Korea	Jung et al. (2012)
Phab	Wheat, wild herbs	Dry, mixed starter to produce *chyang*	Molds, yeasts, LAB	India, China (Tibet), Bhutan, Nepal	Tamang (2010a)
Poo	Rice, herbs	Dry, mixed starter to produce *chyang*	Molds, yeasts, LAB	Bhutan	Tamang (2012b)
Ragi	Rice flour, spices	Starter to produce *tape*	*Rhizopus, Mucor, Amylomyces rouxii, Aspergillus, Saccharomycopsis, Candida parapsilosis, C. melinii, C. lactosa, C. pelliculosa, Sacch. cerevisiae, Hansenula subpelliculosa, H. anomala* and *H. malanga, Enterococcus faecalis, Lb. plantarum* and *Ped. pentosaceus, B. coagulans, B. brevis, B. stearothermophilus*	Indonesia	Hesseltine et al. (1988), Hesseltine and Ray (1988)

Samac	Sugar cane	Basi production	Yeast, bacteria, molds	Philippines	Alexandraki et al. (2013)
Thiat	Rice-herbs	Dry, mixed starter to produce *kiad-lieh*	Molds, yeasts, LAB	India	Tamang (2010a)
Torami	Rice	Fermented rice gruel	*Hansenlu anomala, Candida guilliermondii, C. tropicalis, Geotrichium candidum*	India	Batra and Millner (1974)
Yao Qu (yào qu)	Rice	Starter to make Chinese wine	*Saccharomycopsis fibuligera, Sacch. Cerevisiae, Pichia, Candida, Cryptococcus, Rhodotorula, Sporobolomyces, Rhodosporidium*	China	Lv et al. (2013)

alcohol-producing yeasts, and LAB) with rice or wheat as the base in the form of dry, flat or round balls, for the production of alcoholic beverages in South East Asia including the Himalayan regions of India, Nepal, and Bhutan (Tamang 2010a). Three types of dry, amylolytic and mixed cultures or inocula are traditionally used in Asia as starters to convert cereal starch to sugars and subsequently to alcohol and organic acids (Tamang and Fleet 2009):

1. A consortium of mycelial or filamentous molds, amylolytic and alcohol-producing yeasts and LAB with rice or wheat as the base in the form of dry, flat or round balls of various sizes. The starter is inoculated with a previous starter. This mixed flora is allowed to develop for a short time, then dried, and used to make either alcohol or fermented foods from starchy materials, for example, *marcha, ragi, bubod, loogpang, nuruk, men,* and so on (Tamang 2010c), which are used as starters for a number of fermentations based on rice and cassava or other cereals in Asia (Table 1.12).
2. A combination of *Aspergillus oryzae* and *A. sojae* is used in the form of a starter called *koji* in Japan to produce alcoholic beverages including *saké. Koji* also produces amylases that convert starch into fermentable sugars, which are then used for the second stage yeast fermentation to make nonalcoholic fermented soybean products called *miso* and *shoyu,* while proteases are formed to break down the soybean protein.
3. Whole-wheat flour is moistened and made into large compact cakes, which are incubated to culture yeasts and filamentous molds and are used to ferment starchy material to produce alcohol in China.

Asian amylolytic starters have different vernacular names such as *marcha* in India and Nepal, *hamei, humao, phab* in India (Tamang et al. 1996, 2012; Shrestha et al. 2002), *mana* and *manapu* in Nepal (Nikkuni et al. 1996), *men* in Vietnam (Dung et al. 2007), *ragi* in Indonesia (Uchimura et al. 1991), *bubod* in the Philippines (Hesseltine and Kurtzman 1990), *chiu/chu* in China and Taiwan (Steinkraus 1996), *loogpang* in Thailand (Vachanavinich et al. 1994), and *nuruk* in Korea (Steinkraus 1996).

Microbial profiles of Indian amylolytic starters are filamentous molds—*Mucor circinelloides* forma *circinelloides, Mu. hiemalis, Rhi. chinensis,* and *Rhi. stolonifer* variety *lyococcus* (Tamang et al. 1988), yeasts—*Sacch. cerevisiae, Sacch. bayanus, Saccharomycopsis* (*Sm.*) *fibuligera, Sm. capsularis, Pichia anomala, Pic. burtonii,* and *Candida glabrata* (Tamang and Sarkar 1995, Tsuyoshi et al. 2005, Tamang et al. 2007, Jeyaram et al. 2008b, 2011), and LAB—*Ped. pentosaceus, Lb. bifermentans,* and *Lb. brevis* (Hesseltine and Ray 1988, Tamang and Sarkar 1995, Tamang et al. 2007). Microorganisms in *men* of Vietnam include amylase producers (*Rhi. oryzae, Rhi. microsporus, Absidia corymbifera, Amylomyces rouxii, Saccharomycopsis fibuligera*), ethanol producers (*Sacch. cerevisiae, Issatchenkia* sp., *Pic. anomala, Pic. ranongensis, Candida tropicalis, Clavispora lusitaniae*), yeasts contaminants (*Xeromyces bisporus, Botryobasidium subcoronatum*); LAB (*Ped. pentosaceus, Lb. plantarum, Lb. brevis, Weissella confusa, W. paramesenteroides*), amylase-producing bacilli (*Bacillus subtilis, B. circulans, B. amyloliquefaciens, B. sporothermodurans*), acetic acid bacteria (*Acetobacter orientalis, A. pasteurianus*), and environmental contaminants (*Burkholderia ubonensis, Ralstonia solanacearum, Pelomonas puraquae*) (Dung et al. 2006, 2007, Thanh et al. 2008).

A combination of *Asp. oryzae* and *Asp. sojae* are used in *koji* in Japan to produce alcoholic beverages including *saké* (Zhu and Trampe 2013). *Koji* (Chinese *chu, shi,* or *qu*) also produces amylases that convert starch into fermentable sugars, which are then used for the second stage yeast fermentation to make nonalcoholic fermented soybean *miso* and *shoyu* (Sugawara 2010). *Asp. awamori, Asp. kawachii, Asp. oryzae, Asp. shirousamii,* and *Asp. sojae* have been widely used as the

Table 1.12 Some Common and Uncommon Ethnic Fermented Beverages and Alcohol Drinks of the World

Product	*Substrate*	*Sensory Property and Nature*	*Microorganisms*	*Country*	*References*
Aara	Cereals	Clear distilled liquor	Unknown	India	Tamang (2010a)
Aarak	Barley, millet, *phab*	Distilled from *chyang*, clear liquor	Unknown	India, China (Tibet), Bhutan	Tamang (2010a)
Arrakku	Palm sap, sugar	Palm wine	*Sacch. cerevisiae*	Sri Lanka	
Atingba	Rice, *hamei*	Mild-alcoholic, sweet-sour		India	Jeyaram et al. (2009)
Apong	Rice, *phab*	Mild-alcoholic		India	Chakrabarty et al. (2014)
Bantu beer	Sorghum, millet	Opaque appearance, sour flavor, beer	LAB, yeasts	South Africa	Kutyauripo et al. (2009)
Basi	Sugar cane, *bubod*	Clear or cloudy liquid	Yeasts, molds	Philippines	Tanimura et al. (1978)
Bhaati Jaanr	Glutinous rice, *marcha*	Fermented rice beverage	*Mu. circinelloides, Rhiz. chinensis, Sm. fibuligera, Pic. anomala, Sacch. cerevisiae, Cand. glabrata, Ped. pentosaceus, Lb. bifermentans*	India	Tamang and Thapa (2006)
Bhang-chyang	Maize-rice/barley, *phab*	Extract of *mingri*, alcoholic beverage	Yeasts, molds	India	Thakur
Brem	Glutinous rice, ragi	Alcoholic drink	*Sacch. cerevisiae, Cand. glabrata, Cand. parapsilosis P. anomala, Issatchenkia arientalis, Lactobacillus* sp., *Acetobacter* sp. *Mu. indicus,*	Indonesia	Sujaya et al. (2004)

(*Continued*)

Table 1.12 (*Continued*) Some Common and Uncommon Ethnic Fermented Beverages and Alcohol Drinks of the World

Product	*Substrate*	*Sensory Property and Nature*	*Microorganisms*	*Country*	*References*
Bouza	Wheat, malt	Alcoholic thin gruel, alcoholic drink	LAB	Egypt	Steinkraus (1996)
Boza	Wheat, rye, millet, maize	Cooked slurry, food beverage	LAB, yeasts	Bulgaria, Romania, Turkey, Albania	Steinkraus (1996)
Bussa	Maize, sorghum, finger millet	Alcoholic thin gruel, refreshing drink	Yeasts, LAB	Kenya	Steinkraus (1996)
Bushera	Sorghum, millet	Slurry, food beverage	Yeasts, LAB	Uganda	Steinkraus (1996)
Bupju	Rice, glutinous rice, water, starter (Nuruk)	Alcoholic beverage	*Saccharomyces* sp.	Korea	Jung et al. (2012)
Cauim	Cassava, rice, peanuts, pumpkin, cotton seed, maize	Alcoholic beverage	Lb. plantarum, Lb. fermentum, Lb. paracasei, Lb. brevis; Pic. guilliermondii, K. lactis, Candida sp, Rhi. toruloides, Sacch. cerevisiae	Brazil	Ramos et al. (2010)
Chyang/Chee	Finger millet/barley, *phab*	Mild-alcoholic, slightly sweet-acidic		China (Tibet), Bhutan, Nepal, India	Tamang (2010a)
Chicha	Maize, human saliva	Alcoholic drink	*Sacch. cerevisiae*, *Sacch. apiculata*, *Sacch. pastorianus*, species of *Lactobacillus*, *Acetobacter*	Peru	Vallejo et al. (2013)
Chulli	Apricot	Filtrate, clear, alcoholic drink	Yeast	India	Thakur et al. (2004)

Daru	Cereal	Alcoholic beverages; filtrate, jiggery	Yeast, LAB	India	Thakur et al. (2004)
Emu	Palm	Palm wine, submerged	*Sacch. cerevisiae*, *Schizosaccharomyces pombe*, *Lb. plantarum*, *Leuc. mesenteroides*	West Africa	Odunfa and Oyewole (1997)
Ennog	Rice, paddy husk	Black rice beer	Yeast, LAB	India	Tamang (2010a)
Ewhaju	Rice, *nuruk*	Nondistilled, filtered and clarified, clear liquor	Yeast, LAB	Korea	Jung et al. (2012)
Faapar ko jaanr	Buck wheat, *marcha*	Mild-acidic, alcoholic beverage		India, Nepal	Tamang (2010a)
Feni	Cashew apple	Distilled wine from cashew apples, strong flavor	*Sacch. cerevisiae*	World-wide	Tamang (2010c)
Gahoon ko jaanr	Wheat, *marcha*	Mild-acidic, alcoholic beverage		India, Nepal	Tamang (2010a)
Haria	Rice, *dabai*	Alcoholic beverage	*Sacch. cerevisiae*, *Sacch. boulardii*, *Zygosaccharomyces cidri*, *Candida tropicalis*, *C. musae*, *C. nitratophila*, *Issatchenkia* sp., *Pediococcus* sp., *Lactobacillus* sp.	India	Sha et al. (2012)
Jao ko jaanr	Barley, *marcha*	Mild-acidic, alcoholic beverage	Yeast, molds, *Pediococcus*	India, Nepal	Tamang (2010a)
Jou	Rice	Mild-alcoholic beverage	Yeasts, LAB	India	Tamang (2010a)

(*Continued*)

Table 1.12 (*Continued*) Some Common and Uncommon Ethnic Fermented Beverages and Alcohol Drinks of the World

Product	*Substrate*	*Sensory Property and Nature*	*Microorganisms*	*Country*	*References*
Kaffir beer (same as *Bantu beer)*	Sorghum, millet	Opaque appearance, sour flavor, beer	LAB, yeasts	South Africa	Tamang (2010c)
Kanji	Carrot/beet roots, *Torani*	Strong flavored, alcoholic drink	*Hansenlu anomala, Candida guilliermondii, C. tropicalis, Geotrichium candidum, Leuc. mesenteroides, Pediococcus* spp., *Lb. dextranicum, Lb. paraplantarum, Lb. pentosus*	India	Sura et al. (2001), Kingston et al. (2010)
Khao maak	Rice, *loogpang*	Juicy, white colored, sweet taste, mild alcoholic dessert	LAB, yeasts	Thailand	Phithakpol et al. (1995)
Kiad lieh	Rice, *thiat*	Distilled liquor, clear, alcoholic drink	LAB, yeasts	India	Tamang (2010a)
Krachae	Rice, *loogpang*	Nondistilled and filtered liquor	Molds, yeasts	Thailand	Vachanavinich et al. (1994)
Kodo Ko Jaanr	Millet	Alcoholic liquor	*Mu. circinelloides, Rhiz. Chinensis, Sm. fibuligera, P. anomala, Sacch. cerevisiae, Cand. glabrata, Ped. pentosaceus, Lb. bifermentans*	India, Nepal	Thapa and Tamang (2004)
Judima	Rice	Alcoholic beverage	*Ped. pentosaceous, B. circulans, B. laterosporus, B. pumilus, B. firmus; D. hansenii, Sacch. cerevisiae*	India	Chakrabarty et al. (2014)
Lohpani	Maize-rice, barley	Alcoholic liquor, beverage	Unknown	India	Tamang (2010a)

Lugri	Barley, *phab*	Sweet-sour, mild alcoholic, thick liquid, alcoholic beverage	Yeasts, molds	India, China (Tibet)	Thakur et al. (2004)
Madhu	Rice	Distilled liquor, alcoholic drink	Yeasts, molds	India	Tamang (2010a)
Makai ko jaanr	Maize, marcha	Mild-alcoholic, sweet-sour beverage	Yeast, molds, *Pediococcus*	India, Nepal	Tamang (2010a)
Makgeolli	Rice, *nuruk*	Mild-alcoholic, sweet-sour beverage	Family-Saccharomycetaceae γ-*Proteobacteria* to *Firmicutes*	Korea	Jung et al. (2012)
Mangisi	Maize	Liquor, alcoholic drink	Yeast, LAB	Zimbabwe	Tamang (2010c)
Mbege	Malted millet	Acidic, mild-alcoholic, drink	Yeast, LAB	Tanzania	Tamang (2010c)
Merrisa	Millet, cassava	Turbid drink, beer	Yeasts, LAB	Sudan	Tamang (2010c)
Mingri	Maize-rice/barley	Sweet, mild alcoholic, thick, beverage	*Phab*	India	Thakur et al. (2004)
Nam khao	Rice, *loogpang*	Distilled liquor, alcoholic drink		Thailand	Phithakpol et al. (1995)
Nareli	Coconut palm	Sweet, milky, effervescent, mild alcoholic beverage	Yeasts, LAB	India	Tamang (2010a)
Nchiangne	Red rice, *khekhrii*	Distilled liquor, alcoholic drink	Yeasts, LAB	India	Tamang (2010a)
Oh	Rice-millet	Soft, mild-alcoholic beverage	Unknown	India	Tamang (2010a)
Ou	Rice, *loogpang*	Distilled liquor, alcoholic drink	Yeasts, LAB	Thailand	Phithakpol et al. (1995)

(Continued)

Table 1.12 (*Continued*) Some Common and Uncommon Ethnic Fermented Beverages and Alcohol Drinks of the World

Product	*Substrate*	*Sensory Property and Nature*	*Microorganisms*	*Country*	*References*
Toddy/tari	Palm sap	Palm wine, sweet, milky, effervescent and mild alcoholic beverage	*Sacch. cerevisiae*, *Schizosaccharomyces pombe*, *Acetobacter aceti*, *A. rancens*, *A. suboxydans*, *Leuc. dextranicum*, *Micrococcus* sp., *Pediococcus* sp., *Bacillus* sp., *Sarcina* sp.	India	Shamala and Sreekantiah (1988)
Poko	Rice, *manapu*	Sweet-acidic, mild-alcoholic beverage	Yeasts, molds, LAB	Nepal	Shrestha et al. (2002)
Pona	Rice	Mild-alcoholic, sweet-sour, paste	Molds, yeast, LAB	India	Tamang (2010a)
Pulque	Agave juice	White, viscous, acidic-alcoholic, refreshing drink	*Lc. lactis* subsp. *lactis*, *Lb. acetotolerans*, *Lb. acidophilus*, *Lb. hilgardii*, *Lb. kefir*, *Lb. plantarum*, *Leuc. citreum*, *Leuc. kimchi*, *Leuc. mesenteroides*, *Leuc. pseudomesenteroides*, *Erwinia rhapontici*, *Enterobacter* spp., *Acinetobacter radioresistens*, *Zymomonas mobilis*, *Acetobacter malorum*, *A. pomorium*, *Microbacterium arborescens*, *Flavobacterium johnsoniae*, *Gluconobacter oxydans*, *Hafnia alvei*, *Sacch. bayanus*, *Sacch. cerevisiae*, *Sacch. Paradoxus*, *Candida* spp., *C. parapsilosis*, *Clavispora lusitaniae*, *Hanseniaspora uvarum*, *Kl. lactis*, *Kl. marxianus*, *Pic. membranifaciens*, *Pic.* spp., *Torulaspora delbrueckii*	Mexico	Escalante et al. (2008), Lappe-Oliveras et al. (2008)

Raksi	Cereals, *marcha*	Clear distilled liquor , alcoholic drink	Molds, LAB	India, Nepal	Kozaki et al. (2000)
Ruou de	Rice, *men*	Distilled liquor, clear, alcoholic drink	Molds, LAB	Vietnam	Dung (2004)
Ruou nep	Rice, *men*	Distilled liquor, clear, alcoholic drink	Molds, LAB	Vietnam	Dung (2004)
Ruou nep than	Rice (purple), *men*	Nondistilled, viscous, thick food beverage	Molds, LAB	Vietnam	Dung (2004)
Ruou nep chan	Rice, maize, cassava, *men*	Nondistilled, viscous, thick; or distilled, alcoholic drink	Molds, LAB	Vietnam	Dung (2004)
Ruhi	Rice	Distilled liquor, alcoholic beverage	Yeasts	India	Tamang (2010a)
Roselle wine	Roselle fruit, water, sugar	Roselle wine	*Sacch. ellipsoideus* var. *montrachet*	Philippine	Tamang (2010c)
Saké	Polished rice, glucose, *koji*	Nondistilled, clarified, and filtered liquor, alcoholic drink	*Asp. oryzae, Sacch. cerevisiae, Lb. sakei, Leuc. mesenteroides*	Japan	Kotaka et al. (2008)
Sato	Rice, *loogpang*	Distilled liquor, alcoholic drink	Yeasts, molds	Thailand	Phithakpol et al. (1995)
Seketch	Maize	Alcoholic beverage	*Sacch. cerevisiae, Sacch. chevalieri, Sacch. elegans, Lb. plantarum, Lc. lactis, B. subtilis, Asp. niger, Asp. flavus, Mu. Rouxii*	Nigeria	Blandino et al. (2003)
Shochu/soju	Rice, sweet potato, barley, millet, corn, *koji*	Distilled spirit, alcoholic drink	*Asp. awamorii, Asp. kawachii, Sacch. cerevisiae*	Japan	Steinkraus (1996)

(*Continued*)

Table 1.12 (*Continued*) Some Common and Uncommon Ethnic Fermented Beverages and Alcohol Drinks of the World

Product	*Substrate*	*Sensory Property and Nature*	*Microorganisms*	*Country*	*References*
Soju	Rice, *nuruk*	Distilled liquor	Mold, yeasts	Korea	Steinkraus (1996)
Sura	Finger millet, *dheli*	Alcoholic, staple	Unknown	India	Thakur et al. (2004)
Takju	Rice or barley, wheat flour, sweet potato, starter (*nuruk*)	Lower or diluted concentration of *yakju* is known as *takju*, alcoholic beverage	*Sacch. cerevisiae, Hansenula anomala, Bacillus* sp., *Lactobacillus* sp.	Korea	Lee and Rhee (1970)
Tapai	Rice, cassava, *jui-paing*	Alcoholic beverage	Molds, yeasts	Malayasia	Wong and Jakson (1977)
Tapuy	Rice, bubod	Alcoholic beverage	*Saccharomycopsis fibuligera, Rhodotorula glutinis, Debaromyces hansenii, Candida parapsilosis, Trichosporon fennicum, Leuconostoc*	Philippines	Tanimura et al. (1977)
Tchoukoutou	Red sorghum	Effervescent, sweet, beer	*Sacch. cerevisiae, Hanseniaspora uvarum, H. guillermondii, Kl. marxianus, Clavispora lusitaniae*	Benin	Greppi et al. (2013a,b)
Tej	Honey	Sweet, effervescent, cloudy alcoholic	*Sacch. cerevisiae, Kluyvermyces bulgaricus, K. veronae, Debaromyces phaffi, Lactobacillus, Streptococcus, Leuconostoc, Pediococcus* spp.	Mexico	Bahiru et al. (2006)

Tequila	Agave juice	Effervescent, sweet, distilled alcoholic drink	LAB, *Sacch. cerevisiae, Candida lusitaniae, Kluyvermyces marxianus, Pichia fermentans*	Mexico	De León-Rodŕiguez et al. (2006)
Themsing	Finger millet, barley	Mild-alcoholic, sweet, alcoholic beverage	Molds, yeasts	India	Tamang (2010a)
Tien-chiu-niang	Rice, *chiu-yueh*	Mild-alcoholic, sweet, alcoholic beverage	Molds, yeasts	China, Taiwan	Tamang (2010c)
Tari or *Toddy*	Palmyra and date palm sap	Sweet, milky, effervescent and mild alcoholic, alcoholic beverage	*Sacch. cerevisiae, Schizosaccharomyces pombe, Acetobacter aceti, A. rancens, A. suboxydans, Leuc. dextranicum, Micrococcus* sp., *Pediococcus* sp., *Bacillus* sp., *Sarcina* sp.	India	Shamala and Sreekantiah (1988)
Togwa	Maize	Cooked slurry, alcoholic beverage	Yeasts, LAB	East Africa	Tamang (2010c)
Yakju	Rice, wheat, barley, maize, *nuruk*	Alcoholic beverage	*Sacch. cerevisae, Hansenula* spp.	Korea	Kim and Kim (1993)
Yu	Rice, *hamei*	Distilled from *atingba*, alcoholic drink	Yeasts, LAB	India	Singh and. Singh (2006)
Zu	Rice	Distilled from fermented rice; clear liquor	Yeasts, LAB	India	Tamang (2010a)
Zutho/Zhuchu	Rice, *khekhrii*	Milky white, sweet-sour, mild-alcoholic	*Sacch. cerevisiae*	India	Tamang et al. (2012)

starter in preparation of *koji* for production of *saké, shoyu, miso, shochu* (Lee et al. 2007, Suganuma et al. 2007). The predominant fungi in Chinese *koji* are *Aspergillus* and *Candida* species along with a few species of bacteria *Weissella* and *Staphylococcus* (Yan et al. 2013).

1.6.2 Alcoholic Beverages and Drinks

There are 10 major categories of alcoholic beverages consumed/drunk across the world (Tamang 2010c, Table 1.12):

1. Nondistilled and unfiltered alcoholic beverages produced by amylolytic starters
2. Nondistilled and filtered alcoholic beverages produced by amylolytic starters
3. Distilled alcoholic beverages produced by amylolytic starters
4. Alcoholic beverages produced by human saliva
5. Alcoholic beverages produced by mono-fermentation
6. Alcoholic beverages produced from honey
7. Alcoholic beverages produced from plants
8. Alcoholic beverages produced by malting (germination)
9. Alcoholic beverages prepared from fruits without distillation
10. Distilled alcoholic beverages prepared from fruits and cereals

1.6.3 Nondistilled and Unfiltered Alcoholic Beverages Produced by Amylolytic Starters

Common examples of nondistilled and unfiltered alcoholic beverages produced by mixed amylolytic starters are *lao-chao* of China, *tapé* of Indonesia, *makgeolli* of Korea, *bhaati jaanr* and *kodo ko jaanr* of India and Nepal (Tamang 2010c), *kanji* of India (Tamang 2012b). The biological process of liquefaction and saccharification of cereal starch by filamentous molds and yeasts, supplemented by amylolytic starters, under solid-state fermentation is one of the two major stages of production of alcoholic beverages in Asia. These alcoholic beverages are mostly considered as food beverages and eaten as a staple food with high calories in many parts of Asia, for example, *kodo ko jaanr*, a fermented finger millet beverage of the Himalayan regions in India, Nepal, Bhutan, and China (Tibet) with 5% alcohol content (Thapa and Tamang 2004). *Marcha* used as an amylolytic starter supplements functional microorganisms in *kodo ko jaanr* fermentation. Yeasts *Candida glabrata, Pic. anomala, Sacch. cerevisiae, Sm. fibuligera*, and LAB *Lb. bifermentans* and *Ped. pentosaceus* have been recovered in *kodo ko jaanr* samples (Thapa and Tamang 2004). Saccharifying activities are mostly shown by *Rhizopus* spp. and *Sm. fibuligera* whereas liquefying activities are shown by *Sm. fibuligera* and *Sac. cerevisiae* (Thapa and Tamang 2006). *Bhaati jaanr* is the Himalayan sweet-sour, mild alcoholic food beverage paste prepared from rice and consumed as a staple food (Tamang and Thapa 2006). *Rhizopus, Amylomyces, Torulopsis*, and *Hansenula* are present in *lao-chao*, a popular ethnic fermented rice beverage of China (Wei and Jong 1983). During fermentation of *makgeolli* (a traditional Korean alcoholic beverage prepared by the amylolytic starter *nuruk*) the proportion of family Saccharomycetaceae increased significantly, and the major bacterial phylum of the samples shifted from γ-*Proteobacteria* to *Firmicutes* (Jung et al. 2012).

Kanji is an ethnic Indian strong-flavored but mild alcoholic beverage prepared from beet and carrots by natural fermentation (Batra and Millner 1974). It is drunk as a mild-alcoholic refreshing drink in India. Alcohol content in *kanji* is 2.5% and pH is 4.0 showing the product as mild-alcoholic and acidic in taste (Sura et al. 2001). During its preparation, carrots or beet are washed, shredded and mixed with salt and mustard seeds and placed in earthen pot and allowed to ferment naturally at 26–34°C for 4–7 days. Sometimes, the mixture is inoculated with a portion of a previous batch of *kanji*. After fermentation, a pink alcoholic liquor is drained off and bottled or drunk directly. In north India it is prepared with purple or occasionally orange cultivars of carrots plus beet and spices, whereas in south India *torami*, yeast-containing fermented rice gruel is used as a starter for *kanji* production. *Hansenlu anomala, Candida guilliermondii, C. tropicalis,* and *Geotrichium candidum* are involved in *kanji* fermentation (Batra and Millner 1974). *Leuc. mesenteroides, Pediococcus* spp. and *Lb. dextranicum* were isolated from *kanji* fermentation (Sura et al. 2001). Kingston et al. (2010) reported *Lb. paraplantarum* and *Lb. pentosus* from *kanji* based on rep-PCR identification method.

1.6.4 Nondistilled and Filtered Alcoholic Beverages Produced by Amylolytic Starters

Nondistilled and filtered alcoholic beverages produced by amylolytic starters are *saké* of Japan, *krachae* or *nam-khaao* or *sato* of Thailand, *basi* of the Philippines, *yakju* and *takju* of Korea (Table 1.12). Alcoholic beverages produced by an amylolytic starter (*koji*) is not distilled but the extract of the fermented cereals is filtered into clarified high alcohol-content liquor, for example, *saké* which is the national drink of Japan and is one of the most popular traditional nondistilled alcoholic drinks in the world. It is prepared from rice using *koji* and is clear, pale yellow, containing 15%–20% alcohol (Tamang 2010c). Improved strains of *Asp. oryzae* are used for *saké* production on an industrial scale (Kotaka et al. 2008, Hirasawa et al. 2009).

1.6.5 Distilled Alcoholic Beverages Produced by Amylolytic Starters

This category of alcoholic drinks are the clear, distillate part of high alcohol-content drinks prepared from fermented cereal beverages by using amylolytic starters, for example, *raksi* of India, Nepal, and Bhutan, *shochu* of Japan, *soju* of Korea. *Raksi* is an ethnic alcoholic (22%–27% v/v) drink of the Himalayas with a characteristic aroma, and distilled from traditional fermented cereal beverages (Kozaki et al. 2000).

1.6.6 Alcoholic Beverages Produced by Human Saliva

Traditionally, saliva serves as the source of amylase for conversion of cereal starch to fermentation sugars. *Chicha* is a unique ethnic fermented alcoholic (2%–12% v/v) beverage of the Andes Indians of South America, mostly Peru, and is prepared from maize by the human salivation process (Escobar et al. 1996, Hayashida 2008). *Sacch. cerevisiae, Sacch. apiculata, Sacch. pastorianus,* and species of *Lactobacillus* and *Acetobacter* are present in *chicha* (Escobar 1977). *Sacch. cerevisiae* was isolated from *chicha* and identified using MALDI-TOF (Vallejo et al. 2013).

1.6.7 Alcoholic Beverages Produced by Mono Fermentation

Beer, a fermented extract of malted barley with alcohol content of 2%–8%, is the most common example of mono fermentation (*Sacch. cerevisiae* strain). Strains within *Sacch. carlsbergensis* and *Sacch. uvarum* have been merged into either *Sacch. cerevisiae* or *Sacch. pastorianus* (Kurtzman and Robnet 2003). Species of *Dekkera* produce high levels of acetic acid and esters, *Pichia* and *Hansenula* species give excessive ester production in beer (Dufour et al. 2003).

1.6.8 Alcoholic Beverage Produced from Honey

Some alcoholic beverages are produced from honey, for example, *tej* of Ethiopia. It is a yellow, sweet, effervescent and cloudy alcoholic (7%–14% v/v) beverage (Steinkraus 1996). *Sacch. cerevisiae, Kluyvermyces bulgaricus, Debaromyces phaffi*, and *K. veronae*, and LAB *Lactobacillus, Streptococcus, Leuconostoc*, and *Pediococcus* species were isolated from *tej* fermentation (Bahiru et al. 2006).

1.6.9 Alcoholic Beverages Produced from Plants

Pulque is one of the oldest alcoholic beverages prepared from the juice of the cactus (*Agave*) plant of Mexico (Steinkraus 1996). Bacteria present during the fermentation of *pulque* were LAB—*Lc. lactis* subsp. *lactis, Lb. acetotolerans, Lb. acidophilus, Lb. hilgardii, Lb. kefir, Lb. plantarum, Leuc. citreum, Leuc. kimchi, Leuc. mesenteroides, Leuc. pseudomesenteroides*, the γ-Proteobacteria—*Erwinia rhapontici, Enterobacter* spp. and *Acinetobacter radioresistens*, several α-Proteobacteria—*Zymomonas mobilis, Acetobacter malorum, Acetobacter pomorium, Microbacterium arborescens, Flavobacterium johnsoniae, Gluconobacter oxydans*, and *Hafnia alvei* (Escalante et al. 2004, 2008). Yeasts isolated from *pulque* include *Saccharomyces* (*Sacch. bayanus, Sacch. cerevisiae, Sacch. paradoxus*) and non-*Saccharomyces* (*Candida* spp., *C. parapsilosis, Clavispora lusitaniae, Hanseniaspora uvarum, Kl. lactis, Kl. marxianus, Pichia membranifaciens, Pichia* spp., *Torulaspora delbrueckii*) (Lappe-Oliveras et al. 2008).

Toddy or *tari* is an ethnic alcoholic drink of India prepared from palm juice. There are three types of *toddy* (Batra and Millner 1974): (1) *sendi*, from the palm; (2) *tari*, from the *palmyra* and date palms; and (3) *nareli*, from the coconut palm. *Geotrichum, Saccharomyces* and *Schizosacchoramyces* spp. of yeast are responsible for fermentation (Batra and Millner 1974, 1976). Microorganisms that are responsible in fermenting *toddy* are *Sacch. cerevisiae, Schizosaccharomyces pombe, Acetobacter aceti, A. rancens, A. suboxydans, Leuc. dextranicum, Micrococcus* sp., *Pediococcus* sp., *Bacillus* sp., and *Sarcina* sp. (Shamala and Sreekantiah 1988).

1.6.10 Alcoholic Beverages Produced by Malting or Germination

Malting or germination process allows amylase to break down cereal starch to sugars, which are used as substrates for alcohol fermentation, for example, *Bantu* beer or sorghum beer of the Bantu tribes of South Africa (Taylor 2003). The major part of the sorghum crop (*Sorghum caffrorum* or *S. vulgare*) is malted and used for brewing beer (Kutyauripo et al. 2009).

1.6.11 Alcoholic Beverages Produced from Fruits without Distillation

Wine generally refers to the alcoholic fermentation of grape juice, or other fruits, without distillation. Until 75–100 years ago, most wines were produced by spontaneous or natural alcoholic fermentation of grape juice by indigenous yeast flora (Walker 2014). Wine fermentation is initiated by the growth of various species of *Saccharomyces* and non-*Saccharomyces* yeasts (e.g., *Candida colliculosa, C. stellata, Hanseniaspora uvarum, Kloeckera apiculata, Kl. thermotolerans, Torulaspora delbrueckii, Metschnikowia pulcherrima*) (Versavaud et al. 1995, Pretorius 2000, Moreira et al. 2005, Sun et al. 2014). Using mCOLD-PCR-DGGE method, *Candida* sp. and *Cladosporium* sp. were isolated from fermenting white wine, which were not detected by conventional PCR (Takahashi et al. 2014). *Sacch. cerevisiae* strains develop during wine fermentation which play an active role in the characteristics of wine (Vilanova and Sieiro 2006, Capece et al. 2013).

1.6.12 Distilled Alcoholic Beverages without Amylolytic Starters

Distillate high alcohol-content spirit from fermented cereal is whisky, fermented molasses is rum and fermented grape is brandy. Rum production from molasses fermentation may involve contributions from *Schizosaccharomyces pombe* and *Sacch. cerevisiae* (Fahrasame and Ganow-Parfeit 1998).

1.6.13 Recommendations

- Exchange of LAB strains/cultures from plant-origins with superior functional properties to ferment new animal products (milks, meat, sausages, etc.).
- Every country to establish microbial sequence banks and culture collection centres, of strains/cultures isolated from naturally fermented foods and beverages.
- Basic training on molecular microbial taxonomy and identification.
- Incorporation of published research materials on ethnic fermented foods and beverages into academic programs at master and doctoral level in Food Microbiology/Biotechnology/Food Science and Technology courses in universities following the references of the academic program on fermented foods in Sikkim University (India) and Wageningen University (the Netherlands).

1.7 Conclusion

The sustainable use of microorganisms in food fermentation is based on the interrelationship of indigenous knowledge of food fermentation, modern expertise and information, basic understanding of the microbial background of fermentation and of Good Hygienic Practices (GHP), some experience in handling of microbial strains or cultures, even under crude conditions such as back-slopping, and conservation of microbial strains. The diversity of functional microorganisms in fermented foods and beverages consists of bacteria, yeasts, and fungi. Microorganisms establish on relevant substrates for survival and produce bioactive compounds that enrich the human diet, thereby benefiting the health of consumers. Ethnic fermented foods of the world are considered to be a means to preserve microbial diversity *ex situ* and they are custodians of microbial diversity and play a key role in the storage and supply of authentic reference material for research and development. One of the challenges facing scientists in the future will undoubtedly be to allow the large-scale production of fermented foods without losing the unique flavor and other traits associated with the traditional products from which they are derived.

References

Aagaard, K., Ma, J., Antony, K.M., Ganu, R., and J. Versalovic. 2014. The placenta harbors a unique microbiome. *Science Translational Medicine* 6: 237–265.

Abe, M., Takaoka, N., Idemoto, Y., Takagi, C., Imai, T., and K. Nakasaki. 2008. Characteristic fungi observed in the fermentation process for Puer tea. *International Journal of Food Microbiology* 124: 199–203.

Abimbola, U. 2007. Degradation of dietary fibre from gari by faecal bacteria and bacteria extracellular polysaccharides. *Nigerian Food Journal* 25: 46–58.

Abriouel, H., Omar, N.B., López, R.L., Martínez-Cañamero, M., Keleke, S., and A. Gálvez. 2006. Culture-independent analysis of the microbial composition of the African traditional fermented foods *poto poto* and *dégué* by using three different DNA extraction methods. *International Journal of Food Microbiology* 111: 228–233.

Abriouel, H., Benomar, N., Lucas, R., and A. Gálvez. 2011. Culture-independent study of the diversity of microbial populations in brines during fermentation of naturally-fermented Aloreña green table olives. *International Journal of Food Microbiology* 144: 487–496.

Adams, M.R. 2010. Fermented meat products, In: Tamang JP, Kailasapathy K. eds. *Fermented Foods and Beverages of the World*, CRC Press, Taylor & Francis Group, New York, 309–322.

Adams, M.R. 2014. Vinegar, In: *Encyclopaedia of Food Microbiology*, 2nd edition (Eds: Batt, C. and Tortorello, MA). Elsevier Ltd., Oxford, pp. 717–721.

Adhikari R.R. and H. Ghimirey. 2000. *Nepalese Society and Culture*. Vidharthi Pushtak Bhandar, Kathmandu (Nepali).

Aidoo, K.E. and M.J.R. Nout. 2010. Functional yeasts and molds in fermented foods and beverages, In: Tamang JP, Kailasapathy K. eds. *Fermented Foods and Beverages of the World*, CRC Press, Taylor & Francis Group, New York, 127–148.

Aidoo, K.E., Nout, M.J.R., and P.K. Sarkar. 2006. Occurrence and function of yeasts in Asian indigenous fermented foods. *FEMS Yeast Research* 6: 30–39.

Akabanda, F., Owusu-Kwarteng, J., Tano-Debrah, K., Glover, R.L.K., Nielsen, D.S., and L. Jespersen. 2013. Taxonomic and molecular characterization of lactic acid bacteria and yeasts in *nunu*, a Ghanaian fermented milk product. *Food Microbiology* 34(2): 277–283.

Aksu, M.I., Kaya, M., and H.W. Ockerman. 2005. Effect of modified atmosphere packaging and temperature on the shelf life of sliced Pastirma produced from frozen/thawed meat. *Journal of Muscle Foods* 16(3): 192–206.

Albano, H., van Reenen, C.A., Todorov, S.D., Cruz, D., Fraga, L., Hogg, T., Dicks, L.M., and P. Teixeira. 2009. Phenotypic and genetic heterogeneity of lactic acid bacteria isolated from "Alheira", a traditional fermented sausage produced in Portugal. *Meat Science* 82: 389–398.

Alegría, A., González, R., Díaz, M., and B. Mayo. 2011. Assessment of microbial populations dynamics in a blue cheese by culturing and denaturing gradient gel electrophoresis. *Current Microbiology* 62: 888–893.

Alexandraki, V., Tsakalidou, E., Papadimitriou, K., and W.H. Holzapfel. 2013. Status and trends of the conservation and sustainable use of microorganisms in food processes. Commission on Genetic Resources for Food and Agriculture. FAO Background Study Paper No. 65.

Al-Jedah, J.H., Ali, M.Z., and R.K. Robinson. 1999. Chemical and microbiological properties of *mehiawah*—a popular fish sauce of golf. *Journal of Food Science and Technology* 36(6): 561–564.

Amoa-Awua, W.K., Terlabie, N.N., and E. Sakyi-Dawson. 2006. Screening of 42 *Bacillus* isolates for ability to ferment soybeans into *dawadawa*. *International Journal of Food Microbiology* 106: 343–347.

Aneja, R.P., Mathur, B.N., Chandan, R.C., and A.K. Banerjee. 2002. Cultured/fermented products. Technology of Indian milk products: *Handbook on Process Technology Modernization for Professionals, Entrepreneurs and Scientists*. Dairy India Yearbook.

Angelakis, E., Million, M., Henry, M., and D. Raoult. 2011. Rapid and accurate bacterial identification in probiotics and yoghurts by MALDI-TOF mass spectrometry. *Journal of Food Science* 76: 568–572.

Ardhana, M.M. and G.H. Fleet. 1989. The microbial ecology of tapé ketan fermentation. *International Journal of Food Microbiology* 9: 157–165.

Arroyo, P.T., Ludovico-Pelayo, L.A., Solidium, H.T., Chiu, Y.N., Lero, M.C., and E.E. Alcantara. 1978. Studies on rice-shrimp fermentation, balao-balao. *Philippines Journal of Food Science and Technology* 2(1&2): 106–125.

Asahara, N., Zhang, X.B., and Y. Ohta. 2006. Antimutagenicity and mutagen-binding activation of mutagenic pyrolyzates by microorganisms isolated from Japanese *miso*. *Journal of Science of Food and Agriculture* 58: 395–401.

Astuli, M. 1999. History of the development of *tempeh*. In: *The Complete Handbook of Tempeh*, ed. J. Agranoff, 2–7. Singapore: American Soybean Association.

Azokpota, P., Hounhouigan, D.J., and M.C. Nago. 2006. Microbiological and chemical changes during the fermentation of African locust bean (*Parkia biglobosa*) to produce afitin, iru, and sonru, three traditional condiments produced in Benin. *International Journal of Food Microbiology* 107: 304–309.

Bahiru, B., Mehari, T., and M. Ashenafi. 2006. Yeast and lactic acid flora of *tej*, an indigenous Ethiopian honey wine: Variations within and between production units. *Food Microbiology* 23: 277–282.

Baens-Arega, L. 1977. Patis, a traditional fermented fish sauce and condiment of the Philippines. In: *The Proceeding of the Symposium on Indigenous Fermented Foods,* November 21–27, 1977, GIAM-V, Bangkok.

Batra, L.R. 1986. Microbiology of some fermented cereals and grains legumes of India and vicinity. In: *Indigenous Fermented Food of Non-Western Origin,* eds. C.W. Hesseltine and H.L. Wang, 85–104. Berlin: J. Cramer.

Batra, L.R. and P.D. Millner. 1974. Some Asian fermented foods and beverages and associated fungi. *Mycologia* 66: 942–950.

Batra, L.R. and P.D. Millner. 1976. Asian fermented foods and beverages. *Development in Industrial Microbiology* 17: 117–128.

Behre, K.-E. 1984. Zur Geschichte der Bierwürzen nach Fruchtfunden und Schriftlichen Quellen. In: *Plants and Ancient Man. Studies in Palaeoethnobotany,* eds. W. van Zeist and W.A. Casparie, 115–122. Rotterdam: A.A. Balkema.

Berger, B., Pridmore RD, Barretto C, Delmas-Julien F, Schreiber K, Arigoni, F., and H. Brüssow. 2007. Similarity and differences in the *Lactobacillus acidophilus* group identified by polyphasic analysis and comparative genomics. *Journal of Bacteriology* 189: 1311–1321.

Bernardeau, M., Guguen, M., and J.P. Vernoux. 2006. Beneficial lactobacilli in food and feed: Long-term use, biodiversity and proposals for specific and realistic safety assessments. *FEMS Microbiology Review* 30: 487–513.

Bernardo, E.B., Neilan, B.A., and I. Couperwhite. 1998. Characterization, differentiation and identification of wild-type cellulose-synthesizing *Acetobacter* strains involved in nata de coco production. *Systematic and Applied Microbiology* 21(4): 599–608.

Blandino, A., Al-Aseeri, M.E., Pandiella, S.S., Cantero, D., and C. Webb. 2003. Cereal-based fermented foods and beverages. *Food Research International* 36: 527–543.

Briggiler-Marcó M, Capr, M.L., Quiberoni, A., Vinderola, G., Reinheimer, J.A., and E. Hynes. 2007. Nonstarter *Lactobacillus* strains as adjunct cultures for cheese making: *in vitro* characterization and performance in two model cheese. *Journal of Dairy Science* 90: 4532–4542.

Bo, T.A. 1984a. Origin of douchi and its production technology (Part 1). *Brewing Society of Japan* 79: 221–223.

Bo, T.A. 1984b. Origin of douchi and its production technology (Part 2). *Brewing Society of Japan* 79: 395–402.

Bose, D.K. 1922. *Wine in Ancient India.* Kolkata: Connor.

Bourdichon, F., Casaregola, S., Farrokh, C., Frisvad, J.C., Gerds, M.L., Hammes, W.P., Harnett, J. et al. 2012. Food fermentations: Microorganisms with technological beneficial use. *International Journal of Food Microbiology* 154(3): 87–97.

Campbell-Platt, G. 1987. *Fermented Foods of the World: A Dictionary and Guide.* London: Butterworths.

Carr, F.J., Chill, D., and N. Maida. 2002. The lactic acid bacteria: A literature survey. *Critical Review of Microbiology* 28: 281–370.

Capece, A., Siesto, G., Poeta, C., Pietrafesa, R., and P. Romano. 2013. Indigenous yeast population from Georgian aged wines produced by traditional "Kakhetian" method. *Food Microbiology* 36: 447–455.

Chang, C.H., Chen, Y.S., and F. Yanagida. 2011. Isolation and characterisation of lactic acid bacteria from *yan-jiang* (fermented ginger), a traditional fermented food in Taiwan. *Journal of Science of Food and Agriculture* 91: 1746–1750.

Chang, H.W., Kim, K.H., Nam, Y.D., Roh, S.W., Kim, M.S., Jeon, C.O., Oh, H.M., and J.W. Bae. 2008. Analysis of yeast and archaeal population dynamics in kimchi using denaturing gradient gel electrophoresis. *International Journal of Food Microbiology* 126:159–166.

Chakrabarty, J., Sharma, G.D., and J.P. Tamang. 2014. Traditional technology and product characterization of some lesser-known ethnic fermented foods and beverages of North Cachar Hills District of Assam. *Indian Journal of Traditional Knowledge* 13(4): 706–715.

Chao, S-H., Wu, R-J., Watanabe, K., and Y-C. Tsai. 2009. Diversity of lactic acid bacteria in *suan-tsai* and *fu-tsai,* traditional fermented mustard products of Taiwan. *International Journal of Food Microbiology* 135: 203–210.

Chao, S-H., Tomii, Y., Watanabe, K., and Y-C. Tsai. 2008. Diversity of lactic acid bacteria in fermented brines used to make stinky tofu. *International Journal of Food Microbiology* 123: 134–141.

Chao, S.H., Kudo, Y., Tsai, Y.C., and K. Watanabe. 2012. *Lactobacillus futsaii* sp. nov., isolated from traditional fermented mustard products of Taiwan, *fu-tsai* and *suan-tsai*. *International Journal of Systematic and Evolutionary Microbiology* 62: 489–494.

Chen, Y.S., Yanagida, F., and J.S. Hsu. 2006. Isolation and characterization of lactic acid bacteria from *suan-tsai* (fermented mustard), a traditional fermented food in Taiwan. *Journal of Applied Microbiology* 101: 125–130.

Chen, Y.S., Wu, H.C., Liu, C.H., Chen, H.C., and F. Yanagida. 2010. Isolation and characterization of lactic acid bacteria from jiang-sun (fermented bamboo shoots), a traditional fermented food in Taiwan. *Journal of Science of Food and Agriculture* 90: 1977–1982.

Chang, J.H. 1975. Studies on the origin of Korean vegetable pickles. *Thesis Collection of Sung-Sim Women College* 6: 149–174.

Cheigh, H.S. 2002. *Kimchi Culture and Dietary Life in Korea*. Seoul: Hyoil Publishing Co.

Chettri, R. 2013. *Microbiological Evaluation of turangbai and bekang, ethnic fermented soybean foods of North East India*. Ph.D. thesis, North Bengal University, Siliguri, India, p. 380.

Chettri, R. and J.P. Tamang. 2008. Microbiological evaluation of maseura, an ethnic fermented legume-based condiment of Sikkim. *Journal of Hill Research* 21: 1–7.

Choi, S.H., Lee, M.H., Lee, S.K., and Oh, M.J. 1995. Microflora and enzyme activity of conventional *meju* and isolation of useful mould. *Journal of Agricultural Science Chungnam National University, Korea* 22: 188–197.

Choi, U.K., Kim, M.H., and N.H. Lee. 2007. The characteristics of cheonggukjang, a fermented soybean product, by the degree of germination of raw soybeans. *Food Science and Biotechnology* 16: 734–739.

Chokesajjawatee, N., Pornaem, S., Zo, Y.G., Kamdee, S., Luxananil, P., Wanasen, S., and R. Valysevi. 2009. Incidence of *Staphylococcus aureus* and associated risk factors in Nham, a Thai fermented pork product. *Food Microbiology* 26: 547–551.

Chunhachart, O., Itoh, T., Sukchotiratana, M., Tanimoto, H., and Y. Tahara. 2006. Characterization of γ-glutamyl hydrolase produced by *Bacillus* sp. isolated from Thai thua-nao. *Bioscience, Biotechnology and Biochemistry* 70: 2779–2782.

Cocolin, L., Aggio, D., Manzano, M., Cantoni, C., and G. Comi. 2002. An application of PCR-DGGE analysis to profile the yeast populations in raw milk. *International Dairy Journal* 12: 407–411.

Cocolin, L., Alessandria V., Dolci, P., Gorra, R., and K. Rantsiou. 2013. Culture independent methods to assess the diversity and dynamics of microbiota during food fermentation. *International Journal of Food Microbiology* 167(1): 29–43.

Cocolin, L. and D. Ercolini, (Editors). 2008. *Molecular Techniques in the Microbial Ecology of Fermented Foods*. New York: Springer.

Cocolin, L., Dolci, P., and K. Rantsiou. 2011. Biodiversity and dynamics of meat fermentations: The contribution of molecular methods for a better comprehension of a complex ecosystem. *Meat Science* 89(3): 296–302.

Coppola, S., Fusco, V., Andolfi, R., Aponte, M., Aponte, M., Blalotta, G., Ercolini, D., and G. Moschetti. 2006. Evaluation of microbial diversity during the manufacture of Fior di Latte di Agerola, a traditional raw milk pasta-filata cheese of the Naples area. *Journal of Dairy Research* 73: 264–272.

Corsetti, A. and L. Settanni. 2007. Lactobacilli in sourdough fermentation. *Food Research International* 40: 539–558.

Coton, E., Desmonts, M.H., Leroy, S., Coton, M., Jamet, E., Christieans, S., Donnio, P.Y., Lebert, I., and R. Talon. 2010. Biodiversity of coagulase-negative staphylococci in French cheeses, dry fermented sausages, processing environments and clinical samples. *International Journal of Food Microbiology* 137: 221–229.

Curtis, R.I. 2001. *Ancient Food Technology*. Leiden: Brill.

Dajanta, K., Apichartsrangkoon, A., Chukeatirote, E., Richard, A., and R.A. Frazie. 2011. Free-amino acid profiles of *thua nao,* a Thai fermented soybean. *Food Chemistry* 125: 342–347.

Dalmacio, L.M.M., Angeles, A.K.J., Larcia, L.L.H., Balolong, M., and R. Estacio. 2011. Assessment of bacterial diversity in selected Philippine fermented food products through PCR-DGGE. *Beneficial Microbes* 2: 273–281.

Davis, J.G. 1964. *Cheese, vol 1, Basic Technology.* Edinburg: Churchill Livingstone.

de Bruyne, K., Camu, N., Lefebvre, K., De Vuyst, L., and P. Vandamme. 2008. *Weissella ghanensis* sp. nov., isolated from a Ghanaian cocoa fermentation. *International Journal of Systematic and Evolutionary Microbiology* 58: 2721–2725.

de Bruyne, K., Camu, N, De Vuyst, L., and P. Vandamme. 2009. *Lactobacillus fabifermentans* sp. nov. and *Lactobacillus cacaonum* sp. nov., isolated from Ghanaian cocoa fermentations. *International Journal of Systematic and Evolutionary Microbiology* 59: 7–12.

de Bruyne, K., Camu, N., de Vuyst, L., and P. Vandamme. 2010. *Weissella fabaria* sp. nov., from a Ghanaian cocoa fermentation. *International Journal of Systematic and Evolutionary Microbiology* 60: 1999–2005.

de Bruyne, K., Franz, C.M., Vancanneyt, M., Schillinger, U., Mozzi, F., de Valdez, G.F., de Vuyst, L., and P. Vandamme. 2008. *Pediococcus* argentinicus sp. nov. from Argentinean fermented wheat flour and identification of *Pediococcus* species by pheS, rpoA and atpA sequence analysis. *International Journal of Systematic and Evolutionary Microbiology* 58: 2909–2916.

de Bruyne, K., Schillinger, U., Caroline, L., Boehringer, B., Cleenwerck, I., Vancanneyt, M., De Vuyst, L., Franz C.M., and P. Vandamme. 2007. *Leuconostoc holzapfelii* sp. nov., isolated from Ethiopian coffee fermentation and assessment of sequence analysis of housekeeping genes for delineation of *Leuconostoc* species. *International Journal of Systematic and Evolutionary Microbiology* 57: 2952–2959.

De León-Rodríguez, A., González-Hernández, L., Barba de la Rosa, A., Escalante-Minakata, P., and López, M. 2006. Characterization of volatile compounds of mezcal, an ethnic alcoholic beverage obtained from *Agave salmiana. Journal of Agriculture and Food Chemistry* 54: 1337–1341.

Delong, D. 1992. *How to Dry Foods.* Penquin Group, New York, p. 79.

Denter, J. and B. Bisping. 1994. Formation of B-vitamins by bacteria during the soaking process of soybeans for tempe fermentation. *International Journal of Food Microbiology* 22(1): 23–31.

de Ramesh, C.C., White, C.H., Kilara, A., and Y.H. Hui. 2006. *Manufacturing Yogurt and Fermented Milks.* Blackwell Publishing, Oxford.

de Vuyst, L., Vrancken G, Ravyts F, Rimaux T., and S. Weckx. 2009. Biodiversity, ecological determinants, and metabolic exploitation of sourdough microbiota. *Food Microbiology* 26: 666–675.

Dewan, S. and J.P. Tamang. 2006. Microbial and analytical characterization of *Chhu*, a traditional fermented milk product of the Sikkim Himalayas. *Journal of Scientific and Industrial Research* 65: 747–752.

Dewan, S. and J.P. Tamang. 2007. Dominant lactic acid bacteria and their technological properties isolated from the Himalayan ethnic fermented milk products. *Leeuwenhoek International Journal of General and Molecular Microbiology* 92: 343–352.

Diancourt, L., Passet, V., Chervaux, C., Garault, P., Smokvina, T., and S. Brisse. 2007. Multilocus sequence typing of *Lactobacillus casei* reveals a clonal population structure with low levels of homologous recombination. *Applied Environmental Microbiology* 73: 6601–6611.

Dirar, H.A., Harper, D.B., and M.A. Collins. 2006. Biochemical and microbiological studies on kawal, a meat substitute derived by fermentation of *Cassia obtusifolia* leaves. *Journal of Science of Food and Agriculture* 36: 881–892.

Dirar, H.A. 1993. *The Indigenous Fermented Foods of Sudan.* Wallingford: CAB International.

Dufour, J., Verstrepen, K., and G. Derdelinckx. 2003. Brewing yeasts, In: *Yeast in Foods*, Boekhout T, Rober V. eds. Woodhead, Cambridge, 347–388.

Dung, N.T.P., 2004. Defined fungal starter granules for purple glutinous rice wine, Ph.D. Thesis. Wageningen University, Wageningen, The Netherlands, p. 110.

Dung, N.T.P., Rombouts, F.M., and M.J.R. Nout. 2006. Functionality of selected strains of moulds and yeasts from Vietnamese rice wine starters. *Food Microbiology* 23: 331–340.

Dung, N.T.P., Rombouts, F.M., and Nout, M.J.R. 2007. Characteristics of some traditional Vietnamese starch-based rice wine starters *(Men). LWT—Food Science and Technology* 40: 130–135.

Dušková, M., Šedo, O., Kšicová, K., Zdráhal, Z., and R. Karpíšková. 2012. Identification of lactobacilli isolated from food by genotypic methods and MALDI-TOF MS. *International Journal of Food Microbiology* 159: 107–114.

Encinas, J.P., Lopez-Diaz, T.M., Garcia-Lopez, M.L., Otero, A, and Moreno, B. 2000. Yeast populations on Spanish fermented sausages. *Meat Science* 54: 203–208.

Endo, A., Mizuno, H., and S. Okada. 2008. Monitoring the bacterial community during fermentation of sunki, an unsalted, fermented vegetable traditional to the Kiso area of Japan. *Letters in Applied Microbiology.* 47: 221–226.

Escalante, A., Rodríguez, M.E., Martínez, A., López-Munguía, A., Bolívar, F., and G. Gosset. 2004. Characterization of bacterial diversity in *Pulque*, a traditional Mexican alcoholic fermented beverage, as determined by 16S rDNA analysis. *FEMS Microbiology Letters* 2: 273–279.

Escalante, A.M., Giles-Gómez, G., Hernández, M.S., Córdova-Aguilar, A., López-Munguía, F., Gosset, G., and F. Bolívar. 2008. Analysis of bacterial community during the fermentation of pulque, a traditional Mexican alcoholic beverage, using a polyphasic approach. *International Journal of Food Microbiology* 124: 126–134.

Escobar, A. 1977. The American maize beverage chichi. MSc thesis. New York: Cornell University.

Escobar, A., Gardner, A., and K.H. Steinkraus. 1996. Studies of South American chichi, In: *Handbook of Indigenous Fermented Food*, 2nd edition, ed., Steinkraus K.H., Marcel Dekker, Inc., New York, 402–406.

Fahrasame, L. and B. Ganow-Parfeit. 1998. Microbial flora of rum fermentation media. *Journal of Applied Microbiology* 84: 921–928.

Farhad, M., Kailasapathy, K., and Tamang, J.P. 2010. Health aspects of fermented foods, In: Tamang JP, Kailasapathy K. eds. *Fermented Foods and Beverages of the World*, CRC Press, Taylor & Francis Group, New York, 391–414.

FAO, 1998. Fermented fruits and vegetables. A global perspective. *FAO Agricultural Services Bulletin* 134.

FAO, 1999. Fermented cereals. A global perspective. *FAO Agricultural Services Bulletin* No. 138.

Feng, X.M., Eriksson, A.R.B., and J. Schnürer. 2005. Growth of lactic acid bacteria and *Rhizopus oligosporus* during barley tempeh fermentation. *International Journal of Food Microbiology* 104: 249–256.

Fernandez-Lopez, J., Sendra, E., Sayas-Barbera, E., Navarro, C., and J.A. Perez-Alvarez. 2008. Physicochemical and microbiological profiles of "Salchichon" (Spanish dry fermented sausage) enriched with orange fiber. *Meat Science* 80: 410–417.

Foschino, R., Gallina, S., Andrighetto, C., Rossetti, L., and A. Galli. 2004. Comparisions of cultural methods for the identification and molecular investigations of yeasts from sourdoughs for Italian sweet baked products. *FEMS Yeasts Research* 4: 609–618.

Fujii, T., Wu, Y.C., Suzuk, T., and B. Kimura. 1999. Production of organic acids by bacteria during the fermentation of squid shiokara. *Fisheries Science* 65: 671–672.

Gadaga, T.H., Mutukumira, A.N., and Narvhus, J.A. 2000. Enumeration and identification of yeast isolates from Zimbabwean traditional fermented milk. *International Dairy Journal* 10: 459–466.

Ganasen, P. and S. Benjakul. 2010. Physical properties and microstructure of pidan yolk as affected by different divalent and monovalent cations. *LWT—Food Science and Technology* 43: 77–85.

Gänzle, M.G., Ehmann, M., and W.P. Hammes. 1998. Modeling of growth of *Lactobacillus sanfranciscensis* and *Candida milleri* in response to process parameters of sourdough fermentation. *Applied Environmental Microbiology* 64: 2616–2623.

Garcia-Fontan, M.C., Lorenzo, J.M., Parada, A., Franco, I., and J. Carballo. 2007. Microbiological characteristics of "Androlla", a Spanish traditional pork sausage. *Food Microbiology* 24: 52–58.

Garcia-Varona, M., Santos, E.M., Jaime, I., and J. Rovira. 2000. Characterization of Micrococcaceae isolated from different varieties of chorizo. *International Journal of Food Microbiology* 54: 189–195.

Genccelep, H., Kaban, G., Aksu, M.I., Oz, F., and M. Kaya. 2008. Determination of biogenic amines in sucuk. *Food Control* 19(9): 868–872.

Ghosh, J. and G.S. Rajorhia. 1990. Selection of starter culture for production of indigenous fermented milk product (*Misti dahi*). *Lait* 70: 147–154.

Giraffa, G. and D. Carminati. 2008. Molecular techniques in food fermentation: Principles and applications. In: *Molecular Techniques in the Microbial Ecology of Fermented Foods.* (Eds: Cocolin, L. and Ercolini, D.). Springer Science + Business Media, LCC, New York. Chapter 1, pp. 1–30.

Gode, P.K. 1943. Some notes on the history of Indian dietetics with special reference to the history of jalebi. *New Indian Antique* 169–181.

Goncalves de Lima, O. 1975. *Pulque, balche e pajuaru.* Recife: Universidade Federal de Pernambuco.

Greppi, A., Rantsiou, K., Padonou, W., Hounhouigan, J., Jespersen, L., Jakobsen, M., and L. Cocolin. 2013a. Determination of yeast diversity in ogi, mawè, gowé and tchoukoutou by using culture-dependent and -independent methods. *International Journal of Food Microbiology* 165(2): 84–88.

Greppi, A., Rantisou, K., Padonou, W., Hounhouigan, J., Jespersen, L., Jakobsen, M., and L. Cocolin. 2013b. Yeast dynamics during spontaneous fermentation of mawè and tchoukoutou, two traditional products from Benin. *International Journal of Food Microbiology* 165(2): 200–207.

Gorer, G. 1938. *The Lepchas of Sikkim*. Delhi: Gian Publishing House.

Guan, L., Cho, K.H., and J.H. Lee. 2011. Analysis of the cultivable bacterial community in *jeotgal*, a Korean salted and fermented seafood, and identification of its dominant bacteria. *Food Microbiology* 28: 101–113.

Guarner, F., Perdigon, G., Corthier G, Salminen S, Koletzko, B., and L. Morelli. 2005. Should yoghurt cultures be considered probiotic? *British Journal of Nutrition* 93: 783–786.

Gupta, M., Khetarpaul, N., and B.M. Chauhan. 1992. Preparation, nutritional value and acceptability of barley *rabadi*—an indigenous fermented food of India. *Plant Foods for Human Nutrition* 42: 351–358.

Gupta, R.C., Mann, B., Joshi, V.K., and D.N. Prasad. 2000. Microbiological, chemical and ultrastructural characteristics of misti doi (sweetened dahi). *Journal of Food Science and Technology* 37(1): 54–57.

Guyot, J.P. 2010. Fermented cereal products, In: Tamang, J.P., and Kailasapathy, K. eds. *Fermented Foods and Beverages of the World*, CRC Press, Taylor & Francis Group, New York, 247–261.

Hamad, S.H., Dieng, M.M.C., Ehrmann, M.A., and R.F. Vogel. 1997. Characterisation of the bacterial flora of Sudanese sorghum flour and sorghum sourdough. *Journal of Applied Microbiology* 83: 764–770.

Hammes, W.P., Brandt, M.J., Francis, K.L., Rosenheim, J., Seitter, M.F.H., and S.A. Vogelmann. 2005. Microbial ecology of cereal fermentations. *Trends in Food Science and Technology* 16: 4–11.

Haard, N.F., Odunfa, S.A., Lee, C.H., Quintero-Ramírez, R., Lorence-Quiñones, A., and C. Wacher-Radarte. 1999. *Fermented Cereals: A Global Perspective*. FAO Agricultural Service Bulletin 138, 63–97. Rome: Food and Agriculture Organization.

Han, B.Z., Beumer, R.R., Rombouts, F.M., and Nout, M.J.R. 2001. Microbiological safety and quality of commercial sufu—A Chinese fermented soybean food. *Food Control* 12: 541–547.

Hansen, E.B. 2002. Commercial bacterial starter cultures for fermented foods of the future. *International Journal of Food Microbiology* 78: 119–131.

Hansen, E.B. 2004. Micro-organisms. *In: Handbook of Food and Beverage Fermentation Technology*, Eds. Hui, Y.H., Meunier-Goddik, L., Hansen, Å.S., Josephsen, J., Nip, W.K., Stanfield, P.S., and Toldrá, F., Marcel Dekker, Inc., 270 Madison Avenue, New York, 2, pp. 9–21.

Hao, Y., Zhao, L., Zhang, H., and Z. Zhai. 2010. Identification of the bacterial biodiversity in koumiss by denaturing gradient gel electrophoresis and species-specific polymerase chain reaction. *Journal of Dairy Science* 93: 1926–1933.

Hara, T., Chetanachit, C., Fujio, Y., and S. Ueda. 1986. Distribution of plasmids in polyglutamate-producing *Bacillus* strains isolated from "natto"-like fermented soybeans, "thua nao," in Thailand. *Journal of General and Applied Microbiology* 32: 241–249.

Hara, T., Hiroyuki, S., Nobuhide, I., and K. Shinji. 1995. Plasmid analysis in polyglutamate-producing *Bacillus* strain isolated from nonsalty fermented soybean food, "kinema", in Nepal. *Journal of General and Applied Microbiology* 41: 3–9.

Hara, T., Zhang, J.R., and S. Ueda. 1983. Identification of plasmids linked with polyglutamate production in *Bacillus subtilis (natto)*. *Journal of General and Applied Microbiology* 29: 345–354.

Harun-ur-Rashid, M., Togo, K., Useda, M., and T. Miyamoto. 2007. Probiotic characteristics of lactic acid bacteria isolated from traditional fermented milk "Dahi" in Bangladesh. *Pakistan Journal of Nutrition* 6: 647–652.

Haruta, S., Ueno, S., Egawa, I., Hashiguchi, K., Fujii, A., Nagano, M., and Y.I. Igarashi. 2006. Succession of bacterial and fungal communities during a traditional pot fermentation of rice vinegar assessed by PCR-mediated denaturing gradient gel electrophoresis. *International Journal of Food Microbiology* 109: 79–87.

Hayashida, F.M. 2008. Ancient beer and modern brewers: Ethnoarchaeological observations of *chicha* production in two regions of the North Coast of Peru. *Journal of Anthropological Archaeology* 27(2): 161–174.

Hesseltine, C.W. 1983. Microbiology of oriental fermented foods. *Annual Review of Microbiology* 37: 575–601.

Hesseltine, C.W. 1991. Zygomycetes in food fermentations. *Mycologist* 5: 162–169.

Hesseltine, C.W. and C.P. Kurtzman. 1990. Yeasts in amylolytic food starters. *Annls Inst Biol Uni Nac Antón México Ser Botany* 60: 1–7.

Hesseltine, C.W. and M.L. Ray. 1988. Lactic acid bacteria in murcha and ragi. *Journal of Applied Bacteriology* 64: 395–401.

Hesseltine, C.W., Rogers, R., and F.G. Winarno. 1988. Microbiological studies on amylolytic Oriental fermentation starters. *Mycopathologia* 101: 141–155.

Hirasawa, T., Yamada. K., Nagahisa, K., Dinh, T.N., Furusawa, C., Katakura, Y., SHioya, S., and Shimizu, H. 2009. Proteomic analysis of responses to osmotic stress in laboratory and sake-brewing strains of *Saccharomyces cerevisiae. Process Biochemistry* 44: 647–653.

Holzapfel, W.H. and G. Müller. 2007. Kaffee, In: *Lebensmittel pflanzlicher Herkunft*, Holzapfel, W.H. ed. e Behr's Verlag, Hamburg, 457–467.

Holzapfel, W.H., Schillinger, U., Toit, M.D., and L. Dicks. 1997. Systematics of probiotic lactic acid bacteria with reference to modern phenotypic and genomic methods. *Microecology and Therapy* 26: 1–10.

Hong, S.W., Choi, J.Y., and K.S. Chung. 2012. Culture-based and denaturing gradient gel electrophoresis analysis of the bacterial community from chungkookjang, a traditional Korean fermented soybean food. *Journal of Food Science* 77(10): M572–M578.

Ho, C.C. 1986. Identity and characteristics of *Neurospora intermedia* responsible for *oncom* fermentation in Indonesia. *Food Microbiology* 3: 115–132.

Hooker, J.D. 1854. *Himalayan Journals: Notes of a Naturalist in Bengal, the Sikkim and Nepal Himalayas, the Khasia Mountains*. London: John Murray.

Hounhouigan, D., Nout, M., Nago, C., Houben, J., and F. Rombouts. 1993. Characterization and frequency distribution of species of lactic acid bacteria involved in the processing of mawe, a fermented maize dough from Benin. *International Journal of Food Microbiology* 18: 279–287.

Huang, Y., Luo, Y., Zhai, Z., Zhang, H., Yang, C., Tian, H., Li, Z., Feng, J., Liu, H., and Y. Hao. 2009. Characterization and application of an anti-*Listeria* bacteriocin produced by *Pediococcus pentosaceus* 05–10 isolated from Sichuan Pickle, a traditionally fermented vegetable product from China. *Food Control* 20: 1030–1035.

Hulse, J.H. 2004. Biotechnologies: Past history, present state and future prospects. *Trends in Food Science* 15: 3–18.

Humblot, C. and J.P. Guyot. 2009. Pyrosequencing of tagged 16S rRNA gene amplicons for rapid deciphering of the microbiomes of fermented foods such as pearl millet slurries. *Applied and Environmental Microbiology* 75: 4354–4361.

Hwanhlem, N., Buradaleng, S., Wattanachant, S., Benjakul, S., Tani, A., and Maneerat, S. 2011. Isolation and screening of lactic acid bacteria from Thai traditional fermented fish (*Plasom*) and production of *Plasom* from selected strains. *Food Control* 22: 401–407.

Iacumin, L., Cecchini, F., Manzano, M., Osualdini, M., Boscolo, D., Orlic, S., and G. Comi. 2009. Description of the microflora of sourdoughs by culture-dependent and culture-independent methods. *Food Microbiology* 26: 128–135.

Ijong, F.G. and Y. Ohta. 1996. Physicochemical and microbiological changes associated with bakasang processing—A traditional Indonesian fermented fish sauce. *Journal of the Science of Food and Agriculture* 71: 69–74.

Inatsu, Y., Nakamura N, Yuriko Y, Fushimi T, Watanasritum L, Kawanmoto S. 2006. Characterization of *Bacillus subtilis* strains in Thua nao, a traditional fermented soybean food in northern Thailand. *Letters in Applied Microbiology* 43: 237–242.

Ishige, N. 1993. Cultural aspects of fermented fish products in Asia. In: *Fish Fermentation Technology*, eds. C.-H. Lee, K.H. Steinkraus and P.J. Alan Reilly, 13–32. Tokyo: United Nations University Press.

Itoh, H., Tachi, H., and S. Kikuchi. 1993. Fish fermentation technology in Japan. In: *Fish Fermentation Technology* (Eds: Lee, C.H., Steinkraus, K.H. and Alan Reilly, P.J.), pp. 177–186. United Nations University Press, Tokyo.

Itoh, H., Tong, J., and Y. Li. 1996. Chinese dauchi, from itohiki natto to nonmashed miso. *Miso Science Technology* 44: 224–250.

Iyengar, S.H. 1950. *Lokopakara of Chavundarava*. Madras: Oriental Manuscripts Library.

Jagannath, A., Raju, P.S., and A.S. Bawa. 2010. Comparative evaluation of bacterial cellulose (natta) as a cryoprotectant and carrier support during the freeze drying process of probiotic lactic acid bacteria. *LWT—Food Science and Technology* 43: 1197–1203.

Jeng, K.C., Chen, C.S., Fang, Y.P., Hou, R.C.W., and Y.S. Chen. 2007. Effect of microbial fermentation on content of statin, GABA, and polyphenols in Puerh tea. *Journal of Agriculture and Food Chemistry* 55: 8787–8792.

Jennessen, J., Schnürer, J., Olsson, J., Samson, R.A., and J. Dijiksterhuis. 2008. Morphological characteristics of sporangiospores of the *tempeh* fungus *Rhizopus oligosporus* differentiate it from other taxa of the *R. microsporus* group. *Mycology Research* 112: 547–563.

Jeyaram, J., Anand Singh, Th., Romi, W., Ranjita Devi, A., Mohendro Singh, W., Dayanidhi, H., Rajmuhon Singh, N., and J.P. Tamang. 2009. Traditional fermented foods of Manipur. *Indian Journal of Traditional Knowledge* 8(1): 115–121.

Jeyaram, K., Romi, W., Singh, TAh., Devi, A.R., and S.S. Devi. 2010. Bacterial species associated with traditional starter cultures used for fermented bamboo shoot production in Manipur state of India. *International Journal of Food Microbiology* 143: 1–8.

Jeyaram, K., Mohendro Singh, W., Premarani, T., Ranjita Devi, A., Selina Chanu, K., Talukdar, N.C., and M. Rohinikumar Singh. 2008a. Molecular identification of dominant microflora associated with "Hawaijar" – a traditional fermented soybean (*Glycine max* L.) food of Manipur, India. *International Journal of Food Microbiology* 122: 259–268.

Jeyaram, K., Singh, W.M., Capece, A., and P. Romano. 2008b. Molecular identification of yeast species associated with "Hamei"—A traditional starter used for rice wine production in Manipur, India. *International Journal of Food Microbiology* 124: 115–125.

Jeyaram, K., Tamang, J.P., Capece, A., and P.P. Romano. 2011. Geographical markers for *Saccharomyces cerevisiae* strains with similar technological origins domesticated for rice-based ethnic fermented beverages production in North East India. *Leeuwenhoek International Journal of General and Molecular Microbiology* 100: 569–578.

Jianzhonga, Z., Xiaolia, L., Hanhub, J., and D. Mingshengb. 2009. Analysis of the microflora in Tibetan kefir grains using denaturing gradient gel electrophoresis *Food Microbiology* 26: 770–775.

Jiang, J. J., Zeng, Q.X., Zhu, Z.W., and L.Y. Zhang. 2007. Chemical and sensory changes associated Yu-lu fermentation process—A traditional Chinese fish sauce. *Food Chemistry* 104: 1629–1634.

Johanningsmeier, S., McFeeters, R.F., Fleming, H.P., and R.L. Thompson. 2007. Effects of *Leuconostoc mesenteroides* starter culture on fermentation of cabbage with reduced salt concentrations. *Journal of Food Science* 72: M166–M172.

Josephsen, J. and L. Jespersen L. 2004. Handbook of food and beverage fermentation technology. In: *Starter Cultures and Fermented Products,* Eds. Hui, Y.H., Meunier-Goddik, L., Hansen, Å.S., Josephsen, J., Nip, W.K., Stanfield, P.S., and Toldrá, F., Marcel Dekker, Inc., 270 Madison Avenue, New York, 3, pp. 23–49.

Jung, D.H., 2012. *Great Dictionary of Fermented Food.* Yuhanmunwhasa, Inc., Kayang-dong, Seoul.

Jung, J.Y., Lee, S.H., Kim, J.M., Park, M.S., Bae, J.W., Hahn, Y., Madsen, E.L., and C.O. Jeon. 2011. Metagenomic analysis of kimchi, a traditional Korean fermented food. *Applied and Environmental Microbiology* 77: 2264–2274.

Jung, J.Y., Lee, S.H., Lee, H.J., and C.O. Jeon. 2013. Microbial succession and metabolite changes during fermentation of *saeu-jeot*: Traditional Korean salted seafood. *Food Microbiology* 34(2): 360–368.

Jung, M.J., Nam, Y.D., Roh, S.W., and J.W. Bae. 2012. Unexpected convergence of fungal and bacterial communities during fermentation of traditional Korean alcoholic beverages inoculated with various natural starters. *Food Microbiology* 30: 112–123.

Kahala M., Mäki, M., Lehtovaara, A., Tapanainen, J.M., Katiska, R., Juuruskorpi, M., Juhola, J., and V. Joutsjoki. 2008. Characterization of starter lactic acid bacteria from the Finnish fermented milk product viili. *Journal of Applied Microbiology* 105: 1929–1938.

Karim, M.I.A. 1993. Fermented fish products in Malaysia. In: *Fish Fermentation Technology* (Eds: Lee, C.H., Steinkraus, K.H. and Alan Reilly, P.J.), pp. 95–106. United Nations University Press, Tokyo.

Karki, T., Okada, S., Baba, T., Itoh, H. and M. Kozaki. 1983. Studies on the microflora of Nepalese pickles gundruk. *Nippon Shokuhin Kogyo Gakkaishi* 30: 357–367.

Karagozlu, N., Ergonul, B., and C. Karagozlu. 2008. Microbiological attributes of instant tarhana during fermentation and drying. *Bulgarian Journal of Agricultural Science* 14: 535–541.

Khanh, T.M., May, B.K., Smooker, P.M., Van, T.T.H., and P.J. Coloe. 2011. Distribution and genetic diversity of lactic acid bacteria from traditional fermented sausage. *Food Research International* 44: 338–344.

Khatri, P.K. 1987. *Nepali Samaj ra Sanskriti (Prachin-Madhyakal).* Shaja Prakashan, Kathmandu (Nepali).

Kiers, J.L., Van laeken, A.E.A., Rombouts, F.M., and M.J.R. Nout. 2000. *In vitro* digestibility of *Bacillus* fermented soya bean. *International Journal of Food Microbiology* 60: 163–169.

Kim, J.O. and J.G. Kim. 1993. Microbial and enzymatic properties related to brewing of traditional ewhaju. *Korean Journal of Society of Food Science* 9(4): 266–271.

Kim, T.W., Lee, J.W., Kim, S.E., Park, M.H., Chang, H.C., and H.Y. Kim. 2009. Analysis of microbial communities in *doenjang*, a Korean fermented soybean paste, using nested PCR-denaturing gradient gel electrophoresis. *International Journal of Food Microbiology* 131: 265–271.

Kim, Y.B., Seo, Y.G., and C.H. Lee. 1993. Growth of microorganisms in dorsal muscle of gulbi during processing and their effect on its quality. In: *Fish Fermentation Technology* (Eds: Lee, C.H., Steinkraus, K.H. and Alan Reilly, P.J.), pp. 281–289. United Nations University Press, Tokyo.

Kimura, K. and Y. Itoh. 2007. Determination and characterization of IS*4Bsu1*-insertion loci and identification of a new insertion sequence element of the IS*256* family in a natto starter. *Bioscience, Biotechnology and Biochemistry* 71: 2458–2464.

Kingston, J.J., Radhika, M., Roshini, P.T., Raksha, M.A., Murali, H.S., and H.V. Batra. 2010. Molecular characterization of lactic acid bacteria recovered from natural fermentation of beet root and carrot Kanji. *Indian Journal of Microbiology* 50: 292–298.

Kisworo, D. 2003. Characteristics of lactic acid bacteria from raw milk and white soft cheese. *Philippine Agricultural Scientist* 86: 56–64.

Kitamoto, K. 2002. Molecular biology of the *Koji* molds. *Advances in Applied Microbiology* 51: 129–153.

Kiuchi, K. 2001. Miso and natto. *Food Culture* 3: 7–10.

Kiyohara, M., Koyanagi, T., Matsui, H., Yamamoto, K., Take, H., Katsuyama, Y., Tsuji, A., Miyamae, H., Kondo, T., Nakamura, S., Katayama, T., and H. Kumagai. 2012. Changes in microbiota population during fermentation of Narezushi as revealed by pyrosequencing analysis. *Bioscience, Biotechnology, Biochemistry* 76: 48–52.

Kobayashi, T., Kimura, B., and Fujii, T. 2000a. Strictly anaerobic halophiles isolated from canned Swedish fermented herrings (Suströmming). *International Journal of Food Microbiology* 54: 81–89.

Kobayashi, T., Kimura, B., and T. Fujii. 2000b. *Haloanaerobium fermentans* sp. nov., a strictly anaerobic, fermentative halophile isolated from fermented puffer fish ovaries. *International Journal of Systematic and Evolutionary Microbiology* 50: 1621–1627.

Kobayashi, T., Kimura, B., and T. Fujii. 2000c. Differentiation of *Tetragenococcus* populations occurring in products and manufacturing processes of puffer fish ovaries fermented with rice-bran. *International Journal of Food Microbiology* 56: 211–218.

Kolawole, O.M., Kayode, R.M.O., and Akinduyo, B. 2013. Proximate and microbial analyses of burukutu and pito produced in Ilorin, Nigeria. *African Journal of Microbiology* 1(1): 15–17.

Kosikowski, F.V. and V.V. Mistry. 1997. *Cheese and Fermented Milk Foods.* Connecticut: LLC Westport.

Kotaka, A., Bando, H., Kaya, M., Kato-Murai, M., Kuroda, K., Sahara, H., Hata, Y., Kondo, A., and Ueda, M. 2008. Direct ethanol production from barley β-glucan by sake yeast displaying *Aspergillus oryzae* β-glucosidase and endoglucanase. *Journal of Bioscience and Bioengineering* 105: 622–627.

Kozaki, M. 1976. Fermented foods and related microorganisms in Southeast Asia. *Proceedings of Japanese Association of Mycotoxicology* 2: 1–9.

Kozaki, M., Tamang, J.P, Kataoka, J., Yamanaka, S., and S. Yoshida. 2000. Cereal wine (*jaanr*) and distilled wine (*raksi*) in Sikkim. *Journal of Brewing Society of Japan* 95: 115–122.

Kozaki, M. and T. Uchimura. 1990. Microorganisms in Chinese starter "bubod" and rice wine "tapuy" in the Philippines. *Journal of Brewing Society of Japan* 85(11): 818–824.

Kubo, Y., Rooney, A.P., Tsukakoshi, Y., Nakagawa, R., Hasegawa, H., and K. Kimura. 2011. Phylogenetic analysis of *Bacillus subtilis* strains applicable to natto (fermented soybean) production. *Applied Environmental Microbiology* 77: 6463–6469.

Kurtzman, C.P., Fell JW, and T. Boekhout (Editor), 2011. *The Yeasts: A Taxonomic Study*, 5th edition. Elsevier: London.

Kurtzman, C.P. and C.J. Robnett. 2003. Phylogenetic relationship among yeasts of the "*Saccharomyces* complex" determined from multigene sequence analyses. *FEMS Yeast Research* 3: 417–432.

Kurtzman, C.P., Robnett, C.J., and Basehoar-Powers, E. 2001. *Zygosaccharomyces kombuchaensis*, a new ascosporogenous yeast from "Kombucha tea". *FEMS Yeast Research* 1: 133–138.

Kuda, T., Izawa, Y., Yoshida, S., Koyanagi, T., Takahashi, H., and B. Kimura. 2014. Rapid identification of *Tetragenococcus halophilus* and *Tetragenococcus muriaticus*, important species in the production of salted and fermented foods, by matrix-assisted laser desorption ionization-time of flight mass spectrometry (MALDI-TOF MS). *Food Control* 35(1): 419–425.

Kutyauripo, J., Parawira, W., Tinofa, S., Kudita, I., and C. Ndengu. 2009. Investigation of shelf-life extension of sorghum beer (*Chibuku*) by removing the second conversion of malt. *International Journal of Food Microbiology* 129: 271–276.

Kwon, G.H., Lee, H.A., Park, J.Y., Kim, J.S., Lim, J., Park, C.S., Kwon, D.Y., and J.H. Kim. 2009. Development of a RAPD-PCR method for identification of *Bacillus* species isolated from Cheonggukjang. *International Journal of Food Microbiology* 129: 282–287.

Lactic Acid Bacteria. 2013. http://www.metamicrobe.com/lactobacteria/

Lappe-Oliveras, P., Moreno-Terrazas, R., Arrizón-Gaviño, J., Herrera-Suárez, T., Garcia-Mendoza, A., and A. Gschaedler-Mathis. 2008. Yeasts associated with the production of Mexican alcoholic nondistilled and distilled *Agave* beverages. *FEMS Yeast Research* 8: 1037–1052.

Lee, C.H. 1993. Fish fermentation technology in Korea. In: *Fish Fermentation Technology* (Eds: Lee, C.H., Steinkraus, K.H. and Alan Reilly, P.J.), pp. 187–201. United Nations University Press, Tokyo.

Lee, C.H. 1995. An introduction to Korean food culture. *Korean and Korean American Studies Bulletin* 6(1): 6–10.

Lee, S.W. 1984. *Hankuk sikpum munhwasa (Korean Dietary Culture).* Seoul: Kyomunsa. (in Korean).

Lee, I.H., Hung, Y.H., and C.C. Chou. 2007. Total phenolic and anthocyanin contents, as well as antioxidant activity, of black bean *koji* fermented by *Aspergillus awamori* under different culture conditions. *Food Chemistry* 3: 936–942.

Lee, Z.S. and T.W. Rhee. 1970. Studies on the microflora of Takju brewing. *Korean Journal of Microbiology* 8: 116–133.

Lefeber, T., Janssens, M., Camu, N., and L. De Vuyst. 2010. Kinetic analysis of strains of lactic acid bacteria and acetic acid bacteria in cocoa pulp simulation media toward development of a starter culture for cocoa bean fermentation. *Applied Environmental Microbiology* 76: 7708–7716.

Lepage, P., Leclerc, M.C., Joossens, M., Mondot, S., Blottière, H.M., Raes, J., Ehrlich, D., and J. Doré. 2013. A metagenomic insight into our gut's microbiome *Gut* 62(1): 146–158.

Leroy, F. and L. De Vuyst. 2004. Lactic acid bacteria as functional starter cultures for the food fermentation industry. *Trends in Food Science and Technology* 15: 67–78.

Lindqvist, R. and M. Lindblad. 2009. Inactivation of *Escherichia coli, Listeria monocytogenes* and *Yersinia enterocolitica* in fermented sausages during maturation/storage. *International Journal of Food Microbiology* 129: 59–67.

Longo, M.A. and M.A. Sanromán. 2006. Production of food aroma compounds: Microbial and enzymatic methodologies. *Food Technology and Biotechnology* 44: 335–353.

Lopetcharat, K., Choi, Y.J., Park, J.W., and M.A. Daeschel. 2001. Fish sauce products and manufacturing: A review. *Food Reviews International* 17: 65–88.

Lücke, F.K. 1985. Fermented sausages. In: *Microbiology of Fermented Foods*, vol. 2, ed. B.J.B. Wood, 41–83. London: Elsevier Applied Science Publishers.

Lv, X-C., Huang, X-L., Zhang, W., Rao, P-F., and L. Ni. 2013. Yeast diversity of traditional alcohol fermentation starters for Hong Qu glutinous rice wine brewing, revealed by culture-dependent and culture-independent methods. *Food Control* 34: 183–190.

Mabesa, R.C. and J.S. Babaan. 1993. Fish fermentation technology in the Philippines. In: *Fish Fermentation Technology* (Eds: Lee, C.H., Steinkraus, K.H., and Alan Reilly, P.J.), pp. 85–94. United Nations University Press, Tokyo.

Marsh, A.J., O'Sullivan, O., Hill, C., R. Paul Ross, R.P., and Cotter, D. 2014. Sequence-based analysis of the bacterial and fungal compositions of multiple kombucha (tea fungus) samples. *Food Microbiology* 38: 171–178.

Martín, B., Garriga, M., Hugas, M., Bover-Cid, S., Veciana-Noqués, M.T., and Aymerich, T. 2006. Molecular, technological and safety characterization of Gram-positive catalase-positive cocci from slightly fermented sausages. *International Journal of Food Microbiology* 107: 148–158.

Marty, E., Buchs J, Eugster-Meier E, Lacroix, C., and L. Meile. 2011. Identification of staphylococci and dominant lactic acid bacteria in spontaneously fermented Swiss meat products using PCR–RFLP. *Food Microbiology* 29: 157–166.

Masoud, W., Cesar, L.B., Jespersen, L., and M. Jakobsen. 2004. Yeast involved in fermentation of *Coffea arabica* in East Africa determined by genotyping and direct denaturating gradient gel electrophoresis. *Yeast* 21: 549–556.

Mathara, J.M., Schillinger, U., Kutima, P.M., Mbugua, S.K., and W.H. Holzapfel. 2004. Isolation, identification and characterisation of the dominant microorganisms of kule naoto: The Maasai traditional fermented milk in Kenya. *International Journal of Food Microbiology* 94: 269–278.

Matsushita, M., Tada, S., Suzuki, S., Kusumoto, K., and Y. Kashiwagi. 2009. Deletion analysis of the promoter of *Aspergillus oryzae* gene encoding heat shock protein 30. *Journal of Bioscience and Bioengineering* 107: 345–351.

Mayo, B., Ammor, M.S., Delgado, S., and A. Alegría. 2010. Fermented milk products. In: Tamang JP, Kailasapathy K. eds. *Fermented Foods and Beverages of the World*, CRC Press, Taylor & Francis Group, New York, 263–288.

Meerak, J., Iida, H., Watanabe, Y., Miyashita, M., Sato, H., Nakagawa, Y., and Y. Tahara. 2007. Phylogeny of γ-polyglutamic acid-producing *Bacillus* strains isolated from fermented soybean foods manufactured in Asian countries. *Journal of General and Applied Microbiology* 53: 315–323.

Meerak, J., Yukphan, P., Miyashita, M., Sato, H., Nakagawa, Y., and Y. Tahara 2008. Phylogeny of γ-polyglutamic acid-producing *Bacillus* strains isolated from a fermented locust bean product manufactured in West Africa. *Journal of General and Applied Microbiology* 54: 159–166.

Merican, Z. 1996. Malaysian pickles. In: *Handbook of Indigenous Fermented Food,* 2nd edition, ed. K.H. Steinkraus, 138–141. New York: Marcel Dekker, Inc.

Merican, Z. 1977. Budu (fish sauce). In: *The Proceedings of the Symposium on Indigenous Fermented Foods,* November 21–27, 1977, GIAM-V, Bangkok.

Merican, Z. and Q.L. Yeoh. 1989. Tapai proceeding in Malaysia: A technology in transition. In: *Industrialization of Indigenous Fermented Foods*, ed. K.H. Steinkraus, 169–189. New York: Marcel Dekker, Inc.

Mitsuoka, T. 1992. Intestinal flora and aging. *Nutrition Review* 50: 438–446.

Mo, H., Zhu, Y., and Z. Chen. 2008. Microbial fermented tea—A potential source of natural food preservatives. *Trends in Food Science and Technology* 19: 124–130.

Mohammed, S.I., Steenson, L.R., and A.W. Kirleis. 1991. Isolation and characterization of microorganisms associated with the traditional sorghum fermentation for production of Sudanese kisra. *Applied Environmental Microbiology* 57: 2529–2533.

Mogensen, G., Salminen, S., O'Brien, J., Ouwehand, A., Holzapfel, W., Shortt, C., Fonden, R. et al. 2002. Inventory of micro-organisms with a documented history of use in food. *Bulletin of IDF* 377: 10–19.

Moreira, N., Mendes, F., Hogg, T., and I. Vasconcelos. 2005. Alcohols, esters and heavy sulphur compounds produced by pure and mixed cultures of apiculture wine yeasts. *International Journal of Food Microbiology* 103: 285–294.

Moroni, A.V., Arendt, E.K., and F.D. Bello. 2011. Biodiversity of lactic acid bacteria and yeasts in spontaneously-fermented buckwheat and teff sourdoughs. *Food Microbiology* 28: 497–502.

Mozzi, F., Eugenia Ortiz, M., Bleckwedel, J., De Vuyst, L., and P. Micaela. 2013. Metabolomics as a tool for the comprehensive understanding of fermented and functional foods with lactic acid bacteria. *Food Research International* 54: 1152–1161.

Mshvildadze, M. and J. Neu. 2010. The infant intestinal microbiome: Friend or foe? *Early Human Development* 86: 67–71.

Mugula, J.K., Ninko, S.A.M., Narvhus, J.A., and T. Sorhaug. 2003. Microbiological and fermentation characteristics of *togwa*, a Tanzanian fermented food. *International Journal of Food Microbiology* 80: 187–199.

Murray, M.A. 2000. Viticulture and wine production. In: *Ancient Egyptian Materials and Technology*, eds. P.T. Nicholson and I. Shaw, 577–608. Cambridge: Cambridge University Press.

Nagai, T., Koguchi, K., and Y. Itoh. 1997. Chemical analysis of poly-γ-glutamic acid produced by plasmid-free *Bacillus subtilis (natto)*: evidence that plasmids are not involved in poly-γ-glutamic acid production. *Journal of General and Applied Microbiology* 43: 139–143.

Nagai, T. and J.P. Tamang. 2010. Fermented soybeans and non-soybeans legume foods. In: Tamang JP, Kailasapathy K. eds. *Fermented Foods and Beverages of the World.* New York: CRC Press, Taylor & Francis Group, pp. 191–224.

Nagai, T., Tran, L.S., Inatsu, Y., and Y. Itoh. 2000. A new IS*4* family insertion sequence, IS*4Bsu1*, responsible for genetic instability of poly-γ-glutamic acid production in *Bacillus subtilis*. *Journal of Bacteriology* 182: 2387–2392.

Nakao, S. 1972. Mame no ryori, In: *Ryori no kigen*. Tokyo: Japan Broadcast Publishing, Tokyo (in Japanese), 115–126.

Nam, Y-D., Chang, H.W., Kim, K.H., Roh, S.W., and J.W. Bae. 2009. Metatranscriptome analysis of lactic acid bacteria during *kimchi* fermentation with genome-probing microarrays. *International Journal of Food Microbiology* 130: 140–146.

Nam, Y-D., Lee, So-Y., and S-I. Lim. 2011. Microbial community analysis of Korean soybean pastes by next-generation sequencing. *International Journal of Food Microbiology* 155(1–2): 36–42.

Nam, Y-D., Yi, S-H., and S-I. Lim. 2012. Bacterial diversity of *cheonggukjang*, a traditional Korean fermented food, analyzed by barcoded pyrosequencing. *Food Control* 28(1): 135–142.

Naser, S.M., Thompson, F.L., Hoste, B., Gevers, D., Dawyndt, P., Vancanneyt, M., and J. Swings. 2005. Application of multilocus sequence analysis (MLSA) for rapid identification of *Enterococcus* species based on *pheS* and *rpoA* genes. *Microbiology* 151: 2141–2150.

Ngaba, R.R. and Lee, J.S. 1979. Fermentation of cassava. *Journal of Food Science* 44: 1570–1571.

Nguyen, H., Elegado, F., Librojo-Basilio, N., Mabesa, R., and Dizon, E. 2011. Isolation and characterisation of selected lactic acid bacteria for improved processing of *nem chua*, a traditional fermented meat from Vietnam. *Beneficial Microbes* 1(1): 67–74.

Nguyen, D.T.L., Van Hoorde, K., Cnockaert, M., de Brandt, E., de Bruyne, K., Le, B.T., and P. Vandamme. 2013a. A culture-dependent and -independent approach for the identification of lactic acid bacteria associated with the production of *nem chua*, a Vietnamese fermented meat product. *Food Research International* 50(1): 232–240.

Nguyen, D.T. L., Van Hoorde, K., Cnockaert, M., de Brandt, E., Aerts, M., Thanh, L.B., and P. Vandamme. 2013b. A description of the lactic acid bacteria microbiota associated with the production of traditional fermented vegetables in Vietnam. *International Journal of Food Microbiology* 163(1): 19–27.

Nielsen, D.S., Schillinger, U., Franz, C.M.A.P., Bresciani, J., Amoa-Awua, W., Holzapfel, W.H., and M. Jakobsen. 2007. *Lactobacillus ghanensis* sp. nov., a motile lactic acid bacterium isolated from Ghanaian cocoa fermentations. *International Journal of Systematic and Evolutionary Microbiology* 57: 1468–1472.

Nikkuni, S., Karki, T.B., Terao, T., and C. Suzuki. 1996. Microflora of mana, a Nepalese rice koji. *Journal of Fermentation and Bioengineering* 81: 168–170.

Nishito, Y., Osana, Y., Hachiya, T., Popendorf, K., Toyoda, A., Fujiyama, A., Itaya, M., and Sakakibara, Y. 2010. Whole genome assembly of a *natto* production strain *Bacillus subtilis natto* from very short read data. *BMC Genomics* 11: 243–255.

Norman, J. M., Handley, S. A., and W. Virgin. 2014. Kingdom-agnostic metagenomics and the importance of complete characterization of enteric microbial communities. *Gastroenterology* 146(6): 1459–1469.

Nout, M.J.R. and K.E. Aidoo. 2002. Asian fungal fermented food, In: *The Mycota*, ed. Osiewacz, H.D., Springer-Verlag, New York, 23–47.

Nout, M.J.R. and J.L. Kiers. 2005. Tempeh fermentation, innovation and functionality: Update into the third millenium. *Journal of Applied Microbiology* 98: 789–805.

Odunfa, S.A. 1988. Review: African fermented foods: From art to science. *MIRCEN Journal* 4: 259–273.

Odunfa, S.A. and O.B. Oyewole. 1997. *African Fermented Foods*. Blackie Academic and Professional: London.

Oguntoyinbo, F.A. and C.E.R. Dodd. 2010. Bacterial dynamics during the spontaneous fermentation of cassava dough in *gari* production. *Food Control* 21: 306–312.

Oguntoyinbo, F.A., Huch, M., Cho, G.S., Schillinger, U., Holzapfel, W.H., Sanni, A.I., and C.M.A.P. Franz. 2010. Diversity of *Bacillus* species isolated from okpehe, a traditional fermented soup condiment from Nigeria. *Journal of Food Protection* 73: 870–878.

Oguntoyinbo, F.A., Sanni, A.I., Franz, S.M.A.P., and W.H. Holzapfel. 2007. *In vitro* fermentation studies for selection and evaluation of *Bacillus* strains as starter cultures for the production of okpehe, a traditional African fermented condiment. *International Journal of Food Microbiology* 113: 208–218.

Oguntoyinbo, F.A., Tourlomousis, P., Gasson, M.J., and Narbad, A. 2011. Analysis of bacterial communities of traditional fermented West African cereal foods using culture independent methods. *International Journal of Food Microbiology* 145: 205–210.

Okafor, N. and A.O. Ejiofor. 1990. Rapid detoxifiction of cassava mash fermenting for garri production following inoculation with a yeast simultaneously producing linamarase and amylase. *Proceeding of Biochemical Institute* 25: 82–86.

Oki, K., Dugersuren, J., Demberel, S., and K. Watanabe. 2014. Pyrosequencing analysis of the microbial diversity of *airag, khoormog* and *tarag*, traditional fermented dairy products of Mongolia. *Bioscience of Microbiota, Food and Health* 33(2): 53–64.

Oki, K., Kudo, Y., and K. Watanabe. 2012. *Lactobacillus saniviri* sp. nov. and *Lactobacillus senioris* sp. nov., isolated from human faeces. *International Journal of Systematic and Evolutionary Microbiology* 62: 601–607.

Oki, K., Rai, A.K., Sato, S., Watanabe, K., and J.P. Tamang. 2011. Lactic acid bacteria isolated from ethnic preserved meat products of the Western Himalayas. *Food Microbiology* 28: 1308–1315.

Olasupo, N.A., Odunfa, S.A., and O.S. Obayori. 2010. Ethnic African fermented foods, In: Tamang JP, Kailasapathy K. eds. *Fermented Foods and Beverages of the World*, CRC Press, Taylor & Francis Group, New York, 323–352.

Ongol, M.P. and K. Asano. 2009. Main microorganisms involved in the fermentation of Uganda ghee. *International Journal of Food Microbiology* 133: 286–291.

Ouoba, L., Cantor, M., Diawara, B., Traoré, A., and Jakobsen, M., 2003a. Degradation of African locust bean oil by *Bacillus subtilis* and *Bacillus pumilus* isolated from soumbala, a fermented African locust bean condiment. *Journal of Applied Microbiology* 95: 868–873.

Ouoba, L., Diawara, B., Annan, N., Poll, L., and Jakobsen, M., 2005. Volatile compounds of Soumbala, a fermented African locust bean (*Parkia biglobosa*) food condiment. *Journal of Applied Microbiology* 99: 1413–1421.

Ouoba, L.I.I., Diawara, B., Christensen, T., Dalgaard Mikkelsen, J., and Jakobsen, M., 2007a. Degradation of polysaccharides and non-digestible oligosaccharides by *Bacillus subtilis* and *Bacillus pumilus* isolated from Soumbala, a fermented African locust bean (*Parkia biglobosa*) food Condiment. *European Food Research and Technology* 224: 689–694.

Ouoba, L.I.I., Diawara, B., Jespersen, L., and Jakobsen, M., 2007b. Antimicrobial activity of *Bacillus subtilis* and *Bacillus pumilus* during the fermentation of African locust bean (*Parkia biglobosa*) for Soumbala production. *Journal of Applied Microbiology* 102: 963–970.

Ouoba, L.I., Nyanga-Koumou, C.A., Parkouda, C., Sawadogo, H., Kobawila, S.C., Keleke, S., Diawara, B., Louembe, D., and J.P. Sutherland. 2010. Genotypic diversity of lactic acid bacteria isolated from African traditional alkaline-fermented foods. *Journal of Applied Microbiology* 108: 2019–2029.

Ouoba, L., Parkouda, C., Diawara, B., Scotti, C., and A. Varnam. 2008. Identification of *Bacillus* spp. from Bikalga, fermented seeds of *Hibiscus sabdariffa*: Phenotypic and genotypic characterization. *Journal of Applied Microbiology* 104: 122–131.

Ouoba, L., Rechinger, K., Barkholt, V., Diawara, B., Traore, A., and Jakobsen, M., 2003b. Degradation of proteins during the fermentation of African locust bean (*Parkia biglobosa*) by strains of *Bacillus subtilis and Bacillus pumilus* for production of Soumbala. *Journal of Applied Microbiology* 94: 396–402.

Ouoba, L., Diawara, B., Wk, A.A., Traore, A., and Moller, P., 2004. Genotyping of starter cultures of *Bacillus subtilis* and *Bacillus pumilus* for fermentation of African locust bean (*Parkia biglobosa*) to produce Soumbala. *International Journal of Food Microbiology* 90: 197–205.

Oyewole, O.B., Olatunji, O.O., and S.A. Odunfa. 2004. A process technology for conversion of dried cassava chips into "gari". *Nigeria Food Journal* 22: 65–76.

Papalexandratou, Z., Vrancken, G., De Bruyne, K., Vandamme, P., and L. De Vuyst. 2011. Spontaneous organic cocoa bean box fermentations in Brazil are characterized by a restricted species diversity of lactic acid bacteria and acetic acid bacteria. *Food Microbiology* 28: 1326–1338.

Parente, E. and Cogan, T.M. 2004. Starter cultures: general aspects, In: *Cheese: Chemistry, Physics and Microbiology*, 3rd edition, ed. Fox, P. O., Elsevier, Oxford, 123–147.

Park, E.J., Chang, H.W., Kim, K.H., Nam, Y.D., Roh, S.W., and J.W. Bae. 2009. Application of quantitative real-time PCR for enumeration of total bacterial, archaeal, and yeast populations in kimchi. *Journal Microbiology* 47: 682–685.

Park, C., Choi, J.C., Choi, Y.H., Nakamura, H., Shimanouchi, K., Horiuchi, T., Misono, H., Sewaki, T., Soda, K., Ashiuchi M., and M.H. Sung. 2005. Synthesis of super-high-molecular-weight poly-γ-glutamic acid by *Bacillus subtilis* subsp. *chungkookjang*. *Journal of Molecular Catalysis B: Enzymatic* 35: 128–133.

Park, E.J., Chun, J., Cha, C.J., Park, W.S., Jeon, C.O., and J.W. Bae. 2012. Bacterial community analysis during fermentation of ten representative kinds of *kimchi* with barcoded pyrosequencing. *Food Microbiology* 30: 197–204.

Park, J.M., Shin, J.H., Lee, D.W., Song, J.C., Suh, H.J., Chang, U.J., and J.M. Kim. 2010. Identification of the lactic acid bacteria in kimchi according to initial and over-ripened fermentation using PCR and 16S rRNA gene sequence analysis. *Food Science and Biotechnology* 19: 541–546.

Parkouda C, Nielsen, D.S., Azokpota, P., Ouoba, L.I.I., Amoa-Awua, W.K., Thorsen, L., Houhouigan, J.D., Jensen, J.S., Tano-Debrah, K., Diawara, B., and M. Jakobsen. 2009. The microbiology of alkaline-fermentation of indigenous seeds used as food condiments in Africa and Asia. *Critical Review in Microbiology* 35: 139–156.

Parente, E.S., Di Matteo, M., Spagna Musso, S., and M.A. Crudele. 1994. Use of commercial starter cultures in the production of soppressa lucana, a fermented sausage from Basilicata. *Italian Journal of Science* 6: 59–69.

Parente, E.S., Grieco, S., and M.A. Crudele. 2001a. Phenotypic diversity of lactic acid bacteria isolated from fermented sausages produced in Basilicata (Southern Italy). *Journal of Applied Microbiology* 90: 943–952.

Parente, E., Martuscelli, M., Gardini, F., Grieco, S., Crudele, M.A., and G. Suzzi. 2001b. Evolution of microbial populations and biogenic amine production in dry sausages produced in Southern Italy. *Journal of Applied Microbiology* 90: 882–891.

Patidar, S.K. and J.B. Prajapati. 1998. Standardization and evaluation of lassi prepared using *Lactobacillus acidophilus* and *Streptococcus thermophilus*. *Journal of Food Science and Technology* 35(5): 428–431.

Patil, M.M., Pal, A., Anand, T., and K.V. Ramana. 2010. Isolation and characterization of lactic acid bacteria from curd and cucumber. *Indian Journal of Biotechnology* 9: 166–172.

Patrignani, F., Lanciotti R, Mathara J.M., Guerzoni M.E., and W.H. Holzapfel. 2006. Potential of functional strains, isolated from traditional *Maasai* milk, as starters for the production of fermented milks. *International Journal of Food Microbiology* 107: 1–11.

Pederson, C.S. 1979. *Microbiology of Food Fermentations*, 2nd edition. Westport: AVI Publishing Company.

Pederson, C.S. and M.N. Albury. 1969. The sauerkraut fermentation. *Food Technology* 8: 1–5.

Phithakpol, B. 1993. Fish fermentation technology in Thailand. In: *Fish Fermentation Technology* (Eds: Lee, C.H., Steinkraus, K.H., and Alan Reilly, P.J.), pp. 155–166. United Nations University Press, Tokyo.

Phithakpol, B., Varanyanond, W., Reungmaneepaitoon, S., and H. Wood. 1995. *The Traditional Fermented Foods of Thailand*. Kuala Lumpu: ASEAN Food Handling Bureau.

Picozzi, C., Bonacina, G., Vigentini, I., and Foschino, R. 2010. Genetic diversity in Italian *Lactobacillus sanfranciscensis* strains assessed by multilocus sequence typing and pulsed field gel electrophoresis analyses. *Microbiology* 156: 2035–2045.

Plengvidhya, V., Breidt, F., and H.P. Fleming. 2007. Use of RAPD-PCR as a method to follow the progress of starter cultures in sauerkraut fermentation. *International Journal of Food Microbiology* 93: 287–296.

Prakash, O. 1961. *Food and Drinks in Ancient India*. Delhi: Munshi Ram Monoharlal Publ.

Prajapati, J.B. and B.M. Nair. 2003. The history of fermented foods. In: *Handbook of Fermented Functional Foods*, ed. R. Farnworth, 1–25. New York: CRC Press.

Pretorius, I.S. 2000. Review: Tailoring wine yeast for the new millennium: Novel approaches to the ancient art of wine making. *Yeast* 16: 675–729.

Purchiaroni, F., Tortora, A., Gabrielli, M., Bertucci, F., Gigante, G., Ianiro, G., Ojetti, V., Scarpellini, E., and A. Gasbarrini. 2013. The role of intestinal microbiota and the immune system. *European Review for Medical and Pharmacological Sciences* 17: 323–333.

Puspito, H. and G.H. Fleet. 1985. Microbiology of *sayur asin* fermentation. *Applied Microbiology and Biotechnology* 22: 442–445.

Putro, S. 1993. Fish fermentation technology in Indonesia. In: *Fish Fermentation Technology* (Eds: Lee, C.H., Steinkraus, K.H., and Alan Reilly, P.J.), pp. 107–128. United Nations University Press, Tokyo.

Quigley, L., O'Sullivan, O., Beresford, T.P., Ross, R.P., Fitzgerald, G.F., and P.D. Cotter. 2011. Molecular approaches to analysing the microbial composition of raw milk and raw milk cheese. *International Journal of Food Microbiology* 150: 81–94.

Rai, A.K., Palni, U., and J.P. Tamang. 2009. Traditional knowledge of the Himalayan people on production of indigenous meat products. *Indian Journal of Traditional Knowledge* 8(1): 104–109.

Rai, A.K., Palni, U., and J.P. Tamang. 2010. Microbiological studies of ethnic meat products of the Eastern Himalayas. *Meat Science* 85: 560–567.

Ramakrishnan, C.V. 1979. Studies on Indian fermented foods. *Baroda Journal of Nutrition* 6: 1–54.

Ramos, C.L., de Almeida, E.G., de Melo Pereira, G.V., Cardoso, P.G., Dias, E.S., and R.F. Schwan. 2010. Determination of dynamic characteristics of microbiota in a fermented beverage produced by Brazilian Amerindians using culture-dependent and culture-independent methods. *International Journal of Food Microbiology* 140(2–3): 225–231.

Rani, D.K. and S.K. Soni. 2007. Applications and commercial uses of microorganisms. In: *Microbes: A Source of Energy for 21st Century*, ed. Soni, S.K., Jai Bharat Printing Press, Tohtas Nagar, Shahdara, Delhi. Chapter 2, pp. 71–126.

Rantsiou, K. and L. Cocolin. 2006. New developments in the study of the microbiota of naturally fermented sausages as determined by molecular methods: A review. *International Journal of Food Microbiology* 108: 255–267.

Rasic, J.L. and J.A. Kurmann. 1978. *Yoghurt—Scientific Grounds, Technology, Manufacture and Preparations*. Copenhagen: Technical Dairy Publishing House.

Renfrew, J.W. 1999. Palaeoethnobotany and the archaeology of wine. In: *The Oxford Companion to Wine*, 2nd edition, ed. J. Robinson, 508–509. Oxford: Oxford University Press.

Rhee, S.J., Lee, J.E., and C.H. Lee. 2011. Importance of lactic acid bacteria in Asian fermented foods. *Microbial Cell Factories* 10: 1–13.

Risley, H.H. 1928. *The Gazetteer of Sikkim*. New Delhi: D. K. Publishing Distributors (P) Ltd.

Robert, H., Gabriel, V., and C. Fontagné-Faucher. 2009. Biodiversity of lactic acid bacteria in French wheat sourdough as determined by molecular characterization using species-specific PCR. *International Journal of Food Microbiology* 135: 53–59.

Robinson, R.K. and A.Y. Tamime. 2006. Types of fermented milks, In: *Fermented Milks,* Tamime, A.Y. ed. Tamime, Wiley, Hoboken, 1–10.

Romano, P., Capace, A., and L. Jespersen. 2006. Taxonomic and ecological diversity of food and beverage yeasts, In: Querol, A., Fleet, G.H. eds. *The Yeast Handbook-Yeasts in Food and Beverages*, Springer-Verlag, Berlin, 13–53.

Romano-Keeler, J., Moore, D.J., Wang, C., Brucker, R.M., Fonnesbeck, C., Slaughter, J.C., Li, H., Curran, D.P., Meng, S., and H. Correa et al. 2014. Early life establishment of site-specific microbial communities in the gut. *Gut Microbes* 5: 192–201.

Rossi, L.P.R., Almeida, R.C.C., Lopes, L.S., Figueiredo, A.C.L., Ramos, M.P.P., and P.F. Almeida. 2011. Occurrence of *Listeria* spp. in Brazilian fresh sausage and control of *Listeria monocytogenes* using bacteriophage P100. *Food Control* 22: 954–958.

Ruddle, K. 1993. The availability and supply of fish for fermentation in Southeast Asia. In: *Fish Fermentation Technology*, eds. C.-H. Lee, K.H. Steinkraus and P.J. Alan Reilly, 45–84. Tokyo: United Nations University Press.

Sakai, H., Caldo, G. A., and M. Kozaki. 1983a. Yeast-flora in red *burong-isda* a fermented fish food from the Philippines. *Journal of Agricultural Science* (Tokyo) 28: 181–185.

Sakai, H., Caldo, G. A., and M. Kozaki. 1983b. The fermented fish food, *burong-isda*, in the Philippines. *Journal of Agricultural Science* (Tokyo) 28: 138–144.

Saisithi, P. 1987. Traditional fermented fish products with special reference to Thai products. *ASEAN Food Journal* 3: 3–10.

Saithong, P., Panthavee, W., Boonyaratanakornkit, M., and C. Sikkhamondhol. 2010. Use of a starter culture of lactic acid bacteria in *plaa-som*, a Thai fermented fish. *Journal of Bioscience and Bioengineering* 110: 553–557.

Sakamoto, N., Tanaka, S., Sonomoto, K., and J. Nakayama. 2011. 16S rRNA pyrosequencing-based investigation of the bacterial community in nukadoko, a pickling bad of fermented rice bran. *International Journal of Food Microbiology* 144: 352–359.

Salampessy, J., Kailasapathy, K., and N. Thapa. 2010. Fermented fish products. In: Tamang, J.P. and Kailasapathy, K. eds. *Fermented Foods and Beverages of the World.* New York: CRC Press, Taylor & Francis Group, pp. 289–307.

Salminen, S., Wright, A.V., and A. Ouwehand. 2004. *Lactic Acid Bacteria Microbiology and Functional Aspects,* 3rd edition, New York: Marcel Dekker.

Samuel, D. 1996. Archaeology of ancient Egyptian beer. *Journal of American Society of Brewing Chemists* 54(1): 3–12.

Samuel, D. 2000. Brewing and baking. In: *Ancient Egyptian Materials and Technology*, eds. P.T. Nicholson and I. Shaw, 537–576. Cambridge: Cambridge University Press.

Samuel, D. 2002. Bread in archaeology. *Civilisations* 49: 28–36.

Sarkar, P.K., Hasenack, B., and M.J.R. Nout. 2002. Diversity and functionality of *Bacillus* and related genera isolated from spontaneously fermented soybeans (Indian Kinema) and locust beans (African Soumbala). *International Journal of Food Microbiology* 77: 175–186.

Sarkar, S. 2008. Innovations in Indian fermented milk products—A review. *Food Biotechnology* 22(1): 78–97.

Sarkar, P.K. and J.P. Tamang. 1994. The influence of process variables and inoculum composition on the sensory quality of kinema. *Food Microbiology* 11: 317–325.

Sarkar, P.K., Tamang, J.P., Cook, P.E., and J.D. Owens. 1994. Kinema—A traditional soybean fermented food: Proximate composition and microflora. *Food Microbiology* 11: 47–55.

Sarma, P.J. 1939. The art of healing. *Rigveda Annals of Medical History*, 3rd Series: 1, 538.

Sato, H., Torimura, M., Kitahara, M., Ohkuma, M., Hotta, Y., and H. Tamura. 2012. Characterization of the *Lactobacillus casei* group based on the profiling of ribosomal proteins coded in S10-spc-alpha operons as observed by MALDI-TOF MS. *Systematic and Applied Microbiology* 35: 447–454.

Savadogo, A., Tapi, A., Chollet M, Wathelet B, Traoré A.S., and Jacques, P. 2011. Identification of surfactin producing strains in *Soumbala* and *Bikalga* fermented condiments using polymerase chain reaction and matrix assisted laser desorption/ionization-mass spectrometry methods. *International Journal of Food Microbiology* 151: 299–306.

Sawamura, S. 1906. On the micro-organisms of natto. Bulletin College Agri. Tokyo Imperial University, 7, 107–110.

Schillinger, U. Ban-Koffi, L., and C.M.A.P. Franz. 2010. Tea, coffee and cacao. In: *Fermented Foods and Beverages of the World*, eds. J.P. Tamang and K. Kailasapathy, 353–375. New York: CRC Press, Taylor & Francis Group.

Schillinger, U., Böhringer, B., Wallbaum, S., Caroline, L., Gonfa, A., Kostinek, M., Holzapfel W.H., and Franz, C.M.A.P. 2008. A genus-specific PCR for differentiation between *Leuconostoc* and *Weissella* and its application in identification of heterofermentative lactic acid bacteria from coffee fermentation. *FEMS Microbiology Letters* 286: 222–226.

Schillinger, U., Yousif, N.M.K., Sesar, L., and C.M.A.P. Franz. 2003. Use of group-specific and RAPD-PCR analyses for rapid differentiation of *Lactobacillus* strains from probiotic yogurts. *Current Microbiology* 47: 453–456.

Schuijt, T.J., Poll, T., de Vos, W.M., and W.J. Wiersinga. 2013. Human microbiome: The intestinal microbiota and host immune interactions in the critically ill. *Trends in Microbiology* 21: 221–229.

Schuller, D., Pereira, L., Alves, H., Cambon, B., Dequin, S., and M. Casal. 2007. Genetic characterization of commercial *Saccharomyces cerevisiae* isolates recovered from vineyard environment. *Yeast* 24: 625–636.

Scott, R. 1986. *Cheese Making Practice*, 2nd edition. London: Elsevier.

Sealey, P.R. and P.A. Tyers. 1989. Olives from Roman Spain: A unique amphora find in British waters. *The Antiquaries Journal* 69: 54–72.

Sekwati-Monang, B. and M.G. Gänzle. 2011. Microbiological and chemical characterisation of *ting*, a sorghum-based sourdough product from Botswana. *International Journal of Food Microbiology* 150: 115–121.

Sengun, I.Y. and S. Karabiyikli. 2011. Importance of acetic acid bacteria in food industry. *Food Control* 22: 647–665.

Sengun, I.Y., Nielsen, D.S., Karapinar, M., and M. Jakobsen. 2009. Identification of lactic acid bacteria isolated from Tarhana, a traditional Turkish fermented food. *International Journal of Food Microbiology* 135: 105–111.

Sha, S.P., Thakur, N., Tamang, B., and J.P. Tamang. 2012. *Haria*, a traditional rice fermented alcoholic beverage of West Bengal. *International Journal of Agriculture Food Science and Technology* 3(2): 157–160.

Shi, Z., Zhang, Y., Phillips, G.O., and Yang, G. 2014. Utilization of bacterial cellulose in food. *Food Hydrocolloids* 35: 539–545.

Shin, M.S., Han, S.K., Ryu, J.S., Kim, K.S., and W.K. Lee. 2008. Isolation and partial characterization of a bacteriocin produced by *Pediococcus pentosaceus* K23–2 isolated from kimchi. *Journal of Applied Microbiology* 105: 331–339.

Shin, D., Kwon, D., Kim, Y., and D. Jeong. 2012. *Science and Technology of Korean Gochujang*. Seoul: Public Health Edu, pp. 10–133.

Shon, M.Y., Lee, J., Choi, J.H., Choi, S.Y., Nam, S.H., Seo, K.I., Lee, S.W., Sung, N.J., and S.K. Park. 2007. Antioxidant and free radical scavenging activity of methanol extract of chungkukjang. *Journal of Food Composition and Analysis* 20: 113–118.

Shrestha, H., Nand, K., and E.R. Rati. 2002. Microbiological profile of *murcha* starters and physico-chemical characteristics of *poko*, a rice based traditional food products of Nepal. *Food Biotechnology* 16: 1–15.

Shurtleff, W. and A. Aoyagi. 2010. History of soybeans and soyfoods in South Asia/Indian subcontinent (1656–2010): Extensively annotated, bibliography and sourcebook. www.soyinfocenter.com/books.

Silva, C.F., Batista, L.R., Abreu, L.M., Dias, E.S., and R.F. Schwan. 2008. Succession of bacterial and fungal communities during natural coffee (*Coffea arabica*) fermentation. *Food Microbiology* 25: 951–957.

Shamala, T.R. and K.R. Sreekantiah. 1988. Microbiological and biochemical studies on traditional Indian palm wine fermentation. *Food Microbiology* 5: 157–162.

Simoncini, N., Rotelli, D., Virgili, R., and S. Quuintavalla. 2007. Dynamics and characterization of yeasts during ripening of typical Italian dry-cured ham. *Food Microbiology* 24(6): 577–584.

Singh, P.K. and K.I. Singh. 2006. Traditional alcoholic beverage, *Yu* of *Meitei* communities of Manipur. *Indian Journal of Traditional Knowledge* 5(2): 184–190.

Singh, T.A., Devi, K.R., Ahmed, G., and K. Jeyaram. 2014. Microbial and endogenous origin of fibrinolytic activity in traditional fermented foods of Northeast India. *Food Research International* 55: 356–362.

Solieri, L. and Giudici, P. 2008. Yeasts associated to traditional balsamic vinegar: Ecological and technological features. *International Journal of Food Microbiology* 125: 36–45.

Sonar, R.N. and P.M. Halami. 2014. Phenotypic identification and technological attributes of native lactic acid bacteria present in fermented bamboo shoot products from North-East India. *Journal of Food Science and Technology* DOI 10.1007/s13197-014-1456-x.

Soni, S.K., Sandhu, D.K., Vilkhu, K.S., and N. Kamra. 1986. Microbiological studies on dosa fermentation. *Food Microbiology* 3: 45–53.

Sridevi, J., Halami, P.M., and Vijayendra, S.V.N. 2010. Selection of starter cultures for *idli* batter fermentation and their effect on quality of *idli*. *Journal of Food Science and Technology* 47: 557–563.

Srinivasa, P.T.I. 1930. *Pre-Aryan Tamil Culture*. Madras: University of Madras.

Steinkraus, K.H. 1996. *Handbook of Indigenous Fermented Food*, 2nd edition. New York: Marcel Dekker, Inc.

Steinkraus K.H., 2004. *Industrialization of Indigenous Fermented Foods*. (Eds: Holzapfel, W.H. and Talijaard, J.L.) Marcel Dekker, Inc, New York, Chapter 7, pp. 363–405.

Steinkraus, K.H., van Veer, A.G., and D.B. Thiebeau. 1967. Studies on idli—An Indian fermented black gram-rice food. *Food Technology* 21: 110–113.

Stevens, H.C. and L. Nabors. 2009. Microbial food cultures: A regulatory update. *Food Technolnology (Chicago)* 63: 36–41.

Stiles, M.E. and W.H. Holzapfel. 1997. Lactic acid bacteria of foods and their current taxonomy. *International Journal of Food Microbiology* 36: 1–29.

Suganuma, T., Fujita, K., and K. Kitahara. 2007. Some distinguishable properties between acid-stable and neutral types of α-amylases from acid-producing *koji*. *Journal of Bioscience and Bioengineering* 104: 353–362.

Sugawara, E. 2010. Fermented soybean pastes *miso* and *shoyu* with reference to aroma, In: Tamang JP, Kailasapathy K. eds. *Fermented Foods and Beverages of the World*, CRC Press, Taylor & Francis Group, New York, 225–245.

Sujaya, I., Antara, N., Sone, T., Tamura, Y., Aryanta, W., Yokota, A., Asano, K., and F. Tomita, F. 2004. Identification and characterization of yeasts in brem, a traditional Balinese rice wine. *World Journal of Microbiology and Biotechnology* 20: 143–150.

Sukontasing, S., Tanasupawat, S., Moonmangmee, S., Lee, J.S., and K. Suzuki. 2007. *Enterococcus camelliae* sp. nov., isolated from fermented tea leaves in Thailand. *International Journal of Systematic and Evolutionary Microbiology* 57: 2151–2154.

Sumino, T., Endo, E., Kageyama, A, S., Chihihara, R., and Yamada, K., 2003. Various Components and Bacteria of Furu (Soybean Cheese). *Journal of Cookery Science of Japan* 36: 157–163.

Sun, S.Y., Gong, H.S., Jiang, X.M., and Y.P. Zhao. 2014. Selected non-*Saccharomyces* wine yeasts in controlled multistarter fermentations with *Saccharomyces cerevisiae* on alcoholic fermentation behaviour and wine aroma of cherry wines. *Food Microbiology* 44: 15–23.

Sun, Z., Liu, W., Gao, W., Yang, M., Zhang, J., Wang, J., Menghe, B., Sun, T., and H. Zhang. 2010. Identification and characterization of the dominant lactic acid bacteria from *kurut*: The naturally fermented yak milk in Qinghai, China. *Journal of General and Applied Microbiology* 56: 1–10.

Suprianto, Ohba, R., Koga, T., and S. Ueda. 1989. Liquefaction of glutinous rice and aroma formation in tapé preparation by ragi. *Journal of Fermentation and Bioengineering* 64(4): 249–252.

Sura, K., Garg, S., and F.C. Garg. 2001. Microbiological and biochemical changes during fermentation of *Kanji*. *Journal of Food Science and Technology* 38: 165–167.

Takahashi, M., Masaki, K., Mizuno, A., and N. Goto-Yamamoto. 2014. Modified COLD-PCR for detection of minor microorganisms in wine samples during the fermentation. *Food Microbiology* (39): 74–80.

Takeda, S., Yamasaki K, Takeshita M, Kikuchi Y, Tsend-Ayush C, Dashnyam B, Ahhmed AM, Kawahara, S., and M. Muguet Ruma. 2011. The investigation of probiotic potential of lactic acid bacteria isolated from traditional Mongolian dairy products. *Animal Science Journal* 82: 571–579.

Tamang, J.P. 1998. Role of microorganisms in traditional fermented foods. *Indian Food Industry* 17: 162–167.

Tamang, J.P. 2001. Kinema. *Food Culture* 3: 11–14.

Tamang, J.P. 2003. Native microorganisms in fermentation of *kinema*. *Indian Journal of Microbiology* 43: 127–130.

Tamang, J.P. 2005. *Food Culture of Sikkim*. Sikkim Study Series volume IV. Information and Public Relations Department, Government of Sikkim, Gangtok, p. 120.

Tamang, J.P. 2010a. *Himalayan Fermented Foods: Microbiology, Nutrition, and Ethnic Values*. New: CRC Press, Taylor & Francis Group.

Tamang, J.P. 2010b. Diversity of fermented foods, In: Tamang JP, Kailasapathy K. eds. *Fermented Foods and Beverages of the World*, CRC Press, Taylor & Francis Group, New York, 41–84.

Tamang, J.P. 2010c. Diversity of fermented beverages, In: Tamang JP, Kailasapathy K. eds. *Fermented Foods and Beverages of the World*, CRC Press, Taylor & Francis Group, New York, 85–125.

Tamang, J.P. 2012a. Ancient food culture: History and ethnicity. In: *Globalisation and Cultural Practices in Mountain Areas: Dynamics, Dimensions and Implications*. ed. Lama, M.P., Sikkim University Press and Indus Publishing Company, New Delhi, pp. 43–63.

Tamang, J.P. 2012b. Chapter 4. Plant-based fermented foods and beverages of Asia. In: *Handbook of Plant-Based Fermented Food and Beverage Technology*, Second Edition (Eds: Hui, Y.H. and Özgül, E.). CRC Press, Taylor & Francis Group, New York, pp. 49–90.

Tamang, J.P. 2014. Biochemical and modern identification techniques—microfloras of fermented foods. In: *Encyclopaedia of Food Microbiology*, 2nd edition (Eds: Batt, C. and Tortorello, M.A.). Elsevier Ltd., Oxford, pp. 250–258.

Tamang, J.P., Chettri, R., and R.M. Sharma. 2009. Indigenous knowledge of Northeast women on production of ethnic fermented soybean foods. *Indian Journal Traditional Knowledge* 8: 122–126.

Tamang, J.P., Dewan, S., Tamang, B., Rai, A., Schillinger, U., and W.H. Holzapfel. 2007. Lactic acid bacteria in *Hamei* and *Marcha* of North East India. *Indian Journal of Microbiology* 47: 119–125.

Tamang, J.P., Dewan, S., Thapa, S., Olasupo, N.A., Schillinger, U., Wijaya, A., and W.H. Holzapfel. 2000. Identification and enzymatic profiles of predominant lactic acid bacteria isolated from soft-variety *chhurpi*, a traditional cheese typical of the Sikkim Himalayas. *Food Biotechnology* 14: 99–112.

Tamang, J.P. and G.H. Fleet. 2009. Yeasts diversity in fermented foods and beverages. In: Satyanarayana T, Kunze G. eds. *Yeasts Biotechnology: Diversity and Applications*, Springer, New York, 169–198.

Tamang, J.P. and S. Nikkuni. 1996. Selection of starter culture for production of kinema, fermented soybean food of the Himalaya. *World Journal of Microbiology and Biotechnology* 12: 629–635.

Tamang, J.P. and D. Samuel. 2010. Dietary culture and antiquity of fermented foods and beverages, In: J.P. Tamang and K. Kailasapathy, eds. *Fermented Foods and Beverages of the World*, CRC Press, Taylor & Francis Group, New York, 1–40.

Tamang, J.P. and P.K. Sarkar. 1993. Sinki—A traditional lactic acid fermented radish tap root product. *Journal of General and Applied Microbiology* 39: 395–408.

Tamang, J.P. and P.K. Sarkar. 1995. Microflora of murcha: An amylolytic fermentation starter. *Microbios* 81: 115–122.

Tamang, J.P. and P.K. Sarkar. 1996. Microbiology of mesu, a traditional fermented bamboo shoot product. *International Journal of Food Microbiology* 29: 49–58.

Tamang, J.P., Sarkar, P.K., and C.W. Hesseltine. 1988. Traditional fermented foods and beverages of Darjeeling and Sikkim—A review. *Journal of Science of Food and Agriculture* 44: 375–385.

Tamang, B. and J.P. Tamang. 2007. Role of lactic acid bacteria and their functional properties in *Goyang*, a fermented leafy vegetable product of the Sherpas. *Journal of Hill Research* 20: 53–61.

Tamang, B. and J.P. Tamang. 2009. Lactic acid bacteria isolated from indigenous fermented bamboo products of Arunachal Pradesh in India and their functionality. *Food Biotechnology* 23: 133–147.

Tamang, B. and J.P. Tamang. 2010. *In situ* fermentation dynamics during production of *gundruk* and *khalpi*, ethnic fermented vegetables products of the Himalayas. *Indian Journal of Microbiology* 50(Suppl 1): 93–98.

Tamang, B., Tamang, J.P., Schillinger, U., Franz, C.M.A.P., Gores, M., and W.H. Holzapfel. 2008. Phenotypic and genotypic identification of lactic acid bacteria isolated from ethnic fermented tender bamboo shoots of North East India. *International Journal of Food Microbiology* 121: 35–40.

Tamang, J.P., Tamang, B., Schillinger, U., Franz, C.M.A.P., Gores, M., and W.H. Holzapfel. 2005. Identification of predominant lactic acid bacteria isolated from traditional fermented vegetable products of the Eastern Himalayas. *International Journal of Food Microbiology* 105: 347–356.

Tamang, J.P., Tamang, N., Thapa, S., Dewan, S., Tamang, B.M., Yonzan, H., Rai, A.K., Chettri, R., Chakrabarty, J., and N. Kharel. 2012. Microorganisms and nutritional value of ethnic fermented foods and alcoholic beverages of North East India. *Indian Journal of Traditional Knowledge* 11(1): 7–25.

Tamang, J.P., Thapa, S., Dewan, S., Jojima, Y., Fudou, R., and S. Yamanaka. 2002. Phylogenetic analysis of *Bacillus* strains isolated from fermented soybean foods of Asia: *Kinema, chungkokjang* and *natto*. *Journal of Hill Research* 15: 56–62.

Tamang, J.P. and S. Thapa. 2006. Fermentation dynamics during production of bhaati jaanr, a traditional fermented rice beverage of the Eastern Himalayas. *Food Biotechnology* 20: 251–261.

Tamang, J.P., Thapa, S., Tamang, N., and B. Rai. 1996. Indigenous fermented food beverages of the Darjeeling hills and Sikkim: Process and product characterization. *Journal of Hill Research* 9: 401–411.

Tamime, A.Y. 2005. *Probiotic Dairy Products*. Oxford: Blackwell Publishing.

Tamime, A.Y. and R.K. Robinson. 2007. *Yoghurt Science and Technology*. Cambridge: Woodhead Publishing Ltd.

Tanaka, N., Traisman, E., Lee, M.S., Cassens, R.G., and E.M. Foster. 1980. Inhibition of botulinum toxin formation in bacon by acid development. *Journal of Food Protection* 43: 450–457.

Tanasupawat, S., Pakdeeto, A., Thawai, C., Yukphan, P., and S. Okada. 2007. Identification of lactic acid bacteria from fermented tea leaves (miang) in Thailand and proposals of *Lactobacillus thailandensis* sp. nov., *Lactobacillus camelliae* sp. nov., and *Pediococcus siamensis* sp. nov. *Journal of General and Applied Microbiology* 53: 7–15.

Tanganurat, W., Quinquis, B., Leelawatcharamas, V., and A. Bolotin. 2009. Genotypic and phenotypic characterization of *Lactobacillus plantarum* strains isolated from Thai fermented fruits and vegetables. *Journal of Basic Microbiology* 49: 377–385.

Tanigawa, K., Kawabata, H., and K. Watanabe. 2010. Identification and typing of *Lactococcus lactis* by matrix-assisted laser desorption ionization—time-of-flight mass spectrometry. *Applied and Environmental Microbiology* 76: 4055–4062.

Tanigawa, K. and K. Watanabe. 2011. Multilocus sequence typing reveals a novel subspeciation of *Lactobacillus delbrueckii*. *Microbiology* 157: 727–738.

Tanimura, W., Sanchez, P.C., and M. Kozaki. 1977. The fermented food in the Philippines (Part 1) Tapuy (rice wine). *Journal of Agricultural Science of the Tokyo University of Agriculture* 22(1): 118–134.

Tanimura, W., Sanchez, P.C., and M. Kozaki. 1978. The fermented foods in the Philippines. (Part-II). Basi (sugarcane wine). *Journal of Agricultural Society (Japan)* 22: 118–133.

Taylor, J.R.N. 2003. Beverages from sorghum and millet. In: *Encyclopedia of Food Sciences and Nutrition*, 2nd edition, eds. B. Caballero, L.C. Trugo and P. M. Finglas, 2352–2359. London: Academic Press.

Teoh, A.L., Heard, G., and J. Cox. 2004. Yeasts ecology of Kombucha fermentation. *International Journal of Food Microbiology* 95: 119–126.

Thakur, N., Savitri, and T.C. Bhalla. 2004. Characterisation of some traditional fermented foods and beverages of Himachal Pradesh. *Indian Journal of Traditional Knowledge* 3(3): 325–335.

Thanh, V.N., Mai, L.T., and D.A. Tuan. 2008. Microbial diversity of traditional Vietnamese alcohol fermentation starters (*banh men*) as determined by PCR-mediated DGGE. *International Journal of Food Microbiology* 128: 268–273.

Thapa, N., Pal, J., and J.P. Tamang. 2004. Microbial diversity in *ngari, hentak* and *tungtap,* fermented fish products of Northeast India. *World Journal of Microbiology and Biotechnology* 20: 599–607.

Thapa, N., Pal, J., and J.P. Tamang. 2006. Phenotypic identification and technological properties of lactic acid bacteria isolated from traditionally processed fish products of the Eastern Himalayas. *International Journal of Food Microbiology* 107: 33–38.

Thapa, N., Pal, J., and J.P. Tamang. 2007. Microbiological profile of dried fish products of Assam. *Indian Journal of Fisheries* 54: 121–125.

Thapa, S. and J.P. Tamang. 2004. Product characterization of kodo ko jaanr: Fermented finger millet beverage of the Himalayas. *Food Microbiology* 21: 617–622.

Thapa, S. and J.P. Tamang. 2006. Microbiological and physico-chemical changes during fermentation of *kodo ko jaanr*, a traditional alcoholic beverage of the Darjeeling hills and Sikkim. *Indian Journal of Microbiology* 46: 333–341.

Toldra, F. 2007. Handbook of fermented meat and poultry. Blackwell Publishing, Oxford.

Topisirovic, L., Kojic, M., Fira, D., Golic, N., Strahinic, I., and J. Lozo. 2006. Potential of lactic acid bacteria isolated from specific natural niches in food production and preservation. *International Journal of Food Microbiology* 112: 230–235.

Tou, E.H., Mouquet-River, C., Rochette, I., Traoré. A.S., Treche. S., and J.P. Guyot. 2007. Effect of different process combinations on the fermentation kinetics, microflora and energy density of *ben-saalga*, a fermented gruel from Burkina Faso. *Food Chemistry* 100: 935–943.

Tsuyoshi, N., Fudou, R., Yamanaka, S., Kozaki. M., Tamang. N., Thapa, S., and J.P. Tamang. 2005. Identification of yeast strains isolated from marcha in Sikkim, a microbial starter for amylolytic fermentation. *International Journal of Food Microbiology* 99: 135–146.

Tyn, M.T. 1993. Trends of fermented fish technology in Burma. In: *Fish Fermentation Technology* (Eds: Lee, C.H., Steinkraus, K.H. and Alan Reilly, P.J.), pp. 129–153. United Nations University Press, Tokyo.

Uchimura, T., Okada, S., and M. Kozaki. 1991. Identification of lactic acid bacteria isolated from Indonesian Chinese starter, "ragi". Microorganisms in Chinese starters from Asia (Part-4). *Journal of Brewing Society of Japan* 86: 55–61.

Urushibata, Y., Tokuyama, S., and Y. Tahara. 2002. Characterization of the *Bacillus subtilis ywsC* gene, involved in λ-polyglutamic acid production. *Journal of Bacteriology* 184: 337–343.

van Veen, A.G. 1965. Fermented and dried sea food products in South-East Asia. In: *Fish as Food*, volume 3 ed. Borgstrom, G., pp. 227–250. Academic Press, New York.

Vachanavinich, K., Kim, W.J., and Y.I. Park. 1994. Microbial study on krachae, Thai rice wine, In: *Lactic Acid Fermentation of Non-Alcoholic Dairy Food and Beverages*, Lee CH, Adler-Nissen J, Bärwald G. eds. Ham Lim Won, Seoul, 233–246.

Vallejo, J.A., Miranda, P., Flores-Félix, J.D., Sánchez-Juanes, F., Ageitos, J.M., González-Buitrago, J.M., Velázquez, E., and T.G. Villa. 2013. Atypical yeasts identified as *Saccharomyces cerevisiae* by MALDI-TOF MS and gene sequencing are the main responsible of fermentation of *chicha*, a traditional beverage from Peru. *Systematic and Applied Microbiology* 36(8): 560–564.

van Hijum, S.A.F.T., Vaughan, E.E., and R.F.Vogel. 2013. Application of state-of-art sequencing technologies to indigenous food fermentations. *Current Opinion in Biotechnology* 24(2): 178–186.

Vaughn, R.H. 1985. The microbiology of vegetable fermentations. In: *Microbiology of Fermented Foods*, vol. 1, (Ed: Wood, B.J.B.), pp. 49–109. Elsevier Applied Science Publishers, London.

Veinocchi, P. Valmossi, S., Dalai, I., Torrsani, S., et Gianotti A, Suzzi G, Guerzoni ME, Mastrocola, D., and F. Gardini. 2006. Characterization of the yeast populations involved in the production of a typical Italian bread. *Journal of Food Science* 69: M182–M186.

Versavaud, A., Coucoux, P., Roulland, C., Dulac, L., and J.N. Hallet. 1995. Genetic diversity and geographical distribution of wild *Saccharomyces cerevisiae* strains from the wine producing area of charentes, France. *Applied and Environmental Microbiology* 61: 3521–3529.

Vieira-Dalodé, G., Jespersen L, Hounhouigan J, Moller PL, Nago C.M., and M. Jakobsen. 2007. Lactic acid bacteria and yeasts associated with *gowé* production from sorghum in Bénin. *Journal of Applied Microbiology* 103: 342–349.

Vilanova, M. and C. Sieiro. 2006. Contribution *by Saccharomyces cerevisiae* yeast to fermentative flavour compounds in wines from cv. Albariño. *Journal of Industrial Microbiology and Biotechnology* 33: 929–933.

Vogel, R.F., Hammes, W.P., Habermeyer, M., Engel, K.H., Knorr, D., and G. Eisenbrand. 2011. Microbial food cultures—Opinion of the Senate Commission on Food Safety (SKLM) of the German Research Foundation (DFG). *Molecular Nutrition and Food Research* 55: 654–662.

Von Mollendorff, J.W. 2008. Characterization of bacteriocins produced by lactic acid bacteria from fermented beverages and optimization of starter cultures. MSc thesis, University of Stellenbosch, South Africa.

Wacher, C., Díaz-Ruiz, G., and J.P. Tamang 2010. Fermented vegetable products. In: *Fermented Foods and Beverages of the World*, eds. J.P.Tamang and K. Kailasapathy, 149–190. New York: CRC Press, Taylor & Francis Group.

Walker, G.M. 2014. Microbiology of Winemaking. In: *Encyclopaedia of Food Microbiology*, 2nd edition (Eds: Batt, C. and Tortorello, MA). Elsevier Ltd., Oxford, pp. 787–792.

Wallace, T.C., Guarner, F., Madsen, K., Cabana, M.D., Gibson, G., Hentges, E., and M.E. Sanders. 2011. Human gut microbiota and its relationship to health and disease. *Nutrition Reviews* 69(7): 392–403.

Wang, J. and D.Y.C. Fung. 1996. Alkaline-fermented foods: A review with emphasis on pidan fermentation. *Critical Review in Microbiology* 22: 101–138.

Wang, C.T., Ji, B.P., Li, B., Nout, R., Li, P.L., Ji, H., and L.F. Chen. 2006. Purification and characterization of a fibrinolytic enzyme of *Bacillus subtilis* DC33, isolated from Chinese traditional *Douchi. Industrial Microbiology and Biotechnology* 33: 750–758.

Watanabe, K., Fujimoto, J., Sasamoto, M., Dugersuren, J., Tumursuh, T., and Demberel, S. 2008. Diversity of lactic acid bacteria and yeasts in *airag* and *tarag*, traditional fermented milk products from Mongolia. *World Journal of Microbiology and Biotechnology* 24: 1313–1325.

Watanabe, K., Fujimoto, J., Tomii, Y., Sasamoto, M., Makino, H., Kudo, Y., and Okada, S. 2009a. *Lactobacillus kisonensis* sp. nov., *Lactobacillus otakiensis* sp. nov., *Lactobacillus* rapi sp. nov. and *Lactobacillus sunkii* sp. nov., heterofermentative species isolated from sunki, a traditional Japanese pickle. *International Journal of Systematic and Evolutionary Microbiology* 59: 754–760.

Watanabe, K., Makino, H., Sasamoto, M., Kudo, Y., Fujimoto, J., and S. Demberel. 2009b. *Bifidobacterium mongoliense* sp. nov., from *airag*, a traditional fermented mare's milk product from Mongolia. *International Journal of Systematic and Evolutionary Microbiology* 59: 1535–1540.

Weckx, S., Allemeersch, J., Van der Meulen, R., Vrancken, G., Huys, G., Vandamme, P., Van Hummelen, P., and L. de Vuyst. 2009. Development and validation of a species-independent functional gene microarray that targets lactic acid bacteria. *Applied Environmental Microbiology* 75: 6488–6495.

Weckx, S., Van der Meulen, R., Maes, D., Scheirlinck, I., Huys, G., Vandamme, P., and L. De Vuyst. 2010. Lactic acid bacteria community dynamics and metabolite production of rye sourdough fermentations share characteristics of wheat and spelt sourdough fermentations. *Food Microbiology* 27: 1000–1008.

Wei, D. and S. Jong. 1983. Chinese rice pudding fermentation: Fungal flora of starter cultures and biochemical changes during fermentation. *Journal of Fermentation Technology* 61: 573–579.

Wilson, H. 1999. Origins of viticulture. In: *The Oxford Companion to Wine*, 2nd edition, ed. J. Robinson, 505–506. Oxford: Oxford University Press.

Winarno, F.G., Fardiaz, S., and Daulay, D. 1973. Indonesian Fermented Foods, Department of Agricultural Product Technology, Fatema, Bogor Agricultural University, Indonesia.

Winarno, F.G., Fardiaz, S., and Daulay, D. 1973. Indonesian Fermented Foods, Department of Agricultural Product Technology, Fatema, Bogor Agricultural University, Indonesia.

Wong, P.P. and H. Jakson. 1977. Malaysian belechan. In: *The Proceedings of the Symposium on Indigenous Fermented Foods,* November 21–27, 1977, GIAM-V, Bangkok.

Wongkhalaung, C. 2004. Industrialization of Thai fish sauce (nam pla) In: *Industrialization of Indigenous Fermented Foods.* 2nd edition, Revised and Expanded, ed. K. H. Steinkraus. New York: Marcell Dekker, Inc.

Wu, Y.C., Kimura, B., and T. Fujii. 2000. Comparison of three culture methods for the identification of *Micrococcus* and *Staphylococcus* in fermented squid shiokara. *Fisheries Science* 66: 142–146.

Wu, R., Wang, L., Wang, J., Li, H., Menghe, B., Wu, J., Guo, M., and H. Zhang. 2009. Isolation and preliminary probiotic selection of lactobacilli from Koumiss in Inner Mongolia. *Journal of Basic Microbiology* 49: 318–326.

Yan, Y., Qian, Y., Ji, F., Chen, J., and B. Han. 2013. Microbial composition during Chinese soy sauce *koji*-making based on culture dependent and independent methods. *Food Microbiology* 34(1): 189–195.

Yan, P.M., Xue, W.T., Tan, S.S., Zhang, H., and X.H. Chang. 2008. Effect of inoculating lactic acid bacteria starter cultures on the nitrite concentration of fermenting Chinese paocai. *Food Control* 19: 50–55.

Yegna Narayan Aiyar, A.K. 1953. Dairying in ancient India. *Indian Dairyman* 5: 77–83.

Ying, A., Yoshikazu, A., and Yasuki, O. 2004. Classification of lactic acid bacteria isolated from chigee and mare milk collected in Inner Mongolia. *Animal Science Journal* 75: 245–252.

Yokotsuka, T. 1985. Fermented protein foods in the Orient, with emphasis on shoyu and miso in Japan. In: *Microbiology of Fermented Foods.* Vol 1, ed. B.B. Wood, 197–247. London: Elsevier Applied Sciences.

Yonzan, H. and J.P. Tamang. 2009. Traditional processing of *Selroti*—a cereal-based ethnic fermented food of the *Nepalis. Indian J Traditional Knowledge* 8(1): 110–114.

Yonzan, H. and J.P. Tamang. 2010. Microbiology and nutritional value of *selroti,* an ethnic fermented cereal food of the Himalayas. *Food Biotechnology* 2: 227–247.

Yonzan. H. and J.P. Tamang. 2013. Optimization of traditional processing of *Selroti,* a popular cereal-based fermented food. *Journal of Scientific and Industrial Research* 72: 43–47.

Yoon, M.Y., Kim, Y.J., and H.J. Hwang. 2008. Properties and safety aspects of *Enterococcus faecium* strains isolated from *Chungkukjang,* a fermented soy product. *LWT-Food Science Technology* 41: 925–933.

Yousif, N.M.K., Huch, M., Schuster, T., Cho, G.S., Dirar, H.A. Holzapfel, W.H., and C.M.A.P. Franz. 2010. Diversity of lactic acid bacteria from Hussuwa, a traditional African fermented sorghum food. *Food Microbiology* 27: 757–768.

Yu, J., Wang, W.H., Menghe, B.L., Jiri, M.T., Wang, H.M., Liu, W.J., Bao, Q.H. et al. 2011. Diversity of lactic acid bacteria associated with traditional fermented dairy products in Mongolia. *Journal of Dairy Science* 94: 3229–3241.

Zhang, S. and Y. Liu. 2000. *Prepare Technology of Seasoning in China.* Beijing: South China University of Technology Press (in Chinese).

Zhang, J.H., Tatsumi, E., Fan, J.F., and Li, L.T. 2007. Chemical components of *Aspergillus*-type Douchi, a Chinese traditional fermented soybean product, change during the fermentation process. *International Journal of Food Science and Technology* 42: 263–268.

Zhu, Y.P., Cheng, Y.Q., Wang, L.J., Fan, J.F., and Li, L.T., 2008. Enhanced antioxidative activity of Chinese traditionally fermented Okara (Meitauza) prepared with various microorganism. *International Journal of Food Properties* 11: 519–529.

Zhu, Y. and J. Trampe. 2013. Koji – where East meets West in fermentation. *Biotechnology Advances*31(8): 1448–1457.

Zhu, L., Xu, H., Zhang, Y., Fu, G., Wu, PQ., and Y. Li. 2014. BOX-PCR and PCR-DGGE analysis for bacterial diversity of a naturally fermented functional food (enzymes). *Food Bioscience* 5: 115–122.

Chapter 2

Functionality and Therapeutic Values of Fermented Foods

Namrata Thapa and Jyoti Prakash Tamang

Contents

2.1 Introduction

Microorganisms transform the chemical constituents of raw materials of plant/animal sources during fermentation thereby enhancing the nutrition value of foods, enriching them with improved flavor and texture, prolonging their shelf life, fortifying them with health-promoting bioactive compounds, vitamins and minerals, degrading undesirable compounds and antinutritive factors, producing antioxidant and antimicrobial compounds, and stimulating probiotic functions (Tamang 2007, Farhad et al. 2010). Fermentation plays different roles in food processing (Tamang et al. 2009b, Lee et al. 2011, Bourdichon et al. 2012):

- Biopreservative effects and improved food safety
- Biological enrichment (by improved bioavailability) of nutrients
- Improvement of the sensory quality of the food
- Expansion of the diet for more diversity
- Degradation of toxic components
- Degradation of antinutritive factors
- Functionality of microbial strains, including probiotic features
- Medicinal and therapeutic values

From an initial emphasis on survival, through hunger satisfaction, and a subsequent focus on food safety, food sciences now aim at developing foods to promote well-being and health by conferring beneficial physiological and psychological effects that go beyond adequate nutritional effects. Existing scientific data show that both nutritive and nonnutritive components in foods have the potential to modulate specific target functions in the body, which are relevant to well-being and health and/or reduction of some major chronic and degenerative diseases, such as cardiovascular diseases, obesity, gastrointestinal tract disorders, and cancer (Alexandraki et al. 2013). However, 90% of health-benefitted naturally fermented foods and alcoholic beverages in different countries and regions of the world are still produced at home under traditional conditions.

2.2 Functional Properties of Microorganisms in Fermented Foods

The functional properties of microorganisms isolated from fermented foods are important criteria for the selection of starter cultures to be used in the manufacture of functional foods (Durlu-Ozkaya et al. 2001, Badis et al. 2004). The most remarkable aspect of fermented foods is that they have biological functions enhancing several health-promoting benefits to consumers due to the functional microorganisms associated with them. Today, some of these fermented foods are commercialized and marketed globally as health foods,functional foods, therapeutic foods, nutraceuticals, biofoods, medico-foods, organic foods or as health foods/drinks. Some genera and species of microorganisms used in food fermentation are listed in Table 2.1.

2.2.1 Acidification

Acidification is an important functional logical property relevant for starter culture selection among the lactic acid bacteria (LAB) (de Vuyst 2000). The ability of some species of LAB particularly *Lactobacillus plantarum* in acidification of the substrates is significant in food preservation (Ammor and Mayo 2007). It was found that some LAB strains isolated from ethnic fermented vegetable and bamboo products of India and Nepal (Tamang et al. 2005, 2008) were able to lower the pH to 4.0 showing high acidifying capacity (Tamang et al. 2009b). Lactic acid forms the natural protection of the body against various infections and liver diseases, improves digestion, increases immunity, and protects against physiological infection agents (Karovicova and Kohajdova 2005).

2.2.2 Biological Preservation

Biological preservation refers to extended storage life and implies a significant approach to improve the microbiological safety of foods without refrigeration by lactic acid fermentation (Tamang 2010b). The species of LAB during fermentation produce organic acids (mostly lactic acid) which reduce the pH of the substrate inhibiting the growth of pathogenic microorganisms, thus, the LAB can exert a "biopreservative" effect (Holzapfel et al. 1995). Biological preservation refers to the extension of the shelf life of food products and the improvement of their microbial safety by using two different approaches:

- The inoculation of the food matrix with microorganisms, defined as protective cultures, with consequent *in situ* production of inhibitory molecules and/or a competitive effect against pathogen and spoilage bacteria and
- The use of microbial metabolites in purified form, in particular bacteriocins.

During fermentation of Himalayan ethnic fermented vegetable products (*gundruk, sinki), Lb. plantarum, Lactobacillus brevis, Pediococcus pentosaceus, Leuconostoc fallax* produce lactic acid and acetic acid and lower the pH of the substrates making the products more acidic in nature (Tamang et al. 2005, 2008). Owing to the low pH and high acid content and the sun-drying process of freshly fermented vegetables in the Himalayas, perishable vegetables can be preserved for several years without refrigeration and without the addition of any synthetic preservative. This is a good example of biopreservation of perishable vegetables, which are plentiful in the Himalayan winters. Several other fermented vegetable products preserved by lactic acid fermentation include *kimchi*, the fermented vegetable product of Korea, *sauerkraut* in Germany and Switzerland, and so on.

Table 2.1 Some Genera and Species of Microorganisms Used in Food Fermentation

Group	*Genera/Species*	*Product/Application(s)*
Bacteria		
	Acetobacter	
	A. aceti subsp. aceti	Vinegar
	A. fabarum	Cocoa, coffee
	A. lovaniensis	Vegetables
	A. malorum	Vinegar
	A. orientalis	Vegetables
	A. pasteurianus subsp. *pasteurianus*	Rice vinegar, cocoa
	A. pomorum	Industrial vinegar
	A. suboxidans	Ascorbic acid (food additive)
	A. syzygii	Vinegar, cocoa
	A. tropicalis	Cocoa, coffee
	Arthrobacter	
	Ar. arilaitensis	Dairy
	Ar. bergerei	Dairy
	Ar. globiformis	Citrus fermentation to remove limonin and reduce bitterness
	Ar. nicotianae	Cheese maturation
	Bacillus	
	B. acidopullulyticus	Pullulanases (food additive)
	B. amyloliquefaciens	Fish
	B. coagulans	Cocoa; glucose isomerase (food additive), fermented soybeans
	B. licheniformis	Protease (food additive)
	B. pumilus	Locust beans
	B. subtilis	Fermented soybeans, protease, glycolipids, riboflavin-B_2 (food additive)
	Bifidobacterium	
	Bif. adolescentis	Used in fermented milks; probiotic properties

Table 2.1 (*Continued*) Some Genera and Species of Microorganisms Used in Food Fermentation

Group	*Genera/Species*	*Product/Application(s)*
	Bif. animalis subsp. *animalis*	Used in fermented milks; probiotic properties
	Bif. animalis subsp. *lactis*	Fermented milks with probiotic properties; common in European fermented milks
	Bif. bifidum	Used in fermented milks as probiotic ingredient
	Bif. breve	Used as probiotics in fermented milks and infant formulas soy
	Bif. longum	Fermented milks with probiotic properties
	Bif. pseudolongum subsp. *pseudolongum*	Fermented milk and probiotic for animals
	Bif. thermophilum	Dairy
	Brachybacterium	
	Brachy. alimentarium	Gruyère and Beaufort cheese
	Brachy. tyrofermentants	Gruyère and Beaufort cheese
	Brevibacterium	
	Brevi. ammoniagenes	Nucleosides (food additive)
	Brevi. aurantiacum	Used for cheese production
	Brevi. casei	Used for cheese production
	Brevi. flavum	Malic acid, glutamic acid, lysine, monosodium glutamate (food additives)
	Brevi. linens	Soft cheese ripening
	Carnobacterium	
	Car. divergens	Dairy, meat, fish
	Car. maltaromaticum	Dairy, meat
	Car. piscicola	Meat
	Corynebacterium	
	Coryne. ammoniagenes	Cheese ripening
	Coryne. casei	Cheese ripening
	Coryne. flavescens	Used in cheese ripening cultures

(*Continued*)

Table 2.1 (*Continued*) Some Genera and Species of Microorganisms Used in Food Fermentation

Group	Genera/Species	Product/Application(s)
	Coryne. glutamicum	Glutamic acid, lysine, monosodium glutamate (food additives)
	Coryne. manihot	Cassava root
	Coryne. variabile	Cheese ripening
	Enterobacter	
	Enter. aerogenes	Bread fermentation
	Enterococcus	
	Ent. durans	Cheese and sour dough fermentation
	Ent. faecalis	Dairy, meat, soybean, vegetables
	Ent. faecium	Soybean, dairy, meat, vegetables
	Gluconacetobacter	
	Gluco. azotocaptans	Cocoa, coffee
	Gluco. diazotrophicus	Cocoa, coffee
	Gluco. entanii	Vinegar
	Gluco. europaeus	Vinegar
	Gluco. hansenii	Vinegar
	Gluco. johannae	Cocoa, coffee
	Gluco. oboediens	Vinegar
	Gluco. oxydans	Vinegar
	Gluco. xylinus	Vinegar
	Hafnia	
	Hafnia alvei	Ripening of meat; dairy
	Halomonas	
	Halomonas elongata	Ripening of ham
	Klebsiella	
	Klebsiella aerogenes	Tryptophan (food additive)
	Klebsiella pneumoniae subsp. *ozaenae*	*Tempeh*; production of Vitamin B12

Table 2.1 (*Continued*) Some Genera and Species of Microorganisms Used in Food Fermentation

Group	Genera/Species	Product/Application(s)
	Kocuria	
	Kocuria rhizophila	Dairy, meat
	Kocuria varians	Dairy, meat
	Lactobacillus	
	Lb. acetotolerans	Ricotta cheese, vegetables
	Lb. acidifarinae	Sourdough
	Lb. acidipiscis	Dairy, fish
	Lb. acidophilus	Fermented milks, probiotics, vegetables
	Lb. alimentarius	Fermented sausages; ricotta; meat, fish
	Lb. amylolyticus	Bread fermentation; production of glycoamylase
	Lb. amylovorus	Bread fermentation; production of glycoamylase
	Lb. bavaricus	Meat fermentation and biopreservation of meat
	Lb. brevis	Bread fermentation; wine; dairy, vegetables
	Lb. buchneri	Malolactic fermentation in wine; sourdough
	Lb. cacaonum	Cocoa
	Lb. casei subsp. *casei*	Dairy starter; cheese ripening; green table olives
	Lb. collinoides	Wine, fruits
	Lb. composti	Beverages
	Lb. coryniformis subsp. *coryniformis*	Fermentation of cheese and cassava
	Lb. crispatus	Sourdough
	Lb. crustorum	Sourdough
	Lb. curvatus subsp. *curvatus*	Meat
	Lb. delbruecki subsp. *bulgaricus*	Yogurt and other fermented milks, Mozzarella
	Lb. delbruecki subsp. *delbruecki*	Fermented milks, vegetables
	Lb. delbruecki subsp. *lactis*	Fermented milk and cheese

(*Continued*)

Table 2.1 (*Continued*) Some Genera and Species of Microorganisms Used in Food Fermentation

Group	*Genera/Species*	*Product/Application(s)*
	Lb. dextrinicus	Meat
	Lb. diolivorans	Cereals
	Lb. fabifermentants	Cocoa
	Lb. farciminis	Fermentation of bread; soybean, fish
	Lb. fermentum	Fermented milks, sourdough, urease (food additive)
	Lb. fructivorans	Beverages
	Lb. frumenti	Cereals
	Lb. gasseri	Fermented milk and probiotics, ricotta, sourdough
	Lb. ghanensis	Cocoa
	Lb. hammesii	Sourdough
	Lb. harbinensis	Vegetables
	Lb. helveticus	Starter for cheese; cheese ripening, vegetables
	Lb. hilgardii	Malolactic fermentation of wine
	Lb. homohiachii	Beverages, sourdough
	Lb. hordei	Beverages
	Lb. jensenii	Fermentation of cereals; sourdough
	Lb. johnsonii	Sourdough
	Lb. kefiri	Fermented milk (*kefir*), reduction of bitter taste in citrus juice
	Lb. kefranofaciens subsp. *kefiranofaciens*	Dairy
	Lb. kefranofaciens subsp. *kefirgranum*	Dairy
	Lb. kimchii	Vegetables
	Lb. kisonensis	Vegetables
	Lb. mali	Wine, fruits
	Lb. manihotivorans	Sourdough
	Lb. mindensis	Sourdough
	Lb. mucosae	Sourdough

Table 2.1 (*Continued*) Some Genera and Species of Microorganisms Used in Food Fermentation

Group	*Genera/Species*	*Product/Application(s)*
	Lb. nagelii	Cocoa
	Lb. namurensis	Sourdough
	Lb. nantensis	Sourdough
	Lb. nodensis	Dairy
	Lb. oeni	Wine
	Lb. otakiensis	Vegetables
	Lb. panis	Sourdough, bread
	Lb. parabrevis	Dairy, vegetables
	Lb. parabuchneri	Sourdough
	Lb. paracasei subsp. *paracasei*	Cheese fermentation, probiotic cheese, probiotics, wine, meat
	Lb. parakefiri	Dairy
	Lb. paralimentariums	Sourdough
	Lb. paraplantarum	Ricotta, vegetables
	Lb. pentosus	Meat fermentation and biopreservation of meat; green table olives; dairy, fruits, wine
	Lb. plantarum subsp. *plantarum*	fermentation of vegetables, malolactic fermentation, green table olives; dairy, meat
	Lb. pobuzihii	Vegetables
	Lb. pontis	Sourdough
	Lb. rapis	Vegetables
	Lb. reuteri	Sourdough
	Lb. rhamnosus	Dairy, vegetables, meat
	Lb. rossiae	Sourdough
	Lb. sakei subsp. *carnosus*	Meat fermentation
	Lb. sakei subsp. *sakei*	Fermentation of cheese and meat products; beverages
	Lb. salivarious subsp. *salivarius*	Cheese fermentation
	Lb. sanfranciscensis	Sourdough
	Lb. satsumensis	Vegetables

(*Continued*)

Table 2.1 (*Continued*) Some Genera and Species of Microorganisms Used in Food Fermentation

Group	*Genera/Species*	*Product/Application(s)*
	Lb. secaliphilus	Sourdough
	Lb. senmaizukei	Vegetables
	Lb. siliginis	Sourdough
	Lb. similis	Vegetables
	Lb. spicheri	Sourdough
	Lb. suebicus	Fruits
	Lb. sunkii	Vegetables
	Lb. tucceti	Dairy, meat
	Lb. vaccinostercus	Fruits, vegetables, cocoa
	Lb. versmoldensis	Dry sausages
	Lb. yamanashiensis	Beverages
	Lactococcus	
	Lc. lactis subsp. *cremoris*	Dairy starter
	Lc. lactis subsp. *lactis*	Dairy starter, nisin (food additive)
	Lc. Raffinolactis	Dairy
	Leuconostoc	
	Leuc. carnosum	Meat, bioprotection
	Leuc. citreum	Dairy, fish
	Leuc. fallax	Vegetables
	Leuc. holzapfelii	Coffee
	Leuc. inhae	Vegetables
	Leuc. kimchii	Vegetables
	Leuc. lactis	Dairy starter
	Leuc. mesenteroides subsp. *cremoris*	Dairy starter
	Leuc. mesenteroides subsp. *dextranicum*	Dairy starter
	Leuc. mesenteroides subsp. *mesenteroides*	Dairy starter
	Leuc. palmae	Wine
	Leuc. pseudomesenteroides	Dairy

Table 2.1 (*Continued*) Some Genera and Species of Microorganisms Used in Food Fermentation

Group	Genera/Species	Product/Application(s)
	Macrococcus	
	Macrococcus caseolyticus	Dairy, meat
	Microbacterium	
	Microbacterium gubbeenense	Soft cheese ripening
	Micrococcus	
	Micrococcus luteus	Cheese ripening
	Micrococcus lylae	Meat fermentation
	Micrococcus lysodeikticus	Catalase (food additive)
	Oenococcus	
	Oenococcus oeni	Malolactic fermentation of wine
	Pediococcus	
	Ped. acidilactici	Meat fermentation and biopreservation of meat Cheese starter
	Ped. damnosus	Meat, bioprotection
	Ped. parvulus	Wine
	Ped. pentosaceus	Meat fermentation and biopreservation of meat
	Propionibacterium	
	Prop. acidipropionici	Meat fermentation and biopreservation of meat
	Prop. arabinosum	Cheese fermentation; probiotics
	Prop. freudenreichii subsp. *freudenreichii*	Cheese fermentation (Emmental cheese starter)
	Prop. freudenreichii subsp. *shermanii*	Cheese fermentation (Emmental cheese starter)
	Prop. jensenii	Dairy
	Prop. thoenii	Biopreservation of foods
	Staphylococcus	
	Staphy. carnosus subsp. *carnosus*	Meat fermentation and biopreservation of meat
	Staphy. carnosus subsp. *utilis*	Meat fermentation

(*Continued*)

Table 2.1 (*Continued*) Some Genera and Species of Microorganisms Used in Food Fermentation

Group	*Genera/Species*	*Product/Application(s)*
	Staphy. cohnii	Dairy, meat
	Staphy. condimenti	Soy
	Staphy. equorum subsp. *equorum*	Dairy, meat
	Staphy. equorum subsp. *linens*	Dairy
	Staphy. fleurettii	Dairy
	Staphy. piscifermentans	Fish
	Staphy. saprophyticus	Meat
	Staphy. sciuri subsp. *sciuri*	Cheese fermentation
	Staphy. succinus subsp. *succinus*	Meat
	Staphy. succinus subsp. *casei*	Dairy
	Staphy. vitulinus	Meat fermentation; dairy
	Staphy. warneri	Meat
	Staphy. xylosus	Dairy
	Streptococcus	
	Strep. gallolyticus subsp. *macedonicus*	Dairy
	Strep. salivarius subsp. *salivarius*	Soy, vegetables
	Strep. salivarius subsp. *thermophilus*	Dairy
	Strep. griseus subsp. *griseus*	Meat Cyanocobalamin-B_{12} (food additive)
	Strep. natalensis	Natamycin (food additive)
	Strep. olivaceous	Glucose isomerase (food additive)
	Tetragenococcus	
	Tetragenococcus halophilus	Soy sauce
	Tetragenococcus koreensis	Vegetables
	Weisella	
	W. confusa	Meat, sourdough
	W. beninensis	Vegetables
	W. cibaria	Vegetables
	W. fabaria	Cocoa

Table 2.1 (*Continued*) Some Genera and Species of Microorganisms Used in Food Fermentation

Group	*Genera/Species*	*Product/Application(s)*
	W. ghanensis	Cocoa
	W. hellenica	Meat
	W. koreensis	Vegetables
	W. paramesenteroides	Meat
	W. thailandensis	Fish
	W. halotolerans	Meat
	Zymomonas	
	Zymomonas mobilis subsp. *mobilis*	Beverages
Filamentous Molds		
	Actinomucor	
	Actinomucor elegans	Fresh *tofu*
	Aspergillus	
	Aspergillus acidus	Tea
	Aspergillus flavus	α-Amylases (food additive)
	Aspergillus glaucus	Fermentation of soybean wheat curd
	Aspergillus niger	Beverages; industrial production of citric acid; amyloglucosidases, pectinase, cellulase, glucose oxidase, protease (food additives)
	Aspergillus oryzae	Soy sauce, beverages; α-amylases, amyloglucosidase, Lipase (food additives)
	Aspergillus sojae	Soy sauce
	Fusarium	
	Fusarium solani	Cheese production
	Fusarium domesticum	Dairy
	Fusarium venenatum	Dairy
	Lecanicillium	
	Lecanicillium lecanii	Dairy
	Mucor	
	Mu. circinelloides	Amylolytic starter of Asia

(*Continued*)

Table 2.1 (*Continued*) Some Genera and Species of Microorganisms Used in Food Fermentation

Group	*Genera/Species*	*Product/Application(s)*
	Mu. hiemalis	Fresh *tofu*, amylolytic starter of Asia
	Mu. indicus	Rice fermentation
	Mu. mucedo	Dairy
	Mu. plumbeus	Dairy
	Mu. racemosus	Dairy
	Mu. rouxianus	Rice fermentation
	Neurospora	
	Neurospora sitophila	Vegetables
	Penicillium	
	P. camemberti	White mold cheeses (camembert type)
	P. caseifulvum	Dairy
	P. chrysogenum	Dairy, glucose oxidase (food additive)
	P. citrinum	Nuclease (food additive)
	P. commune	Dairy
	P. nalgiovense	Meat (sausage) fermentation; dairy
	P. notatum	Glucose oxidases (food additive)
	P. roqueforti	Blue mold cheeses
	P. solitum	Meat
	Rhizopus	
	Rhi. chinensis	Fermentation of rice, amylolytic starter of Asia
	Rhi. microspores	Vegetables
	Rhi. niveus	Amyloglucosidases (food additive)
	Rhi. oligosporus	Soybean fermentation
	Rhi. oryzae	Soy sauce, *koji*
	Rhi. stolonifer	Soybean fermentation
	Scopulariopsis	
	Scopulariopsis flava	Dairy
	Sporendonema	
	Sporendonema casei	Dairy

Table 2.1 (*Continued*) Some Genera and Species of Microorganisms Used in Food Fermentation

Group	*Genera/Species*	*Product/Application(s)*
Yeasts		
	Candida	
	C. etchellsii	Dairy, soy, vegetables
	C. famata	Fermentation of blue vein cheese and biopreservation of citrus; meat
	C. friedricchi	*Kefir* fermentation
	C. guilliermondii	Citric acid (food additive)
	C. holmii	Kefir fermentation
	C. krusei	Kefir fermentation; sourdough fermentation
	C. lipolytica	Citric acid (food additive)
	C. milleri	Sourdough
	C. oleophila	Wine
	C. pseudotropicalis	Lactase (food additive)
	C. rugosa	Dairy
	C. tropicalis	Vegetables
	C. utilis	Fortification of corn meal by fermentation
	C. valida	Used for cheese ripening
	C. versatilis	Dairy, soy
	C. zemplinina	Wine
	C. zeylanoides	Dairy
	Cyberlindnera	
	Cyberlindnera jadinii	Dairy
	Cyberlindnera mrakii	Wine
	Cystofilobasidium	
	Cystofilobasidium infirmominiatum	Dairy
	Debaryomyces	
	Debaryomyces hansenii	Ripening of smear cheeses; meat
	Dekkera	
	Dekkera bruxellensis	Beverages

(*Continued*)

Table 2.1 (*Continued*) Some Genera and Species of Microorganisms Used in Food Fermentation

Group	Genera/Species	Product/Application(s)
	Hanseniaspora	
	Hanseniaspora guilliermondii	Wine
	Hanseniaspora osmophila	Wine
	Hanseniaspora uvarum	Wine
	Kazachstania	
	Kazachstania exigua	Dairy, sourdough
	Kazachstania unispora	Dairy
	Galactomyces	
	Galactomyces candidum	Dairy
	Geotrichum	
	Geotrichum candidum	Ripening of soft and semisoft cheeses or fermented milks; meat
	Guehomyces	
	Guehomyces pullulans	Vegetables
	Kluyveromyces	
	Kl. lactis	Cheese ripening; lactase (food additive)
	Kl. marxianus	Fermentation of soy milk; fortification of soft cheese Flavor enhancer
	Lachancea	
	Lachancea fermentati	Wine
	Lachancea thermotolerans	Wine
	Metschnikowia	
	Metschnikowia pukcherrima	Wine
	Pichia	
	Pic. kudriavzevii	Diary, cocoa
	Pic. occidentalis	Dairy, vegetables
	Pic. fermentans	Isolated from fermented olives; dairy, wine
	Pic. kluyverii	Wine
	Pic. membranifaciens	Dairy
	Pic. pijperi	Wine

Table 2.1 (*Continued*) Some Genera and Species of Microorganisms Used in Food Fermentation

Group	*Genera/Species*	*Product/Application(s)*
	Saccharomyces	
	Sacch. bayanus	*Kefir* fermentation; juice and wine fermentation
	Sacch. cerevisiae	Beer, bread, invertase (food additive)
	Sacch. cerevisiae subsp. *Boulardii*	Used as probiotic culture
	Sacch. florentius	*Kefir* fermentation
	Sacch. pastorianus	Beer
	Sacch. sake	Fermentation of rice
	Sacch. unisporus	*Kefir* fermentation
	Saccharomycopsis	
	Saccharomycopsis fibuligera	Asian amylolytic starter
	Saccharomycopsis capsularis	Asian amylolytic starter
	Schizosaccharomyces	
	Schizosaccharomyces pombe	Wine
	Schwanniomyces	
	Schwanniomyces vanrijiae	Wine
	Starmerella	
	Starmerella bombicola	Wine
	Torulopsis	
	Torulopsis candida	Vegetables
	Torulopsis holmii	Vegetables
	Torulaspora	
	Torulaspora delbrueckii	Dairy, wine
	Trigonopsis	
	Trigonopsis cantarellii	Wine
	Wickerhamomyces	
	Wickerhamomyces anomalus	Wine
	Yarrowia	
	Yarrowia lipolytica	Dairy

(*Continued*)

Table 2.1 (*Continued*) Some Genera and Species of Microorganisms Used in Food Fermentation

Group	*Genera/Species*	*Product/Application(s)*
	Zygosaccharomyces	
	Zygosaccharomyces rouxii	Soy sauce
	Zygotorulaspora	
	Zygotorulaspora florentina	Dairy

Source: Amended and compiled from Bernardeau, M., Guguen, M., and J.P. Vernoux. 2006. *FEMS Microbiology Review* 30: 487–513; Mogensen, G. et al. 2002. *Bulletin of IDF* 377: 10–19; Tamang, J.P. 2010a. *Himalayan Fermented Foods: Microbiology, Nutrition, and Ethnic Values*. New York: CRC Press, Taylor & Francis Group; Tamang, J.P. 2010b. *Fermented Foods and Beverages of the World*. New York: CRC Press, Taylor & Francis Group, pp. 41–84; Tamang, J.P. 2010c. *Fermented Foods and Beverages of the World*. New York: CRC Press, Taylor & Francis Group, pp. 85–125; Bourdichon, F. et al. 2012. *International Journal of Food Microbiology* 154(3): 87–97; Alexandraki, V. et al. 2013. Status and trends of the conservation and sustainable use of microorganisms in food processes. Commission on Genetic Resources for Food and Agriculture. FAO Background Study Paper No. 65.

Pickled vegetables, cucumbers, radishes, carrots, even some green fruits such as olives, papaya, and mango are acid fermented in the presence of salt (Wacher et al. 2010).

2.2.3 Biotransformation of Bland Substrates

One of the major roles functionality of fermented foods is the biological transformation of bland raw substrates of plant/animal origins during fermentation into edible, flavored, and sensorially acceptable foods by consumers. The biological transformation of bland vegetable protein into meat-flavored amino acid sauces and pastes by mold fermentation is common in Japanese *miso* and *shoyu*, Chinese soy sauce, and Indonesian *tauco* (Steinkraus 1996). *Monascuspurpureus* produces a purple–red water-soluble color in *angkak*, an ethnic fermented rice food of South-East Asia, which is used as a colorant (Beuchat 1978). Halophilic bacteria contribute flavor and quality to fermented fish products of South-East Asia (Itoh et al. 1993). Fermentation improves the taste of otherwise bland foods, imparts a typical flavor and texture to fermented soybean products such as *tempeh, kinema, natto, chungkokjang*, and so on (Nagai and Tamang 2010). In fermented milks, LAB produce diacetyl and other desirable flavors (Kosikowski 1997). During *tempeh* fermentation, mycelia of *Rhizopus oligosporus* knit the soybean cotyledons into a compact cake which when sliced resemble nontextured bacon (Steinkraus 1994). Similarly, in *ontjom*, an Indonesian fermented peanut product, *Neurospora sitophila* knits the particles into firm cakes imparting a meat-like texture (Steinkraus 1996).

2.2.4 Biological Enhancement of Nutritional Value

During fermentation, biological enrichment of food substrates with essential amino acids, vitamins, and various bioactive compounds occur spontaneously. In *tempeh*, the levels of niacin, nicotinamide, folic acids, riboflavin, and pyridoxine are increased by *Rhi. oligosporus*, whereas cyanocobalamine or vitamin B12 is synthesized by nonpathogenic strains of *Klebsiellapneumoniae* and *Citrobacter freundii* during fermentation. Liem et al. (1977), Keuth and Bisping (1994), Okada (1989), Ginting and Arcot (2004) reported that folic acid in unfermented soybeans was 71.6 μg/100 g and increased to 416.4 μg/100 g in *tempeh*. Thiamine, riboflavin, and methionine contents in *idli*, the fermented rice-legume food of India and Sri Lanka, are increased during fermentation (Rajalakshmi and Vanaja 1967, Steinkraus et al. 1967, Ghosh and Chattopadhyay 2011). There is an increase in vitamin B complex and vitamin C, lysine and tryptophane, and bioavailable iron during fermentation of *pulque*, the fermented agave beverage of Mexico (Steinkraus 1996, Ramírez et al. 2004). In fermented milks, LAB largely converts the lactose into more digestible lactate and the proteins into free amino acids imparting digestibility to the product (Campbell-Platt 1994). *Kimchi* has been selected as one of the world's healthiest foods in 2006 by the Health Magazine due to its various functional properties (Nam et al. 2009).

During the process of *kinema* production, soy proteins, which have been denatured by cooking, are hydrolyzed by proteolytic enzymes produced by *Bacillus subtilis* into peptides and amino acids, which enhance digestibility (Tamang and Nikkuni 1998, Kiers et al. 2000). A remarkable increase in water-soluble nitrogen and trichloroacetic acid (TCA)-soluble nitrogen contents is observed during *kinema* fermentation (Sarkar and Tamang 1995). Total amino acids, free amino acids, and mineral contents increases during *kinema* fermentation, and subsequently enrich the nutritional value of the product (Nikkuni et al. 1995, Sarkar et al. 1997a, Tamang and Nikkuni 1998). *Kinema* contains all essential amino acids and its essential amino acids score is as high as that of egg and milk proteins (Sarkar et al. 1997a). Degradation of oligosaccharides has been reported in *kinema* (Sarkar et al. 1997b). *Kinema* is rich in linoleic acid, an essential fatty acid in foods (Sarkar et al. 1996). Traditionally prepared *kinema* contains 8 mg thiamine, 12 mg riboflavin, and 45 mg niacin per kilogram dry matter (Sarkar et al. 1998). The content of riboflavin and niacin increases in *kinema*, while thiamine decreases during fermentation (Sarkar et al. 1998). An increase in total phenol content (TPC) has also been reported in the Korean fermented soybean food *chungkokjang* (Shon et al. 2007) and in the Chinese fermented soybean food *douchi* (Wang et al. 2007a). Compared with nonfermented soybeanflour, *kinema* flour has a higher viscosity and nitrogen solubility index (Shrestha and Noomhorn 2001). The recipe for *kinema* has been modified and it is now made into biscuits containing higher protein with an improved organoleptic property (Shrestha and Noomhorn 2002). *Tungrymbai* contains protein (45.9 g/100 g), fat (30.2 g/100 g), fiber (12.8 g/100 g), carotene (212.7 μg/100 g) and folic acid (200 μg/100 g) (Agrahar-Murugkar and Subbulaksmi 2006). During the fermentation of *chungkokjang* vitamin B_2 and vitamin K are increased 5–10 times (Kim and Hahm 2002, Wu and Ahn 2011). Production of riboflavin by *Leuconostoc mesenteroides* and folic acid by *Lactobacillus sakei* during *kimchi* fermentation was reported thus making *kimchi* a potential source of dietary vitamins (Jung et al. 2013). Several strains of *Saccharomyces cerevisiae*, *Candida tropicalis*, *Aureobasidium* sp., and *Pichia manschuria* isolated from *idli* and *jalebi* batter were found to produce vitamin B12 (Syal and Vohra 2013).

2.2.5 Biodegradation of Undesirable Compounds

The enzymes produced by functional microorganisms present in fermented foods degrade unsatisfactory or antinutritive compounds and thereby convert the substrates into consumable products with enhanced flavor and aroma. Bitter varieties of cassava tubers contain the cyanogenic glycoside linamarin, which can be detoxified by species of *Leuconostoc, Lactobacillus,* and *Streptococcus* in *gari* and *fufu*, and thereby be rendered safe to eat (Westby and Twiddy 1991). The trypsin inhibitor is inactivated during *tempeh* fermentation by *Rhi. oligosporus* which eliminates the flatulence-causing indigestible oligosaccharides such as stachyose and verbascose into absorbable monosaccharides and disaccharides (Hesseltine 1983). Microorganisms associated with *idli* batter fermentation reduce the phytic acid content of the substrates (Reddy and Salunkhe 1980). Reduction of phytic acid has also been reported in *rabadi*, a fermented cereal food of India (Gupta et al. 1992). Raw soybeans contain some allergenic proteins, a major one is Gly m Bd 30 K (Ogawa et al. 1991), which is also found in nonfermented soybean foods (Tsuji et al. 1995). *B. subtilis* (*natto*) is found to degrade Gly m Bd 30 K in raw soybeans during fermentation and makes *natto* a suitable food for persons allergic to raw soybeans (Yamanishi et al. 1995).

2.2.6 Probiotic Properties

The term probiotic has been defined as live microorganisms which when administered in adequate amounts confer a health benefit on the host (FAO/WHO 2002, Lee and Salminen 2009). The development of probiotics during the past decade has signaled an important advance in the food industry moving toward the development of such foods (Ouwehand et al. 2002, Saad et al. 2013). Probiotic organisms used in foods must be able to survive the passage through the gut; that is, they must have the ability to resist gastric juices and exposure to bile. Furthermore, they must be able to proliferate and colonize the digestive tract (Saad et al. 2013). In addition, they must be safe and effective, and maintain their effectiveness and potency for the duration of the shelf life of the product (FAO/WHO 2002). The most commonly used probiotic strains belong to the heterogeneous group of LAB (*Lactobacillus, Enterococcus*) and to the genus *Bifidobacterium* (Ouwehand et al. 2002). However, other microbes and even yeasts have been developed as potential probiotics during recent years (Ouwehand et al. 2002). The global market for probiotic ingredients, supplements, and foods is expected to reach $19.6 billion in 2013, with more than 500 probiotic products introduced in the past decade alone (Ghishan and Kiela 2011). Probiotics have been added to drinks and marketed as supplements which include tablets, capsules, and freeze-dried preparations (Shah 2007). Some commercial probiotic (Lee and Salminen 2009) cultures are *Bacillus coagulans* BC30 marketed by Ganeden Biotech Inc., Cleveland, Ohio, *Lactobacillus acidophilus* NCFM, *Lactobacillus rhamnosus* HN001 (DR20) and *Bifidobacterium (Bif.) lactis* HN019 (DR10) marketed by Danisco (Madison, Wisconsin), *Lactobacillus casei* strain Shirota and *Bifidobacterium breve* strain Yakult marketed by Yakult (Tokyo, Japan), *Lactobacillus fermentum* VRI003 (PCC) marketed by Probiomics (Eveleigh, Australia), *Lb. rhamnosus* R0011 marketed by Institut Rosell (Montreal, Canada), *Streptococcus oralis* KJ3 marketed by Oragenics Inc. (Alachua, Florida), and *Sacch. cerevisiae* (*boulardii*) marketed by Biocodex (Creswell, Oregon) (USProbiotics Home 2011, www.usprobiotics.org). The beneficial effects of probiotic foods on human health and nutrition are increasingly recognized by health professionals. The number and type of probiotic foods and drinks that are available to consumers, and marketed as having health benefits has increased considerably (FAO/WHO 2002, de LeBlanc et al. 2007).

Fermented dairy products are the most traditional source of probiotic strains of lactobacilli (Bernardeau et al. 2006); probiotic lactobacilli have been added to cooked pork meat products, snacks, fruit juice, chocolate, and chewing gum (Ouwehand et al. 2002, Ranadheera et al. 2010). It is important to develop probiotic products with food and beverages that are a part of the normal daily diet to easily maintain the minimum therapeutic level (Ranadheera et al. 2010). Beverages will be the next food category where healthy bacteria will make their mark. Likely candidates are chilled fruit juices, bottled water, or fermented vegetable juices (Prado et al. 2008). Fruit juice has been suggested as a novel, appropriate medium for fortification with probiotic cultures because it is already positioned as a healthy food product, and is consumed frequently and loyally by a large percentage of the consumer population (Siró et al. 2008). Ingestion of probiotic yoghurt has been reported to stimulate cytokine production in blood cells and enhance the activities of macrophages (Solis and Lemonnier 1996). Probiotic strain *Lb. acidophilus* La-5 produces conjugated linoleic acid (CLA), an anticarcinogenic agent (Macouzet et al. 2009).

Himalayan fermented yak milks have probiotic properties (Tamang et al. 2000, Dewan and Tamang 2007). *Lactobacillus johnsonii* (= *Lb. acidophilus*) which is used in the production of acidophilus milk is considered an important representative of probiotic bacterium which is used in the production of novel yoghurt-like products (Stiles and Holzapfel 1997). The probiotic strain of *Lb. plantarum*, isolated from *kimchi*, inhibits the growth and adherence of *Helicobacter pylori* in MKN-45 cell line with small peptides as the possible inhibitors (Lee and Lee 2006). Yakult is a Japanese commercial probiotic milk product which has several health-promoting benefits such as modulation of the immune system, maintenance of gut flora, regulation of bowel habits, alleviation of constipation, and curing of gastrointestinal infections (Kiwaki and Nomoto 2009). *Ped. pentosaceus* CIAL-86 isolated from wine showed a high percentage of adhesion to intestinal cells (>12%), and a high antiadhesion activity against *Escherichia coli* CIAL-153 (>30%), all of which support the wine LAB strain as a potential probiotic (García-Ruiz et al. 2014).

Probiotics are becoming more and more acceptable in clinical practice, where they are successfully employed in the management of a variety of diarrheal disorders, including rotavirus diarrhea, antibiotic-associated diarrhea, *Clostridium difficile* diarrhea (McFarland 2006), and traveller's diarrhea (McFarland 2007). Probiotics bacteria are used as biotherapeutic agents for protection against diarrhea, stimulation of the immune system, alleviation of lactose intolerance symptoms, and reduction of serum cholesterol (Shah 2007), as adjuvant in controlling inflammatory diseases (Ewaschuk and Dieleman 2006), treating and preventing allergic diseases (Kalliomäki et al. 2010), and preventing cancer (Kumar et al. 2010). Genomic and proteomic approaches will help to identify key molecules and define novel targets of probiotic action (Schiffrin and Blum 2001, Vanderhoof 2001). Different modes of administering probiotics are currently being investigated, which may ultimately lead to the widespread use of probiotics in functional foods (Vanderhoof 2001). Controlled human studies are essential for the success of probiotic functional foods, and they should be tailored for specific population groups such as the elderly and babies (Coman et al. 2012).

Current industrial probiotic foods are basically dairy products, which may represent inconveniences due to their lactose and cholesterol content (Rivera-Espinoza and Gallardo-Navarro 2010). Meat has been shown to be an excellent vehicle for probiotics (Rivera-Espinoza and Gallardo-Navarro 2010). Technological advances have made possible to alter some structural characteristics of fruit and vegetables matrices by modifying food components in a controlled way which could make them ideal substrates for the culture of probiotics, since they already contain beneficial nutrients such as minerals, vitamins, dietary fibers, and antioxidants (Rivera-Espinoza and Gallardo-Navarro 2010). With microencapsulation technologies, probiotics can become an important ingredient in functional foods (Prado et al. 2008, Chávarri et al. 2010).

The characteristics of probiotics to be tested include acidification ability of LAB strains (Tamang et al. 2009b), and the resistance to pH 3 is often used in *in vitro* assays to determine the resistance to stomach pH (Prasad et al. 1998), tolerance against bile, the mean intestinal bile concentration is believed to be 0.3% (w/v) and the staying time of food in the small intestine is suggested to be 4 h (Prasad et al. 1998), lysozyme tolerance (Brennan et al. 1986), antimicrobial activity of LAB isolates against some Gram-positive and Gram-negative bacteria (Schillinger et al. 1993); nonproduction of biogenic (Bover-Cid and Holzapfel 1999); bacterial adhesion to hydrocarbons known as hydrophobicity assay (Tamang et al. 2009b); *in vitro* adherence assay using HT-29 human colon adenocarcinoma epithelial cells (Tamang et al. 2009b); *in vitro* cholesterol lowering test (Rudel and Morris 1973); antioxidant activities such as 1,1-diphenyl-2-picryl hydrazyl (DPPH) radical scavenging activity (Abubakr et al. 2012), 2, 2′-azino-bis (3-ethylbenzothiazoline-6-sulfonic acid) (ABTS) radical scavenging activity (Re et al. 1999), TPC estimation (Waterhouse 2005), reducing power assay (Liu and Pan 2010); and the ability of different peptides generated by LAB to chelate ferrous ions (Nielsen et al. 2009).

2.2.7 Bioproduction of Peptides

Bioactive peptides are formed by (i) hydrolysis of food protein by gastrointestinal enzymes, (ii) through hydrolysis by proteolytic enzymes derived from microorganisms and plants, and (iii) through hydrolysis by proteolytic microorganisms during fermentation (Erdmann et al. 2008, de Mejia and Dia 2010). Peptides are specific fragments of protein formed on hydrolysis which have a positive impact on body functions (Saito et al. 2000). Some peptides have multifunctional activities and can exert more than one of the functional properties (Erdmann et al. 2008). Once absorbed in the small intestine bioactive peptides exert a beneficial effect on the various systems of the body such as the nervous system, the cardiovascular, endocrine, and immune systems (Erdmann et al. 2008). Peptides exhibit various biological functions such as antimicrobial (Meira et al. 2012), immunomodulatory (Qian et al. 2011), antioxidant (Sabeena et al. 2010, Perna et al. 2013), antithrombic (Singh et al. 2014), hypocholesterimic (Hartmann and Meisel 2007), and antihypertensive properties (Chen et al. 2010, Phelan and Kerins 2011). Soysauce, *chungkokjang, natto,* and *kinema* are involved in the process of enzymatic hydrolysis of protein, produce peptides and amino acids, which confer health benefits (Tamang and Nikkuni 1998).

2.2.8 Bioproduction of Enzymes

During fermentation, microorganisms produce enzymes on the substrates to break down complex compounds into simple biomolecules for several biological activities. Microorganisms in fermented foods show a wide spectrum of enzymatic activities such as amylase, glucoamylase, protease, lipase, and so on. Some of these strains produce a high amount of enzymes, which may be exploited for commercial production. *B. subtilis* produces enzymes such as proteinase, amylase, mannase, cellulase, and catalase during *natto* (Ueda 1989), and *kinema* fermentation (Tamang and Nikkuni 1996), and the fermentation of *tungrymbai,* and *bekang* (Chettri and Tamang 2014). Species of *Actinomucor, Amylomyces, Mucor, Rhizopus, Monascus, Neurospora, and Aspergillus* produce various carbohydrases (enzymes) such as α-amylase, amyloglucosidase, maltase, invertase, pectinase, ß-galactosidase, cellulase, hemicellulase; pentosan degrading enzymes; acid and alkaline proteases; and lipases (Nout and Aidoo 2002). Taka-amylase A (TAA), a major enzyme produced by *A. oryzae* (present in *koji*) is well-known worldwide to be a leading enzyme for industrial utilization (Suganuma et al. 2007). *Saccharomycopsis fibuligera, Saccharomycopsis capsularis*and *Pichia burtonii* have high amylolytic activities as shown in *marcha,* an ethnic amylolytic starter for alcohol production in the Himalayas (Tsuyoshi et al. 2005, Tamang et al. 2007). A considerable amount of glucomaylase is produced by *Rhizopus* spp. (Ueda and Kano 1975) and *Sm. fibuligera* (Ueda and Saha 1983).

Nattokinase produced by *B. subtilis* subsp. *natto* is the origin of this fibrinolytic activity in *natto* (Sumi et al. 1987). Fujii et al. (1975) demonstrated that nattokinase could pass through the intestinal track by showing its availability in plasma and simultaneously degradation of fibrinogen after intraduodenal administration of nattokinase to rats. Various fermented foods were reported with fibrinolytic activity namely the fermented soybean foods of India (*tungrymbai, hawaizar, bekang*) and Indian fermented fish products (*ngari, shedal, tungtap, hentak*) (Singh et al. 2014), *chungkokjang, douchi* (Chinese fermented soybean), *jeotgal* (Korean fermented fish), and *tempeh* (Mine et al. 2005, Kotb 2012). Fermented soybean and fish products were found to be a potential source of fibrinolytic enzymes (Kotb 2012). *B. subtilis* and *Bacillus amyloliquefaciens* isolated from fermented soybean products have fibrinolytic activity (Peng et al. 2003, Zeng et al. 2013, Singh et al. 2014). Chang et al. (2012) purified and characterized fibrinolytic enzymes from the *B. subtilis* fermented red bean. Fibrinolytic enzymes myulchikinase reported from Korean pickled anchovy (Jeong et al. 2004) and katsuwokinase from Japanese *skipjack shiokara* (Sumi et al. 1995) showed a similar amino acids sequence to endogenous trypsin of starfish and dogfish, respectively, used as raw material for fermentation. Montriwong et al. (2012) isolated novel fibrinolytic enzymes from *Virgibacillus halodenitrificans* SK1-3-7 isolated from fish sauce fermentation. Novel fibrinolytic enzymes from *Bacillus* sp. KA38 isolated from *jeotgal* was purified and characterized (Kim et al. 1997). LAB with fibrinolytic activity in the fermented foods included *Vagococcus carniphilus*, *Vagococcus lutrae*, *Enterococcus faecalis*, *Enterococcus faecium*, *Enterococcus gallinarum*, and *Pediococcus acidilactici* (Singh et al. 2014).

The use of the API ZYM technique has been reported (Arora et al. 1990) as a rapid and simple means of evaluating and localizing 19 different hydrolases of microorganisms associated with dairy fermentations. This method is also of relevance for the selection of strains as potential starter cultures based on superior enzyme profiles, especially peptidases and esterases, for accelerated maturation and flavor development of fermented products (Tamang et al. 2000, Kostinek et al. 2005). Enzymatic profiles of bacteria mostly LAB isolated from the naturally fermented milks of the Himalayas (Tamang et al. 2000, Dewan and Tamang 2006, 2007), fermented vegetables (Tamang et al. 2005, 2008, Tamang and Tamang 2010), fermented fish (Thapa et al. 2004), fermented meat (Rai et al. 2010), fermented cereal food (Yonzan and Tamang 2010), and fermented soybeans (Chettri and Tamang 2014) were recorded using API ZYM.

2.2.9 Antimicrobial Properties

Lactic acid bacteria compete with other microbes by screening antagonistic compounds and modifying the microenvironment by their metabolism (Lindgren and Dobrogosz 1990). Consumption of LAB in fermented foods without any adverse health effects is taken as their "GRAS" (generally recognized as safe) status and therefore their bacteriocins might have potential as biopreservatives (Adams 1999). Bacteriocins are defined as proteinaceous compounds (usually peptides) that have bactericidal action against a range of organisms, which are usually closely related to the producer organism (Barnby-Smith 1992). Bacteriocidal peptides or proteins produced by bacteria are labeled as bacteriocins (Hoover and Chen 2005). The site of bacteriocins action is the cytoplasmic membrane (Holzapfel et al. 1995). The inhibitory spectrum includes *Listeria monocytogenes* and the Gram-negative organisms *Pseudomonas fragi* and *Pseudomonas fluorescens*. Pediocin PA-1, produced by *Ped. acidilactici* strain PAC 1.0, displays antimicrobial activity against a wide spectrum of Gram-positive bacteria, many of them responsible for food spoilage or food-borne diseases, and shows a particularly strong activity against *Lis. monocytogenes* (Rodríguez et al. 2002). Pediocin AcH, from *Ped. acidilactici*, has been shown to inhibit *Lis. monocytogenes*, *Staphylococcus aureus,* and *Clostridium perfringens.* Pediocin A, produced by *Ped. pentosaceus,* has potential as a food preservative, owing to its relatively wide spectrum of activity, which includes *Clostridium* spp. and *Staph. aureus* (Barnby-Smith 1992). Another example are the bacteriocins produced by *Enterococcus,* called the enterocins which are found to be active against *Lis. monocytogenes,* and a few have also been reported to be active even against Gram-negative bacteria (Khan et al. 2010).

Kimchi has strong antimicrobial activity against *Lis. monocytogenes, Staphy. aureus, E. coli,* and *Salmonella typhimurium* (Lee et al. 2009). Many strains of LAB isolated from *kimchi* produce antimicrobial compounds such as leuconocin J by *Leuconostoc* sp. J2 (Choi et al. 1999), bacteriocin by *Leuc. Lactis* BH5 (Hur et al. 2000), *Leuc. Citreum* GJ7 (Chang et al. 2008), and pediocin by *Ped. pentosaceus* (Shin et al. 2008). Bacteriocins inhibit *Lis. Monocytogenes* in fermented sausages, cottage cheese, and smoked salmon (McAuliffe et al. 1999). An exopolysaccharide producing *Weissella cibaria* 92 isolated from fermented cabbage was found to have considerable antimicrobial activity against Gram-positive and Gram-negative pathogens (Patel et al. 2014). Several LAB isolated from Romanian traditional fermented fruits and vegetables have antimicrobial activity against *Lis. monocytogenes, E. coli, Salmonella,* and *Bacillus* (Grosu-Tudor and Zamfir 2013). Species of LAB strains isolated from several global fermented vegetable products show strong antimicrobial activities (Rubia-Soria et al. 2006, Tamang et al. 2009b, Lee et al. 2011, Jiang et al. 2012).

2.2.10 Angiotensin-Converting Enzymes (ACE) Inhibitory Properties

The ACE-inhibitory peptides derived from food protein are gaining much importance for treating hypertension (Haque and Chand 2008, Hartmann and Meisel 2007). These peptides inhibit ACE which is a key enzyme responsible for the conversion of angiotensin I to angiotensin II, a strong vasoconstrictor (Hartmann and Meisel 2007). Angiotensin II causes vasoconstriction, reabsorption of water and sodium ions, which affects the electrolyte balance, volume, and pressure of blood (Hartmann and Meisel 2007). Inhibition of ACE by peptides is considered to be a first line of therapy for the treatment of hypertension (Hartmann and Meisel 2007). ACE-inhibitory properties have been studied in various fermented milk products such as fermented sour milk (Nakamura et al. 1995), *dahi,* Indian curd (Harun-ur-Rashid et al. 2007), *kefir* (Quiros et al. 2005), *koumiss,* fermented mare milk (Chen et al. 2010), sheep milk yogurt (Papadimitriou et al. 2007), fermented camel milk (Moslehishad et al. 2013), fermented goat milk (Minervini et al. 2009), and cheese (Meyer et al. 2009).

Several novel ACE-inhibitory peptides were purified from milk fermented with *Ent. faecalis* strains (Quiros et al. 2005). The antihypertensive properties of fermented milk products have been validated by various animal studies and clinical trials (Sipola et al. 2002, Seppo et al. 2002, 2003). *Calpis,* the fermented sour milk of Japan containing two potent tripeptides VPP and IPP, have shown hypotensive effect in spontaneous hypotensive rats (Nakamura et al. 1995) and in human subjects (Hata et al. 1996). Nakamura et al (1996) also showed a decrease in the activity of tissue ACE upon feeding sour milk in spontaneously hypertensive rats. Fermented milk with *Lactobacillus helvetius* reduces elevated blood pressure in subjects with normal high blood pressure as well as mild hypertension without any adverse effect (Aihara et al. 2005).

Consumption of fermented soybean foods has generated much interest because of the evidence that their consumption lowers the risk of cardiovascular diseases (Liu and Pan 2010). A peptide including amino acids Ala, Phe, and His showing ACE-inhibitory properties have been isolated from soybeans fermented by *Bacillus natto* and *chungkokjang* fermented with *B. subtilis* (Korhonen and Pihlanto 2003). ACE-inhibitory properties have also been reported from several fermented fish products such as fermented fish sauce prepared from salmon, sardine, and anchovy (Okamoto et al. 1995), fermented blue mussel and oyster sauce (Je et al. 2005a,b), and fish sauce (Ichimura et al. 2003).

2.2.11 Nonproduction of Biogenic Amines

Biogenic amines are organic basic compounds which occur in different kinds of foods such as sauerkraut (Taylor et al. 1978), fish products, cheese, wine, beer, dry sausages, other fermented foods (Ten Brink et al. 1990, Halász et al. 1994), and fruits and vegetables (Suzzi and Gardini 2003). In foods, biogenic amines are mainly generated by decarboxylation of their precursor amino acids, either as a result of the action of decarboxylase activity (Halász et al. 1994) or by the growth of decarboxylase positive microorganisms (Silla-Santos 2001). The major biogenic amine producers in foods are enterobacteriaceae and enterococci (Nout 1994). Most LAB do not produce significant levels of biogenic amines (Nout 1994). Halász et al. (1994) indicated a maximum limit of 100 mg/kg of histamine as a safe level in foods. High levels (>100 mg/kg) of histamine and tyramine can cause adverse effects to human health (Rauscher-Gabernig et al. 2009). Several toxicological problems resulting from the ingestion of food containing relatively high levels of biogenic amines have been reported (Ten Brink et al. 1990). In susceptible humans, biogenic amines can lead to a variety of cutaneous, gastrointestinal, hemodynamic, and neurological symptoms (Taylor 1986). In homemade and commercially prepared *tarhana*, an average of 92.8 and 55.0 mg/kg, respectively, of tyramine production is reported (Özdestan and Üren 2013). Fermentation of cabbage with certain lactic starters such as *Lb. casei* subsp. *casei, Lb. plantarum,* and *Lactobacillus curvatus* could reduce the biogenic amine content of *sauerkraut* (Rabie et al. 2011). None of the strains of LAB-produced biogenic amines in Himalayan fermented vegetables (Tamang et al. 2009b), fermented bamboo shoots of India (Tamang and Tamang 2009), and naturally fermented milks (Dewan and Tamang 2007), which is a good indication of their potential for the possible development as a starter culture. Samples with moderate, high, or very high levels of biogenic amines could be considered as products of less quality and their consumption could be unhealthy for sensitive individuals (Latorre-Moratalla et al. 2007).

2.2.12 Degree of Hydrophobicity

Bacterial adherence to hydrocarbons, such as hexadecane, proved to be a simple and rapid method to determine cell surface hydrophobicity (Rosenberg et al. 1980, van Loosdrecht et al. 1987). Adherence is one of the most important selection criteria for probiotic bacteria (Shah 2001). The adherence of microorganisms to various surfaces seemed to be mediated by hydrophobic interactions (Rosenberg 1984). The functional effects of probiotic bacteria include adherence to the intestinal cell wall for colonization in the gastrointestinal tract with the capacity to prevent pathogenic adherence or pathogen activation (Bernet et al. 1993, Salminen et al. 1996). The high degree of hydrophobicity shown by LAB isolated from Himalayan ethnic fermented milk products (Dewan and Tamang 2006, 2007), and fermented vegetables (Tamang et al. 2009b) indicate the potential of adhesion to the gut epithelial cells of the human intestine, advocating their probiotic character (Holzapfel et al. 1998).

2.2.13 Reduction in Serum Cholesterol

Consumption of fermented milks containing very large populations of probiotic bacteria (~10^9 bacteria/g) by hypercholesterolemic persons has resulted in lowering cholesterol level from

3.0 to 1.5 g/L (Homma 1988). Several animal studies have shown that administration of fermented milks or specific strains of LAB are effective in lowering blood cholesterol levels (Agerholm-Larsen et al. 2000). Fermented whole-grain foods have the potential positive role to alter the following risk factors: serum LDL-cholesterol values, serum HDL-cholesterol values, hypertriacylglycerolaemia, hypertension, diabetes, obesity, coronary heart disease (CHD), insulin resistance, antioxidant status, hyperhomocysteinemia, vascular reactivity, and the inflammatory state (Anderson 2003). Fermented soybean products reduce the blood cholesterol level, and increase digestibility and nutritional value (Lee 2001, Lee 2004). Acidophilus milk reduces the serum total and LDL-cholesterol, but remains unchanged on serum HDL-cholesterol or triacylglycerols (Danielson et al. 1989). *Kefir* plays an important role in controlling high cholesterol levels and in this way it protects us from cardiovascular damage (Otes and Cagindi 2003). Phytosterols which have a cholesterol-lowering effect are increased during *kinema* fermentation (Sarkar et al. 1996). Consumption of *tempeh* reduces the cholesterol level which is due to the inhibition of hydroxymethylglutaryl coenzyme A reductase, a key enzyme in cholesterol biosynthesis, by oleic acid and linoleic acid during fermentation (Hermosilla et al. 1993).

2.2.14 Protective Cultures

The term protective cultures has been applied to microbial food cultures exhibiting a metabolic activity contributing to inhibit or control the growth of undesired microorganisms in food (EFFCA 2011). Those starter culture species apart from being used in fermentation processes have also been applied to food in order to make use of their bioprotective potential with or without sensory impact (Holzapfel et al. 1995). Use of microorganisms as protective cultures, for example, bacteriocin producers, may have several advantages, as microorganisms can not only be the source of antimicrobial peptides but also of a wide spectrum of molecules such as organic acids, carbon dioxide, ethanol, hydrogen peroxide, and diacetyl, whose antimicrobial action is well-known (EFFCA 2011). They can contribute to the flavor, texture, and nutritional value of the product besides producing bacteriocins (Gaggia et al. 2011). Protective cultures should in the first instance be considered as an additional safety factor, with the potential of improving the microbiological safety of food (Liong 2008), and supporting good manufacturing practices, thereby reducing risks of growth and survival of pathogens and spoilage organisms (Holzapfel et al. 2003).

Health traits, such as stabilization of the gastrointestinal tract, anticarcinogenic action, and tumor control, may serve as an important additional advantage for future selection and application of protective cultures (Gaggia et al. 2011). In fresh fermented products, soft cheeses, cured, cooked, and ground meat protective cultures are used to control *Listeria, Cambylobacter,* and *Salmonella* (www.pathogencombat.com/workshop/~/media/Adtomic/PatComBilleder/Articles/Brussels/BrusselsBiavati.ashx). A strain combination of LAB and propionic acid bacteria (PAB), used as a protective culture, was found to be the most active against yeasts, molds, and *Bacillus* spp. in fermented milks and in bakery products (Suomalainen and Mäyär-Mäkinen 1999).

Industrial starters like SafePro® (CHR Hansen, DK) and Bovamine Meat Culture™ (NPC, US) have been developed for *Lis. monocytogenes* control for the meat industry (Pilet and Leroi 2011). Protective culture manufactured by HOLDBACTM (Danisco, DK) is used for growth control of yeasts and molds and some heterofermentative lactic bacteria in fresh fermented foods, for growth control of leuconostoc, heterofermentative lactobacilli, and enterococci in hard and semi-hard cheese and for growth control of *Listeria* in soft and smear cheese, dry and semi-dry cured meats, cooked and fresh ground meats (www.danisco.com/product-range/cultures/holdbactm/). Other branded commercial protective cultures are Microgard™ (Wesman Foods, Inc. Beaverton, USA), Bioprofit™ (Valio, Helsinki, Finland), ALTA™ 2341, and FARGO™ 23 (Quest International, USA) (Kesenkas et al. 2006).

Nisin is commercially made in a partially purified form, and a marketed preparation with the pediocin PA-1 (AcH) producer is available (de Vuyst and Leroy 2007). Nisin is produced by strains of *Lc. lactis* subsp. *lactis* and inhibits Gram-positive and Gram-negative bacteria and also the outgrowth of spores of bacilli and clostridia (de Arauz et al. 2009). Nisin may also be added to low-acid (higher than pH 4.5) canned foods, such as vegetables, to prevent the growth of heat-resistant spores of *Clostridium (Cl.) thermosaccharolyticum* and *Bacillus stearothermophilus*, both of which can survive the heat treatment designed to kill *Clostridium botulinum* spore (de Arauz et al. 2009). Nisin can also be added to wines to control the malolactic fermentation by preventing the growth of the natural LAB (Barnby-Smith 1992).

2.2.15 LAB as Live Vaccines

Edible vaccines are mucosal-targeted vaccines, which cause stimulation of both systematic and mucosal immune response (Mishra et al. 2008). Food LAB usage would overcome the problem since these bacteria have a long history of safe use and could possibly be delivered safely at a high dose (Renault 2002). The LABVAC European research network is presently comparing the vaccine potential of *Lc. lactis, Strep. gordonii,* and *Lactobacillus* spp. (Mercenier et al. 2000). More specifically, *Lc. lactis* is a potential candidate for the production of biologically useful proteins and application as an antigen delivery vehicle for the development of live mucosal vaccines (Anderson et al. 2010). The advantage of live bacterial vaccines is that they mimic natural infection, have intrinsic adjuvant properties, and can be given orally (Amdekar et al. 2010).

2.2.16 Degradation of Undesirable Compounds

Microorganisms present in fermented foods produce desirable amounts of enzymes that may degrade unsatisfactory or antinutritive compounds and thereby convert the substrates into consumable products with enhanced flavor and aroma (Tamang 2010b). Bitter varieties of cassava tubers, the main staple crop in West Africa contain the cyanogenic glycoside linamarin, which can be detoxified by natural fermentation into a product called *gari* by species of *Leuconostoc, Lactobacillus,* and *Streptococcus* and thus the fermented cassava is rendered safe to eat (Westby and Twiddy 1991, Abimbola 2007). During *tempeh* fermentation, the trypsin inhibitor is inactivated by *Rhi. oligosporus* and eliminates the flatulence-causing indigestible oligosaccharides such as stachyose and verbascose into absorbable monosaccharides and disaccharides (Hesseltine 1983). Species of *Lactobacillus, Lactococcus, Leuconostoc,* and *Pediococcus* isolated from fermented vegetables and tender bamboo shoots of the Eastern Himalayaswere found to degrade antinutritive factors such as phytic acids and flatulence-causing oligosaccharides (Tamang et al. 2009b). Microorganisms associated with *idli* batter fermentation reduce the phytic acid content of the substrates (Reddy and Salunkhe 1980). *Lb. brevis, Ent. faecium, Enterococcus durans, Enterococcus hirae, Enterococcus raffinossus,* and *Enterococcus cecorum,* isolated from Indian fermented soybean foods are able to degrade phytic acid and oligosaccharides, showing their ability to degrade antinutritive factors (Chettri and Tamang 2014).

2.2.17 Isoflavones and Saponin

The main isoflavones found in soybeans are daidzein, genistein, and glycitein, each of which exists in four chemical forms: aglycones, β and glycitein, each of which exists in four chemical forms: aglycones. Isoflavone glucosides are hydrolyzed into their corresponding aglycones during the fermentation of soybean foods such as *sufu* (Yin et al. 2004), *miso* (Chiou and Cheng 2001), *natto* (Ibe et al. 2001), and *tempeh* (Murakami et al. 1984, Lu et al. 2009), while b-glucosidase has been considered to be a key enzyme for the conversion of isoflavone forms in *sufu* processing (Yin et al. 2004). In *douchi*, a Chinese fermented soybean food, isoflavones in the form of aglycones exceeded 90% of the total content following fermentation (Wang et al. 2007b). During *tempeh* fermentation, isoflavone particularly factor-II and aglycone contents are found to increase (Pawiroharsono 2002). Newly improved methods for *tempeh* production have been developed that raise levels of aminobutyric acid (Aokiet al. 2003) and isoflavones (Nakajima et al. 2005). The isoflavones suppress the onset of arteriosclerosis because they improve the metabolism of lipids such as cholesterol (Stein 2000). Isoflavones included in soybeans are presented as genistin, daidzin, and glycitin, which are increased about 21 times in *chungkokjang* (Lee et al. 2007). *Doenjang* shows an increase in isoflavones (Choi et al. 2010).

Saponins of soybean are oleanane triterpenoid glycosides, which are present in about 0.2%–0.9% of seed weight (Paucar-Menacho et al. 2010). Soybean saponins are divided into Group A and DDMP (2,3-dihydro-2,5-dihydroxy-6-metyl-4*H*-pyran-4-one)-conjugated saponins according to their type of aglycone (Berhow et al. 2006). DDMP and their derivatives, Groups B and E saponins show health-beneficial effects such as the prevention of dietary hypercholesterolemia (Murata et al. 2006), the suppression of colon cancer cell proliferation (Ellington et al. 2006), and the anti-peroxidation of lipids and liver-protecting action by the acceleration of secretion of thyroid hormones (Ishii and Tanizawa 2006). *Natto* contains saponin, isoflavones, fibrinolytic enzyme, vitamin K2, and dipicolinic acid, which are generated by soybeans and *natto* bacteria (Yanagisawa and Sumi 2005). *Kinema* has many health benefits due to the high content of Group B saponin (Omizu et al. 2011).

2.2.18 Production of Poly-Glutamic Acid

PGA is one of the few naturally occurring polyamides which are not synthesized by ribosomal proteins (Oppermann-Sanio and Steinbüchel 2002). Some strains of *B. subtilis* produce λ-PGA which is an amino acid polymer commonly present in Asian fermented soybean foods giving the characteristic sticky texture to the product (Urushibata et al. 2002, Meerak et al. 2007, Nishito et al. 2010). The γ-PGA produced by *B. subtilis* (*natto*) has a very large molecular mass of over 10^5 Da and both L- and D-glutamic acids (Saito et al. 1974). *B. subtilis* and *Bacillus licheniformis* are the most widely used industrial producers of γ-PGA (Stanley and Lazazzera 2005). The γ-PGA product is secreted into the medium and may protect the organism from harsh environmental conditions or serve as a carbon, nitrogen, energy source, or a biofilm formation enhancer (Stanley and Lazazzera 2005). *Chungkokjang* contains γ-PGA generated by *Bacillus* in *chungkokjang* (Lee et al. 2010). It is safe for eating as the viscosity element of fermented soybean products such as *chungkokjang* and *natto*. PGA is completely biodegradable and watersoluble and nontoxic to humans (Yoon et al. 2000). *B. subtilis* TS1:B25 (isolated from *tungrymbai*) and *B. subtilis* BT:B9 (isolated from *bekang*) accounted for the highest production of PGA (Chettri and Tamang 2014).

2.2.19 Antioxidant Activity

Antioxidant activities mostly DPPH radical scavenging activity (Abubakr et al. 2012); ABT Sradical scavenging activity (Re et al. 1999); TPC estimation(Waterhouse 2005); and reducing power assay

(Liu and Pan 2010) are estimated in fermented foods. Antioxidant activities have been reported in many ethnic fermented foods such as in *natto* (Iwai et al. 2002), *chungkokjang* (Shon et al. 2007), *douchi* (Wang et al. 2007a), *kinema* (Moktan et al. 2008; Tamang et al. 2009a), *tungrymbai* and *bekang* (Chettri and Tamang 2014), *tempeh* (Horii 2008), *kimchi* (Sim and Han 2008, Sun et al. 2009, Park et al. 2011), *kefir* (Güven et al. 2003), and yoghurt (Sabeena et al. 2010). Fermented whole grains are an excellent sources of antioxidant, vitamins, and phytochemicals (Anderson 2003).

2.2.20 Functional Foods

Functional food is natural or processed food that contains known biologically active compounds which when in defined quantitative and qualitative amounts provides a clinically proven and documented health benefit, and thus, an important source in the prevention, management, and treatment of chronic diseases of the modern age (Martirosyan 2011). A functional food has proven health benefits that reduce the risk of specific chronic diseases or beneficially affect target functions beyond its basic nutritional functions (Doyon 2008). Today, functional foods constitute the fastest growing sector in the food industry worldwide. In 2013 milk formula, energy drinks, probiotic yogurt, juice drinks, sports drinks, cereal, and biscuits were among the top-performing functional foods in global markets (Euromonitor 2014). The top 10 functional foods in global markets listed in 2013 are Dannon Light & Fit Greek yogurt, with first-year sales of $144.9 million, the best-selling new food product of 2013, followed by Yoplait Greek 100 yogurt, $135.1 million; Kellogg's Special K Pastry Crisps snack bars, $100.6 million; Tostitos Cantina Tortilla Chips, $100.3 million; Bud Light Lime Lime-A-Rita, $97.4 million; Müller yogurt, $95.8 million; Eight O'Clock K Cups coffee, $89.8 million; Pepsi NEXT, $83.2 million; Kellogg's Special K Flatbread Breakfast Sandwiches, $77.9 million; and Atkins frozen meals, $74.0 million (Sloan 2014).

Functional foods are closely associated with claims on foods (Hilliam 2000). Regulation 1924/2006 of the European Union identifies two categories of claims on foods: nutrition claims and health claims (Verhagen et al. 2010). Nutrition claims are claims that state, suggest, or imply that a food has particular beneficial nutritional properties due to the energy it provides or the nutrients it contains while health claims are claims that state, suggest, or imply a relationship between a food or food category and health (Verhagen et al. 2010). The EU-project "Process for the Assessment of Scientific Support for Claims on Foods (PASSCLAIM)" resulted in a set of criteria for the scientific substantiation of health claims on foods which emphasized the need for direct evidence of benefits to humans, recognized the usefulness of markers of intermediate effects, and emphasized that effects should be both statistically and biologically meaningful (Asp and Bryngelsson 2008).

In the United States, claims on food and dietary supplement labels fall into three categories: nutrient content claims, structure/function claims, and health claims (Alexandraki et al. 2013). Those claims that are not substantiated on evidence that meets the level of Significant Scientific Agreement (SSA) standard, include a qualifying statement intended to convey to the consumer the level of evidence for the claim (Rowlands and Hoadley 2006). The current Japanese foods with health claims include two categories. For the first category, "Food with Nutrient Function Claims," the label may be freely used if a product satisfies the standard for the minimum and maximum levels per daily portion usually consumed (Yamada et al. 2008). The second category is defined as food for specified health uses (FOSHU) which contains dietary ingredients that have beneficial effects on the physiological functions of the human body, maintain and promote health, and improve health-related conditions (http://www.mhlw.go.jp/english/topics/foodsafety/fhc/02.html).

2.3 Therapeutic and Medicinal Values of Fermented Foods

Most ethnic foods, both fermented and non-fermented, have therapeutic values and are eaten for the prevention of illness. The food culture of many ethnic people in the world, whether they belong to industrialized or underdeveloped countries, traditionally do not require additional medicines or supplementary drugs. This may be due to the healthbenefits of their ethnic fermented foods and beverages such as antioxidants, antimicrobials, probiotics, low-cholesterol values, essential amino acids, bionutrients, and the production of bioactive compounds during fermentation (Tamang 2007, Farhad et al. 2010). It is also suggested that ethnic Himalayan fermented milk products have protective and probiotic properties which stimulate the immune system, and may cure stomach-related diseases (Dewan and Tamang 2006, 2007, Tamang et al. 2000, 2009b). *Gundruk* and *sinki* are used during indigestion and commonly eaten as appetizers (Tamang 2010a). *Kinema* is highly nutritive and has several health-promoting benefits (Tamang 2010a, Omizu et al. 2011). Ethnic mild-alcoholic beverages of the Himalayas such as *kodo ko jaanr/chyang, bhaati jaanr, poko,* and so on have been consumed for their therapeutic uses (Tamang 2010a). Ailing persons and postnatal women consume the extract of *kodo ko jaanr* and *bhaati jaanr* due to its high calorie content, to regain their strength (Thapa and Tamang 2004, Tamang and Thapa 2006). Chinese fermented soybean food *douchi* reduces high blood pressure (Zhang et al. 2006). Drinking of the fermented *puer* tea of China prevents cardiovascular disease (Mo et al. 2008). In Korea, the popular fermented vegetable *kimchi* has several therapeutic uses (Park et al. 2006, Kim et al. 2008a,b, Lee and Lee 2009). *Kimchi* has several health-promoting benefits (Park et al. 2014) such as its antiobesity effect (Kim et al. 2011), probiotic property (Lee et al. 2011), antioxidant activity (Park et al. 2011), and antistress effect (Lee and Lee 2009).

Koumiss, a fizzy gray acidic–alcoholic beverage prepared from horse or donkey milk in Russia, contains *Lc. lactis, Lactobacillus bulgaricus* along with some yeasts *Candida kefyr* and *Torulopsis* sp. (Kosikowski 1997). *Koumiss* is not only regarded as a food high in nutritional quality, but is also considered therapeutic, particularly in the treatment of pulmonary tuberculosis (Auclair and Accolas 1974). *Kvass*, a rye or wheat-based sour alcoholic beverage of the Ukraine is fermented by *Sacch. cerevisiae* and *Lactobacillus* spp. and is suggested to provide protection to the digestive tract against cancer (Wood and Hodge 1985). Consumption of *natto* in Japan prevents hemorrhage caused by vitamin K deficiency in infants (Ueda 1989). Several health-benefit effects of *kimchi* have been reported such as prevention of constipation, colon cancer, reduction of serum cholesterol (Park et al. 2006), possession of antistress principles (Lee and Lee 2009), S-adenosyl-L-methionine, a bioactive material used in the treatment of depression, osteoarthritis, and liver disease (Lee et al. 2008), antiobesity effect (Kong et al. 2008), inhibition of atherosclerosis (Kim et al. 2008a), anticarcinogenic effects (Cheigh and Park 1994, Park 1995), reducing blood cholesterol, stabilizing blood sugar, and regulating bowel movements (Lee et al. 2008).

Puer tea extract is known to prevent cardiovascular disease and mortality of patients (Mo et al. 2008). Acidophilus milk is used therapeutically (Kosikowski 1997). *Kombucha* is a sweetened tea beverage that, as a consequence of fermentation, contains ethanol, carbon dioxide, a high concentration of acid (gluconic, acetic, and lactic) as well as a number of other metabolites and is thought to contain a number of health-promoting components (Schillinger et al. 2010). *Kvass* of the Ukraine provides protection to the digestive tract against cancer (Wood and Hodge 1985). Intake of *natto* increases serum level of MK-7 and γ-carboxylated osteocalcin in normal individuals (Tsukamoto et al. 2000). Content of γ-aminobutyric acid in *tempeh* can improve the brain bloodstream and retard high blood pressure (Aoki et al. 2003). There are reports that LAB isolated from *dahi* can be used to cure intestinal disease such as diarrhea (Agarwal and Bhasin 2002), and the intake of *dahi* has anticholesteremic effects (Sinha and Sinha 2000). One-month of rinsing with a mouthwash using the culture extract of *B. subtilis* (*natto*) isolated from *natto*, which is commercially supplied, could reduce the swelling of gums and drive out microorganisms in plaque from periodontitis patients (Tsubura 2012).

Though clinical studies of 90% of naturally fermented foods and beverages are still to be conducted, people have a customary belief in the therapeutic values of some of their foods, which have been in use both as foods and as therapy for centuries. Such ethnic foods, if studied properly, may be presented even in global markets. Some major health benefits of fermented foods and beverages (Table 2.2) are mentioned below.

2.3.1 Prevention of Cardiovascular Disease

Alcohol consumption at a moderate level of two drinks or so per day may have protective effects, and cardiovascular benefits have been claimed for wine (Klatsky et al. 1997). Those who consume wine in moderation are healthier than those who drink other alcoholic beverages or those who abstain from alcoholic beverages (Walker 2014). The Mediterranean diet, which also includes moderate wine consumption, has its cardiovascular benefits (Menotti et al. 1999). Ogborne and Smart (2001) showed that the moderate consumption of wine in the majority of adults in Canada (57%) had cardiovascular health benefits. People who consume as little as one alcoholic drink per day may significantly reduce their risk of stroke, but drinking more does not increase the benefit (Berger et al. 1999).

CHD is a multifactorial disease characterized by long-term degenerative changes in the walls of arteries, which result in the narrowing of the lumen of blood vessels and limiting the blood supply to vital organs such as the heart (Subbiah 1998). Fermented whole-grain intake appears to protect from the development of CHD and diabetes (Anderson et al. 2000). Low intakes of antioxidants and vitamins (mainly vitamin E) appear to be associated with high risk for CHD (Regnstrom et al. 1996). Whole grains also may provide phytoestrogens that are likely to have similar protective effects on blood vessels (Slavin et al. 1997). Intake of soybean protein tends to increase serum HDL-cholesterol slightly but not significantly (Anderson 1995). The isoflavones in *doenjang* increase the activation of an LDL-C receptor, which becomes a cause factor in vascular diseases, and increase the HDL-C level, which is beneficial to prevent vascular diseases and which plays an important role in preventing cardiovascular diseases (Kwak et al. 2012). The polyphenols of red wine are probably synergists of tocopherol (vitamin E) and ascorbic acid (vitamin C), thus they inhibit lipid peroxidation (Feher et al. 2007) and prevent cardiovascular disease (Wallerath et al. 2005).

2.3.2 Prevention of Cancer

Fermented foods may influence intestinal detoxification and immune status, which may be associated with colon cancer and thus it is believed that probiotics play a protective role in colon cancer risk reduction (Saikali et al. 2004, Cabana et al. 2006). LAB-fermented foods may confer a variety of important nutritional and therapeutic benefits to consumers, including antimutagenic and anticarcinogeinc activity (Lee et al. 2004).

Kefir has been used for the treatment of tuberculosis and cancer when modern medical treatment was not available (Otes and Cagindi 2003). Fermented cabbage, cabbage juice, and sauerkraut contain s-methylmethionine which reduces tumourigenesis risk in the stomach (Kris-Etherton et al. 2002). Cabbage contains the isothiocyananins and indoles that are responsible for anticancer effects against cancer of the colon, breast, lung, fore stomach, and liver (Karovicova and Kohajdova 2005). Some peptides produced from soybean sauce and paste exert a number of health benefits such as ACE inhibition, antithrombotic, and anticancer effects (Shon et al. 1996). Consumption

Table 2.2 Some Bioactive Compounds Synthesized in Fermented Foods and Their Health Benefits to Consumers

Bioactive Compounds	*Synthesized in Fermented Foods*	*Health Benefits*	*References*
Mevinolin citrinin ($C_{13}H_{14}O_5$)	*Angkak*	Prohibits creation of cholesterol by blocking a key enzyme, HMG-CoA reductase	Pattanagul et al. (2008)
Lactobacillus	*Dahi*	Probiotic Anticarcinogenic effect against colorectal cancer hepatocarcinogenesis	Mohania et al. (2013)
Genistein	*Doenjang*	Facilitates β-oxidation of fatty acid, reducing body weight	Kwak et al. (2012)
LAB Vitamin K	Fermented vegetables	Probiotics Blood clotting normally Intracellular electrolyte for reducing blood pressure Appetite stimulant	Breidt et al. (2013)
Phenolics, flavonoids, tannin, crude fibre	Fermented bamboo shoots	Antioxidants, anti-free radicals, anticancer, and antiaging activity	Tamang and Tamang (2009), Sonar and Halami (2014)
Lipoteichoic acid from *Lb. rhamnosus* GG	Fermented milk	Oral photoprotective agent against UV-induced carcinogenesis	Weill et al. (2013)
Organic acids	*Gundruk*	Appetizer, improves milk efficiency	Tamang et al. (2009b)
LAB	*Inziangsang*	Probiotics, appetizers	Tamang et al. (2009b)
LAB	*Khalpi*	Biopreservative, probiotics	Tamang et al. (2009b)
Minerals, Betacyanin	*Kanji*	Prevention of infection, anticancer	Winkler et al. (2005)
Isocyanate and sulfide Indole-3-carbinol	*Kimchi*	Prevention of cancer, detoxification of heavy metals in liver, kidney, and small intestine	Park and Kim (2010)
Ornithine		Antiobesity efficacy	Park et al. (2012)
Vitamin A, vitamin C, fibers		Suppression of cancer cells	Cheigh (1999)

Table 2.2 (*Continued*) Some Bioactive Compounds Synthesized in Fermented Foods and Their Health Benefits to Consumers

Bioactive Compounds	*Synthesized in Fermented Foods*	*Health Benefits*	*References*
Lactobacillus, organic acids		Suppression of harmful bacteria, stimulation of beneficial bacteria, prevention of constipation, cleaning the intestine, prevention of colon cancer	Cheigh (1999)
Capsaicin, allicin		Prevention of cancer, suppression of *H. pylori*	An et al. (2014)
Chlorophyll		Helps in prevention of absorbing carcinogens	Ferruzzi and Blakeslee (2007)
Vitamin U		Inhibition of free radical production	Lee et al. (2014a)
S-adenosyl-L-methionine (SAM)		Treatment of depression	Lee and Lee (2009)
β-Sitosterol		Antiproliferative mechanism	Choi et al. (2004)
HDMPPA (an antioxidant)		Therapeutic application in human atherosclerosis	Kim et al. (2007)
Nattokinase, antibiotics, vitamin K	*Natto*	Antitumor, immunomodulating	Nagai and Tamang (2010)
GABA (nonprotein amino acid)	*Nham*	Reducing hypertension, diuretic effect, inhibiting the proliferation of cancer cells and preventing diabetes	Ratanaburee et al. (2013)
Bioactive substance	*Puer* tea	Prevents cardiovascular disease	Mo et al. (2008)
LAB	*Saurkraut*	Probiotics	Beganović et al. (2011)
Vitamin C		Scurvy	Peñas et al. (2013)
Isothiocynate		Prevention of cancer	Higdon et al. (2007)
Glucosinolates		Activation of natural antioxidant enzymes.	Martinez-Villaluenga et al. (2012)

(*Continued*)

Table 2.2 (*Continued*) Some Bioactive Compounds Synthesized in Fermented Foods and Their Health Benefits to Consumers

Bioactive Compounds	*Synthesized in Fermented Foods*	*Health Benefits*	*References*
LAB	*Sinki*	Biopreservative, probiotics, antidiarrheal, stomach pain.	Tamang et al. (2009b)
Antioxidant genestein, daidzein, tocopherol, superoxide dismutase	*Tempe*	Prevents oxidative stress-causing noncommunicable disease such as hyperlipidemia, diabetes mellitus type 2, cancer (breast and colon), cognitive decline and dementia, prevents the damage of pancreatic beta cell.	Kiriakidis et al. (1997), Lu et al. (2009)
Phenolics-resveratrol	*Wine (red)*	Anti-inflammatory	Jeong et al. (2010)
Phenolics (activates release of saliva) succinic acid (activates release of gastric juice) Ethanol (activates release of bile in intestine)		Digestive aid	Jackson (2008)
Phenolics-resveratrol, Flavonoids-quercitin, ethanol, vitamins C and E, mineral selenium		Prevent cardiovascular diseases, reduced incidence of heart attacks, and mortality rate	Truelsen et al. (1998)
Melatonin, resveratrol		Antioxidant and antiaging property	Corder et al. (2006)
Resveratol		Antidiabetic	Ramadori et al. (2009)
Lactic acid by probiotic LAB	Yogurt	Decreases pH in colon leading to suppression of pathogens. Reduces yeast infection. Protection and cure of vaginitis in women.	Shah et al. (2013)

Table 2.2 (*Continued*) Some Bioactive Compounds Synthesized in Fermented Foods and Their Health Benefits to Consumers

Bioactive Compounds	*Synthesized in Fermented Foods*	*Health Benefits*	*References*
Yogurt culture and probiotics		Improvement of digestive health, curb the growth of undesirable organisms, prevents irritable bowel syndrome, Crohn's disease, ulcerative colitis, and infant gastroenteritis.	Chandan and Kilara (2013)
Biomarkers of cancer initiation		Reduction of harmful fecal enzymes. Prevention of bladder and colon cancer, cervical cancer.	Chandan and Kilara (2013)

of fermented foods containing viable cells of *Lb. acidophilus* decreased the enzymes, ß-glucuronidase, azoreductase, and nitroreductase (that catalyze conversion of procarcinogens to carcinogens), thus possibly removing procarcinogens, and activating the immune system of consumers (Goldin and Gorbach 1984). The removal of procarcinogens by probiotic bacteria might involve a reduction in the rate at which nitrosamines are produced, due to the fact that certain species of *Bif. breve* have high absorbing properties for carcinogens such as those produced upon the charring of meat products (Mitsuoka 1990). Indian *dahi* has anticarcinogenic properties (Arvind et al. 2010). Glycoprotein antimutagenic substances have been isolated from *Lb. plantarum* isolated from *kimchi* (Rhee and Park 2001). Kiriakidis et al. (1997) demonstrated that glucolipids in *tempeh* inhibit the proliferation of tumor cell in mice.

2.3.3 Prevention of Hepatic Disease

Hepatic disease is a liver disease, also known as hepatic encephalopathy (HE) and its effects can be life threatening (Cunningham-Rundles et al. 2000). The probiotics (*Strep. thermophilus*, bifidobacteria, *Lb. acidophilus, Lb. plantarum, Lb. casei, Lb. delbrueckii bulgaricus,* and *Ent. faecum*) with therapeutic effect have multiple mechanisms of action that could disrupt the pathogenesis of HE by lowering the portal pressure with a reduction in the risk of bleeding and thus may make them superior to conventional treatment (Shanahan 2001, Solga 2003).

2.3.4 Prevention against Gastrointestinal Disorders and Inflammatory Bowel Disease

A number of studies involving humans suggest that LAB in fermented foods can decrease the incidence, duration, and severity of some gastric and intestinal illnesses such as diarrhea (Marteau et al. 2002). Bunte et al. (2000) reported that the ingested bacteria (*Lb. paracasei* LTH 2579) in dry-fermented sausage can be recovered from human feces and it suggested that the fermented bacteria may contribute to the microbial ecosystem of the gastrointestinal tract (Farnworth 2003). Fermented meat products such as dry sausages are considered to be a suitable carrier for probiotics into the human gastrointestinal tract (Rebucci et al. 2007).

Consumption of probiotic-fermented foods is reported to be beneficial for alleviating many types of diarrhea such as antibiotic associated, infantile, and traveller's diarrhea and diarrheal diseases in young children caused by rotaviruses (Marteau et al. 2002). Probiotic therapy is reported to shorten the duration of acute diarrheal illness in children (Gill and Guarner 2004). The consumption of certain strains of lactobacilli improved the symptoms of inflammatory bowel disease (IBD), paucities, and ulcerative colitis (Parvez et al. 2006). LAB may also improve intestinal mobility and relieve constipation possibly through the reduction of gut pH (Sanders and Klaenhammer 2001). The combination therapy with probiotics may benefit patients with IBD (Shanahan 2001). Modulation of the intestinal flora may be helpful in the treatment of Crohn's disease (Cabana et al. 2006). It was also reported that *Saccharomyces boulardii* can decrease diarrhea in irritable bowel syndrome, but was not effective in alleviating other symptoms of the syndrome (Marteau et al. 2001). In a double-blind clinical trial, administration of *Lb. plantarum* strain reduces abdominal pain, bloating, flatulence, and constipation in patients with irritable bowel syndrome (MacFarlane and Cummings 2002). There are reports that LAB isolated from *dahi* can be used to cure intestinal disease such as diarrhea (Agarwal and Bhasin 2002). LAB from *kimchi* may be used as a therapeutic to control inflammatory disorders such as atopic dermatitis and IBD (Lim et al. 2011). *Lb. rhamnosus* GG and other probiotic strains are effective in the treatment of acute diarrhea (Szajewska et al. 2007). Consumption of fermented milks containing live bacteria may account by their immunomodulation capacity (Granier et al. 2013).

2.3.5 Protection from Hypertension

Hypertension is the main cause of several cardiovascular diseases such as heart failure, stroke, CHD, and myocardial infarction (FitzGerald et al. 2004). Elderly patients with hypertensive disease who consumed fermented milk with a starter containing *Lactobacillus helveticus* and *Sacch. cerevisiae* experienced reduced systolic and diastolic blood pressure (Hata et al. 1996, Aihara et al. 2005). Whole-grain foods are rich in fiber and provide complex carbohydrates, phytochemicals, minerals, and vitamins (Anderson et al. 2000). Fermented foods rich in fibrinolytic enzymes can be a potential weapon for the treatment of cardiovascular diseases (Mine et al. 2005). *Douchi* produces angiotensin I-converting enzyme inhibitors with the potential to lower blood pressure (Zhang et al. 2006). Fermented soybean products such as *douchi* (Zhang et al. 2006), *sufu* (Iwamik and Buki 1986), *natto* (Okamoto et al. 1995), *tempeh* (Gibbs et al. 2004), soy sauce (Kinoshita et al. 1993), and *doengjong* (Rho et al. 2009) have been found to possess antihypertensive properties.

2.3.6 Prevention of Thrombosis

More than 20 enzymes are produced by the human body to assist in blood clotting, while only one is involved in the breakdown of the blood clot and is called "plasmin" (Mine et al. 2005). Imbalance in the circulatory system leads to fibrin accumulation in the blood vessels, slows down blood flow, and increases blood viscosity contributing to the elevation of blood pressure, which leads to myocardial infarction and other cardiovascular diseases (Mine et al. 2005). To prevent thrombosis, daily intake of fibrinolytic enzymes from a fermented food source is recommended (Singh et al. 2014). If a fibrinolytic enzyme is produced by food grade microorganisms isolated from fermented food, it can be directly consumed daily for the prevention of cardiovascular diseases (Mine et al. 2005, Singh et al. 2014). Fermented foods rich in fibrinolytic enzymes are useful for thrombolytic therapy to prevent rapidly emerging cardiovascular diseases in the modern world

(Mine et al. 2005). Thrombolytic activity (average 450 IU/g dry weight) has been observed in *tempeh* (Sumi and Okamoto 2003).

2.3.7 Protection from Osteoporosis

Vitamin K2 in *natto* stimulates the formation of bone, which might help to prevent osteoporosis in older women in Japan (Yanagisawa and Sumi 2005). Yogurt nutrients calcium, magnesium, phosphorus, potassium, and protein function together to promote strong healthy bones (Chandan and Kilara 2013).

2.3.8 Protection from Spoilage and Toxic Pathogens

LAB are used for fermentation to produce functional foods and have been added as starter cultures in dairy, meat, vegetable, and beverage products (Campbell-Platt 1987). These fermented food products have an extended shelf life, new aromas, and consistencies (Nordvi et al. 2007). The preservation of LAB-fermented foods is due to the production of lactic acid and other organic acids, which contribute to the reduction of pH and thus inhibit the growth of a wide range of pathogenic and spoilage organisms (Chokesajjawatee et al. 2009, Tamang et al. 2009b). Mitra et al. (2010) isolated *Lc. lactis* from *dahi* which produced a *nisin* like (Nisin Z) bacteriocin that inhibited important food pathogens *Lis. monocytogenes* and *Staph. aureus*. The hazard analysis and critical control points (HACCP) is the science-based system which identifies specific hazards and measures for their control to ensure the safety of foods (Gupta et al. 2010). An HACCP model for optimized production of *kinema* has been proposed to reduce the pathogenic load to an acceptable level (Rai et al. 2014).

2.3.9 Protection from Allergic Reactions

Fermented foods may exert a beneficial effect on allergic reactions, on lactose intolerance, in decreasing serum cholesterol concentrations, in increasing nutrient bioavailability, and in improving urogenital health (Galdeano and Perdigon 2006). Soy sauce contains certain bioactive components and also reported various biological activities, including anticarcinogenic, antimicrobial, antioxidative, and antiplatelet activities, and the inhibition of an angiotensin I-converting enzyme (Ando et al. 2003). New immunological functions of soy sauce are also reported with respect to allergy such as hypoallergenicity and antiallergic activity (Kobayashi 2005). It was shown that heat-inactivated *Lactobacillus kefiranofaciens* M1 isolated from *kefir* grains had an antiallergic effect on ovalbumin sensitized BABL/c mice (Hong et al. 2010). Probiotics modulate allergic reactions and exert beneficial effects by improving mucosal barrier functions and microbial stimulation of the immune system (MacFarlane and Cummings 2002).

In view of the worldwide increase in gluten-related food allergies, such as celiac disease, the development of natural baking aids for producing gluten-free bread is highly desirable (Waldherr and Vogel 2009). Rühmkorf et al. (2012) investigated the influence of flour type and various other factors on the *in situ* production of different exopolysaccharides (EPS) in sourdough by three *Lactobacillus* strains (*Lactobacillus animalis* TMW 1.971, *Lactobacillus reuteri* TMW 1.106 and *Lb. curvatus* TMW 1.624). High amounts of EPS could be achieved in gluten-free (buckwheat and quinoa) sourdough under optimized conditions, and by using carefully selected LAB strains (Rühmkorf et al. 2012). EPS are produced by several food grade bacteria, and can act as hydrocolloids to improve bread qualities, in particular for preparing gluten-free bread (Galle et al. 2012) and also in Indian *dahi* (Vijayendra et al. 2008). Gerez et al. (2012) evaluated the gliadin hydrolysis during wheat dough fermentation by a combination of *Lb. plantarum* CRL 775 and *Ped. pentosaceus* CRL 792, and found that gliadins, along with glutenin, play a role in the formation of gluten, and may be the cause of food allergies resulting in severe immune response also known as celiac disease. Oral administration of *Lb. sakei* proBio65 in mice treated with DNCB (1-chloro-2,4-dinitro-benzene) showed a more rapid recovery from allergic dermatitis compared with control mice through the regulation of both elevated IgE and IL-4 (Kim et al. 2013). Digestion of caseins during the maturation of fermented milk products has been shown to facilitate loss of allergenic reactivity during gut digestion, thus increasing tolerance (Alessandri et al. 2012). *Chungkokjang* has an antiallergic effect against atopic dermatitis in mice, improving common allergic responses such as decreased ear thickness, dermis thickness, auricular lymph node, and infiltrating mast cells (Lee et al. 2014b). *Lactobacillus* species isolated from *kimchi* were also found to modulate Th1/Th2 balance by producing a large amount of IL-12 and IFN-γ but less IL-4 with the ability to alleviate atopic dermatitis and food allergy (Won et al. 2011). Natural fish oil and fermented fish oil, rich in omega-3 polyunsaturated fatty acids such as eicosapentaenoic acid and docosahexaenoic acid, have been reported to have antiallergic effects including reducing sensitization to allergens and alleviation of symptoms of atopic dermatitis, eczema, and asthma (Han et al. 2012a). External application of fermented olive flounder fish oil has an antiallergy effect (Han et al. 2012b).

2.3.10 Protection from Diabetes

Recent studies have indicated that a high fiber intake is associated with a significant reduction in the prevalence of diabetes (Meyer et al. 2000). Clinical studies indicated that the increased whole-grain intake increases the insulin sensitivity (Pereira et al. 2002) and has a favorable impact on guthormone and insulin responses after meals (Juntunen et al. 2000). It is also possible that the increased intake of whole grains would decrease the prevalence of diabetes and improve the blood glucose values in diabetic individuals (Anderson 2003). Several studies indicated that the high carbohydrate intakes together with high fiber (mostly fermented cereals) intakes decrease the insulin requirements in diabetic individuals and increase the sensitivity to insulin for nondiabetic individuals (Fukagawa et al. 1990). The probiotic dahi-supplemented diet significantly delayed the onset of glucose intolerance, hyperglycemia, hyperinsulinemia, dyslipidemia, and oxidative stress in high fructose-induced diabetic rats, indicating a lower risk of diabetes and its complications (Yadav et al. 2007). Consumption of *chungkokjang* prevents and improves diabetes by improving the insulin resistivity (Shin et al. 2011, Tolhurst et al. 2012).

2.3.11 Synthesis of Nutrient and Bioavailability

The probiotic activity in fermented foods or in the digestive tract has been shown to improve the quantity, availability, and digestibility of some dietary nutrients (Parvez et al. 2006). Fermentation with LAB increases the level of folic acid, niacin, and riboflavin levels in yogurt; and also increases the folic acid in bifidus milk and *kefir* (Deeth and Tamime 1981). The enzymatic hydrolysis of probiotic bacteria may enhance the bioavailability of protein and fat and also may increase the production of free amino acids, short-chain fatty acids (SCFAs), lactic acid, propionic acid, and butyric acid (Fernandes et al. 1987). When absorbed, these SCFAs contribute available energy to the host and thus may protect the host against pathological changes in the colonic mucosa

(Leopold and Eileler 2000). Tongnual and Fields (1979) reported that lactic acid fermented rice improves the nutritional value and the available lysine content in rice. Probiotics are also used in fermented meat products to improve the nutritional value of these products as functional foods (Leroy et al. 2006).

2.3.12 Reduction of Obesity

Approximately last 30 years' epidemiological data, observational studies, human experimental research, and clinical trials supported the role of dietary fiber in the development and management of obesity (Anderson and Bryant 1986). Lactic acid produced by *kimchi* is found to prevent fat accumulation and to reduce the risk of obesity-induced cardiovascular diseases (Park et al. 2008). Several researchers have reported the antiobesity activities of *kimchi* including clinical trials (Kang et al. 2011, Kim et al. 2011, Moon et al. 2012, Park et al. 2012) and *doenjang* (Lee et al. 2012). *Doenjang* is more effective for antiobesity than unfermented soybeans through various animal (Kwak et al. 2012) and clinical tests (Cha et al. 2012, Jung et al. 2014).

2.3.13 Increase in Immunity

The translocation of a small number of *Lb. acidophilus* and bifidobacteria via M cells to the Payer's patches of the gut-associated lymphoid tissue in the small intestine is responsible for enhancing immunity (Marteau et al. 2002). Many gut-related inflammatory diseases occur due to altered gut microecology and inflammation and are accompanied by imbalances in the intestinal microbiota (Gill and Guarner 2004). The consumption of fermented foods containing viable cells of *Lb. acidophilus* decrease ß-glucuronidase, azoreductase, and nitroreductase (which catalyze conversion of procarcinogens to carcinogens), thus possibly removing procarcinogens, and activating the immune system of consumers (Goldin and Gorbach 1984).

2.3.14 Alleviation of Lactose Intolerance

People suffer from lactose intolerance or lactose malabsorption, a condition in which lactose, the principal carbohydrate of milk, is not completely digested into glucose and galactose (Onwulata et al. 1989). Since lactose is cleaved into its constituent monosaccharides by ß-D-galactosidase, lactose malabsorption results from a deficiency of this enzyme (Shah and Jelen 1991). It is well known that probiotic bacteria incorporated with a starter culture in yogurt improves lactose digestion in many lactose intolerant people, and the beneficial effect is due to the presence of microbial β-galactosidase (lactase enzyme) (Oberhelman et al. 1999). *Lb. delbrueckii* sub-sp. *bulgaricus* and *Strep. thermophilus*, the cultures used in making yoghurt, contain substantial quantities of ß-D-galactosidase, and it has been observed that the consumption of yoghurt may assist in alleviating the symptoms of lactose malabsorption (Shah 1993). Yoghurt or probiotic yoghurt is tolerated well by lactose-intolerant consumers, may be due to some lactose hydrolyzed by lactics and bifids during fermentation, the bacterial enzyme autodigests lactose intracellularly before reaching the intestine, or it may be due to slower oral–cecal transit time (Shah et al. 1992). In different human studies the consumption of fresh yogurt (with live yogurt cultures) demonstrated better lactose digestion and absorption than with the consumption of a pasteurized product (with heat killed bacteria) (Pedone et al. 2000, Marteau et al. 2002). Fermented acidophilus milk may be better tolerated than sweet acidophilus milk, as coagulated milk because of its viscous nature may pass more slowly through the gut than unfermented milk (Shah 2004). Consumption of *kefir* minimizes symptoms of lactose intolerance by providing an extra source of β-galactosidase (Hertzler and Clancy 2003).

2.3.15 Antiaging Effects

Kimchi contains antioxidative compounds that show antiaging effects on the skin (Ryu et al. 2004a). Some components of mustard leaf *kimchi* may have a large effect on skin rejuvenescence (Ryu et al. 2004b). Kim et al. (2002a,b) reported that the concentration of total free radicals and hydroxyl radicals in the plasma of elderly persons who consume more than 112 g of *kimchi* per day was lower than that of the elderly who consume less *kimchi*, indicating role of *kimchi* in inhibiting the production of free radicals or in discarding the free radicals more efficiently.

Red wine contains melatonin which regulates the body clock, which may help one sleep, it also has antiaging properties (Corder et al. 2006).

2.3.16 Recommendations

- More clinical trials and validation of health claims of ethnic fermented foods may be focused on.
- Establishment of more national or international research and extension centers of some common ethnic fermented foods and beverages of the world as being already established: World Institute of *Kimchi* in South Korea, Kikkoman International Institute for *shoyu* in Japan, and so on.
- Basic training in determination of functional properties and extraction of important bioactive compounds from fermented foods.
- Development of new strains and thereby novel foods to fulfill the needs of specific consumer groups.
- Introduction of new fermented food products containing good bacteria such as cereals, energy bars, cheese, juices, disease-specific medical foods, and infant foods.

2.4 Conclusion

The health benefits of fermented foods are expressed either directly through the interaction of ingested live microorganisms or indirectly because of ingestion of microbial metabolites produced during the fermentation process. New research evidence supports the effectiveness of fermented food products or probiotics for the treatment and prevention of infectious and antibiotic-associated diarrhea. Fermented food therapyhas also been applied to a wide range of health disorders such as immune compromise and gastrointestinal disorders. Increased understanding of the viability of probiotic bacteria, interactions between gut microbiota, diet, and the host will open up new possibilities of producing new ingredients for nutritionally optimized foods, which promote consumer health through microbial activities in the gut. In addition, industry-based probiotic research will focus on increasing the shelf life of fermented food and increasing the survival rate of probiotics through the intestinal tract by introducing new stress-tolerant strains and by improving handling and packaging procedures to ensure that the desired health benefits are delivered to the consumer. The establishment of a standard identity of friendly bacteria, will serve to accelerate the new development and availability of a range of new healthy fermented food products from bacterial fermented food.

References

Abimbola, U. 2007. Degradation of dietary fibre from gari by faecal bacteria and bacteria extracellular polysaccharides *Nigerian Food Journal* 25: 46–58.

Abubakr, M.A.S., Hassan, Z., Imdakim, M.M.A., and N.R.S. Sharifah. 2012. Antioxidant activity of lactic acid bacteria (LAB) fermented skim milk as determined by 1,1-diphenyl-2-picrylhydrazyl (DPPH) and ferrous chelating activity (FCA). *African Journal of Microbiology Research* 6(34): 6358–6364.

Adams, M.R. 1999. Safety of industrial lactic acid bacteria. *Journal of Biotechnology* 63: 17–78.

Agarwal, K.N. and S.K. Bhasin. 2002. Feasibility studies to control acute diarrhoea in children by feeding fermented milk preparations actimel and Indian dahi. *European Journal of Clinical Nutrition* 56(4): S56–S59.

Agrahar-Murugkar, D. and G. Subbulakshmi. 2006. Preparation techniques and nutritive value of fermented foods from the Khasi tribes of Meghalaya. *Ecology of Food and Nutrition* 45: 27–38.

Agerholm-Larsen, L., Bell, M.L., Grunwald, G.K., and A. Astrup. 2000. The effect of probiotic milk product on plasma cholesterol: A meta-analysis of short-term intervention studies. *European Journal of Clinical Nutrition* 54: 856–60.

Aihara, K., Kajimoto, O., Hirata, H.,Takahashi, R., and Y. Nakamura. 2005. Effect of powdered fermented milk with *Lactobacillus helveticus* on subjects with high-normal blood pressure or mild hypertension. *Journal of AmericanCollege of Nutrition* 24: 257–265.

Alessandri, C., Sforza, S., Palazzo, P., Lambertini, F., Paolella, S., Zennaro, D. et al. 2012. Tolerability of a fully maturated cheese in cow's milk allergic children: Biochemical, immunochemical, and clinical aspects. *PLoS One* 7: e40945.

Alexandraki, V., Tsakalidou, E., Papadimitriou, K., and W.H. Holzapfel. 2013. Status and trends of the conservation and sustainable use of microorganisms in food processes. Commission on Genetic Resources for Food and Agriculture. FAO Background Study Paper No. 65.

Amdekar, S., Dwivedi, D., Roy, P., Kushwah, S., and V. Singh. 2010. Probiotics: Multifarious oral vaccine against infectious traumas. *Immunology and Medical Microbiology* 58(3): 299–306.

Ammor, M.S. and B. Mayo. 2007. Selection criteria for lactic acid bacteria to be used as functional starter cultures in dry sausage production: An update. *Meat Science* 76(1): 138–146.

An, J., Jung, S.M., Chan, K., and C.F. Tam. 2014. Development of a 28-day *kimchi* cyclic menu for health. *Journal of Culinary Science and Technology* 12: 43–66.

Anderson, J.W. 1995. Dietary fibre, complex carbohydrate and coronary artery. *Canadian Journal of Cardiology* 11: 55G–62G.

Anderson, J.W. 2003.Whole grains protect against atherosclerotic cardiovascular disease. *Proceedings of the Nutrition Society* 62: 135–142.

Anderson, J. and C.A. Bryant. 1986. Dietary fibre: Diabetes and obesity. *American Journal of Gastroenterology* 81: 898–906.

Anderson, J.W., T.J. Hanna, B.S. Xuejun Peng, and R.J. Kryscio. 2000. Whole grain foods and heart disease risk. *Journal of the American College of Nutrition* 19: 291S–299S.

Anderson, M., Bermüdez-Humarán, L.G., Sabtiago Pacheco de Azevedo, M., Langella, P., and V. Azevedo. 2010. Lactic acid bacteria as live vectors: Heterologous protein production and delivery systems. In: F. Mozzi, R.R. Raya, and G.M.Vignolo (Eds.), *Biotechnology of Lactic Acid Bacteria Novel Applications.* Iowa: Blackwell Publishing.

Ando, M., Harada, K., Kitao, S., Kobayashi, M., and Y. Tamura. 2003. Relationship between peroxyl radical scavenging capability measured by the chemiluminescence method and an aminocarbonyl reaction product in soy sauce. *International Journal of Molecular Medicine* 12: 923–928.

Aoki, H., Uda, I., Tagami, K., Furuta, Y., Endo, Y., and K. Fujimoto. 2003. The production of a new tempeh-like fermented soybean containing a high level of γ-aminobutyric acid by anaerobic incubation with *Rhizopus. Bioscience, Biotechnology and Biochemistry* 67: 1018–1023.

Arora, G., Lee, B.H., and M. Lamoureux. 1990. Characteristics of enzyme profiles of *Lactobacillus casei* species by a rapid API-ZYM system. *Journal of Dairy Sciences* 73: 264–273.

Arvind, K., Nikhlesh, K.S., and R.S. Pushpalata. 2010. Inhibition of 1,2-dimethylhydrazineinduced colon genotoxicity in rats by the administration of probiotic curd. *MolecularBiology Reports* 37: 1373–1376.

Asp, N.-G. and Bryngelsson, S. 2008. Health claims in Europe: New legislation and PASSCLAIM for substantiation. *Journal of Nutrition* 138(6): 1210–1215.

Auclair, J. and J.P. Accolas. 1974. Koumiss (koumiss, coomys). In: A.H. Johnson and M.S. Peterson (Eds.), *Encyclopedia of Food Technology.* Westport, CT: AVI, pp. 537–538.

Badis, A., Guetarni, D., Moussa-Boudjemaa, B., Henni, D.E., Tornadijo, M.E., and M. Kihal. 2004. Identification of cultivable lactic acid bacteria isolated from Algerian raw goat's milk and evaluation of their technological properties. *Food Microbiology* 21: 343–349.

Barnby-Smith, F.M., 1992. Bacteriocins: applications in food preservation. *Trends in Food Science and Technology* 3: 133–137.

Beganović, J., A.L. Pavunc, K. Gjuračić, M. Špoljarec, Šušković, J., and B. Kos. 2011. Improved sauerkraut production with probiotic strain *Lactobacillus plantarum* L4 and *Leuconostoc mesenteroides* LMG 7954. *Journal of Food Science* 76: M124–M129.

Berger, K., U.A. Anjani, C.A. Kase, and M.J. Gaziano. 1999. Light-to-moderate alcohol consumption and the risk of stroke among U.S. male physicians. *The New England Journal of Medicine* 341: 1557–1564.

Berhow, M.A., Kong, S.B., Vermillion, K.E., and S.M. Duval. 2006. Complete quantification of group A and group B soyasaponins in soybeans. *Journal of Agricultural and Food Chemistry,* 54, 2035–2044.

Bernardeau, M., Guguen, M., and J.P. Vernoux. 2006. Beneficial lactobacilli in food and feed: Long-term use, biodiversity and proposals for specific and realistic safety assessments. *FEMS Microbiology Review* 30: 487–513.

Bernet, F.M., Brassart, D., Nesser, J.R. and A. Servin. 1993. Adhesion of human bifidobacterial starters to cultured human intestinal epithelial cells and inhibition of enteropathogen cell interaction. *Applied and Environmental Microbiology* 59: 4121–4128.

Beuchat, L.R. 1978. Traditional fermented food products. In: L.R. Beuchat (Ed.), *Food and Beverage Mycology.* Westport, CT: AVI, pp. 224–253.

Bourdichon, F., Casaregola, S., Farrokh, C., Frisvad, J.C., Gerds, M.L., Hammes et al. 2012. Food fermentations: Microorganisms with technological beneficial use. *International Journal of Food Microbiology* 154(3): 87–97.

Bover-Cid, S. and W.H. Holzapfel. 1999. Improved screening procedure for biogenic amine production by lactic acid bacteria. *International Journal of Food Microbiology* 53: 33–41.

Breidt, F., McFeeters, R.F., Perez-Diaz, I., and C.H. Lee. 2013. Fermented vegetables. In: M.P. Doyle and R.L. Buchanan (Eds.), *Food Microbiology: Fundamentals and Frontiers,* 4th ed. Washington, DC: ASM Press, pp. 841–855, doi:10.1128/9781555818463.ch33.

Brennan, M., Wanismail, B., Johnson, M.C., and B. Ray. 1986. Cellular damage in dried *Lactobacillus acidophilus. Journal of Food Protection* 49: 47–53.

Bunte, C., Hertel, C., and W.P. Hammes. 2000. Monitoring and survival of *Lactobacillus paracasei* LTH 2579 in food and the human intestinal tract. *Systematic and Applied Microbiology* 23: 260–266.

Cabana, M.D., Shane, A.L., Chao, C., and M. Oliva-Hemke. 2006. Probiotics in primary care pediatrics. *Clinical Pediatrics* 45: 405–410.

Campbell-Platt, G. 1987. *Fermented Foods of the World: A Dictionary and Guide.* London: Butterworths.

Campbell-Platt, G. 1994. Fermented foods—A world perspective. *Food Research International* 27: 253–257.

Cha, Y.S., Yang, J.A., Back, H.I., Kim, S.R., Kim, M.G., Jung, S.J., Song, W.O., and S.W. Chae. 2012. Visceral fat and body weight are reduced in overweight adults by the supplementation of *Doenjang,* a fermented soybean paste. *Nutrition Research Practice* 6: 520–526.

Chandan, R.C. and A. Kilara (Eds.). 2013. *Manufacturing Yogurt and Fermented Milks,* 2nd ed. Chichester, West Sussex, UK: John Wiley & Sons, 477pp.

Chang, C.T., Wang, P.M., Hung, Y.F., and Y.C. Chung. 2012. Purification and biochemical properties of a fibrinolytic enzyme from *Bacillus subtilis*—Fermented red bean. *Food Chemistry* 133: 1611–1617.

Chang, J.Y., Lee, H.J., and H.C. Chang. 2008.Identification of the agent from *Lactobacillus plantarum* KFRI464 that enhances bacteriocin production by *Leuconostoc citreum* GJ7. *Journal of Applied Microbiology* 103(6): 2504–2515.

Chávarri, M., Marañón, I., Ares, R., Ibáñez, F.C., Marzo, F., and M.C. Villarán. 2010. Microencapsulation of a probiotic and prebiotic in alginate-chitosan capsules improves survival in simulated gastro-intestinal conditions. *International Journal of Food Microbiology* 142: 185–189.

Cheigh, H. 1999. Production, characteristics and health functions of *kimchi*. *Acta Horticulture* (ISHS) 483: 405–420.

Cheigh, H.S. and K.Y. Park. 1994. Biochemical, microbiological, and nutritional aspects of kimchi (Korean fermented vegetable products). *Critical Reviews in Food Science and Nutrition* 34(2): 175–203.

Chen, Y., Wang, Z., Chen, X., Liu, Y., Zhang, H., and T. Sun. 2010. Identification of angiotensin I-converting enzyme inhibitory peptides from koumiss, a traditional fermented mare's milk. *Journal of Dairy Science* 93: 884–892.

Chettri, R. and J.P. Tamang. 2014. Functional properties of *tungrymbai* and *bekang*, naturally fermented soybean foods of North East India. *International Journal of Fermented Foods* 3: 87–103.

Chiou, R.Y.Y. and S.L. Cheng. 2001. Isoflavone transformation during soybean koji preparation and subsequent miso fermentation supplemented with ethanol and NaCl. *Journal of Agricultural and Food Chemistry* 49: 3656–3660.

Chokesajjawatee, N., Pornaem,S., Zo, Y-G., Kamdee, S., Luxananil, P., Wanasen, S., and R. Valyasevi. 2009. Incidence of *Staphylococcus aureus* and associated risk factors in Nham, a Thai fermented pork product. *Food Microbiology* 26: 547–551.

Choi, H.J., Lee, H.S., Her, S., Oh, D.H., Yoon, S.S., and S.-S. Yoon.1999. Partial characterization and cloning of leuconocin J, a bacteriocin produced by *Leuconostoc* sp. J2 isolated from the Korean fermented vegetable Kimchi. *Journal of Applied Microbiology* 86(2): 175–181.

Choi, J., Kwon, S.H., Park, K.Y., Yu, B.P., Kim, N.D., Jung, J.H., and H.Y. Chung. 2010. The anti-inflammatory action of fermented soybean products in kidney of high-fat-fed rats. *Journal of Medicinal Food* 14: 232–239.

Choi, Y.H., Kim, Y.A., Park, C., Choi, B.T., Lee, W.H., Hwang, K.M.H., Jung, K.O., and K.Y. Park. 2004. β-sitosterol induced growth inhibition is associated with up-regulation of Cdk Inhibitor p21WAF1/CIP1 in human colon cancer cells. *Journal of the Korean Society of Food Science and Nutrition* 33: 1–6.

Coman, M.M., Cecchini, C., Verdenelli, M.C., Silvi, S., Orpianesi, C., and A. Cresci. 2012. Functional foods as carriers for SYNBIO®, a probiotic bacteria combination. *International Journal of Food Microbiology* 157: 346–352.

Corder, R., Mullen, W., Khan, N.Q., Marks, S.C., Wood, E.G.,Carrier, M.J., and A. Crozier. 2006. Oenology: Red wine procyanidins and vascular health. *Nature* 444: 566.

Cunningham-Rundles, S., Ahrne, S., Bengmark, S., Johann- Liang, R., Marshall, F., Metakis, L., Califano, C., and A.M. Dunn. 2000. Probiotics and immune response. *American Journal of Gastroenterology* 95: S22–S25.

Danielson, A.D., Peo, E.R., Shahani, K.M., Lewis, A.J., Whalen, P.J., and M.A. Amer. 1989. Anticholesteremic property of *Lactobacillus acidophilus* yogurt fed to mature boars. *Journal of Animal Science* 67: 966–974.

de Arauz, L.J., Jozala, A.F., Mazzola, P.G., and T.C.V. Penna. 2009. Nisin biotechnological production and application: A review. *Trends in Food Science and Technology* 20: 146–154.

Deeth, H.C. and A.Y. Tamime. 1981. Yogurt, nutritive and therapeutic aspects. *Journal of Food Protection* 44: 78–86.

de LeBlanc, A.M., Matar, C., and G. Perdigón. 2007. The application of probiotics in cancer. *British Journal of Nutrition* 98: S105–S110.

de Mejia, E.G. and V.P. Dia. 2010. The role of nutraceutical proteins and peptides in apoptosis, angiogenesis, and metastasis of cancer cells. *Cancer Metastasis Review* 29: 511–528.

Dewan, S. and J.P. Tamang. 2006. Microbial and analytical characterization of Chhu-A traditional fermented milk product of the Sikkim Himalayas. *Journal of Scientific and Industrial Research* 65: 747.

Dewan, S. and J.P. Tamang. 2007. Dominant lactic acid bacteria and their technological properties isolated from the Himalayan ethnic fermented milk products. *Antonie van Leeuwenhoek International Journal of General and Molecular Microbiology* 92 (3): 343–352.

de Vuyst, L. 2000. Technology aspects related to the application of functional starter culture. *Food Technology and Biotechnology* 38(2): 105–112.

de Vuyst, L. and F. Leroy. 2007. Bacteriocins from lactic acid bacteria: Production, purification, and food applications. *Journal of Molecular Microbiology and Biotechnology* 13: 194–199.

Doyon, M. 2008. Functional foods: A conceptual definition. *British Food Journal* 110(11): 1133–1149.

Durlu-Ozkaya, F., Xanthopoulos, V., Tunaï, N., and E. Litopoulou-Tzanetaki. 2001. Technologically important properties of lactic acid bacteria isolated from Beyaz cheese made from raw ewes' milk. *Journal of Applied Microbiology* 91: 861–870.

EFFCA, 2011. Protective cultures. European Food and Feed Cultures Association/2011/52. Brussels, October 17, 2011.

Ellington, A.A., Berhow, M.A., and K.W. Singletary. 2006. Inhibition of Akt singaling and enhanced ERK1/2 activity are involved in induction of macroautophagy by triterpenoid B-group soyasaponins in colon cancer cells. *Carcinogenesis* 27(2): 298–306.

Erdmann, K., Cheung, B.W.Y., and H. Schroder. 2008. The possible role of food derived bioactive peptides in reducing the risk of cardiovascular diseases. *Journal of Nutritional Biochemistry* 19: 643–654.

Euromonitor. 2014. Health and wellness performance overview 2013. London, UK. www.euromonitor.com.

Ewaschuk, J.B. and L.A. Dieleman. 2006. Probiotics and prebiotics in chronic inflammatory bowel diseases. *World Journal of Gastroenterology* 12(37): 5941–5950.

FAO/WHO. 2002. Joint FAO/WHO (Food and Agriculture Organization/World Health Organization) working group report on drafting guidelines for the evaluation of probiotics in food. London, Ontario, Canada.

Farhad, M., Kailasapathy, K., and J.P. Tamang. 2010. Health aspects of fermented foods. In: J.P. Tamang and K. Kailasapathy (Eds.), *Fermented Foods and Beverages of the World*. New York: CRC Press, Taylor & Francis Group, pp. 391–414.

Farnworth, E.R. 2003. *Handbook of Fermented Functional Foods*. Food Research andDevelopment Centre, Agriculture and Agri-Food Canada. CRC Press: BocaRaton, FL, pp. 251–275.

Feher, J., Lengyel, G., and A. Lugasi. 2007. The cultural history of wine—Theoretical background to wine therapy. *Central European Journal of Medicine* 2(4): 379–391.

Fernandes, C.F., Shahani, K.M., and M.A. Amer. 1987. Therapeutic role of dietary *lactobacilli* and *lactobacillic* fermented dairy products. *FEMS Microbiology Review* 46: 343–356.

Ferruzzi, M.G. andJ. Blakeslee. 2007. Digestion, absorption, and cancer preventative activity of dietary chlorophyll derivatives. *Nutrition Research* 27: 1–12.

FitzGerald, R.J., Murray, B.A., and D.J. Walsh. 2004. Hypotensive peptides from milk protein. *Journal of Nutrition* 34: 9805–9885.

Fujii, H., Shiraishi, A., Kaba, H., Shibagaki, M., Takahashi, S., and A. Honda. 1975. Abnormal fermentation in natto production and *Bacillus natto* phages. *Journal of Fermentation Technology* 53: 424–428 (in Japanese).

Fukagawa, N.K., Anderson, J., Young, V.R., and K.L. Minaker. 1990. High-carbohydrate, high-fiber diets increase peripheral insulin sensitivity in healthy young and old adults. *American Journal of Clinical Nutrition* 52: 524–528.

Gaggia, F., Di Gioia, D., Baffoni, L., and B. Biavati. 2011. The role of protective and probiotic cultures in food and feed and their impact in food safety. *Trends in Food Science and Technology* 22(1): 58–66.

Galdeano, C.M. and G. Perdigon. 2006. Probiotic bacterium *Lactobacillus casei* induces activation of the gut mucosal immune system through innate immunity. *Clinical and Vaccine Immunology* 13: 219–226.

Galle, S., Schwab, C., Dal Bello, F., Coffey, A., Ganzle, M.G., and E.K. Arendt. 2012. Influence of in-situ synthesized exopolysaccharides on the quality of gluten-free sorghum sourdough bread. *International Journal of Food Microbiology* 155: 105–112.

García-Ruiz, A., de Llano, Esteban-Fernández, D.G.A., Requena, T., Bartolomé, B., and M.V. Moreno-Arribas. 2014. Assessment of probiotic properties in lactic acid bacteria isolated from wine. *Food Microbiology* 44: 220–225.

Gerez, C.L., Dallagnol, A., Rollán, G., and G. Font de Valdez. 2012. A combination of two lactic acid bacteria improves the hydrolysis of gliadin during wheat dough fermentation. *Food Microbiology* 32: 427–430.

Ghishan, F.K. and P.R. Kiela. 2011. From probiotics to therapeutics: Another step forward? *Journal of Clinical Investigation* 121(6): 2149–2152.

Ghosh, D. and P. Chattopadhyay. 2011. Preparation of *idli* batter, its properties and nutritional improvement during fermentation. *Journal of Food Science and Technology* 48(5): 610–615.

Gibbs, B.F., Zougman, A., Masse, R., and C. Mulligan. 2004. Production and characterization of bioactive peptides from soy hydrolysate and soy-fermented food. *Food Research International* 37: 123–131.

Gill, H.S. and F. Guarner. 2004. Probiotics and human health: A clinical perspective. *Postgraduate Medical Journal* 80: 516–526.

Ginting, E. and J. Arcot. 2004. High-performance liquid chromatographic determination of naturally occurring folates during *tempeh* preparation. *Journal of Agricultural and Food Chemistry* 52: 7752–7758.

Goldin, B.R. and S.L. Gorbach. 1984. The effect of milk and lactobacillus feeding on human intestinal bacterial enzyme activity. *American Journal of Clinical Nutrition* 39: 756–761.

Granier, A., Goulet, O., and C. Hoarau. 2013. Fermentation products: Immunological effects on human and animal models. *Pediatric Research* 74: 238–244.

Grosu-Tudor, S.S. and M. Zamfir. 2013. Functional properties of LAB isolated from Romanian fermented vegetables. *Food Biotechnology* 27: 235–248.

Gupta, M., Khetarpaul, N., and B.M. Chauhan. 1992. Rabadi fermentation of wheat: Changes in phytic acid content and *in vitro* digestibility. *Plant Foods for Human Nutrition* 42: 109–116.

Gupta, A., Sharma, P.C., and A.K. Verma. 2010. Application of food safety management system (HACCP) in food industry. *Indian Food Industry* 29(2): 39–46.

Güven, A., Güven, A., and M. Gülmez. 2003. The effect of kefir on the activities of GSH-Px, GST, CAT, GSH and LPO levels in carbon tetrachloride-induced mice tissues. *Journal of Veterinary Medicine* Series B 50: 412–416.

Halász, A., Baráth, A., Simon-Sarkadi, L., and Holzapfel, W.H. 1994. Biogenic amines and their production by microorganisms in food. *Trends in Food Science and Technology* 5: 42–49.

Han, S., Kang, G., Ko, Y., Kang, H., Moon, S., Ann, Y., and E. Yoo. 2012a. Fermented fish oil suppresses T helper 1/2 cell response in a mouse model of atopic dermatitis via generation of $CD4^+CD25^+Foxp3^+$ T cells. *BMC Immunology* 13: 44.

Han, S., Kang, G., Ko, Y., Kang, H., Moon, S., Ann, Y., and E. Yoo. 2012b. External application of fermented olive flounder (*Paralicthys olivaceus*) oil alleviates inflammatory responses in 2,4-dinitrochlorobenzene-induced atopic dermatitis mouse model. *Toxicology Research* 28(3): 159–164.

Haque, E. and R. Chand. 2008. Antihypertensive and antimicrobial bioactive peptides from milk protein. *European Food Research Technology* 227: 7–15.

Hartmann, R. and H. Meisel. 2007. Food-derived peptides with biological activity: From research to food applications. *Current Opinion in Biotechnology* 18: 163–169.

Harun-ur-Rashid, M., Togo, K., Ueda, M., and T. Miyamoto. 2007. Identification and characterization of dominant lactic acid bacteria isolated from traditional fermented milk Dahi in Bangladesh. *World Journal of Microbiology and Biotechnology* 23: 125–133.

Hata, Y., Yamamoto, M., Ohni, M., Nakajima, K., Nakamura, Y., and T. Takano. 1996. A placebo-controlled study of the effect of sour milk on blood pressure in hypertensive subjects. *American Journal of Clinical Nutrition* 64: 767–771.

Hermosilla, J.A.G., Jha, H.C., Egge, H., and M. Mahmud. 1993. Isolation and characterization of hydroxymethylglutaryl coenzyme A reductase inhibitors from fermented soybean extracts. *Journal of Clinical Biochemistry and Nutrition* 15: 163–174.

Hertzler, S.R. and S.M. Clancy. 2003. Kefir improves lactose digestion and tolerance in adults with lactose maldigestion. *Journal of American Diet Association* 103: 582–587.

Hesseltine, C.W. 1983. Microbiology of oriental fermented foods. *Annual Review of Microbiology* 37: 575–601.

Higdon, J.V., Delage, B.,Williams, D.E., and R.H. Dashwood. 2007. Cruciferous vegetables and human cancer risk: Epidemiologic evidence and mechanistic basis. *Pharmacological Research* 55: 224–236.

Hilliam, M. 2000. Functional food: How big is the market? *The World of Food Ingredients* 12: 50–53.

Holzapfel, W.H., Giesen, R., and U. Schillinger. 1995. Biological preservation of foods with reference to protective cultures, bacteriocins and food-grade enzymes. *International Journal of Food Microbiology* 24: 343–362.

Holzapfel, W.H., Harberer, P., Snel, J., Schillinger, U., and J.H.J. Huis in't Veld. 1998. Overview of gut flora and probiotics. *International Journal of Food Microbiology* 41: 85–101.

Holzapfel, W.H., Giesen, R.,Schillinger, U., and F.K. Lücke. 2003. Starter and protective cultures. In: N.J. Russell, and G.W. Gould (Eds.), *Food Preservatives*, 2nd ed. New York: Kluwer Academic/Plenum Publishers, pp. 291–319.

Hong, W., Chen, Y., and M. Chen. 2010. The antiallergic effect of kefir *Lactobacilli*. *Journal of Food Science* 75(8): H244–H253.

Hoover, D.G. and Chen, H. 2005. Bacteriocins with potential for use in foods. In: P.M. Davidson, J.N. Sofos, and L. Branen (Eds.), *Antimicrobials in Foods*, 3rd ed. New York: CRC Press, Taylor & Francis, pp. 389–428.

Homma, N. 1988. Bifidobacteria as a resistance factor in human beings. *Bifidobacterium Microflora* 7: 35–43.

Horii, M. 2008. Tempeh. In: K. Kiuchi, T. Nagai, and K. Kimura (Eds.), *Advanced Science on Natto*. Tokyo: Kenpakusha, pp. 234–237 (in Japanese).

Hur, J.-W., Hyun, H.-H., Pyun, Y.-R., Kim, T.-S., Yeo, I.-H., and H.-D. Park. 2000. Identification and partial characterization of lacticin BH5, a bacteriocin produced by *Lactococcus lactis* BH5 Isolated from kimchi. *Journal of Food Protection* 63(12): 1707–1712.

Ibe, S., Kumada, K., Yoshiba, M., and T. Onga. 2001. Production of *natto* which contains a high level of isoflavone aglycons. *Nippon Shokuhin Kagaku Kogaku Kaishi* 48: 27–34.

Ichimura, T., Hu, J., Aita, D.O., and S. Maruyama. 2003. Angiotensin I-converting enzyme inhibitory activity and insulin secretion stimulative activity of fermented fish sauce. *Journal of Bioscience and Bioengineering* 96: 496–499.

Ishii, Y. and H. Tanizawa. 2006. Effects of soya saponins on lipid peroxidation through the secretion of thyroid hormones. *Biological and Pharmaceutical Bulletin* 29(8): 1759–1763.

Itoh, H., Tachi, H., and S. Nikkuni. 1993. Halophilic mechanism of isolated bacteria from fish sauce. In: C.H. Lee, K.H. Steinkraus, and P.J.A. Reilly (Eds.), *Fish Fermentation Technology*. Tokyo: United Nations University Press, pp. 249–258.

Iwai, K., Nakaya, N., Kawasaki, Y., and H. Matsue. 2002. Antioxidative function of Natto, a kind of fermented soybeans: Effect on LDL oxidation and lipid metabolism in cholesterol-fed rats. *Journal of Agricultural and Food Chemistry* 50: 3597–3601.

Iwamik, S.K. and F. Buki. 1986. Involvement of post-digestion hydropholic peptides in plasma cholesterol-lowing effect of dietary plant proteins. *Agricultural and Biological Chemistry* 50: 1217–1222.

Jackson, R.S. 2008. *Wine Science: Principles and Applications*, 3rd ed. San Diego: Academic Press, pp. 686–706.

Je, J.Y, Park, P.J., Byun, H.G., Jung, W.K., and S.K. Kim. 2005a. Angiotensin I converting enzyme (ACE) inhibitory peptide derived from the sauce of fermented blue mussel, *Mytilus edulis*. *Bioresource Technology* 6: 1624–1629.

Je, J.Y., Park, J.Y., Jung, W.K., Park, P.J., and S.K. Kim. 2005b. Isolation of angiotensin I converting enzyme (ACE) inhibitor from fermented oyster sauce, *Crassostrea gigas*. *Food Chemistry* 90: 809–814.

Jeong, J., Junga, H., Leea, S., Leea, H., Hwanga, K.T., and T. Kimb. 2010. Anti-oxidant, anti-proliferative and anti-inflammatory activities of the extracts from black raspberry fruits and wine. *Food Chemistry* 123: 338–344.

Jeong, Y., Yang, W.S., Kim, K.H., Chung, K.T., Joo, W.H., Kim, J.H., Kim, D.E., and J.U. Park. 2004. Purification of a fibrinolytic enzyme (*myulchikinase*) from pickled anchovy and its cytotoxicity to the tumor cell lines. *Biotechnology Letters* 26: 393–397.

Jiang, J., Shi, B., Zhu, D., Cai, Q., Chen, Y., Li, J., Qi, K., and M. Zhang. 2012. Characterization of a novel bacteriocin produced by *Lactobacillus sakei* LSJ618 isolated from traditional Chinese fermented radish. *Food Control* 23: 338–344.

Jung, J.Y., Lee, S.H., Jin, H.M., Hahn, Y., Madsen, E.L., and C.O. Jeon. 2013. Metatranscriptomic analysis of lactic acid bacterial gene expression during *kimchi* fermentation. *International Journal of Food Microbiology* 163: 171–179.

Jung, S.J., Park, S.H., Choi, E.K., Cho, B.H., Cha, Y.S., Kim, Y.K. et al. 2014. Beneficial effects of Korean traditional diets in hypertensive and type 2 diabetic patients. *Journal of Medicinal Food* 17:161–171.

Juntunen, K.S., Mazur, W.M., Liukkonen, K.H., Uehara, M., Poutanen, K.S., Adlercreutz, H.C., and H.M. Mykkanen. 2000. Consumption of wholemeal rye bread increases serum concentrations and urinary excretion of enterolactone compared with consumption of white wheat bread in healthy Finnish men and women. *British Journal of Nutrition* 84: 839–846.

Kalliomäki, M., Antoine, J.-M., Herz, U., Rijkers, G.T., Wells, J.M., and A. Mercenier. 2010. Guidance for substantiating the evidence for beneficial effects of probiotics: Prevention and management of allergic diseases by probiotics. *Journal of Nutrition* 140: 713–721.

Kang, J.H., Tsuyoshi, G., Le Ngoc, H., Kim, H.M., Tu, T.H., Noh, H.J. et al. 2011. Dietary capsaicin attenuates metabolic dysregulation in genetically obese diabetic mice. *Journal of Medicinal Food* 14: 310–315.

Karovicova, J. and Z. Kohajdova. 2005. Lactic acid-fermented vegetable juices-palatable and wholesome foods. *Chemical Papers* 59: 143–148.

Kesenkas, H., Gursoy, O., Kinik, O., and N. Akbulut. 2006. Extension of shelf life of dairy products by biopreservation: Protective cultures. *GIDA* 31: 217–223.

Keuth, S. and B. Bisping. 1994. Vitamin B12production by *Citrobacter freundii* or *Klebsiella pneumoniae* during tempeh fermentation a proof of enterotoxin absence by PCR. *Applied and Environmental Microbiology* 60: 1495–1499.

Khan, H., Flint, S., and P.-L. Yu. 2010. Enterocins in food preservation. *International Journal of Food Microbiology* 141: 1–10.

Kiers, J.L., Van laeken, A.E.A., Rombouts, F.M., and M.J.R. Nout. 2000. *In vitro* digestibility of *Bacillus* fermented soya bean. *International Journal of Food Microbiology* 60: 163–169.

Kim, E.K., An, S.Y., Lee, M.S., Kim, T.H., Lee, H.K., Hwang, W.S. et al. 2011. Fermented kimchi reduces body weight and improves metabolic parameters in overweight and obese patients. *Nutrition Research* 31: 436–443.

Kim, K.Y. and Y.T. Hahm. 2002. Recent studies about physiological functions of *Chungkkokjang* and functional enhancement with genetic engineering. *The Institute of Molecular Biology and Genetic* 16: 1–18.

Kim, H.K., Kim, G.T., Kim, D.K. et al. 1997. Purification and characterization of a novel fibrinolytic enzyme from *Bacillus*sp. KA38 originated from fermented fish. *Journal of Fermentation and Bioengineering* 84: 307–312.

Kim, D.H., Kim, S.H., Kwon, S.W., Lee, J.K., and S.B. Hong. 2013. Fungal diversity of rice straw for *meju* fermentation. *Journal of Microbiology and Biotechnology* 23: 1654–1663.

Kim, H.J., Lee, J.S., Chung, H.Y., Song, S.H., Suh, H., Noh, J.S., and Y.O. Song. 2008a. 3-(4'-hydroxyl-3',5'-dimethoxyphenyl) propionic acid, an active principle of kimchi, inhibits development of atherosclerosis in rabbits. *Journal of Agricultural and Food Chemistry* 55(25): 10486–10492.

Kim, H.J., Lee, J.S., Chung, H.Y., Song, S.H., Suh, H., Noh, J.S., and Y.O. Song. 2007. 3-(4′-Hydroxyl-3′, 5′-dimethoxyphenyl) propionic acid, an active principle of kimchi, inhibits development of atherosclerosis in rabbits. *Journal of Agricultural and Food Chemistry* 55: 10486–10492.

Kim, J.H., Ryu, J.D., Lee, H.G., Park, J.H., Moon, G.S., Cheigh, H.S., and Y.O. Song. 2002a. The effect of kimchi on production of free radicals and anti-oxidative enzyme activities in the brain of SAM. *Journal of the Korean Society of Food Science and Nutrition* 31: 117–123.

Kim, J.H, Ryu, J.D., and Y.O. Song. 2002b. The effect of kimchi intake on free radical production and the inhibition of oxidation in young adults and the elderly people. *Korean Journal of Community Nutrition* 7: 257–265.

Kim, J.Y., Park, B.K., Park, H.J., Park, Y.H., Kim, B.O., and S. Pyo. 2013. Atopic dermatitis-mitigating effects of new *Lactobacillus* strain, *Lactobacillus sakei* probio 65 isolated from Kimchi. *Journal of Applied Microbiology* 115: 517–526.

Kim, Y-S., Zheng, Z-B., and D-H. Shin. 2008b. Growth inhibitory effects of kimchi (Korean traditional fermented vegetable product) against *Bacillus cereus, Listeria monocytogenes,* and *Staphylococcus aureus. Journal of Food Protection* 71(2): 325–332.

Kinoshita, E., Yamakashi, J., and M. Kikuchi. 1993. Purification and identification of an angiotensin I-converting enzyme inhibitor from soy sauce. *Bioscience Biotechnology and Biochemistry* 57: 1107–1110.

Kiriakidis, S., Stathi, S., Jha, H.C., Hartmann, R., and H. Egge. 1997. Fatty acid esters of sitosterol 3β-glucoside from soybeans and *tempe* (fermented soybeans) as antiproliferative substances. *Journal of Clinical Biochemistry and Nutrition* 22: 139–147.

Kiwaki, M. and K. Nomoto. 2009. *Lactobacillus casei* Shirota. In: Y.K. Lee and S. Salminen (Eds.), *Handbook of Probiotics and Prebiotics*, 2nd ed. Hoboken: Wiley, pp. 449–457.

Klatsky, A., Armstrong, M.A., and G.D. Friedman. 1997. Red wine, white wine, liquor, beer and the risk of coronary artery hospitalizations. *The American Journal of Cardiology* 80: 416–420.

Kobayashi, M. 2005. Immunological functions of soy sauce: Hypoallergenicity and antiallergic activity of soy sauce. *Journal of Bioscience and Bioengineering* 100: 144–151.

Kong, Y.-H., Cheigh, H.-S., Song, Y.-O., Jo, Y.-O., and S.Y. Choi. 2008. Anti-obesity effects of kimchi tablet composition in rats fed high-fat diet. *Journal of the Korean Society of Food Science and Nutrition* 36(12): 1529–1536.

Korhonen, H. and A. Pihlanto. 2003. Food-derived bioactive peptides—opportunities for designing future foods. *Current Pharmaceutical Design* 9: 1297–1308.

Kosikowski, F.V. 1997. *Cheese and Fermented Milk Foods*. Westport, Connecticut: LLC (CRC).

Kostinek, M., Specht, I., Edward, V.A., Schillinger, U., Hertel, C., Holzapfel, W.H., and C.M.A.P. Franz. 2005. Diversity and technological properties of predominant lactic acid bacteria from fermented cassava used for the preparation of Gari, a traditional African food. *Systematic and Applied Microbiology* 28: 527–540.

Kotb, E. 2012. Fibrinolytic bacterial enzymes with thrombolytic activity. *Fibrinolytic Bacterial Enzymes with Thrombolytic Activity.* Berlin Heidelberg: Springer, pp. 1–74.

Kris-Etherton, P.M., Hecker, K.D., Bonanome, A., Coval, S.M., Binkoski, A.E., Hilpert, K.F., Griel, A.E., and T.D. Etherton. 2002. Bioactive compounds in foods: Their role in the prevention of cardiovascular disease and cancer. [Review] *American Journal of Medicine* 113: 71S–88S.

Kudou, S., Fleury, Y., Welti, D., Magnolato, D., Uchida, T., Kitamura, K. et al. 1991. Malonyl isoflavone glycosides in soybean seeds (*Glycine max* Merrill). *Agricultural and Biological Chemistry* 55: 2227–2233.

Kumar, M., Kumar, A., Nagpal, R., Mohania, D., Behare P., Verma, V. et al. 2010. Cancer-preventing attributes of probiotics: An update. *International Journal of Food Science and Nutrition* 61(5): 473–496.

Kwak, C.S., Park, S., and K.Y. Song. 2012. *Doenjang,* a fermented soybean paste, decreased visceral fat accumulation and adipocyte size in rats fed with high fat diet more effectively than nonfermented soybeans. *Journal of Medicinal Food* 15: 1–9.

Latorre-Moratalla, M.L., Bover-Cid, S., Aymerich, T., Marcos, B., Vodal-Carou, M.C., and M. Garrig. 2007. Aminogenesis control in fermented sausages manufactured with pressurized meat batter and starter culture. *Meat Science* 75(3): 460–469.

Lee, C.H. 2001. *Fermentation Technology in Korea.* Seoul: KoreaUniversity Press.

Lee, C.H. 2004. Creative fermentation technology for the future. *Journal of Food Science* 69: 33–34.

Lee, H.M. and Y. Lee. 2006. Isolation of *Lactobacillus plantarum* from kimchi and its inhibitory activity on the adherence and growth of *Helicobacter pylori. Journal of Microbiology and Biotechnology* 16(10): 1513–1517.

Lee, H.R. and J.M. Lee. 2009. Anti-stress effects of kimchi. *Food Science and Biotechnology* 18(1): 25–30.

Lee, H., M.J. Chang, and S.H. Kim. 2010. Effects of poly-gamma-glutamic acid on serum and brain concentrations of glutamate and GABA in diet-induced obese rats. *Nutrition Research Practice* 4: 23–29.

Lee, J.W., Shin, J.G., Kim, E.H., Kang, H.E., Yim, I.B., Kim, J.Y., Joo, H.G., and H.J. Woo. 2004. Immunomodulatory and antitumor effects *in vivo* by the cytoplasmic fraction of *Lactobacillus casei* and *Bifidobacterium longum. Journal of Veterinary Science* 5: 41–48.

Lee, J.K., Jung, D.W., Kim, Y.-J., Cha, S.K., Lee, M.-K., Ahn, B.-H., Kwak, N.S. and S.W. Oh. 2009. Growth inhibitory effect of fermented kimchi on food-borne pathogens. *Food Science and Biotechnology* 18(1): 12–17.

Lee, Y.K. and S. Salminen. 2009. *Handbook of Probiotics and Prebiotics,* 2nd ed. Hoboken: Wiley.

Lee, Y., Lee, H.J., Lee, H-S., Jang, Y-A., and C-I. Kim. 2008 Analytical dietary fiber database for the National Health and Nutrition Survey in Korea. *Journal of Food Composition and Analysis* 21: S35–S42.

Lee, Y.W., Kim, J.D., Zheng, J.Z., and K.H. Row. 2007. Comparisons of isoflavones from Korean and Chinese soybean and processed products. *Biochemical Engineering Journal* 36: 49–53.

Lee, H., Yoon, H., Ji, Y., Kim, H., Park, H., Lee, J., Shin, H., and W.H. Holzapfel. 2011. Functional properties of *Lactobacillus* strains isolated from kimchi. *International Journal of Food Microbiology* 145: 155–161.

Lee, M., Chae, S., Cha, Y., and Y. Park. 2012. Supplementation of Korean fermented soy paste *doenjang* reduces visceral fat in overweight subjects with mutant uncoupling protein-1 allele. *Nutrition Research* 32(1): 8–14.

Lee, H.R., Cho, S.D., Lee, W.K., Kim, G.H., and S.M. Shim. 2014a. Digestive recovery of sulfur-methyl-l-methionine and its bio-accessibility in *Kimchi* cabbages using a simulated *in vitro* digestion model system. *Journal of Science Food and Agriculture* 94: 109–112.

Lee, Y.J., Kim, J.E., Kwak, M.H., Go, J., Kim, D.S., Son, H.J., and D.Y. Hwang. 2014b. Quantitative evaluation of the therapeutic effect of fermented soybean products containing high concentration of GABA on phtalic anhydride-induced atopic dermatitis in IL4/Luc/CNS-1 Tg mice. *International Journal of Molecular Medicine* 33(5): 1185–1194.

Leopold, C.S. and D. Eileler. 2000. Basic coating polymer for the colon-specific drug delivery in inflammatory bowel disease. *Drug Development and Industrial Pharmacy* 26: 1239–1246.

Leroy, F., Verluyten, J., and L. De Vuyst. 2006. Functional meat starter cultures for improved sausage fermentation. *International Journal of Food Microbiology* 106: 270–285.

Liem, I.T.H., Steinkraus, K.H., and T.C. Cronk. 1977. Production of vitamin B12 in tempeh, a fermented soybean food. *Applied and Environmental Microbiology* 34: 773–776.

Lim, J., Seo, B.J., Kim, J.E., Chae, C.S., Im, S.H., Hahn, Y.S., and Y.H. Park. 2011. Characteristics of immunomodulation by a *Lactobacillus sakei* proBio65 isolated from Kimchi. *Korean Journal of Microbiology and Biotechnology* 39: 313–316.

Lindgren, S.E. and W.J. Dobrogosz. 1990. Antagonistic activities of lactic acid bacteria in food and feed fermentations. *FEMS Microbiology Review* 87: 149–164.

Liong, M.T. 2008. Safety of probiotics: Translocation and infection. *Nutrition Review* 66: 192–202.

Liu, C.-F. and T.-M. Pan. 2010. *In vitro* effects of lactic acid bacteria on cancer cell viability and antioxidant activity. *Journal of Food and Drug Analysis* 18(2): 77–86.

Lu, Y., Wang, W., Shan, Y., Zhiqiang E., and L. Wang. 2009. Study on the inhibition of fermented soybean to cancer cells. *Journal of Northeast Agricultural University* 16(1): 25–28.

Macouzet, M., Lee, B.H., and N. Robert. 2009. Production of conjugated linoleic acid by probiotic *Lactobacillus acidophilus* La-5. *Journal of Applied Microbiology* 106: 1886–1891.

MacFarlane, G.T. and J.H. Cummings. 2002. Probiotics, infection and immunity. *Current Opinion in Infectious Diseases* 15: 501–506.

Marteau, P., deVrese, M., Cellier, C.J., and J. Schrezenmeir. 2001. Protection from gastrointestinal diseases with the use of probiotics. *American Journal of Clinical Nutrition* 73: 430S–436S.

Marteau, P., Seksik, P., and R. Jian. 2002. Probiotics and intestinal health effects: A clinical perspective. *British Journal of Nutrition* 88: 51–57.

Martirosyan, D.M. 2011. *Functional Foods and Chronic Diseases: Science and Practice*. Dallas: Food Science Publisher.

Martinez-Villaluenga, C., Peñas, E., Sidro, B., Ullate, M., Frias, J., and C. Vidal-Valverde. 2012. White cabbage fermentation improves ascorbigen content, antioxidant and nitric oxide production inhibitory activity in LPS-induced macrophages. *LWT-Food Science and Technology* 46: 77–83.

McAuliffe, O., Hill, C., and R.P. Ross. 1999. Inhibition of *Listeria monocytogenes* in cottage cheese manufactured with a lacticin 3147-producing starter cultures. *Journal of Applied Microbiology* 86: 251–256.

McFarland, L.V. 2006. Meta-analysis of probiotics for the prevention of antibiotic associated diarrhea and the treatment of *Clostridium difficile* disease. *The American Journal of Gastroenterology* 101: 812–822.

McFarland, L.V. 2007. Meta-analysis of probiotics for the prevention of traveler's diarrhea. *Travel Medicine and Infectious Disease* 5: 97–105.

Meerak, J., Lida, H., Watanabe, Y., Miyashita, M., Sato, H., Nakagawa, Y., and Y. Tahara. 2007. Phylogeny of poly-γ-glutamic acid-producing *Bacillus* strains isolated from fermented soybean foods manufactured in Asian countries. *Journal of General and Applied Microbiology* 53: 315–323.

Meira, S.M.M., Daroit, D.J., Helfer, V.E. et al. 2012. Bioactive peptides in water soluble extract of ovine cheese from southern Brazil and Uruguay. *Food Research International* 48: 322–329.

Menotti, A., Kromhout, D., Blackburn, H., Fidanza, F., Buzina, R., and A. Nissinen. 1999. Food intake patterns and 25 years mortality from coronary heart disease: Cross cultural correlations in the seven countries study. *European Journal of Epidemiology* 15: 507–515.

Mercenier, A., Müller-Alouf, H., and C. Grangette. 2000. *Lactic* acid bacteria as live vaccines. *Currrent Issues in Molecular Biology* 2(1): 17–25.

Meyer, K., Kushi, L., Jacobs, D., Slavin, J., Sellers, T., and A. Folsom. 2000. Carbohydrates, dietary fiber, and incidence of type 2 diabetes in older women. *American Journal of Clinical Nutrition* 71: 921–930.

Meyer, J., Butikofer, U., Walther, B., Wechsler, D., and R. Sieber. 2009. Hot topic: Changes in angiotensin-converting enzyme inhibition and concentration of the teripeptides Val-Pro-Pro and Ile-Pro-Pro during ripening of different Swiss cheese varieties. *Journal of Dairy Science* 92: 826–836.

Mine, Y., Wong, A.H.K., and B. Jiang. 2005. Fibrinolytic enzymes in Asian traditional fermented foods. *Food Research International* 38: 243–250.

Minervini, F., Bilanca, M.T., Siragusa, S., Gobbetti, M., and F. Caponio. 2009. Fermented goat milk produced with selected multiple starters as a potentially functional food. *Food Microbiology* 26: 559–564.

Mishra, N., Gupta, P.N., Khatri, K., Goyal A.K., and S.P. Vyas. 2008. Edible vaccines: A new approach to oral immunization. *Indian Journal of Biotechnology* 7: 283–294.

Mitra, S., Chakrabartty, P.K., and S.R. Biswas. 2010. Potential production and preservation of dahi by *Lactococcus lactis* W8, a nisin-producing strain. *LWT-Food Science and Technology* 43(2): 337–342.

Mitsuoka, T. 1990. Bifidobacteria and their role in human health. *Journal of Industrial Microbiology* 6: 263–268.

Mo, H., Zhu, Y., and Z. Chen. 2008. Review. Microbial fermented tea—A potential source of natural food preservatives. *Trends in Food Science and Technology* 19: 124–130.

Mogensen, G., Salminen, S., O'Brien, J., Ouwehand, A., Holzapfel, W., Shortt, C. et al. 2002. Inventory of micro-organisms with a documented history of use in food. *Bulletin of IDF* 377: 10–19.

Mohania, D., Kansal, V.K., Sagwal, R., and D. Shah. 2013. Anticarcinogenic effect of probiotic dahi and piroxicam on DMH-induced colorectal carcinogenesis in Wister rats. *America Journal of Cancer Therapy and Pharmacology* 1(1): 8–24.

Moktan, B., Saha, J., and P.K. Sarkar, P.K. 2008. Antioxidant activities of soybean as affected by *Bacillus*-fermentation to Kinema *Food Research International* 4(6): 586–593.

Montriwong, A., Kaewphuak, S.,Rodtong, S., and S. Roytrakul. 2012. Novel fibrinolytic enzymes from *Virgibacillus halodenitrificans* SK1–3–7 isolated from fish sauce fermentation. *Process Biochemistry* 47: 2379–2387.

Moon, Y.J., Soh, J.R., Yu, J.J., Sohn, H.S., Cha, Y.S., and S.H. Oh. 2012. Intracellular lipid accumulation inhibitory effect of *Weissella koreensis* OK1-6 isolated from Kimchi on differentiating adipocyte. *Journal of Applied Microbiology* 113: 652–658.

Moslehishad, M., Ehsani, M.R., and M. Salami.2013. The comparative assessment of ACE- inhibitory and antioxidant activities of peptide fractions obtained from fermented camel and bovine milk by *Lactobacillus rhamnosus* PTCC1637. *International Dairy Research* 29: 82–87.

Murakami, H., Asakawa, T., Terao, J., and S. Matsushita. 1984. Antioxidative stability of tempeh and liberation of isoflavones by fermentation. *Agricultural and Biological Chemistry* 48: 2971–2975.

Murata, M., Houdai, T., Yamamoto, H., Matsumori, M., and T. Oishi. 2006. Membrane interaction of soyasaponins in association with their antioxidation effect—Analysis of biomembrane interaction. *Soy Protein Research* 9: 82–86.

Nagai, T. and J.P. Tamang. 2010. Fermented soybeans and non-soybeans legume foods. In: J.P. Tamang and K. Kailasapathy (Eds.), *Fermented Foods and Beverages of the World*. New York: CRC Press, Taylor & Francis Group, pp. 191–224.

Nakajima, N., Nozaki, N., Ishihara, K., Ishikawa, A., and H. Tsuji. 2005. Analysis of isoflavone content in *tempeh*: A fermented soybean product, and preparation of a new isoflavone-enriched *tempeh*. *Journal of Bioscience and Bioengineering* 100: 685–687.

Nakamura, Y., Masuda, O., and T. Takano. 1996. Decrease of tissue angiotensin I-converting enzyme activity upon feeding sour milk in spontaneously hypertensive rats. *Bioscience Biotechnology and Biochemistry* 60: 488–489.

Nakamura, Y., Yamamoto, N., Sakai, K., Okubo, A., Yamazaki, S., and T. Takano. 1995. Purification and characterization of angiotensin I-converting enzyme inhibitors from sour milk. *Journal of Dairy Science* 78: 777–783.

Nam, Y.D., Chang, H.W., Kim, K.H., Roh, S.W., and J.W. Bae. 2009. Metatranscriptome analysis of lactic acid bacteria during kimchi fermentation with genome-probing microarrays. *International Journal of Food Microbiology* 130(2): 140–146.

Nielsen, M.S., Martinussen, T., Flambard, B., Sorensen, K.I. and J. Otte. 2009. Peptide profiles and angiotensin-I-converting enzyme inhibitory activity of fermented milk products: Effect of bacterial strain, fermentation pH, and storage time. *International Dairy Journal* 19: 155–165.

Nikkuni, S., Karki, T.B., Vilku, K.S., Suzuki, T., Shindoh, K., Suzuki, C., and N. Okada. 1995. Mineral and amino acid contents of *kinema*, a fermented soybean food prepared in Nepal. *Food Science and Technology International* 1(2): 107–111.

Nishito, Y., Osana, Y., Hachiya, T., Popendorf, K., Toyoda, A., Fujiyama, A., Itaya, M. and Y. Sakakibara. 2010. Whole genome assembly of a natto production strain *Bacillus subtilis natto* from very short read data. *BMC Genomics* 11: 243. doi: 10.1186/1471-2164-11-243.

Nout, M.J.R. 1994. Fermented foods and food safety. *Food Research International* 27: 291–298.

Nout, M.J.R. and K.E. Aidoo. 2002. Asian fungal fermented food. In H.D.Osiewacz (Ed.), *The Mycota*. New York: Springer-Verlag, pp. 23–47.

Nordvi, B., Egelandsdal, B., Langsrud, O., Ofstad, R., and E. Slinde. 2007. Development of a novel, fermented and dried saithe and salmon product. *Innovative Food Science and Emerging Technologies* 8: 163–171.

Oberhelman, R.A., Gilman, R.H., Sheen, P., Taylor, D.N., Black, R.E., Cabrera, L., Lescano, A.G., Meza, R., and G. Madico. 1999. A placebo-controlled trial of *Lactobacillus* GG to prevent diarrhea in undernourished Peruvian children. *Journal of Pediatrics* 134: 15–20.

Ogborne, A. and R.G. Smart. 2001. Public opinion on the health benefits of moderate drinking: results from a Canadian National Population Health Survey. *Addiction (Abingdon, England)* 96: 641–9.

Okada, N. 1989. Role of microorganism in *tempe*h manufacture. Isolation of vitamin B12 producing bacteria. *Japan Agricultural Research Quarterly* 22(4): 310–316.

Okamoto, A., Hanagata, H., Matsumoto, E., Kawamura, Y., Koizumi, Y., and F. Yanagida. 1995. Angiotensin I converting enzyme inhibitory activities of various fermented foods. *Bioscience Biotechnology and Biochemistry* 59: 1147–1149.

Ogawa, T., Bando, N., Tsuji, H., Okajima, H., Nishikawa, K., and K. Sasaoka. 1991. Investigation of the IgE-binding protein in soybeans by immunoblotting with the sera of the soybean-sensitive patients with atopic dermatitis. *Journal of Nutritional Science and Vitaminology* 37: 555–565.

Omizu, Y., Tsukamoto, C., Chettri, R., and J.P. Tamang. 2011. Determination of saponin contents in raw soybean and fermented soybean foods of India. *Journal of Scientific and Industrial Research* 70: 533–538.

Onwulata, C.I., Ramkishan, R.D., and P. Vankineni. 1989. Relative efficiency of yoghurt, sweet acidophilus milk, hydrolysed-lactose milk, and a commercial lactase tablet in alleviating lactose maldigestion. *American Journal of Clinical Nutrition* 49: 1233–1237.

Oppermann-Sanio, F.B. and A. Steinbüchel. 2002. Occurence, functions and biosynthesis of polyamides in microorganisms and biotechnological productions. *Naturwissenschaften* 89: 11–22.

Otes, S. and O. Cagindi. 2003. Kefir: A probiotic dairy-composition, nutritional and therapeutic aspects. *Pakistan Journal of Nutrition* 2: 54–59.

Ouwehand, A.C., Salminen, S., and E. Isolauri, E. 2002. Probiotics: An overview of beneficial effects. *Antonie Van Leeuwenhoek* 82: 279–289.

Özdestan, Ö. and A. Üren. 2013. Biogenic amine content of *Tarhana*: A traditional fermented food. *International Journal of Food Properties* 16: 416–428.

Papadimitriou, C.G., Vafopoulou-Mastrojiannaki, A., Silva, S.V., Gomes, A.M., Malcata, F.X., and E. Alichanidis. 2007. Identification of peptides in traditional and probiotic sheep milk yoghurt with angiotensin I-converting enzyme (ACE)-inhibitory activity. *Food Chemistry* 105: 647–656.

Park, K.Y. 1995. The nutritional evaluation, and antimutagenic and anticancer effects of Kimchi. *Journal of the Korean Society of Food and Nutrition (KoreaRepublic)* 24(1): 169–182.

Park, K.Y. and B.K. Kim. 2010. *Kimchi* lactic acid bacteria and health benefits. *FASEB Journal* 24: (Meeting Abstract Supplement) No. 340.6.

Park, K.-Y., Kil, J.-H., Jung, K.O., Kong, C.S., and J. Lee. 2006. Functional properties of kimchi (Korean fermented vegetables). *Acta Horticulturae* 706: 167–172.

Park, J.-E., Moon, Y.J., and Y.-S. Cha. 2008. Effect of functional materials producing microbial strains isolated from Kimchi on antiobesity and inflammatory cytokines in 3T3-L1 preadipocytes. *The FASEB Journal* 23:111.2.

Park, J.M., Shin, J.H., Gu, J.G., Yoon, S.J., Song, J.C., Jeon, W.M., Suh, H.J., Chang, U.J., Yang, C.Y., and J.M. Kim. 2011. Effect of antioxidant activity in kimchi during a short-term and over-ripening fermentation period. *Journal of Bioscience and Bioengineering* 112: 356–359.

Park, J.A., TirupathiPichiah, P.B., Yu, J.J., Oh, S.H., Daily, J.W. 3rd, and Cha, Y.S. 2012. Anti-obesity effect of kimchi fermented with *Weissella koreensis* OK1–6 as starter in high-fat diet-induced obese C57BL/6 J mice. *Journal of Applied Microbiology*113: 1507–1516.

Park, K.Y., Jeong, J.K., Lee, Y.E., and Daily, J.W. 3rd. 2014. Health benefits of kimchi (Korean fermented vegetables) as a probiotic food. *Journal of Medicine Foods* 17(1): 6–20.

Parvez, S., Malik, K.A., Ah Kang, S., and H.Y. Kim. 2006. Probiotics and their fermented food products are beneficial for health. *Journal of Applied Microbiology* 100: 1171–1185.

Patel, A., Prajapati, J.B., Holst, O., and A. Ljungh. 2014. Determining probiotic potential of exopolysaccharide producing LAB isolated from vegetables and traditional Indianfermented food products. *Food Bioscience* 5: 27–33.

Pattanagul, P., Pinthong, R., Phianmongkhol, A., and S. Tharatha. 2008. Mevinolin, citrinin and pigments of adlay *angkak* fermented by *Monascus* sp. *International Journal of Food Microbiology* 126(1): 20–23.

Paucar-Menacho, L.M., Amaya-Farfan, J., Berhow, M.A., Mandarino, J.M.G., Gonzalez de Mejia, E., and Y.K. Chang. 2010. A high-protein soybean cultivar contains lower isoflavones and saponins but higher minerals and bioactive peptides than a low-protein cultivar. *Food Chemistry* 120: 15–21.

Pawiroharsono, S. 2002. Tempe fermentation: products, technologies, and improvement of bioactive contents. In: K. Liu, J. Gui, R. Tschang, N. Zhuo and Y. Yu (Eds.), *The Proceedings of China and International Soybean Conference* 2002, CCOA and AOCS, Beijing. November 6–9, 2002, pp. 222–223.

Pedone, C.A., Arnaud, C.C., Postaire, E.R., Bouley, C.F., and P. Reinert. 2000. Multicentric study of the effect of milk fermented by *Lactobacillus casei* on the incidence of diarrhoea. International *Journal of Clinical Practice* 54: 568–571.

Peñas, E., Limón, R.I.,Vidal-Valverde, C., and J. Frias. 2013. Effect of storage on the content of indole-glucosinolate breakdown products and vitamin C of sauerkrauts treated by high hydrostatic pressure. *LWT-Food Science and Technology* 53: 285–289.

Pereira, M.A., Jacobs, D.R. Jr., Pins, J.J., Raatz, S.K., and M.D. Gross. 2002. Effect of whole grains on insulin sensitivity in overweight hyper insulinemic adults. *American Journal of Clinical Nutrition* 75: 848–855.

Perna, A., Intaglietta, I., Simonetti, A., and E. Gambacorta. 2013. Effect of genetic type and casein halotype on antioxidant activity of yogurts during storage. *Journal of Dairy Science* 96: 1–7.

Phelan, M. and D. Kerins. 2011. The potential role of milk derived peptides in cardiovascular diseases. *Food and Function* 2: 153–167.

Peng, Y., Huang, Q., Zhang, R., and Y. Zhang. 2003. Purification and characterization of a fibrinolytic enzyme produced by *Bacillus amyloliquefaciens* DC-4 screened from *douchi*, a traditional Chinese soybean food. *Comparative Biochemistry and Physiology-B Biochemistry and Molecular Biology* 134: 45–52.

Pilet, M.-F. and F. Leroi. 2011. Applications of protective cultures, bacteriocins and bacteriophages in fresh seafood and seafood products. In: C. Lacroix (Ed.), *Protective Cultures, Antimicrobial Metabolites and Bacteriophages for Food and Beverage Biopreservation*. Cambridge: Woodhead Publishing Limited.

Prasad, J., Gill, H., Smart, J., and P.K. Gopal. 1998. Selection and characterization of *Lactobacillus* and *Bifidobacterium* strains for use as probiotic. *International Dairy Journal* 8: 993–1002.

Prado, F.C., Parada, J.L., Pandey, A., and C.R. Soccol. 2008. Trends in non-dairy probiotic beverages. *Food Research International* 41: 111–123.

Qian, B., Xing, M., Cui, L., Deng, Y., Xu, Y., Huang, M., and S. Zhang. 2011. Antioxidant, antihypertensive, and immunomodulatory activities of peptide fraction from fermented skim milk with *Lactobacillus delbrueckii* ssp *bulgaricus* LB340. *Journal of Dairy Research* 78: 72–79.

Quiros, A., Hernandez-Ledesma, B., Ramos, M., Amigo, L., and I. Recio. 2005. Angiotensin-converting enzyme inhibitory activity of peptides derived from *caprinekefir*. *Journal of Dairy Science* 88: 3480–3487.

Rabie, M.A., Siliha, H., El-Saidy, S., El-Badawy, A.A., and F.X. Malcata. 2011. Reduced biogenic amine contents in sauerkraut via addition of selected LAB. *Food Chemistry* 129:1778–1782.

Rai, A.K., Palni, U., and J.P. Tamang. 2010. Microbiological studies of ethnic meat products of the Eastern Himalayas. *Meat Science* 85: 560–567.

Rai, R., Kharel, N., and J.P. Tamang. 2014. HACCP model of *kinema*, a fermented soybean food. *Journal of Scientific and Industrial Research* 73: 588–592.

Rajalakshmi, R. and K. Vanaja. 1967. Chemical and biological evaluation of the effects of fermentation on the nutritive value of foods prepared from rice and grams. *British Journal of Nutrition* 21: 467–473.

Ramadori, G., Gautron, L., Fujikawa, T., Claudia, R., Vianna, J., Elmquist, E., and R. Coppari. 2009. Central administration of resveratrol improves diet-induced diabetes. *Endocrinology* 150: 5326–5333.

Ramírez, J.F., Sánchez-Marroquín, A., Aívarez, M.M., and R. Valyasebi. 2004. Industrialization of Mexican pulque. In: K. Steinkraus (Ed.), *Industrialization of Indigenous Fermented Foods*, 2nd ed. New York: Marcel Deckker, pp. 547–586.

Ranadheera, R., Baines, S., and M. Adams. 2010. Importance of food in probiotic efficacy. *Food Research International* 43: 1–7.

Ratanaburee, A., Kantachote, D., Charernjiratrakul, W., and A. Sukhoom. 2013. Selection of γ-aminobutyric acid-producing lactic acid bacteria and their potential as probiotics for use as starter cultures in Thai fermented sausages (Nham). *International Journal of Food Science and Technology* 48(7): 1371–1382.

Rauscher-Gabernig, E., Grossgut, R., Bauer, F., and P. Paulsen. 2009. Assessment of alimentary histamine exposure of consumers in Austria and development of tolerable levels in typical foods. *Food Control* 20: 423–429.

Re, R., Pellegrini, N., Proteggente, A., Pannala, A., Yang, M., and C. Rice Evans. 1999. Antioxidant activity applying an improved ABTS radical cation decolorization assay. *Free-Radical Biology Medicine* 26: 1231–1237.

Rebucci, R., Sangalli, L., Fava, M., Bersani, C., Cantoni, C., and A. Baldi. 2007. Evaluation of functional aspects in *Lactobacillus strains* isolated from dry fermented sausages. *Journal of Food Quality* 30: 187–201.

Reddy, N.R. and D.K. Salunkhe. 1980. Effect of fermentation on phytate phosphorus, and mineral content in black gram, rice, and black gram and rice blends. *Journal of Food Science* 45: 1708–1712.

Regnstrom, J., Nilsson, J., Strom, K., Bavenholm, P., Tornvall, P., and A. Hamsten. 1996. Inverse relationship between concentration of vitamin E and severity of coronary artery disease. *American Journal of Clinical Nutrition* 63: 377–385.

Renault, P. 2002. Genetically modified lactic acid bacteria: Applications to food or health and risk assessment. *Biochemistry* 84: 1073–1087.

Rhee, C.H. and H.-D. Park. 2001. Three glycoproteins with antimutagenic activity identified in *Lactobacillus plantarum* KLAB21. *Applied and Environmental Microbiology* 67: 3445–3449.

Rho, S.J., Lee, J.S., Chung, Y.L., Kim, Y.W., and H.G. Lee. 2009. Purification and identification of an angiotensing I-converting enzyme inhibitory peptide from fermented soybean extract. *Process Biochemistry* 44: 490–493.

Rivera-Espinoza, Y. and Y. Gallardo-Navarro. 2010. Non-dairy probiotic products. *Food Microbiology* 27: 1–11.

Rodríguez, J.M., Martínez, M.I., and J. Kok. 2002. Pediocin PA-1, a wide-spectrum bacteriocin from lactic acid bacteria. *Critical Review in Food Science and Nutrition* 42(2): 91–121.

Rosenberg, M. 1984. Bacterial adherence to hydrocarbons: A useful technique for studying cell surface hydrophobicity. *FEMS Microbiology Letters* 22: 289–295.

Rosenberg, M., Gutnick, D., and E. Rosenberg. 1980. Adherence of bacteria to hydrocarbons: A simple method for measuring cell-surface hydrophobicity. *FEMS Microbiology Letters* 9: 29–33.

Rowlands, J.C. and J.E. Hoadley. 2006. FDA perspectives on health claims for food labels. *Toxicology* 221: 35–43.

Rubia-Soria, A., Abriouel, H., Lucas, R., Omar, N.B., Martinez-Caõamero, M. and A. Gálvez. 2006. Production of antimicrobial substances by bacteria isolated from fermented table olives. *World Journal of Microbiology and Biotechnology* 22(7): 765–768.

Rudel, L.L. and M.D. Morris. 1973. Determination of cholesterol using *o*-phthalaldehyde. *Journal of Lipid Research* 14: 364–366.

Rühmkorf, C., Jungkunz, S., Wagner, M., and R.F. Vogel. 2012. Optimization of homoexopolysaccharide formation by lactobacilli in gluten-free sourdoughs. *Food Microbiology* 32: 286–294.

Ryu, B.M., Ryu, S.H., Jeon, Y.S., Lee, Y.S., and G.S. Moon. 2004a. Inhibitory effect of solvent fraction of various kinds of kimchi on ultraviolet B induced oxidation and erythema formation of hairless mice skin. *Journal of the Korean Society of Food Science and Nutrition* 33: 785–790.

Ryu, B.M., Ryu, S.H., Lee, Y.S., Jeon, Y.S., and G.S. Moon. 2004b. Effect of different kimchi diets on oxidation and photooxidation in liver and skin of hairless mice. *Journal of the Korean Society of Food Science and Nutrition* 33: 291–298.

Saad, N., Delattre, C., Urdaci, M., Schmitter, J.M., and P. Bressollier. 2013. An overview of the last advances in probiotic and prebiotic field. *LWT Food Science and Technology* 50: 1–16.

Sabeena, F.K.H., Baron, C.P., Nielsen, N.S., and C. Jacobsen. 2010. Antioxidant activity of yoghurt peptides: Part 1-in vitro assays and evaluation in ω-3 enriched milk. *Food Chemistry* 123: 1081–1089.

Saikali, J., Picard, V., Freitas, M., and P. Holt. 2004. Fermented milks, probiotic cultures, and colon cancer. *Nutrition and Cancer* 49: 14–24.

Saito, T., Iso, N., Mizuno, H., Kaneoa, H., Suyama, Y., Kawamura, S., and S. Osawa. 1974. Conformational change of a natto mucin in solution. *Agricultural and Biological Chemistry* 38: 1941–1946.

Saito, T., Nakamura, T., Kitazawa, H., Kawai, Y., and T. Itoh. 2000. Isolation and structural analysis of antihypertensive peptides that exist naturally in Gouda cheese. *Journal of Dairy Cheese* 83: 1434–1440.

Salminen, S., Isolauri, E., and E. Salminen. 1996. Clinical uses of probiotics for stabilizing the gut mucosal barrier: Successful strains for future challenges. *Antonie van Leeuwenhoek* 70: 347–358.

Sanders, M.E. and T.R. Klaenhammer. 2001. Invited review: The scientific basis of *Lactobacillus acidophilus* NCFM functionality as a probiotic. *Journal of Dairy Science* 84: 319–331.

Sarkar, P.K. and J.P. Tamang. 1995. Changes in the microbial profile and proximate composition during natural and controlled fermentations of soybeans to produce kinema. *Food Microbiology* 12: 317–325.

Sarkar, P.K., Jones, L.J., Craven, G.S., and S.M. Somerset. 1997a. Oligosaccharides profile of soybeans during kinema production. *Letters in Applied Microbiology* 24: 337–339.

Sarkar, P.K., Jones, L.J., Craven, G.S., Somerset, S.M., and C. Palmer. 1997b. Amino acid profiles of kinema, a soybean-fermented food. *Food Chemistry* 59(1): 69–75.

Sarkar, P.K., Jones, L.J., Gore, W., Craven, G.S., and S.M. Somerset. 1996. Changes in soyabean lipid profiles during kinema production. *Journal of Science of Food and Agriculture* 71: 321–328.

Sarkar, P.K., Morrison, E., Tingii, U., Somerset, S.M., and G.S. Craven. 1998. B-group vitamin and mineral contents of soybeans during kinema production. *Journal of Science of Food and Agriculture* 78: 498–502.

Schillinger, U., Stiles, M.E., and W.H. Holzapfel. 1993. Bacteriocin production by *Carnobacterium piscicola* LV 61. *International Journal of Food Microbiology* 20: 131–147.

Schillinger, U., Ban-Koffi, L., and C.M.A.P. Franz. 2010. Tea, coffee and cacao. In: J.P. Tamang and K. Kailasapathy (Eds.), *Fermented Foods and Beverages of the World*. New York: CRC Press, Taylor & Francis Group, pp. 353–375.

Schiffrin, E.J. and S. Blum. 2001. Food processing: Probiotic microorganisms for beneficial foods. *Current Opinion in Biotechnology* 12: 499–502.

Seppo, L., Jauhiainen, T., Poussa, T., and R. Korpela. 2003. A fermented milk high in bioactive peptides has a blood pressure-lowering effect in hypertensive subjects. *American Journal of Clinical Nutrition* 77: 326–330.

Seppo, L., Kerojoki, O., Suomalainen, T., and R. Korpela. 2002. The effect of a Lactobacillus helveticus LBK-16 H fermented milk on hypertension—A pilot study on humans. *Milchwissen* 57: 124–127.

Shah, N.P. 2001. Functional foods from probiotics and prebiotics. *Food Technology* 55(11): 46–53.

Shah, N.P. 1993. Effectiveness of dairy products in alleviation of lactose intolerance. *Food Australia* 45: 268–271.

Shah, N.P. 2004. Probiotics and prebiotics. *Agro Food Industry HiTech* 15(1): 13–16.

Shah, N.P. 2007. Functional cultures and health benefits. *International Dairy Journal* 17: 1262–1277.

Shah N.P. and P. Jelen. 1991. Lactose absorption by post-weanling rats from yoghurt, quarg, and quarg whey. *Journal of Dairy Science* 74: 1512–1520.

Shah, N.P., Fedorak, R.N., and P. Jelen. 1992. Food consistency effects of quarg in lactose absorption by lactose intolerant individuals. *International Dairy Journal* 2: 257–269.

Shah, N.P., da Cruz, A.G., and Faria, J.d.A.F. (Eds.). 2013. *Probiotics and Probiotic Foods: Technology, Stability and Benefits to Human Health*. New York: Nova Science Publishers.

Shanahan, F. 2001. Inflammatory bowel disease: Immunodiagnostics, immunotherapeutics, and ecotherapeutics. *Gastroenterology* 120: 622–635.

Shin, M.S., Han, S.K., Ryu, J.S., Kim, K.S., and W.K. Lee. 2008. Isolation and partial characterization of a bacteriocin produced by *Pediococcus pentosaceus* K23-2 isolated from kimchi. *Journal of Applied Microbiology* 105(2): 331–339.

Shin, S.K., Kwon, J.H., Jeon, M., Choi, J., and M.S. Choi. 2011. Supplementation of *Cheonggukjang* and Red Ginseng *Cheonggukjang* can improve plasma lipid profile and fasting blood glucose concentration in subjects with impaired fasting glucose. *Journal of Medicinal Food* 14: 108–113.

Shon, D.H., Lee, K.E., Ahn, C.W., Nam, H.S., Lee, H.J., and J.K. Shin. 1996. Screening of antithrombotic peptides from soybean paste by the microplate method. *Korean Journal of Food Science and Technology* 28: 684–688.

Shon, M-Y., Lee, J., Choi, J-H., Choi, S-Y., Nam, S-H., Seo, K-I., Lee, S-W., Sung, N-J., and S-K. Park. 2007. Antioxidant and free radical scavenging activity of methanol extract of chungkukjang. *Journal of Food Composition and Analysis* 20: 113–118.

Shrestha, A.K. and Noomhorn, A. 2001. Composition and functional properties of fermented soybean flour (*Kinema*). *Journal of Food Science and Technology* 38 (5): 467–470.

Shrestha, A.K. and Noomhorm, A. 2002. Composition and physicochemical properties supplemented with soy and *kinema* flour. *International Journal of Food Science and Technology* 37: 361–368.

Silla-Santos, M.H. 2001. Toxic nitrogen compounds produced during processing: Biogenic amines, ethyl carbamides, nitrosamines. In: M.R. Adams and M.J.R. Nout (Eds.), *Fermentation and Food Safety*. Gaithersburg, Maryland: Aspen Publishers, Inc. pp. 119–140.

Sim, K.H. and Y.S. Han. 2008. Effect of red pepper seed on kimchi antioxidant activity during fermentation. *Food Science and Biotechnology* 17(2): 295–301.

Singh, T.A., Devi, K.R., Ahmed, G., and K. Jeyaram. 2014. Microbial and endogenous origin of fibrinolytic activity in traditional fermented foods of Northeast India. *Food Research International* 55: 356–62.

Sinha, P.R. and Sinha, R.N. 2000. Importance of good quality dahi in food. *Indian Dairyman* 52: 45–47.

Sipola, M., Finckenberg, P., Korpela, R., Vapaatalo, H., and M. Nurminen. 2002. Effect of long-term intake of milk products on blood pressure in hypertensive rats. *Journal of Dairy Research* 69: 103–111.

Siró, I., Kapolna, E., Kapolna, B., and A. Lugasi. 2008. Functional food: Product development, marketing and consumer acceptance—A review. *Appetite* 51: 456–467.

Slavin, J., Jacobs, D., and L. Marquart. 1997. Whole-grain consumption and chronic disease: Protective mechanisms. *Nutrition and Cancer* 27: 14–21.

Sloan, A.E. 2014. The top ten functional food trends. *Food Technology* 68(4): 24, 26, 28, 30–32, 36–41.

Solga, S.F. 2003. Probiotics can treat hepatic encephalopathy. *Medical Hypotheses* 61: 307–313.

Solis, P. and D. Lemonnier. 1996. Induction of human cytokines by bacteria used in dairy foods. *Nutrition Research* 13: 1127–1140.

Sonar, N.R. and P.M. Halami. 2014. Phenotypic identification and technological attributes of native lactic acid bacteria present in fermented bamboo shoot products from North-East India. *Journal of Food Science and Technology* 51(12): 4143–4148.

Stanley, N.R. and Lazazzera, B.A. 2005. Defining the genetic differences between wild and domestic strains of *Bacillus subtilis* that affect poly-γ-dl-glutamic acid production and biofilm formation, *Molecular Microbiology* 57: 1143–1158.

Stein, K. 2000. FDA approves health claim labeling for foods containing soy protein. *Journal of the American Dietetic Association* 100: 292–298.

Steinkraus, K.H. 1994. Nutritional significance of fermented foods. *Food Research International* 27: 259–267.

Steinkraus, K.H. 1996. *Handbook of Indigenous Fermented Food*, 2nd ed. New York: Marcel Dekker, Inc.

Stiles, M.E. and W.H. Holzapfel. 1997. Lactic acid bacteria of foods and their current taxonomy. *International Journal of Food Microbiology* 36: 1–29.

Steinkraus, K.H., van Veer, A.G., and D.B. Thiebeau. 1967. Studies on idli-an Indian fermented black gram-rice food. *Food Technology* 21(6): 110–113.

Subbiah, M. 1998. Mechanisms of the cardioprotection of estrogens. *Experimental Biology and Medicine* 217: 23–52.

Suganuma, T., Fujita, K.,and K. Kitahara. 2007. Some distinguishable properties between acid-stable and neutral types of α-amylases from acid-producing *Koji*. *Journal of Bioscience and Bioengineering* 104: 353–362.

Sumi, H., Hamada, H., S. Tsushima, Mihara, H., and H. Muraki. 1987. A novel fibrinolytic enzyme (nattokinase) in the vegetable cheese natto, a typical and popular soybean food of the Japanese diet. *Experientia* 43: 1110–1111.

Sumi, H., Nakajima, N., and C. Yatagai. 1995. A unique strong fibrinolytic enzyme (*katsuwokinase*) in skipjack *"shiokara"*, a Japanese traditional fermented food. *Comparative Biochemistry and Physiology—B Biochemistry and Molecular Biology* 112: 543–547.

Sumi, H. and T. Okamoto. 2003. Thrombolytic activity of an aqueous extract of *tempe*. *Journal of Home Economics of Japan* 54: 337–342 (in Japanese).

Sun, Y.P., Chou, C.C., and R.C. Yu. 2009. Antioxidant activity of lactic-fermented Chinese cabbage. *Food Chemistry* 115(3): 912–917.

Suomalainen, T.H. and A.M. Mäyär-Mäkinen. 1999. Propionic acid bacteria as protective cultures in fermented milks and breads. *Lait* 79: 165–174.

Suzzi, G. and Gardini, F. 2003. Biogenic amines in dry fermented sausages: A review. *International Journal of Food Microbiology* 88(1): 41–54.

Syal, P. and A. Vohra. 2013. Probiotic potential of yeasts isolated from traditional Indian fermented foods. *International Journal of Microbiology Research* 5: 390–398.

Szajewska, H., Skorka, A., Ruszczynski, M., and D. Gieruszczak-bialek. 2007. Meta-analysis: *Lactobacillus* GG for treating acute diarrhoea in children. *Alimentary Pharmacology and Therapeutics* 25: 871–881.

Tamang, J.P. 2007. Fermented foods for human life. In: A.K. Chauhan, A. Verma, and H. Kharakwal (Eds.), *Microbes for Human Life*. New Delhi: I.K. International Publishing House Pvt. Limited, pp. 73–87.

Tamang, J.P. 2010a. *Himalayan Fermented Foods: Microbiology, Nutrition, and Ethnic Values*. New York: CRC Press, Taylor & Francis Group.

Tamang, J.P. 2010b. Diversity of fermented foods. In: J.P. Tamang and K. Kailasapathy (Eds.), *Fermented Foods and Beverages of the World*. New York: CRC Press, Taylor & Francis Group, pp. 41–84.

Tamang, J.P. 2010c. Diversity of fermented beverages. In: J.P. Tamang and K. Kailasapathy (Eds.), *Fermented Foods and Beverages of the World*. New York: CRC Press, Taylor & Francis Group, pp. 85–125.

Tamang, J.P., Chettri, R., and R.M. Sharma. 2009a. Indigenous knowledge of Northeast women on production of ethnic fermented soybean foods. *Indian Journal of Traditional Knowledge* 8 (1): 122–126.

Tamang, J.P., Dewan, S., Tamang, B., Rai, A., Schillinger, U., and W.H. Holzapfel. 2007. Lactic acid bacteria in *Hamei* and *Marcha* of North East India. *Indian Journal of Microbiology* 47 (2): 119–125.

Tamang, J.P., Dewan, S., Thapa, S., Olasupo, N. A., Schillinger, U., and W.H. Holzapfel. 2000. Identification and enzymatic profiles of predominant lactic acid bacteria isolated from soft-variety *chhurpi*, a traditional cheese typical of the Sikkim Himalayas. *Food Biotechnology* 14(1&2): 99–112.

Tamang, J.P. and S. Nikkuni. 1996. Selection of starter culture for production of kinema, fermented soybean food of the Himalaya. *World Journal of Microbiology and Biotechnology* 12(6): 629–635.

Tamang, J.P. and S. Nikkuni. 1998. Effect of temperatures during pure culture fermentation of Kinema. *World Journal of Microbiology and Biotechnology* 14(6): 847–850.

Tamang, B. and J.P. Tamang. 2009. Lactic acid bacteria isolated from indigenous fermented bamboo products of Arunachal Pradesh in India and their functionality. *Food Biotechnology* 23: 133–147.

Tamang, B. and J.P. Tamang. 2010. *In situ* fermentation dynamics during production of *gundruk* and *khalpi*, ethnic fermented vegetables products of the Himalayas. *Indian Journal of Microbiology* 50(Suppl 1): 93–98.

Tamang, B., Tamang, J.P., Schillinger, U., Franz, C.M.A.P., Gores, M., and W.H. Holzapfel. 2008. Phenotypic and genotypic identification of lactic acid bacteria isolated from ethnic fermented tender bamboo shoots of North East India. *International Journal of Food Microbiology* 121: 35–40.

Tamang, J.P. and S. Thapa. 2006. Fermentation dynamics during production of bhaati jaanr, a traditional fermented rice beverage of the Eastern Himalayas. *Food Biotechnology* 20(3): 251–261.

Tamang, J.P., Tamang, B., Schillinger, U., Franz, C.M.A.P., Gores, M., and W.H. Holzapfel. 2005. Identification of predominant lactic acid bacteria isolated from traditional fermented vegetable products of the Eastern Himalayas. *International Journal of Food Microbiology* 105(3): 347–356.

Tamang, J.P., Tamang, B., Schillinger, U., Guigas, C., and W.H. Holzapfel. 2009b. Functional properties of lactic acid bacteria isolated from ethnic fermented vegetables of the Himalayas. *International Journal of Food Microbiology* 135: 28–33.

Taylor, S.L. 1986. Histamine food poisoning: toxicology and clinical aspects. *CRC Critical Review in Toxicology* 17: 91–128.

Taylor, S.L., Leatherwood, M., and E.R. Lieber. 1978. Histamine in sauerkraut. *Journal of Food Science* 43: 1030–1032.

ten Brink, B., Damink, C., Joosten, H.J., and J. Huis in't Veld. 1990. Occurrence and formation of biologically active amines in foods. *International Journal of Food Microbiology* 11: 73–84.

Thapa, N., Pal, J., and J.P. Tamang. 2004. Microbial diversity in *ngari, hentak* and *tungtap,* fermented fish products of Northeast India. *World Journal of Microbiology and Biotechnology* 20: 599–607.

Thapa, S. and J.P. Tamang. 2004. Product characterization of kodo ko jaanr: Fermented finger millet beverage of the Himalayas. *Food Microbiology* 21: 617–622.

Tolhurst, G., Heffron, H., Lam, Y.S., Parker, H.E., Habib, A.M., Diakogiannaki, E., Cameron, J., Grosse, J., Reimann, F., and F.M. Gribble. 2012. Short-chain fatty acids stimulate glucagon-like peptide-1 secretion via the g-protein-coupled receptor FFAR2. *Diabetes* 61: 364–371.

Tongnual, P. and M.L. Fields. 1979. Fermentation and relative nutritive value of rice meal and chips. *Journal of Food Science* 44: 1784–1785.

Truelsen, T., Gronbaek, M., Schnohr, P., and G. Boysen. 1998. Intake of beer, wine, and spirits and risk of stroke: The Copenhagen city heart study. *Stroke* 29: 2467–2472.

Tsubura, S. 2012. Anti-periodontitis effect of *Bacillus subtilis* (*natto*). *Shigaku (Odontology)* 99: 160–164.

Tsuji, H., Okada, N., Yamanishi, R., Bando, N., Kimoto, M., and T. Ogawa. 1995. Measurement of Gly m Bd 30 K, a major soybean allergen, in soybean products by a sandwich enzyme-linked immunosorbent assay. *Bioscience, Biotechnology, and Biochemistry* 59: 150–151.

Tsukamoto, Y., Ichise, H., Kakuda, H., and M. Yamaguchi. 2000. Intake of fermented soybean (natto) increases circulating vitamin K_2 (menaquinone-7) and γ-carboxylated osteocalcin concentration in normal individuals. *Journal of Bone and Mineral Metabolism* 18: 216–222.

Tsuyoshi, N., Fudou, R., Yamanaka, S., Kozaki, M., Tamang, N., S. Thapa, and J.P. Tamang. 2005. Identification of yeast strains isolated from marcha in Sikkim, a microbial starter for amylolytic fermentation. *International Journal of Food Microbiology* 99(2): 135–146.

Ueda, S. 1989. Bacillus subtilis. In: B. Maruo and H. Yoshikawa (Eds.), *Molecular Biology and Industrial Applications.* Elsevier and Kodansha Ltd, Amsterdam pp. 143–161.

Ueda, S. and S. Kano. 1975. Multiple forms of glucoamylase of *Rhizopus* species. *Die Stärke* 27(4): 123–128.

Ueda, S. and B.C. Saha. 1983. Behavior of *Endomycopsis fibuligera* glucoamylase towards raw starch. *Enzyme and Microbial Technology* 5: 196–198.

Urushibata, Y., Tokuyama, S., and Tahara, Y. 2002. Characterization of the *Bacillus subtilis ywsC* gene, involved in λ–polyglutamic acid production. *Journal of Bacteriology* 184(2): 337–343.

Vanderhoof, J.A., 2001. Probiotics: Future directions. *American Journal of Clinical Nutrition* 73: 1152–1155.

van Loosdrecht, M.C.M., Lyklema, J., Norde, W., Schraa, G., and Zehnder, A.J.B. 1987. The role of bacterial cell wall hydrophobicity in adhesion. *Applied and Environmental Microbiology* 53(8): 1893–1897.

Verhagen, H., Vos, E., Francl, S., Heinonen, M., and van Loveren, H. 2010. Status of nutrition and health claims in Europe. *Arch. Biochemistry and Biophysics* 501: 6–15.

Vijayendra, S.V.N., Palanivel, G., Mahadevamma, S., and R.N. Tharanathan. 2008. Physico-chemical characterization of an exopolysaccharide produced by a non-ropy strain of *Leuconostoc* sp. CFR 2181 isolated from *dahi*, an Indian traditional lactic fermented milk product. *Carbohydrate Polymers* 72: 300–307.

Wacher, C., Díaz-Ruiz, G., and J.P. Tamang. 2010. Fermented vegetable products. In: J.P. Tamang and K. Kailasapathy (Eds.), *Fermented Foods and Beverages of the World.* New York: CRC Press, Taylor & Francis Group, pp. 149–190.

Waldherr, F.W. and R.F. Vogel. 2009. Commercial exploitation of homo-exopolysaccharides in non-dairy food systems. In: M. Ullrich (Eds.), *Bacterial Polysaccharides: Current Innovations and Future Trends* Norfolk: Caister Academic Press, pp. 313–329.

Wallerath, T., Li, H., Godtel-Ambrust, U., Schwarz, P.M., and U. Forstermann. 2005. A blend of polyphenolic compounds explains the stimulatory effect of red wine on human endothelial NO synthase. *Nitric Oxide* 12(2): 97–104.

Walker, G.M. 2014. Microbiology of winemaking. In: C. Batt and M.A. Tortorello (Eds.), *Encyclopaedia of Food Microbiology*, 2nd ed.). Oxford: Elsevier Ltd., pp. 787–792.

Wang, L.-J., Li, D., Zou, L., Chen, X.D., Cheng, Y.-Q., Yamaki, K., and L.-T. Li. 2007a. Antioxidative activity of *douchi* (a Chinese traditional salt-fermented soybean food) extracts during its processing. *International Journal of Food Properties* 10: 1–12.

Wang, L.-j., Yin, L.-j., Li, D., Zou, L., Saito, M., Tatsumi, E., and Li, L.-T. 2007b. Influences of processing and NaCl supplementation on isoflavone contents and composition during douchi manufacturing. *Food Chemistry* 101: 1247–1253.

Waterhouse, A. 2005. Folin-Ciocalteau micro method for total phenol in wine. Retrieved May 4, 2005, from http://waterhouse.ucdavis.edu/phenol/folinmicro.htm.

Weill, F.S., Cela, E.M., Paz, M.L., Ferrari, A., Leoni, J., and D.H. Gonzalez Maglio. 2013. Lipoteichoic acid from *Lactobacillus rhamnosus GG* as an oral photoprotective agent against UV-induced carcinogenesis. *British Journal of Nutrition* 109: 457–466.

Westby, A. and D.R. Twiddy. 1991. Role of microorganisms in the reduction of cyanide during traditional processing of African cassava products. In: A. Westby and P.J.A. Reilly (Eds.), *Proceeding of Workshop on Traditional African Foods—Quality and Nutrition*. Stockholm: International Foundation for Science, pp. 127–131.

Winkler, C., Wirleitner, B., Schroecksnadel, K., Schennach, H., and D. Fuchs. 2005. *In vitro* effects of beetroot juice on stimulated and unstimulated peripheral blood mononuclearcells. *American Journal of Biochemistry and Biotechnology* 1: 180–185.

Wood, B.J.B. and M.M. Hodge. 1985. Yeast-lactic acid bacteria interactions and their contribution to fermented foodstuffs. In: B.J.B. Wood (Ed.), *Microbiology of Fermented Foods*, Vol I. London: Elsevier Applied Science Publication, pp. 263–293.

Won, T.J., Kim, B., Song, D.S., Lim, Y.T., Oh, E.S., Lee, D.I., Park, E.S., Min, H., Park, S., and K.W. Hwang. 2011. Modulation of Th1/Th2 balance by *Lactobacillus* strains isolated from *kimchi* via stimulation of macrophage cell line J774A.1 *in vitro*. *Journal of Food Science* 76(2): H55–H61.

Wu, W.J. and B.Y. Ahn. 2011. Improved menaquinone (Vitamin K2) production in *cheonggukjang* by optimization of the fermentation conditions. *Food Science and Biotechnology* 20: 1585–1591.

Yadav, H., Jain, S., and P.R. Sinha. 2007. Antidiabetic effect of probiotic dahi containing *Lactobacillus acidophilus* and *Lactobacillus casei* in high fructose fed rats. *Nutrition* 23(1): 62–68.

Yamada, K., Sato-Mito, N., Nagata, J., and Umegaki, K., 2008. Health claim evidence requirements in Japan. *Journal of Nutrition* 138: 1192–1198.

Yamanishi, R., Huang, T., Tsuji, H., Bando, N., and T. Ogawa. 1995. Reduction of the soybean allergenicity by the fermentation with *Bacillus natto*. *Food Science and Technology International* 1: 14–17.

Yanagisawa, Y. and H. Sumi. 2005. *Natto* bacillus contains a large amount of water-soluble vitamin K (menaquinone-7). *Journal of Food Biochemistry* 29: 267–277.

Yin, L. J., Li, L.T., Li, Z.G., Tatsumi, E., and M. Saito. 2004. Changes in isoflavone contents and composition of *sufu* (fermented tofu) during manufacturing. *Food Chemistry* 87: 587–592.

Yoon, S., Do, J., Lee, S., and H. Chag. 2000. Production of poly-δ-glutamic acid by fed-batch culture of *Bacillus lichenifomis.Biotechnology Letters* 22: 585–588.

Yonzan, H. and J.P. Tamang. 2010. Microbiology and nutritional value of *selroti*, an ethnic fermented cereal food of the Himalayas. *Food Biotechnology* 2: 227–247.

Zeng, W., Li, W.,Shu, L.,Yi, J., Chen, G., and Z. Liang. 2013. Non-sterilized fermentative co-production of poly (γ-glutamic acid) and fibrinolytic enzyme by a thermophilic *Bacillus subtilis* GXA-28. *Bioresource Technology* 142: 697–700.

Zhang, J-H., Tatsumi, E., Ding, C-H., and L-T. Li. 2006. Angiotensin I- converting enzyme inhibitory peptides in douche, a Chinese traditional fermented soybean product. *Food Chemistry* 98: 551–557.

Chapter 3

Role of Lactic Acid Bacteria in Anticarcinogenic Effect on Human Health

Moumita Bishai, Sunita Adak, Lakshmishri Upadrasta, and Rintu Banerjee

Contents

3.1 Introduction

Fermented food, considered to be one of the major classes of health-promoting foods, is found worldwide. It was Elie Metchnikoff who first reported that the consumption of fermented foods could be beneficial to human health (Praveesh et al. 2011). The Food Safety Unit of the World Health Organization (WHO) has also given high priority for the acceptability of fermented food on the global map. The term "fermentation" is derived from a Latin word "*fervere*" meaning "to boil." It has been described as the action of microorganisms on food grain causing desirable biochemical changes along with significant modifications during the process. As a technique for preparation/storage, the process of food fermentation has achieved acceptability pertaining to its nutritional values, therapeutic potential, and sensory attributes. Food scientists and consumers have long recognized fermentation as a relatively efficient, low-energy preservation process, which increases shelf life and decreases the need for refrigeration or other forms of food preservation.

Currently, fermented foods are increasing in popularity (60% of the diet in industrialized countries) and, to assure the homogeneity, quality, and safety of fermented products, they are produced by their intentional application in raw foods using different microbial systems (individually/concoction) (Holzapfel et al. 1998). During fermentation, the activities of the microbes extend the shelf life of the food by producing acids, change the flavor and texture of the food by producing certain compounds such as alcohol, improve the nutritive value of the product by synthesizing vitamins and release nutrients, that is, bound nutrients by decomposing indigestible materials (Gilliland 1990, O'Sullivan et al. 1992). Amongst the various microbes used in fermented foods, lactic acid bacteria (LAB) are the most profoundly used group. LAB that play a key role in the development and microbiological safety of the final product can be used singly or in combination for fermentation of food products. LAB has a generally recognized as safe (GRAS) status and it has been estimated that 25% of the European diet and 60% of the diet in many developing countries consists of LAB derived fermented foods (Stiles 1996). Some LAB organisms which are successfully used in fermented food processing are *Bacillus*, *Lactobacillus*, *Pseudomonas*, *Bifidobacterium*, *Streptococcus*, and so on. Most importantly, such organisms reside in the human system and provide an impact on human health. Surprisingly, many recent researches have indicated that the interactions between LAB and the human system have greater impact than in those systems where interaction is feeble. Thus, the impact of LAB in the human system has gained greater interest. Widened studies on LAB have further enriched the knowledge of their mechanism of action as well as their intermediate metabolites produced during the different metabolic activities and growth resulting in a diverse range of biological activities on health issues.

3.2 LAB-Induced Fermented Food and Its Health Benefits

Lactic acid bacterial cultures and their fermented products provide several nutritional and therapeutic benefits to consumers. Strains of the genera *Lactobacillus*, *Bifidobacterium* (Yateem et al. 2008) and *Enterococcus* (Ljungh and Wadstrom 2006) are the most widely used and commonly studied microorganisms in Indian fermented food. These bacteria perform an essential role in the preservation and production of wholesome fermented foods and are associated with increasing the level of proteins, vitamins, essential amino acids, and fatty acids. The beneficial effect of LAB on the host, their nonpathogenicity and ability to survive through the gastrointestinal (GI) tract stipulate their candidature for incorporation in present processing technologies (Saito 2004, Crittenden et al. 2005). Based upon the basic ingredients used, fermented foods can be divided into five major types based on their impact on health benefits: (i) milk based, (ii) cereal based, (iii) vegetable based, (iv) pulse based, and (v) fish and meat based fermented food as given in Table 3.1.

3.2.1 Milk-Based Fermented Food

Storage life is one of the important parameters for any milk-derived product. As milk is rich in protein and phospholipid along with other macro and micronutrients, scientists were successful in the development of different products/processes. Milk has been recommended for regular consumption by all age groups but its bioabsorbability is hampered due to the deficiency of different minerals, vitamins, or essential nutrients. Say, for example, calcium absorption is inhibited if vitamin D3 is absent in the system (Holick 2003). Thus, it has been recommended to go for the fermentation of milk or milk-derived products for improved functionality. During this process it was further observed that fermentation is an effective means for extending the storage life of milk. Fermented milk/milk derived products are found to be easier to digest for lactose intolerant people, because of the presence of LAB. Fermentation also provides enhanced benefits on health issues by improving/utilizing the initial nutrients present in the food ingredient, making it an appropriate, balanced one. These bacteria are mostly found adhering to the lining of the intestine, producing different metabolites preventing harmful bacterial multiplication. The organisms also decrease the levels of the different regulatory enzymes responsible for the conversion of procarcinogens into cancer-causing agents. Several research groups have reported the functional properties of LAB species isolated from fermented products suitable for starter cultures. Thus, the research emphasis is on standardization and scaling up studies on traditional fermented milk products.

A series of bacteria belonging to the major group of LAB such as *Streptococcus cremoris, Streptococcus lactis, Streptococcus thermophilus, Lactobacillus bulgaricus, Lactobacillus acidophilus, Lactobacillus helveticus, Lactobacillus cremoris, Lactobacillus plantarum, Lactobacillus curvatus, Lactobacillus fermentum, Lactobacillus paracasei* ssp. *pseudoplantarum, Lactobacillus alimentarius, Lactobacillus kefir, Lactobacillus hilgardii, Enterococcus. faecium, Leuconostoc mesenteroides, Lactobacillus farciminis, Lactobacillus brevis, Lactococcus lactis* ssp. *cremoris, Lactobacillus casei* ssp. *casei,* and *Lactobacillus bifermentans* probiotics have been reported to be present in dairy-based fermented food. These organisms can act either individually or in concoction with different microbes.

Fermented milks from different sources have antimicrobial, antitumor, and antileukemic activities (Esser et al. 1983, Reddy et al. 1983, Shahani et al. 1983). The study reveals that daily consumption of these products increases the ratio of LDL and HDL (Kiessling et al. 2002). Saavedra et al. (1994) has reported protection against nosocomial diarrhea in infants by supplementing their milk with *Bifidobacterium lactis* and *Strep. thermophilus.* To support the research findings, clinical studies of fermented milk have been conducted to evaluate the effect of fermented milk product with a starter culture (*Lb. fermentum* ME-3), that resulted in a significant antioxidant rich product which has a positive effect on human health (Kullisaar et al. 2003, Songisepp et al. 2005). Sour milk compared to nonfermented milk proved to have improved antioxidant status while extending resistance of the lipoprotein fraction to oxidation and reducing the ratio of peroxide lipoproteins and glutathione redox. The majority of milk bacteria produces superoxide dismutase thus eliminating excess oxygen-free radicals.

Similar studies have also been carried out with *dahi* or curd. Intake of *dahi* comprises anticholesteremic, anticarcinogenic, antidiabetic, angiotensin-converting enzyme inhibitory and antiatopic dermatitis effects as discovered by different research groups all over the world (Sinha and Sinha 2000, Harun-ur-Rashid et al. 2007, Yadav et al. 2007, Watanabe et al. 2009, Arvind et al. 2010). Agarwal and Bhasin (2002) isolated LAB from *dahi* and used it to cure intestinal disease

Table 3.1 Lactic Acid Bacterial Fermented Food Having a Role in Health Benefits

Fermented Foods				
Types	*Products*	*LAB*	*Beneficial Effect*	*Reference*
Milk fermented food	*Yoghurt*	*Lactobacillus gasseri, Bifi. longum, Bifi. bifidum, Bifidobacterium. adolescentis, Bifi. infantis, Lb. acidophilus, Lb. casei, Lb. plantarum, Lb. delbrueckii*	Increase number of total T cells, NK cells, and MHC class II+ cells and CD4-CD8+ T cells, some indigenous LAB exert tumor-suppressing effects	Lee et al. (2004), Parvez et al. (2006), Yuan et al. (2013)
	Butter Milk	*Strep. thermophilus* DPC 4694, *Lc. lactis* DPC 4268, *Lb. helveticus* DPC TH3 and *Lb. lactis diacetylactis* DPC 911	Inhibit growth of SW480 human colon cancer cells	Kuchta (2011)
	Curd	*Lb. acidophilus, Lb. helveticus, Lb. cremoris, Ped. pentosaceus, Ped. acidilactici, Lb. fermentum, Lb. plantarum, Lb. bulgaricus, Lb. delbrueckii, Strep. cremoris, Strep. lactis, Strep. thermophilus*	Digestibility of some nutrients, hindgut health characteristics, intestinal microbial balance, and hematology of canine model of Labrador dogs	Patil et al. (2010), Kore et al. (2012)
	Kefir	*Lc. lactis* ssp. *lactis, Lc. lactis* ssp. *cremoris, Lc. lactis* ssp. *diacetylactis Lb. parakefir, Lb. kefir, Lb. kefiranofaciens* sp. *kefiranofaciens, Lb. kefiranofaciens* sp. *kefirgranum*	Increase the number of IgA (+) cells in the mammary gland, increase the number of apoptotic cells and decrease Bcl-2(+) cells in the mammary gland	LeBlanc et al. (2007)
	Fermented milk	*Lb. acidophilus, Lb. paracasei* ssp. *paracasei Bifi. infantis, Bifi. Bifidum, and Bifi. animalis*	Growth inhibition of MCF7 breast cancer cell line	Biffi et al. (1997)
	Fermented cow milk	*Lb. plantarum, Lb. casei*	*In vitro* anticancerous activity in T-HeLa cell lines	Praveesh et al. (2011)

Fermented leafy vegetable foods	*Gundruk*	*Ped. pentosaceus, Lb. fermentum, Lb. casei, Lb. casei* ssp *pseudoplantarum, Lb. plantarum*	Probiotics, acidification, used as good appetizers	Tamang and Tamang (2009), Singh et al. (2007)
	Ingiansang	*Lb. brevis, Ped. acidilactici, Lb. plantarum,*	Food used as a remedy for indigestion	Tamang and Tamang (2009)
	Sinki	*Leuc. fallax, Lb. casei, Lb. brevis, Lb. plantarum, Lb. fermentum*	Used as a good appetizers	Tamang and Tamang (2009)
Legume fermented food	*Kinema*	*Bacillus* spp.	Antioxidant properties, possess digested protein, essential amino acids, vitamin B Complex and low cholesterol content	Sarkar et al. (2002), Tamang and Nikkuni (1996)
	Tungrymbai	*Ent. faecium*	Sensitive many antibiotics, increases carotene and folic acid content.	Murughar and Subbulakshmi (2006)
	Wadi	*Lb. mesenteroides, Lb. fermentum*	Responsible for acidification	Aidoo et al. (2006)
	Wari	*Lb. bulgaricus Strep. thermophilus*	Reduces flatulence-causing oligosaccharides	Kulkarni et al. (1997), Tewary and Muller (1992)
Fermented fish food	*Ngari*	*Ent. faecium, Lb. fructosus, Lb. amylophilus, Lb. plantarum*	Antimicrobial, nonbiogenic producer	Thapa et al. (2004)
	Tungtap	*Lc. lactis* ssp. *cremoris, Lc. plantarum, Ent. faecium, Lb. fructosus, Lb. coryniformis* ssp. *torquens*	Antimicrobial, nonbiogenic producer	Thapa et al. (2004)
	Hentak	*Lc. lactis* ssp., *Lc. cremoris, Lc. plantarum, Ent. faecium, Lb. fructosus, Lb. amylophilus*	Antimicrobial, nonbiogenic producer	Thapa et al. (2004)
Meat fermented food	*Sourdough*	*Lb. sanfrancisco, Lb. brevis,*	Acts as a carrier for probiotic into the human gastrointestinal tract	Tyopponen et al. (2003)
	Yak kargyong	*Lb. plantarum, Lb. sake, Lb. casei, Lb. curvatus, Lb. carnis, Lb. divergens, Lb. sanfrancisco, Lb. mesenteroides, Ent. faecium*	High hydrophobicity	Rai et al. (2010)

such as diarrhea. Later, Mitra et al. (2007) isolated *Lc. lactis* from *dahi* which produced *nisin* bacteriocin that inhibited the important food pathogens *Listeria monocytogenes* and *Staphylococcus aureus* that are the probable major causative factors for colorectal cancer. Thus, *dahi* proved to have very high therapeutic potential. *Yoghurt* fermentation with *Strep. thermophilus* and *Ent. faecium* has showed a reduced level of cholesterol in the serum (Agerholm-Larsen et al. 2000). *Yoghurt* bacteria *Lactobacillus delbrueckii* spp. *Bulgaricus* and *Strep. thermophilus* inhibited peroxidation of lipids through reactive scavenging activity (Ling and Yen 1999).

Different scientists have been working on the health beneficiary effect of the LAB organism on fermented milk based products. Kawamura et al. (1981) and Lambert and Hull (1996) have reported that *Lb. casei* ssp. *rhamnosus* and several strains of *Lb. acidophilus* produce some biocompounds which might be the cause of the inhibition of helicobacter. The secreted metabolites also inhibit the growth of *Helicobacter pylori* which is the major causal agent of anal gastritis. LAB have also demonstrated significant antioxidant and antimicrobial effects. Songisepp et al. (2004) have reported the antioxidant and antimicrobial benefit of Estonian cheese *picante* from which *Lb. fermentum* ME-3 was isolated. Satish et al. (2010) reported that *Lb. plantarum* AS1 isolated from *mor kuzhambhu,* a fermented cheese that showed antibacterial activities toward food-borne pathogens *Salmonella typhi* and *L. monocytogenes*. Some of the other milk fermented foods which have health benefits have been mentioned in Table 3.1.

3.2.2 Cereal-Based Fermented Food

Cereals occupy a major portion of our regularly consumed food. They contain important components such as dietary fibers, carbohydrates, vitamins, minerals, proteins, and so on, instantly present in them. It has been further noticed that upon fermentation with LAB organisms most of the major and minor wall bound macro/micromolecules become available upon consumption. Thus, LAB fermentation has been considered to be an alternative protocol for cereal processing. It was further noticed that with controlled fermentation the following benefits have resulted from cereal fermentation (Blandino et al. 2003):

- Fermentation increases the biological availability of essential amino acids while reducing the starch content.
- The hydrolysis of the chelating agents such as phytic acid improves the bioavailability of minerals. The B group vitamin content of the cereals also increases during fermentation.
- The cooking or the heating time required for preparation is reduced and in the process, the flatus producing carbohydrates and the trypsin inhibitor are lowered.
- Fermentation has been reported to reduce aflatoxin B_1 by opening the ring of lactone which results in complete detoxification.

These advantages directed the researchers toward identifying the benefits and risks associated with specific indigenous fermented cereals; elucidating the contributions of microorganisms, enzymes, and other cereal constituents in the fermentation process (Table 3.1).

Traditional fermented foods prepared from the most common types of cereals are well-known in many parts of the world. Cereals such as rice (*Oryza sativum*), ragi flour *(Eleusine coracana)*, wheat flour (*Triticum* sp.), and barley flour (*Hordeum vulgare)* are predominantly used during the fermentation process. Such cereals contain water-soluble fibers such as β-glucan, arabinoxylan, galactooligosaccharides, and fructooligosaccharides, which are prebiotics (Swennen et al. 2006). Cereals rich in cysteine and methionine, are deficient in lysine. In general, the natural fermentation of cereals leads to a decrease in the level of carbohydrates as well as some nondigestible poly and oligosaccharides. Certain amino acids may be synthesized and the availability of B group vitamins may be improved. Fermentation also provides optimum pH conditions for the enzymatic degradation of phytate which is present in cereals in the form of complexes with polyvalent cations such as iron, zinc, calcium, magnesium, and proteins. Such a reduction in phytate may increase the amount of soluble iron, zinc, and calcium several fold (Chavan et al. 1989, Khetarpaul and Chauhan 1990, Haard et al. 1999). *Lactobacillus fermentum, Lactobacillus buchneri, Lb. plantarum, Lb. acidophilus, Leuc. mesenteroides, Lc. lactis, Strep. lactis,* and *Streptococcus faecalis* were isolated from these classes of fermented foods. Other common fermenting bacterial species are of *Leuconostoc, Pediococcus, Micrococcus,* and *Bacillus.*

Certain preliminary work has been carried out on the potential of cereal-based food. *Lactobacillus plantarum* AS1, isolated from the South Indian fermented food *kallappam* has successfully prevented the colonization of enterovirulent bacterium *Vibrio parahaemolyticus* in the HT-29 cell line (Satish et al. 2011). In another study, it induces the production of 1,2-dimethylhydrazine (DMH), thus suppressing the colorectal cancer in male Wistar rats. LAB fermented cereals need to be further investigated to validate their acceptability by end users.

3.2.3 Vegetable-Based Fermented Food

Vegetables are eaten on the side at every meal. Originally, vegetables contain nutrients, vitamins, minerals, fiber, and enzymes. Upon fermentation these vegetables become enriched with live, healthy bacteria that help to strengthen the host immune system, heal the gut, and aid in digestion. Fermentation also regulates the sugars contained naturally in vegetables. Different fermented vegetables include *gundruk, sinki, khalpi,* and *inziangsang.* Bamboo shoot products are *meso, soidon, soibum, soijum, ekung, eup, hiring,* and *lung-siaj* (Tamang et al. 2012). The dominant LAB microorganisms in fermented vegetables and bamboo shoot products are *Pediococcus pentosaceus, Lactobacillus cellobiosus, Lb. plantarum, Lb. fermentum, Lb. brevis, Lb. mesenteroides, Lc. lactis, Ent. faecium,* and *Pediococcus acidilactici* (Tamang et al. 2005, 2008, 2012, Tamang and Tamang 2009).

To establish the health benefit of vegetable-based fermented food, researchers have isolated *Lb. plantarum* from *inziangsang,* a fermented leafy vegetable product which depicted inhibitory effect toward *Staph. aureus* and *Pseudomonas aeruginosa* by producing bacteriocin. Several other LAB strains isolated from different fermented vegetable products show antimicrobial activities by producing bacteriocins and *nisin.* Some of them are fermented olives, *sauerkraut,* fermented carrots, cucumbers, and organic leafy vegetables (Daeschel and Fleming 1987, Uhlman et al. 1992, Tolonen et al. 2004, Rubia-Soria et al. 2006, Ponce et al. 2008). Fermented vegetables consist of oligosaccharides such as raffinose, stachyose, and verbascose that cause flatulence, diarrhea, and indigestion (Abdel-Gawad 1993, Holzapfel 1997). Enzymatic activities, which have been shown by LAB strains, such as alkaline phosphatase, esterase, lipase, leucine arylamidase, valine arylamidase, cysteine-arylamidase, acid phosphatase, napthol-AS-B1-phosphohydrolase, α-galactosidase, β-galactosidase, α-glucosidase, β-glucosidase, and N-acetyl-β-glucosaminidase cause degradation of such oligosaccharides thereby promoting their antimicrobial effect. Due to these nutritional consequences, the degradation of antinutritive factors in food products by fermentation is desirable (Chavan et al. 1989, Mbugua et al. 1992). The high activity of phosphatase by LAB strains showed their role in phytic acid degradation. Professor J.P. Tamang's research group has worked long in the area of LAB fermentation technology and they have reported about 77% degradation of raffinose using *Lb. plantarum* strains. Also such vegetables usually contain low levels of biogenic amines (Tamang and Tamang 2009).

Bacterial adherence to hydrocarbons, such as hexadecane, proved to be a simple and rapid method to determine their hydrophobicity advocated by their probiotic character (Vinderola et al. 2004). A few strains of LAB isolated from fermented vegetables show more than 75% hydrophobicity (Tamang and Tamang 2009) indicating the potential of their adhesion to the gut epithelial cells of the human intestine (Holzapfel et al. 1998). In view of the above fact, it can be said that vegetable-based fermented food has contributed to our food security through preservation by consequently improving its clinical quality.

3.2.4 Legume-Based Fermented Food

Protein malnutrition is a serious problem in India where the diet consists mainly of cereal or starchy food leading to a limited supply of high-quality protein for the average person. Also, in the current scenario of rising prices, there is an urgent need to utilize low-cost sources of protein in the world economy. Legumes or pulses are second only to cereals as important sources of calories and proteins. Fermented pulses have improved digestibility for humans, their detoxification has led to their acceptance in the global market. Hence, developing healthier fermented food products by incorporating pulses may prove beneficial for mankind while modifying the outlook of the Indian market to the global world. Black gram, Bengal gram, red gram, and green gram are most commonly used pulses in this type of fermented food (Table 3.1).

LAB reported in pulse-based fermented foods include *Ent. faecium, Leuc. mesenteroides, Lb. fermentum, Lb. bulgaricus, Strep. thermophilus, Ped. pentosaceus,* and *Ped. acidilactici.* These isolates exhibited sensitivity to most of the common antibiotics tested and were found to be resistant to cloxacillin, cephalexin, and cephalothin at certain concentrations. These probiotic properties, together with the possibility of antibiotic resistance gene transfer, reveal that *Lactobacillus* sp. and *Lactococcus* sp. characterized from the marketed traditionally fermented soybean food are potent health beneficial organisms. Soybean (*Glycine max*) is a summer leguminous crop. Food researchers have documented a number of soya bean-based Indian fermented foods (Tamang and Tamang 2009). Other reported fermented foods include *wadi, masyaura,* and *wari* that have been found in different parts of the Indian subcontinent. *Kinema* is a sticky fermented soybean food with an ammoniacal flavor. During *kinema* production, soya-proteins are hydrolyzed by proteolytic enzymes produced by *Bacillus subtilis* into peptides and amino acids which enhance their digestibility. A remarkable increase in water-soluble nitrogen and trichloroacetic acid (TCA)-soluble nitrogen contents have been observed during *kinema* fermentation. Total amino acids, mineral content, and vitamin B complex have been reported to increase during *Kinema* fermentation, and thus enriching the food value of the product (Tamang and Tamang 2009). Recently, an increase in the antioxidant activities in *kinema* has also been observed.

Tungrymbai is yet another fermented soybean food having cultures of *Enterococcus* sp., *Lactobacillus* sp., and *Lactococcus* sp. *Tungrymbai* can be considered as a potent probiotic product due to its acid and bile tolerance as well as its antibacterial activity against both Gram-positive and Gram-negative bacteria (Thokchom and Joshi 2012). The isolates from this fermented food were found to be sensitive to most antibiotics reducing the antibiotic resistance gene transfer to pathogenic microbes (Thokchom and Joshi 2012). Fermentation caused an increase in carotene and folic acid in *tungrymbai* (Murughar and Subbulakshmi 2006).

A study was also conducted at IIT Kharagpur in the authors' laboratory (Microbial Biotechnology and Downstream Processing Laboratory), for development of a probiotic-based soy whey dietary adjunct. The fermentation was carried out using a probiotic mixed culture of *Lb. acidophilus, Lb. rhamnosus, Bifidobacterium longum, Bifidobacterium bifidum,* and *Saccharomyces boulardii*. Prior to this, a curdling experiment was performed. The ANN-GA based optimized condition for probiotic fermentation of soy whey was found to be; 9.6 h of incubation at 34.5°C with 7.9% of inoculum volume. The probiotic fermented whey showed improved protein content of 33.51 mg/mL and polyphenolic content of 2.67 mg/mL (Singh 2009). It also showed better radical scavenging, reducing power and metal chelation in comparison to the unfermented whey, which may be due to the antioxidant peptides and phenolics produced during fermentation that reacted with free radicals to stabilize and terminate the radical chain reactions.

To widen its applicability and acceptability among consumers of varied age groups, the above-mentioned soy whey-based food adjunct was mixed with fruit (pineapple and dates) and a spices extract (cardamom, black pepper, fennel seeds, salt, etc.). The final formulation for soy whey-based probiotic fruit juice was found to have naturally enriched bioavailable elements (iron, 41.3 ppm, calcium, 51.5 ppm, zinc, 8.2 ppm, and potassium, 2300 ppm). It also contained natural vitamin C of 26.4 mg/100 mL and a high amount of antioxidant showing 54%–91% of DPPH radical scavenging activity (Gulati 2009). Thus, the produced fruit juice can further be used as an original blend or as a probiotic added drink. Therefore, fermentation technology in pulses has improved their acceptability in different groups of people.

3.2.5 Meat and Fish-Based Fermented Food

Meat and fish are considered to be a rich source of a wide range of nutrients, and are highly susceptible to microbial spoilage. The fermentation of meat is found to be a process of extending its shelf life by changing significant characteristics of the initial product through complex biochemical and physical reactions during fermentation. It is a low energy, biological acidulation and preservation method, which results in unique and distinctive meat properties such as flavor, palatability, color, and microbiological safety. Researchers are now exploring the potentiality of these indigenous meat and fish fermented products. Moreover, LAB colonies responsible for meat fermentation facilitated the conversion of nitrate to nitrite, thus improving the flavor, increasing acidity by producing lactic acid and helping in the growth of mold which is highly desirable.

Some of the common as well as lesser-known traditionally processed ethnic meat products are *kargyong, ngari, hentak, kheuri, satchu, geema, arijia,* and *chartyshya* of the Himalayas. Fermented meat products of other countries are *nham, mam-neua* (beef), *mam-moo* (pork), *sai-krork-prieo, som-neua* (Thailand); *uratan* (Balinese); *kulen, zimska salaq* (Yugoslavia), *longaniza, salame milan* (Uruguay); *pizza and veneto salami* (Argentina); *kantwurst, lanjager* (Australia); *ardenner, boulogna* (Belgium); *figatelli, chorizo* (France); *rindfleischsalami* (Germany); *salame genovese, salame milano* (Italy); and so on (Ockerman and Basu 2010) (Table 3.1). *Lactobacillus curvatus, Lactobacillus divergens, Lactobacillus carnis, Lactobacillus sanfrancisco, Leuc. mesenteroides, Ent. faecium, Lb. plantarum, Lb. brevis, Ped. pentosaceus* are the predominant *Lactobacilli* employed in these group of foods that are responsible for their probiotic effect (Rai et al. 2010, Oki et al. 2011). Rai et al. (2010) demonstrated probiotic characters such as enzymes production and hydrophobicity causing weak lipolytic activity in fermented meats. They predicted the absence of proteinases (trypsin and chymotrypsin) and the presence of strong peptidase (leucine-, valine-, and cystine-arylamidase) activities, which are some of the other characteristics of the microbes (Rai et al. 2010). Fermentation of dry sausages resulted in an increase in small peptides and free amino acids, which further improved the flavor of the fermented meat products. LAB isolated from meat products shows strong antimicrobial activity against a group of potentially pathogenic Gram-positive and Gram-negative bacteria (Rai et al. 2010). LAB in fermented sausages were reported to decrease the duration and severity of some gastric and intestinal illnesses (Marteau et al. 2002), while contributing to the microbial ecosystem of the GI tract (Farnworth 2003). The sausage matrix protects the survival of probiotic *Lactobacilli* through the GI tract (Klingberg and Budde 2006). Daily consumption of 50 g of probiotic sausage containing *Lb. paracasei* LTH 2579 was found to modulate various aspects of host immunity. Moreover, in Northern European sausages the presence of potential probiotic strains of *Lb. rhamnosus* and *Lb. plantarum* confirmed the nontoxic effect on the technological and sensory properties of the end-product (Erkkilä et al. 2001). Also the application of *Lb. paracasei* L26 and *Bifi. lactis* B94 in conjunction with a traditional meat starter culture, showed a positive impact on the sensory properties of the product (Pidcock et al. 2002).

The predominant LAB species generally used for fish fermented food in North East India are *Lc. lactis* ssp. *cremoris*, *Lc. plantarum*, *Ent. faecium*, *Lactobacillus fructosus*, *Lactobacillus amylophilus*, *Lactobacillus coryniformis* ssp. *torquens* (Thapa et al. 2004, 2006) which have been isolated from fish fermented food, that is, *gnuchi*, *tungtap*, *bordia*, and so on. Other fish fermenting LAB organisms are from *sikhae* (Korean); *narezushi* (Japanese); *burong-isda*, *balao-balao* (Philippines); *pla-ra*, *kungchao* (Thailand); *nem-chua* (Vietnam) are *Leuc. mesenteroides*, *Lb. plantarum*, *Lb. brevis*, *Streptococcus* sp., *Pediococcus* sp., *Pediococcus cerevisiae*, and so on. (Rhee et al. 2011). Some of these LAB organisms showed low protease activity, while some strains shows amylolytic activity. The proteolysis and liquefaction occurring during fish fermentation is due to the autolysis taking place inside the fish tissues. The organisms also show antagonistic properties against many pathogenic bacteria (Thapa et al. 2004). There are reports of production of biogenic amines in many fish fermented products (Halasz et al. 1994). They can produce histamine and tyramine in processed fish (Leisner et al. 1994). Some strains of LAB isolated from Himalayan fish products show high degrees of hydrophobicity (>75%), among which *Ped. pentosaceus* shows the highest degree of hydrophobicity of 94% (Thapa et al. 2006). All strains indicate their adherence abilities. Low moisture content prolonged the shelf life of the product. Fermented fish products are generally high in protein and amino compounds (Puwastien et al. 1999).

Thus, fermentation using LAB is found to have many therapeutic effects. Later, with serendipity in "probiotic" research, it was pointed out that all fermented foods were derived from products containing probiotic bacteria which forced us to explore their residence in human beings and their underlying mechanisms. The "probiotic concept" will only be accepted if these mechanisms are properly elucidated.

3.3 LAB Microbiome in Human System

A variety of microbial communities and their genes (the microbiome) exist throughout the human body, with fundamental roles to play in human health and disease. Many researches were performed which described the interactions between the innate and adaptive immune systems and the tens of trillions of microbes that live in our GI and urogenital tracts. LAB, one of those organisms, are collectively represented as a major part of the commensal microbial flora of the human GI and the urogenital tract and are frequently used as probiotics either singly or in combination for the fermentation of food products (Shigwedha and Jia 2013). Amongst all, the best known LAB microorganisms are strains belonging to the *Lactobacillus* and *Bifidobacterium* genera. However, other microorganisms, such as *Enterococcus* sp., and *Streptococcus* sp., have also been considered for use as probiotics. They not only act on the large intestine by affecting the intestinal flora but also affect other organs by modulating the immunological parameters and intestinal permeability and by producing bioactive or regulatory metabolites which have a potent role in human health benefit (de Vrese and Schrezenmeir 2008).

The human GI tract harbors a diverse microflora representing several hundred different species. The colonization of the GI tract begins immediately after birth. Colonization pattern is affected by factors such as mode of delivery, initial diet, and geographical location (Fanaro et al. 2003). In breast-fed infants, *Bifidobacteria* are predominant, accumulating 10^{10}–10^{11} CFU/mL (Lourens-Hattingh and Viljoen 2001). The main species of the genus *Bifidobacterium* of infant intestinal flora are *Bifi. bifidum, Bifidobacterium infantis, Bifidobacterium breve*, and *Bifi. longum*. The predominant *Bifidobacteria* species in both breast-fed and formula-infants differ by geographic region. *Bifidobacterium bifidum* was found to predominate in the fecal flora of breast-fed infants, while *Bifi. breve* was the predominant *Bifidobacteria* species among the fecal flora of non-breast-fed infants (Fanaro et al. 2003). The major species in the oral cavity are LAB of the genera *Streptococcus, Lactobacillus*, and *Bifidobacterium*. The main source of nutrients and energy for oral bacteria is ingested food, especially carbohydrates, which are rapidly metabolized to lactic and acetic acids by the predominant LAB, leading to a rapid drop in the pH of the saliva after ingestion of carbohydrates. Food from the oral cavity passes on to the esophagus and stomach which carries the lightest microbial loads in the human GI tract (Figure 3.1).

The predominant bacteria are *Streptococci* and *Lactobacilli*. The human stomach has a remarkably low pH. The normal resting pH of gastric juice is below 3.0, which prevents virtually all bacterial growth, and is bactericidal for most transient species, especially LAB. It increases to values

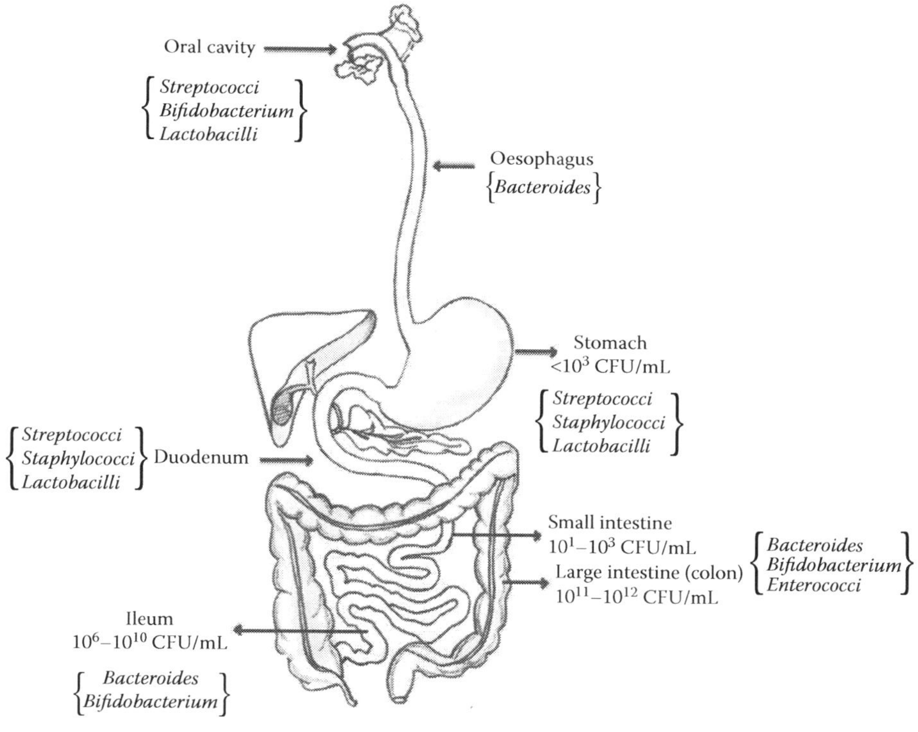

Figure 3.1 Presence of LAB inside human microbiome. (Modified from Sartor, R. B. and S. K. Mazmanian. 2012. *American Journal of Gastroenterology Supplements* 1:15-21; Shigwedha, N. and L. Jia. 2013. *Lactic Acid Bacteria- R and D for Food, Health and Livestock Purposes*, 281–308, Croatia: InTech.)

around 6.0 after a meal. During this *Bifidobacteria* are transported through the zone, surviving the gastric juice, to proceed to the small intestine (Shigwedha and Jia 2013).

Digested food, on entering the small intestine, is mixed with intestinal secretions, such as bile, pancreatic enzymes, and bicarbonates. The bile has a strong bactericidal effect which prevents extensive colonization of bacterial biomass in the small intestine. Colonization usually takes place in crypts and blind loops. Some species of *Streptococcus* and *Lactobacillus* are found in the duodenum which is the uppermost part of the small intestine. The microflora of this proximal small bowel is similar to that of the stomach with bacterial concentrations of 10^3–10^4 CFU/mL (Campieri and Gionchetti 1999). In this lower part, the movement of food is slightly reduced, the bile is diluted, the pH becomes more neutral, and the oxygen tension drops rapidly. In the distal ileum, Gram-negative, anaerobic bacteria, and aerobic organisms are present which include the *Bacteroides, Bifidobacterium, Clostridium,* and *Fusobacterium* sp. This favors the growth and/or transit of different bacteria in the ileum and finally to the large intestine. The dominant floras in the large intestine (colon) are relatively stable, and they include *Bifidobacterium, Bacteriodes,* and anaerobic cocci. The numbers of dominant species are also comparable in different populations. Within the colon, the bacterial counts range from 10^{11} to 10^{12} CFU/mL, and the anaerobic bacteria outnumber aerobes by a factor of 10^2–10^4 CFU/mL (Shigwedha and Jia 2013).

Apart from these, LAB also reside in the urinogenital tract of humans. *Lactobacilli* are the predominant microorganisms in the lower genital tract of healthy premenopausal women. The predominant species isolated from vaginal fluid were *Lb. acidophilus, Lb. fermentum, Lb. plantarum, Lb. brevis, Lactobacillus jensenii, Lb. casei, Lb. delbrueckii,* and *Lactobacillus salivarius* (Wylie and Henderson 1969). Particular strains of LAB showed adjuvant properties by stimulating specific antibodies after infection with pathogenic microorganisms (Pouwels et al. 1996). Another intriguing development is that certain LAB can strengthen the gut mucosal barrier and thereby influence gut mucosal permeability and possible diarrhea. Often, the symbiotic association may also support the fact of its potential as gut and genital tract flora.

3.3.1 Individual Organisms Influencing the Human Health

Several individual probiotic strains were found to be effective in the treatment of different types of intestinal disorders. A significant reduction in either the duration or severity of gastroenteritis was achieved when using two main groups of LAB strains i.e *Lactobacillus* and *Bifidobacterium* (de Vrese and Marteau 2007). Among *Lactobacillus*, important probiotics are *Lb. casei, Lb. plantarum, Lb. acidophilus,* and *Lb. bulgaricus*. Similarly, *Bifi. breve* and *Bifi. bifidum* are known to be therapeutically beneficial as probiotics (Kaila et al. 1992). Some reports related to *Lactobacillus* are quite interesting to note. *Lactobacillus casei* originating from yogurt, proved to be the most studied species among researchers. *Lactobacillus casei* reduces lactose intolerance and make symptoms of constipation disappear, all leading to a better functioning of the immune system. Research has demonstrated increased levels of circulating immunoglobulin A (IgA) by *Lb. casei* in response to rotavirus infection in children. It proved beneficial for people suffering from Crohn's disease and also for children who experience critical diarrhea (Hamne et al. 2001). *Lactobacillus plantarum* which is derived from sourdough, sauerkraut, and salami, has been demonstrated to improve the recovery of patients with enteric bacterial infections. This bacterium adheres to reinforce the barrier function of the intestinal mucosa, thus preventing the attachment of the pathogenic bacteria to the intestinal wall. A bacteriocin isolated from *Lb. plantarum* ST31, a probiotic derived from sourdough, has 20 amino acid peptides (Todorov et al. 1999). A different bacteriocin was isolated from another strain of *Lb. plantarum* having 27 amino acids and containing lanthionine residues. Such type of bacteriocin is classified as a lantibiotic (Bron et al. 2004). *Lactobacillus acidophilus* inhabits the human mouth, the small and large intestine, and the vagina. It can adhere to the human enterocyte while exhibiting a high calcium independent adhesive property. As a result of adhesion, it suppresses hostile invaders including *Candida albicans* through the production of natural antibiotics and other inhibitory substances such as lactic acid, and H_2O_2. In addition to this, these bacteria cultures were found to support intestinal integrity during radiotherapy (Salminen et al. 1988).

Lactobacillus bulgaricus found in yoghurt and cheese encourages a more acidic environment by producing H_2O_2 and antibiotic substances to inhibit harmful bacteria (Balotescu and Roumanian 2004). Apart from *Lactobacillus* sp., Camarri et al. (1981) reported the successful treatment of acute enteritis in double-blind controlled trials along with *Ent. faecium*. It also found effective response in the treatment of recurrent *C. difficile clottis*. *Lactobacillus johnsonii* LA1 was found to increase the frequency phagocytic activity and of interferon-gamma-producing peripheral blood monocytes (Danikas et al. 2008). While studying the antagonistic activity of LAB against pathogens, Balotescu and Roumanian (2004) reported that *Lb. rhamnosus* was found to scavenge superoxide anion radicals, while inhibiting lipid peroxidation and iron chelation *in vitro*. Among the *Bifidobacterium*, *Bifi. breve* was found to eradicate *Campylobacter jejuni* from the stools of children with enteritis, although less rapidly than in those treated with erythromycin. These species were supplemented as infant formula milk along with *Bifi. bifidum* to prevention diarrhea in infants. Along with *Strep. thermophilus* they reduced rotavirus shedding and episodes of diarrhea in hospitalized children (Joshi 2007). The name of several organisms along with their clinical effects are given in Table 3.2.

3.3.2 Beneficial Effect of Concoctions of Probiotics

Lactobacillus and *Bifidobacteria* induce changes in the intestinal flora and modulate the immune response in humans. *Lactobacillus acidophilus* and *Bifi. bifidum* appear to enhance the nonspecific immune phagocytic activity of circulating blood granulocytes which might stimulate the IgA responses in infants infected with rotavirus (Roberfroid 2000).

In healthy individuals, *Lb. salivarius* UCC118 and *Lb. johnsonii* LA1 were demonstrated to produce an increase in the phagocytic activity of peripheral blood monocytes and granulocytes (Miler et al. 1985). These probiotics when colonizing the colon, proved helpful in the management of food allergies by reinforcing the barrier function of the intestinal mucosa. Other LAB, including strains of *Lb. acidophilus*, *Lb. bulgaricus*, *Bifi. longum*, and *Strep. thermophilus*, have also demonstrated antioxidative ability because of the mechanism of toxin neutralization (Joshi 2007).

3.4 Mechanisms behind the Health Benefits Caused by LAB Organisms in the Human System

Probiotics have been found to reinforce and impart beneficial properties apart from indigenous microbes in animals and humans. LAB-based probiotics show a wide range of health-promoting effects which have been well documented. These effects include: alleviation of lactose intolerance, hypocholesterolemic effect, prevention and reduction of diarrhea, antiinflammatory, immunomodulatory, and antimutagenic effects (Havenaar and Spanhaak 1994, Rafter 2002). The type of response generated is found to be strain specific and not all strains of the

Table 3.2 Different LAB with Their Clinical Role

Organism	*Clinical Effect*	*Reference*
Lb. casei	Cause decreased mutation during AMES tests, suppress the growth of MT-2, MT-4 cells from adult T-cell leukemia, Molt-4 cells from acute lymphoblastic leukemia, and U-937 cells from promonocytic leukemia.	Pool-Zobel et al. (1993)
Lb. rhamnosus	Induce mitochondrial pathway of apoptosis in human colonic carcinoma cells (Caco-2).	Altonsy et al. (2010)
Lb. gasseri	Increase the proportion of natural killer (NK) cells and in IgA concentrations.	Olivares et al. (2006)
Lb. paracasei	Show negative effect on the MTT test of K562 cell line.	Riki (2013)
Lb. acidophilus	Stimulate immunity by increasing SCFA, pH decreased, suppress the formation of cancer-causing amines and cancer-promoting enzymes in the intestines of humans.	Wollowski et al. (2001)
Bifi. infantis	Induce MCF7 breast cancer cell line.	Biffi et al. (1997)
Bifi. animalis	Adhere to colon cancer cells, improve lymphocyte transformation, macrophages phagocytic activity, natural killer cell activity, also improve immunity.	Saavedra (2007)
Bifi. longum	Significant reduction in mutagen-induced chromosome aberrations and micronuclei.	Pool-Zobel et al. (1993)
Bifi. bifidium	Cause DNA damage in the colonic cells, decreases the procarcinogenic enzyme activities	Wollowski et al. (2001)
Bifi. breve	Reduce activity of β-glucuronidase, tryptophanase and lysine decarboxylase in feaces and indican, phenols, ammonia and cadaverin in urine, cause treatment of infantile intractable diarrhea, beneficial for the treatment of liver cirrhosis.	Mitsuoka (1990)

same species act against defined health problems (Vasiljevic and Shah 2008). LAB and their cell components (cell wall and cytoplasmic fractions) can bring about health protective effects as described by Miettinen et al. (1996) and Sato et al. (1988). Biffi et al. (1997) reported the active inhibition of tumor cell growth by *ex novo* soluble compounds released by LAB. The immunomodulatory effect includes the proliferation of immune cells, and the enhanced synthesis of cytokines and antibodies to microbial pathogens. Some of the suggested mechanisms have been discussed in this section.

1. Disruption of host and pathogen interaction—In case of diarrhea caused by antibiotic treatment, administration of probiotics helps to restore the balance of intestinal microflora by promoting the growth of indigenous microbes. This in turn helps to eradicate harmful pathogens from the lumen and cure the condition. LAB containing probiotics have been reported to prevent and reduce microbial infections such as in case of diarrhea induced by

rotavirus, enteroinvasive *Escherichia coli,* and so on by competitive exclusion and enhancement of the epithelial barrier function. This averts adhesion of pathogenic organisms to the gut epithelium and the secretion of electrolytes from epithelial cells (Freitas et al. 2003, Resta-Lenert and Barrett 2003). Similarly suppression of *H. pylori* has been found to be strain dependent and the probable mechanisms involve enhanced gut barrier function and competition for adhesion sites (Vasiljevic and Shah 2008).

2. Role of enzymes—Enzymes derived from probiotic bacteria also play an important role in counteracting many unpleasant physiological conditions such as lactose intolerance, hypercholesterolemic effect, and so on. β-Galactosidase from probiotic microbes helps to breakdown lactose which in turn alleviates lactose intolerance. In case of serum cholesterol level, Mann and Spoerry (1974) suggested the production of hydroxymethyl-glutarate by LAB which inhibits the hydroxymethylglutaryl-CoA required for the synthesis of cholesterol, thus leading to a hypocholesterolemic effect.
3. Role of secreted metabolites—Different metabolites involved in antimicrobial activity exert their effect by decreasing luminal pH, making nutrients unavailable to pathogens, decreasing redox potential of lumen, and producing inhibitory compounds (Naidu et al. 1999). Some of the common metabolites include CO_2 and H_2O_2 which prevent the growth of pathogenic microbes by general mechanisms. Other potent metabolites and their mechanisms have been listed below:
   a. Bacteriocins—Bacteriocins are bactericidal proteins produced by LAB, for example, *nisin, lactosin, pediocin,* etc. Generally, these substances are cationic peptides that display hydrophobic or amphiphilic properties and exert their lethal action through binding to the bacterial membrane. Upon binding they bring about bacterial cell death via metabolic, biological, and morphological changes. They have been classified as: Class I, lantibiotics; class II, small heat stable non lantibiotics; and class III, large heat labile bacteriocins. A fourth class is composed of an undefined protein, lipid, and carbohydrate mixture (Savadogo et al. 2006).
   b. Diacetyl and acetaldehyde—Diacetyl (2,3-butanedione), an end product of pyruvate metabolism by citrate-fermenting LAB, interferes with arginine utilization by reacting with the arginine-binding protein of Gram-negative bacteria. Diacetyl elicits a potent antimicrobial activity against various food-borne pathogens and spoilage microorganisms like Gram-negative bacteria.
   c. Small chain fatty acids—LAB, for example, *Bifidobacteria* produce acetic acid and 2-hydroxypropionic acid as a major end-product of carbohydrate metabolism which reduces the pH of the lumen and results in a broad-spectrum inhibition of Gram-positive and Gram-negative bacteria. Control of intestinal pH restricts the production of phenols, ammonia, steroid metabolites, bacterial toxins, vasoconstriction amines, and putrefactive products which cause diarrhea, liver disorders, and malfunction of the circulatory system (Naidu et al. 1999).
   d. Exopolysaccharides (EPS)—EPS produced by LAB have various functional roles in human health including immunomodulatory properties, and antioxidant, antiviral, and antihypertensive activities. They also function as potent prebiotics which help in the growth of beneficial bacteria (Harutoshi 2013).
      i. Immunomodulation—The gut-associated lymphatic tissues (GALT) play a major role in both the local and systemic immunological responses (Havenaar and Spanhaak 1994). The mucosal immune system is responsible for 60% of the daily

production of immunoglobulins (Mestecky and McGhee 1987). The ability of LAB to induce both innate and adaptive immunity vastly depends on the pathway of internalization in the gut. The interaction of LAB with M cells (specialized intestinal epithelial cells) induces mainly specific immune responses, while the interaction with follicle associated epithelium (FAE) cells induces a nonspecific or inflammatory response (Perdigon et al. 2002). Through these interactions they bring about the release of certain cytokines, TNF-α, IL-6, IL-4, IL-10, and so on, and upregulation of phagocytic activity as well as regulation of Th1/Th2 balance (Miettinen et al. 1996, Vasiljevic and Shah 2008). The immunomodulative activity of LAB depends on dosage, cell viability, and mode of ingestion. LAB applied in fermented food induces a higher response compared to that supplied in nonfermented food. Other factors include age and physiological status of the host (Perdigon et al. 2002).

ii. Antioxidant activity—Oxidative damage can cause various diseases including cancer, cirrhosis, arthritis, and so on. Ling and Yen (1999) reported that LAB also has antioxidative ability. Although superoxide dismutase (SOD) activity was not found in this study, strains of *Lb. bulgaricus, Lb. acidophilus, Strep. thermophilus,* and *Bifi. longum* were found to be capable of chelating metal ions, scavenging reactive oxygen species and possessed reducing activity.

Apart from these mechanisms, the role of LAB in cancer treatment is yet another area of study which is proving to have immense potential.

3.5 Role of LAB in Cancer Treatment and Its Mechanism

Cancer being one of the deadliest and most challenging diseases has been the focus of intense research throughout the world. According to an immunological perspective, cancer cells could be defined as altered self-cells that are devoid of the growth regulating mechanisms usually found in normal cells (Goldsby et al. 2002). Out of the different factors responsible for the genesis of cancer some are found to be preventable in nature such as infection, inflammation, smoking, and diet (Lee et al. 2004). Many studies have focused on treatment employing dietary supplements such as prebiotics and probiotics. Though infallible evidence on the ability of LAB-based probiotics for complete cancer suppression/treatment in human is missing, there is still a wealth of evidence available of its probabilistic role as a potential cancer therapy based on various *in vitro, in vivo,* and epidemiological studies.

3.5.1 Evidences of Potent Anticancerous Effect of LAB

Biffi et al. (1997) observed fermented milk containing five LAB strains (*Bifi. infantis, Bifi. bifidum, Bifidobacterium animalis, Lb. acidophilus,* and *Lb. paracasei*) inhibited growth of the MCF7 breast cancer cell line. Several other research works on the role of LAB in inducing metabolic, biological, and genomic level changes in human cancer cell lines have shown promising effect. *Bifidobacterium* sp. was found to decrease growth rate and stimulate differentiation in the HT-29 human colon adenocarcinoma cell line by enhancing the activity of two enzymes—dipeptidyl peptidase IV and alkaline phosphatase (Baricault et al. 1995). Cytoplasmic fractions of *Lactobacillus lactis* ssp. *lactis* inhibited the proliferation of the SNUC2 human colon cancer cell line by inducing S-phase cell-cycle arrest (Kim et al. 2003). The same organism was found to induce apoptosis in the SNU-1 human adenocarcinoma cell line in a study by Kim et al. (2004). Cousin et al. (2012) developed a fermented milk product by the action of *Propionibacterium freudenreichii* which demonstrated pro-apoptotic potential toward HGT-1 human gastric cancer cells and enhanced the cytotoxicity of camptothecin, a drug used in gastric cancer chemotherapy.

Along with studies on *in vitro* condition using cell lines, various researches on animal models have been carried out specially focusing on rats. Colon cancer being a highly researched area, where the effect of dietary factors on tumors and/or early lesions such as aberrant crypt foci (ACF) in rat models have demonstrated a protective role against colon tumor development. McIntosh et al. (1999) fed rats with *Lb. acidophilus* (Delvo Pro LA-1), which showed 25% reduced colon cancer. Challa et al. (1997) conducted an anticancer trial on male Fisher 344 rats using *Bifi. longum*. Feeding *Bifi. longum* reduced the number of aberrant crypt foci to 143 ± 9 as against untreated carcinogen controls with 187 ± 9 aberrant crypts. The administration of *Lb. acidophilius* NCFM in tumor implanted BALB/cByJ mice down regulated expression of CXCR4 mRNA and MHC class I and enhanced apoptosis of CT-26 cells in colon cancer (Chen et al. 2012). Similar effect was shown by *Lb. acidophilus* KFRI342, isolated from the Korean traditional food *kimchi*, on chemically induced precancerous changes (aberrant crypts) of the colon in F344 rats (Chang et al. 2012). Leu et al. (2005) used symbiotic combination of *Lb. acidophilus* and *Bifi. lactis* (1×10^{10} CFU/g) on Sprague-Dawley rats as their animal model and observed a significantly high apoptotic response to a genotoxic carcinogen in the distal colon of rats thus reducing colon cancer. Combined effect of probiotics *Lb. rhamnosus* and *Bifi. lactis* on azoxymethane-induced colon carcinogenesis in male F344 rats showed a positive response (Femia et al. 2002). Similarly the symbiotic combination of *Bifidobacterium* and oligofructose reduced aberrant crypt numbers in five of the six experimental rats (Gallaher and Khil 1999). In a study by Lim et al. (2002) bladder cancer induced mice, when fed with *Lb. rhamnosus* exhibited reduced tumor formation and growth, which was attributed to increased spleen CD3, CD4, and CD8 T lymphocytes and natural killer cells. *Lactobacillus rhamnosus* and *Lb. acidophilus* have also exhibited the protection of the liver against injury caused by alcohol, carbontetracholride, and tert-butyl hydroxide in a rat model (Nanji et al. 1994). The oral administration of fermented foods has also shown a beneficial anticancerous effect. BALB/c mouse injected with 4T1 mouse mammary adenocarcinoma cells used as a breast cancer model, showed reduced tumor growth and enhanced cytokines in response to feeding with fermented milk containing *Lb. helveticus* R389 (Han et al. 2005). Helmy (2012) reported that yoghurt and fermented kidney beans, when fed to female Swiss albino mice with intra-peritoneal cancer, reduced the number and size of tumor cells, along with degradation and necrosis. In studies conducted on Wister rats, feeding of probiotic *dahi* and probiotic fermented milk, both containing *Lactobacillus* sp. showed an anticarcinogenic effect against colorectal cancer and hepatocarcinogenesis, respectively, in combination with an antioxidant (Mohania et al. 2013, Kumar et al. 2012).

Further evidence of the anticancerous effect modulated by LAB has been obtained via epidemiological studies. In a study involving 48 Japanese patients, daily intake of viable *Lb. casei* postponed the recurrence of bladder tumors (Aso and Akazan 1992). A lower incidence of colon cancer in Finland compared to other countries was observed because of the high consumption of milk, yoghurt, and other dairy products in spite of the high fat intake (Rafter 2002). Similarly a case–control study conducted in the Netherlands exhibited lower occurrence of breast cancer in women with a high intake of fermented milk products compared to controls with a low intake of fermented milk products (Veer et al. 1989). Another epidemiological study on 45,241 subjects in EPIC-Italy showed a high yoghurt intake lowered the risk of colorectal cancer (Pala et al. 2011). Apart from this Sharma et al. (2012) showed administration of

Lb. brevis CD2 lozenges reduced the incidence of anticancer therapy-induced oral mucositis in patients with head and neck cancer. Thus, the positive effect of LAB administration in reduction of cancer occurrences supports the hypothesis of its anticancerous function. The above obtained results further encouraged researchers to investigate the plausible mechanisms underlying these effects.

3.5.2 Mechanisms Involved in the Anticancerous Effect of LAB

Currently, the precise mechanism by which LAB inhibits/reduces the occurrences of cancer is not fully known, but the most probable ones include: alteration of GI microflora, binding of potential carcinogens or mutagens, decrease in enzyme activity involved in generation of carcinogens, mutagens or tumor-promoting agents, and enhancement of host immune response.

1. Alteration of GI microflora—the human gut hosts many microbes out of which some are found to have a pathogenic effect such as *Clostridium perfringens* which can produce genotoxic, carcinogenic, and tumor-promoting components (nitrosamines, heterocyclic amines, aglycones, etc.). These microbes are generally less in number compared to the beneficial microbes in healthy humans. Under certain physiological conditions the healthy balance between beneficial and pathogenic microbes is lost, leading to an increase in pathogens in the gut. This can act as a probable causative agent of colon cancer. LAB administration proves to restore the lost balance in the gut microflora. The LAB enter the gut along with consumed food and are known to have beneficial effects on the resident bacteria of the GI microflora. They compete with other bacteria in the human body by producing inhibitory compounds or competitively adhering to the epithelium. Mizutani and Mitsuoka (1979, 1980) reported the promotion of liver tumorigenesis in C3H/He male mice in the presence of *Strep. faecalis, E. coli,* and *Clostridium paraputrificum* in the intestinal lumen. The administration of certain intestinal bacteria such as *Bifi. longum* and *Lb. acidophilus* in the gut suppressed the tumor. Thus, from this study the authors were able to support the role of LAB in cancer cell inhibition indirectly through action on gut microflora.
2. Binding of potential carcinogens or mutagens—many mutagenic compounds are found in food especially in the Western meat-rich diet, such as heterocyclic amines (Felton et al. 1994). These mutagens act as potential cancer causative agents and hence their removal from the system could be a probable cancer preventive method. LAB can mediate the cancer-preventive effect by binding carcinogens as proved by the work of Orrhage et al. (1994). The mutagens PhIP, Trp-P-2, IQ and MeIQx were very efficiently bound by the bacteria. The binding of carcinogens or mutagens leads to reduced urinary excretion and in case these compounds are not metabolized by the LAB then fecal excretion increases (Roos and Katan 2000). Hayatsu and coworkers (1993) observed 50% reduction in the urinary excretion of mutagens in six human volunteers fed with freeze-dried *Lb. casei.* Works of several other researches on similar lines proves the same but reduction in the occurrence of cancer due to this mechanism needs to be further established.
3. Decrease in enzyme activity involved in the generation of carcinogens or mutagens—various procarcinogenic enzymes are produced by intestinal microflora, which include β-glucuronidase, azoreductase, nitroreductase, 7-alpha-dehydroxylase, and 7-alpha-dehydrogenase. These enzymes convert several procarcinogens into carcinogens, enhancing the risk of cancer genesis. The presence of such enzymes and their activity has been found to be the lowest in strains of *Lactobacilli* and *Bifidobacteria* (Naidu et al. 1999). Probiotics

might help overcome the risk of cancer genesis by suppressing the growth of those bacteria that generate such enzymes. Various human trials have shown the effectiveness of LAB in reducing the activity of these enzymes. Goldin et al. (1980) observed reduction in the fecal nitroreductase and β-glucuronidase activities by supplementation of viable *Lactobacillus* cultures in the diet of adult omnivorous volunteers. Similarly, consumption of fermented milk containing *Lb. casei* and *Bifidobacterium* species in two separate trials showed reduced β-glucuronidase activity in healthy volunteers compared to that of the controls (Spanhaak et al. 1998, Bouhnik et al. 1996). These studies do establish the potential role of LAB in reducing the activity of enzymes responsible for the synthesis of carcinogens or mutagens but the direct relationship between such enzymes and cancer risk needs further probing to prove the correctness of the proposed mode of cancer prevention by LAB.

4. Enhancement of host immune response—stimulation of the host immune response is one of the most potent targets of cancer therapy. Many cancer treatments mainly focus on this aspect of the human system. LAB has been found to generate both the innate and adaptive immune responses, which in turn leads to enhanced release of cytokines, antibodies, and high phagocytic and apoptotic activities. Sekine et al. (1985) postulated that tumor suppression or regression by *Bifi. infantis* is via stimulation of the host's immune response. Intrapleural administration of *Lb. casei* strain *shirota* into tumor-bearing mice inhibited tumor growth and increased survival, because it was found to induce the production of several cytokines such as interferon (IFN)-γ, IL-1, and necrosis (TNF)-α (Matsuzaki 1998). Increase in macrophage and lymphocyte activities in mice after the administration of a mixed culture of *Lb. acidophilus* and *Lb. casei* was reported by Perdigon et al. (1986). Similar results were obtained by Kim et al. (2006) on oral administration of heat-killed *Lb. lactis* ssp. *lactis* in male Balb/c mice.

3.6 Conclusion

Fermented foods being an intrinsic part of Indian cuisine have been a source of nutrition and are often linked to many health-promoting effects. Current research on probiotic LAB has proved their multifaceted role in a wide range of Indian traditional fermented foods and their respective health benefits. Not only have these organisms actively participated in maintaining general health and immunity, they have also shown a suggestive role in cancer suppression. The LAB organism during fermentation is assumed to release some metabolites from the food or causes some reactions, which in turn, improves the potential of its health-promoting effect. Also, being present in the human microbiota, these organisms stabilize the natural flora of the human system. In spite of the extensive in vitro, in vivo, clinical, and epidemiological studies on the health effects of LAB, the evidence focusing on the exact mechanism of their action is limited, thus establishing their precise role as health protective and anticancerous agents is an area of active research. Further exhaustive knowledge regarding their biogenic properties, safety, and dosage among different age groups needs to be explored. This will help us to produce new target specific products with extended storage life, ease of delivery within the host system with improved bioabsorbability and bioactivity. The development of proper regulatory norms based on scientific studies for such fermented products is mandatory for their validation, application, and effectiveness. Moreover, the approach for their wider acceptability in the global market in future demands scientific support along with public awareness. With proper research and development probiotic-based fermented foods may become a potential panacea in the near future.

References

Abdel-Gawad, A. S. 1993. Effect of domestic processing on oligosaccharide content of some dry legume seeds. *Food Chemistry* 46: 25–31.

Agarwal, K. N. and S. K. Bhasin. 2002. Feasibility studies to control acute diarrhoea in children by feeding fermented milk preparations Actimel and Indian Dahi. *European Journal of Clinical Nutrition* 56(4): S56–S59.

Agerholm-Larsen, L., A. Raben, N. Haulrik, A. S. Hansen, M. Manders, and A. Astrup. 2000. Effect of 8 week intake of probiotic milk products on risk factors for cardiovascular diseases. *European Journal of Clinical Nutrition* 54: 288–289.

Aidoo, K. E., M. J. R. Nout, and P. K. Sarkar. 2006. Occurrence and function of yeasts in Asian indigenous fermented foods. *FEMS Yeast Research* 6: 30–39.

Altonsy, M. O., S. C. Andrews, and K. M. Tuohy. 2010. Differential induction of apoptosis in human colonic carcinoma cells (Caco-2) by commensal, probiotic and enteropathogenic bacteria is mediated by the mitochondrial pathway and is FAS independent. *International Journal of Food Microbiology* 137: 190–203.

Arvind, K., K. S. Nikhlesh, and R. S. Pushpalata. 2010. Inhibition of 1,2-dimethylhydrazine induced colon genotoxicity in rats by the administration of probiotic curd. *Molecular Biology Reports* 37: 1373–1376.

Aso, Y. and H. Akazan. 1992. Prophylactic effect of a *Lactobacillus casei* preparation on the recurrence of superficial bladder cancer. *Urology International* 49: 125–129.

Balotescu, M. C. and L. M. P. Roumanian. 2004. Adherence of lactobacilli to intestinal mucosa and their antagonistic activity against pathogens. *Biotechnology Letters* 9(4): 1737–1749.

Baricault, L., G. Denariaz, J. J. Houri, C. Bouley, C. Sapin, and G. Trugnan. 1995. Use of HT-29, a cultured human colon cancer cell line, to study the effect of fermented milks on colon cancer cell growth and differentiation. *Carcinogenesis* 16: 245–252.

Biffi, A., D. Coradini, R. Larsen, L. Riva, and G. Di Fronzo. 1997. Antiproliferative effect of fermented milk on the growth of a human breast cancer cell line. *Nutrition and Cancer* 28: 93–99.

Blandino, A., M. E. Al-Aseeri, S. S. Pandiella, D. Cantero, and C. Webb. 2003. Cereal-based fermented foods and beverages. *Food Research International* 36: 527–543.

Bouhnik, Y., B. Flourié, C. Andrieux, N. Bisetti, F. Briet, and J. C. Rambaud. 1996. Effects of *Bifidobacterium* sp. fermented milk ingested with or without inulin on colonic bifidobacteria and enzymatic activities in healthy humans. *European Journal of Clinical Nutrition* 50: 269–273.

Bron, P. A., C. Grangette, A. Mercennier, W. M. de Vos, and M. Kleerebezem. 2004. Identification of *Lactobacillus plantarum* genes that are induced in the gastrointestinal tract of mice. *Journal of Bacteriology* 186: 721–729.

Camarri, E., A. Belvisi, G. Guidoni, G. Marini, and G. Frigerio. 1981. A double-blind comparison of two different treatments for acute enteritis in adults. *Chemotherapy,* 27: 466–470.

Campieri, M. and P. Gionchetti. 1999. Manipulation of intestinal microflora. In *Advances in Inflammatory Bowel Diseases,* ed. P. Rutgeerts, 297–300, Netherland: Kluwer Academic Publisher.

Challa, A., D. R. Rao, C. B. Chawan, and L. Shackleford. 1997. *Bifidobacterium longum* and lactulose suppress azoxymethane-induced colonic aberrant crypt foci in rats. *Carcinogenesis* 18: 517–521.

Chang, J. H., Y. Y. Shim, S. K. Cha, M. J. T. Reaney, and K. M. Chee. 2012. Effect of *Lactobacillu acidophilus* KFRI342 on the development of chemically induced precancerous growths in the rat colon. *Journal of Medical Microbiology* 61: 361–368.

Chavan, J. K., S. S. Kadam, and L. R. Beuchat. 1989. Nutritional improvement of cereals by fermentation. *Critical Reviews in Food Science and Nutrition* 28(5): 349–400.

Chen, C. C., W. C. Lin, M. S. Kong, H. N. Shi, W. A. Walker, C. Y. Lin, C. T. Huang, Y. C. Lin, S., M. Jung, and T. Y. Lin. 2012. Oral inoculation of probiotics *Lactobacillus acidophilus* NCFM suppresses tumor growth both in segmental orthotopic colon cancer and extra-intestinal tissue. *British Journal of Nutrition* 107: 1623–1634.

Cousin, F. J., S. Jouan-Lanhouet, M. T. Dimanche-Boitrel, L. Corcos, and G. Jan. 2012. Milk fermented by *Propionibacterium freudenreichii* induces apoptosis of HGT-1 human gastric cancer cells. *PloS ONE* 7(3): e31892. Doi:10:1371/journal.pone.0031892.

Crittenden, R., A. R. Bird, P. Gopal, A. Henriksson, Y. K. Lee, and M. J. Playne. 2005. Probiotic research in Australia, New Zealand and the Asia-Pacific region. *Current Pharmaceutical Design* 11: 37–53.

Daeschel, M. A. and H. P. Fleming. 1987. Achieving pure culture cucumber fermentations: a review. In *Developments in Industrial Microbiology*, ed. G. Pierce, 28: 141–148. Arlington, VA: Society for Industrial Microbiology.

Danikas, D. D., M. Karakantza, G. L. Theodorou, G. C. Sakellaropoulos, and C. A. Gogos. 2008. Prognostic value of phagocytic activity of neutrophils and monocytes in sepsis. Correlation to CD64 and CD14 antigen expression *Clinical & Experimental Immunology* 154: 87–97.

De Vrese, M. and J. Schrezenmeir. 2008. Probiotics, prebiotics, and synbiotics. *Advances in Biochemical Engineering/Biotechnology* 111: 1–66.

De Vrese, M. and P. R. Marteau. 2007. Probiotics and prebiotics: Effects on diarrhea. *The Journal of Nutrition* 137: 803S–811S.

Erkkilä, S., E. Petäjä, S. Eerola, L. Lilleberg, T. Mattila-Sandholm, and M. L. Suihko. 2001. Flavour profiles of dry sausages fermented by selected novel meat starter cultures. *Meat Science* 58: 111–116.

Esser, P., C. Lund, and J. Clemensen. 1983. Antileukemic effects in mice from fermentation products of *Lactobacillus bulgaricus. Milchwissenschaft* 38: 257–260.

Fanaro, S., R. Chierici, P. Guerrini, and V. Vigi. 2003. Intestinal microflora in early infancy: composition and development. *Acta Paediatrica* 91: 48–55.

Farnworth, E. R. 2003. *Handbook of Fermented Functional Foods*. Food Research and Development Centre, Agriculture and Agri-Food Canada, 251–275. Boca Raton, FL: CRC Press.

Felton, J. S., M. G. Knize, F. A. Dolbeare, and F. Wu. 1994. Mutagenic activity of heterocyclic amines in cooked foods. *Environmental Health Perpectives* 102(6): 201–204.

Femia, A. P., C. Luceri, P. Dolara, A. Giannini, A. Biggeri, M. Salvadori, Y. Clune, , J. K. Collins, M. Paglierani, and G. Caderni. 2002. Antitumorigenic activity of the prebiotic inulin enriched with oligofructose in combination with the prebiotics *Lactobacillus rhamnosus* and *Bifidobacterium lactis* on azoxymethane induced colon carcinogenesis. *Carcinogenesis* 23: 1953–1960.

Freitas, M., E. Tavan, C. Cayuela, L. Diop, C. Sapin, and G. Trugnan. 2003. Host–pathogens cross-talk. Indigenous bacteria and probiotics also play the game. *Biology of Cell* 95: 503–506.

Gallaher, D. G. and J. Khil. 1999. The effect of synbiotics on colon carcinogenesis in rats. *Journal of Nutrition* 129: 1483S–1487S.

Gilliland, S.E. 1990. Health and nutritional benefits from lactic acid bacteria. *FEMS Microbiology Reviews* 87: 175–188.

Goldsby, R. E., L. E. Hays, X. Chen , E. A. Olmsted , W. B. Slayton, G. J. Spangrude, and B. D. Preston. 2002. High incidence of epithelial cancers in mice deficient for DNA polymerase proofreading *Proceedings of the National Academy of Sciences* 99(24): 15560–15565.

Goldin, B. R., L. Swenson, J. Dwyer, M. Sexton, and S. L. Gorbach. 1980. Effect of diet and *Lactobacillus acidophilus* supplements on human fecal bacterial enzymes. *Journal of National Cancer Institute* 64: 255–261.

Gulati, T. 2009 Development of fruit juices and performance evaluation of their nutritional values. BTech thesis, IIT Kharagpur, India.

Haard, N. F., S. A. Odunfa, C. H. Lee, R. Quintero-Ramirez, A. Lorence- Quinones, and C. Wacher-Radarte. 1999. Fermented cereals. A global perspective. *FAO Agricultural Services Bulletin* 138. http://www.fao.org/docrep/x2184e/x2184e06.htm

Halasz, A., A. Barath, L. Simon-Sarkadi, and W. Holzapfel. 1994. Biogenic amines and their production by micro-organisms in food. *Trends in Food Science & Technology* 5: 42–49.

Hamne, J., A. Cuthbert, P. J. Croucher, M. M. Mirza, S. Mascheretti, K. Frenzel, King et al. 2001. Association between insertion mutation in NOD2 gene and Crohn's disease in German and British populations. *The Lancet* 357(9272): 1925–1928.

Han, S. Y., C. S. Huh, Y. T. Ahn, K. S. Lim, Y. J. Baek, and D. H. Kim. 2005. Hepatoprotective effect of lactic acid bacteria, inhibitors of beta-glucuronidase production against intestinal microflora. *Archives of Pharmacal Research* 28: 325–329.

Harun-ur-Rashid, M., K. Togo, M. Useda, and T. Miyamoto. 2007. Probiotic characteristics of lactic acid bacteria isolated from traditional fermented milk "Dahi" in Bangladesh. *Pakistan Journal of Nutrition* 6: 647–652.

Harutoshi, T. 2013. Exopolysaccharides of lactic acid bacteria for food and colon health applications. In *Lactic Acid Bacteria-R and D for Food, Health and Livestock Purposes*, ed. M. Kongo, 515–538, Croatia: InTech.

Havenaar, R. and S. Spanhaak. 1994. Probiotics from an immunological point of view. *Current Opinion in Biotechnology* 5: 320–325.

Hayatsu, H. and T. Hayatsu. 1993. Suppressing effect of *Lactobacillus casei* administration on the urinary mutagenicity arising from ingestion of fried ground beef in the human. *Cancer Letters* 73: 173–179.

Helmy, S. A., 2012. Histopathological effect of probiotics after intra-peritoneal injection of ehrlith ascites tumor cells. *Scientific Reports* 1: 531 doi:10.4172/scientificreports.531.

Holick, M. F. 2003. Vitamin D: A millenium perspective. *Journal of Cellular Biochemistry* 88(2): 296–307.

Holzapfel, W. H. 1997. Use of starter cultures in fermentation on a household scale. *Food Control* 8: 241–258.

Holzapfel, W. H., P. Haberer, J. Snel, U. Schillinger, and J. H. Huis in't Veld. 1998. Overview of gut flora and probiotics. *International Journal of Food Microbiology* 41: 85–101.

Joshi, S. R. 2007. *Microbes: Redefined Personality*. India: APH Publishing Corporation.

Kaila, M., E. Isolauri, and E. Sopi. 1992. Enhancement of the circulating antibody secreting cell response in human diarrhea by a human *Lactobacillus* strain. *Pediatric Research* 32: 141–144.

Kawamura, T., K. Ohnuki, and H. Ichida. 1981. A clinical study on a *Lactobacillus casei* preparation (LBG-01) in patients with chronic irregular bowel movement and abdominal discomfort. *Japanese Pharmacology and* Therapeutics 9: 4361–70.

Khetarpaul, N. and B. M. Chauhan. 1990. Effect of fermentation by pure cultures of yeasts and lactobacilli on the available carbohydrate content of pearl millet. *Tropical Science* 31: 131–139.

Kiessling, G., J. Schneider, and G. Jahreis. 2002. Long-term consumption of fermented dairy products over 6-months increases HDL cholesterol. *European Journal of Clinical Nutrition* 56: 843–849.

Kim, J. Y., H. J. Woo, Y. S. Kim, K. H. Kim, and H. J. Lee. 2003. Cell cycle dysregulation induced by cytoplasm of *Lactococcus lactis* ssp. *lactis* in SNUC2A, a colon cancer cell line. *Nutrition and Cancer* 46: 197–201.

Kim, J. Y., S. Lee, D. W. Jeong, S. Hachimura, S. Kaminogawa, and H. J. Lee. 2006. *In vivo* immunopotentiating effects of cellular components from *Lactococcus lactis* ssp. *lactis*. *Journal of Microbiology and Biotechnology* 16: 786–790.

Kim, S. Y., K. W. Lee, J. Y. Kim, and H. J. Lee. 2004. Cytoplasmic fraction of *Lactococcus lactis* ssp. *lactis* induces apoptosis in SNU-1 stomach adenocarcinoma cells. *Biofactors* 22: 119–122.

Klingberg, T. D. and B. B. Budde. 2006. The survival and persistence in the human gastrointestinal tract of five potential probiotic lactobacilli consumed as freeze dried cultures or as probiotic sausage. *International Journal of Food Microbiology* 109: 157–159.

Kore, K. B., A. K. Pattanaik, K. Sharma, and P. P. Mirajkar. 2012. Effect of feeding traditionally prepared fermented milk dahi (curd) as a probiotics on nutritional status, hindgut health and haematology in dogs. *Indian Journal of Traditional Knowledge* 11(1): 35–39.

Kuchta, A. 2011. Investigations of the health benefits of buttermilk fat globule membrane lipid components. PhD thesis. School of Biotechnology, Dublin City University.

Kulkarni, S. G., J. K. Manan, M. D. Agarwal, and I. C. Shukla. 1997. Studies on physico-chemical composition, packaging and storage of black gram and green gram Wari prepared in Uttar Pradesh. *Journal of Food Science and Technology* 34(2): 119–122.

Kullisaar, T., E. Songisepp, M. Mikelsaar, K. Zilmer, T. Vihalemm, and M. Zilmer. 2003. Antioxidative probiotic fermented goats' milk decreases oxidative stress-mediated atherogenicity in human subjects. *British Journal of Nutrition* 90: 449–456.

Kumar, M., V. Verma, R. Nagpal, A. Kumar, P. V. Behare, B. Singh, and P.K. Aggarwal. 2012. Anticarcinogenic effect of probiotic fermented milk and chlorophyllin on aflatoxin-B_1-induced liver carcinogenesis in rats. *British Journal of Nutrition* 107: 1006–1016.

Lambert, J. and R. Hull. 1996. Upper gastrointestinal tract diseases and probiotics. *Asian Pacific Journal of Clinical Nutrition* 5(1): 31–35.

LeBlanc, A. D. M., C. Matar, E. Farnworth, and G. Perdigon. 2007. Study of immune cells involved in the antitumor effect of kefir in a murine breast cancer model. *Journal of Dairy Science* 90: 1920–1928.

Lee, J. W., J. G. Shin, E. H. Kim, H. E. Kang, I. B. Yim, J. Y. Kim, H. G. Joo, and H. J. Woo. 2004. Immunomodulatory and antitumor effects *in vivo* by the cytoplasmic fraction of *Lactobacillus casei* and *Bifidobacterium longum*. *Journal of Veterinary Science* 5: 41–48.

Leisner, J. J., J. C. Millan, H. H. Huss, and L. M. Larsen. 1994. Production of histamine and tyramine by lactic acid bacteria, isolated from vacuum-packed sugar-salted fish. *Journal of Applied* Bacteriology 76: 417–423.

Leu, R. K. L., I. L. Brown, Y. Hu, A. R. Bird, M. Jackson, and A. Esterman. 2005. A synbiotic combination of resistant starch and *Bifidobacterium lactis* facilitates apoptotic deletion of carcinogen-damaged cells in rat colon. *Journal of Nutrition* 135: 996–1001.

Lim, B. K., R. Mahendran, Y. K. Lee, and B. H. Bay. 2002. Chemopreventive effect of *Lactobacillus rhamnosus* on growth of a subcutaneously implanted bladder cancer cell line in the mouse. *Japanese Journal of Cancer Research* 93: 36–41.

Ling, M. Y. and C. L. Yen. 1999. Antioxidative ability of lactic acid bacteria. *Journal of Agricultural and Food Chemistry* 47: 1460–1466.

Ljungh, A. and T. Wadstrom. 2006. Lactic acid bacteria as probiotics. *Current Issues in Intestinal Microbiology* 7: 73–89.

Lourens-Hattingh, A. and B. C. Viljoen. 2001. Yogurt as probiotic carrier food. *International Dairy Journal* 11: 1–17.

Mann, G. V. and A. Spoerry. 1974. Studies of a surfactant and cholesteremia in the Maasai. *The American Journal of Clinical Nutrition* 27: 464–469.

Marteau, P., P. Seksik, and R. Jian. 2002. Probiotics and intestinal health effects: A clinical perspective. *British Journal of Nutrition* 88: 51–57.

Matsuzaki, T. 1998. Immunomodulation by treatment with *Lactobacillus casei* strain *Shirota*. *International Journal of Food Microbiology* 41: 133–140.

Mbugua, S. K., R. H. Ahrens, H. N. Kigutha, and V. Subramanian. 1992. Effect of fermentation, malted flour treatment and drum drying on nutritional quality of uji. *Ecology of Food and Nutrition* 28: 271–277.

McIntosh, G. H., P. J. Royle, and M. J. Playne. 1999. A probiotic strain of *Lb. acidophilus* reduces DMH-induced large intestinal tumors in male Sprague–Dawley rats. *Nutrition and Cancer* 35: 153–159.

Mestecky, J. and J. McGhee. 1987. Immunoglobulin A (IgA) molecular and cellular interactions involved in IgA biosynthesis and immune response. *Advances in Immunology* 40: 153–245.

Miettinen, M., J. Vuopio-Varkila, and K. Varkila. 1996. Production of human tumor necrosis factor alpha, interleukin-6, and interleukin-10 is induced by lactic acid bacteria. *Infection and Immunity* 64(12): 5403–5405.

Miler, I., V. Vetvicka, P. Síma, and L. Táborský. 1985. The effect of bilirubin on the phagocytic activity of mouse peripheral granulocytes and monocytes in vivo. *Folia Microbiologica* 30(3): 267–271.

Mitra, S., P. K. Chakrabartty, and S. R. Biswas. 2007. Production of Nisin Z by *Lactococcus lactis* isolated from dahi. *Applied Biochemistry and Biotechnology* 143: 41–53.

Mitsuoka, T. 1990. Bifidobacteria and their role in human health. *Journal of Industrial Microbiology* 6: 263–268.

Mizutani, T. and T. Mitsuoka. 1979. Effect of intestinal bacteria on incidence of liver tumors in gnotobiotic C3H/He male mice. *Journal of the National Cancer Institute* 63: 1365–1370.

Mizutani, T. and T. Mitsuoka. 1980. Inhibitory effect of some intestinal bacteria on liver tumorigenesis in gnotobiotic C3H/He male mice. *Cancer* Letters 11: 89–95.

Mohania, D., V. K. Kansal, R. Sagwal, and D. Shah. 2013. Anticarcinogenic effect of probiotic dahi and piroxicam on DMH-induced colorectal carcinogenesis in Wister rats. *America Journal of Cancer Therapy and Pharmacology* 1(1): 8–24.

Murughar, D. A. and G. Subbulakshmi. 2006. Preparation techniques and nutritive value of fermented foods from the khasi tribes of Meghalaya. *Ecology of Food and Nutrition* 45: 27–38.

Naidu, A. S., W. R. Bidlack, and R. A. Clemens. 1999. Probiotic spectra of lactic acid bacteria (LAB). *Critical Reviews in Food Science and Nutrition* 38(1): 13–126.

Nanji, A. A., U. Khettry, and S. M. Sadrzadeh. 1994. Lactobacillus feeding reduces endotoxemia and severity of experimental alcoholic liver (disease). *Proceedings of the Society for Experimental Biology and Medicine* 205: 243–247.

Ockerman, H. W. and L. Basu. 2010. Fermented meat products production and consumption https://kb.osu.edu/dspace/bitstream/handle/1811/45275/fermented?sequence=1 Accessed on June 20th, 2014.

Oki, K., A. K. Rai, S. Sato, K. Watanabe, and J. P. Tamang. 2011. Lactic acid bacteria isolated from ethnic preserved meat products of the Western Himalayas. *Food Microbiology* 28: 1308–1315.

Olivares, M., M. P. Diaz-Ropero, N. Gomez, F. Lara-Villoslada, S. Sierra, J. A. Maldonado, R. J. Martin, M. Rodriguez, and J. Xaus. 2006. The consumption of two new probiotic strains, *Lactobacillus gasseri* CECT 5714 and *Lactobacillus coryniformis* CECT 5711, boosts the immune system of healthy humans. *International Microbiology* 9: 47–52.

Orrhage, K., E. Sillerström, J. A. Gustafsson, C. E. Nord, and J. Rafter. 1994. Binding of mutagenic heterocyclic amines by intestinal and lactic acid bacteria. *Mutation Research* 311(2): 239–248.

O'Sullivan, M. G., G. Thornton, G. C. O'Sullivan, and J. K. Collins. 1992. Probiotic bacteria: Myth or reality. *Trends in Food Science and Technology* 3: 309–314.

Pala, V., S. Sieri, F. Berrino, P. Vineis, C. Sacerdote, D. Palli, G. Masala et al. 2011. Yogurt consumption and risk of colorectal cancer in the Italian European prospective investigation into cancer and nutrition cohort. *International Journal of Cancer* 129: 2712–2719.

Parvez, S., K. A. Malik, S. Ah Kang, and H. Y. Kim. 2006. Probiotics and their fermented food products are beneficial for health. *Journal of Applied Microbiology* 100: 1171–1185.

Patil, M. M., A. Pal, T. Anand, and K. V. Ramana. 2010. Isolation and characterisation of lactic acid bacteria from curd and cucumber. *Indian Journal of Biotechnology* 9: 166–172.

Perdigon, G., C. M. Galdeano, J. C. Valdez, and M. Medici. 2002. Interaction of lactic acid bacteria with the gut immune system. *European Journal of Clinical Nutrition* 56(4): S21–S26.

Perdigon, G., M. E. Macias, S. Alvarez, G. Oliver, and A. A. R. Holgado. 1986. Effect of perorally administered lactobacilli on macrophage activation in mice. *Infection and Immunity* 53: 404–410.

Pidcock, K., G. M. Heard, and A. Henriksson. 2002. Application of nontraditional meat starter cultures in production of Hungarian salami. *International Journal of Food Microbiology* 76: 75–81.

Ponce, A. G., M. R. Moreira, C. E. del Velle, and S. I. Roura. 2008. Preliminary characterization of bacteriocin-like substances from lactic acid bacteria isolated from organic leafy vegetables. *LWT-Food Science and Technology* 41(3): 432–441.

Pool-Zobel, B. L., R. Münzner, and W. H. Holzapfel. 1993. Antigenotoxic properties of lactic acid bacteria in the *S. typhimurium* mutagenicity assay. *Nutrition and Cancer* 20: 261–270.

Pouwels, P. H., R. J. Leer, and W. J. Boersma. 1996. The potential of *Lactobacillus* as a carrier for oral immunization: Development and preliminary characterization of vector systems for targeted delivery of antigens. *Journal of Biotechnology* 44: 183–192.

Praveesh, B. V., J. Angayarkanni, and M. Palaniswamyint. 2011. Antihypertensive and anticancer effect of cow milk fermented by *Lactobacillus plantarum* and *Lactobacillus casei*. *Journal of Pharmacy and Pharmaceutical Science* 3(5): 452–456.

Puwastien, P., K. Judprasong, E. Kettwan, K. Vasanachitt, Y. Nakngamanong, and L. Bhattacharjee. 1999. Proximate composition of raw and cooked Thai freshwater and marine fish. *Journal of Food Composition and Analysis* 12: 9–16.

Rafter, J. 2002. Lactic acid bacteria and cancer: Mechanistic perspective. *British Journal of Nutrition* 88(1): S89–S94.

Rai, A. K., J. P. Tamang, and U. Palni. 2010a. Microbiological studies of ethnic meat products of the Eastern Himalayas. *Meat Science* 85: 560–567.

Rai, K., S. Sarkar, T. Broadbent, M. Voas, K. F. Grossman, L. D. Nadauld, S. Dehghanizadeh et al. 2010b. DNA demethylase activity maintains intestinal cells in an undifferentiated state following loss of APC. *Cell* 142(6): 930–942.

Reddy, G. V., B. A. Friend, K. M. Shahani, and R. Farmer. 1983. Antitumor activity of yogurt components. *Journal of Food Protection* 46: 8–11.

Resta-Lenert, S. and K. E. Barrett. 2003. Live probiotics protect intestinal epithelial cells from the effects of infection with enteroinvasive *Escherichia coli* (EIEC). *Gut* 52: 988–997.

Rhee, S. J., J. E. Lee, and C. H. Lee. 2011. Importance of lactic acid bacteria in Asian fermented foods. *Microbial Cell Factories* 10: 55–68.

Riki, M., F. Farokhi, and A. Tukmechi. 2013. The best time of cytotoxicity for extracted cell wall from *Lactobacillus casei* and *paracasei* in K562 cell line. *Tehran University Medical Journal* 70(11): 691–699.

Roberfroid, B. 2000. Prebiotics and probiotics: Are they functional foods? *American Journal of Clinical Nutrition* 71(6): 1682S–1687S.

Roos, N. M. and M. B. Katan. 2000. Effects of probiotic bacteria on diarrhea, lipid metabolism, and carcinogenesis: A review of papers published between 1988 and 1998. *American Journal of Clinical Nutrition* 71: 405–411.

Rubia-Soria, A., H. Abriouel, R. Lucas, N. B. Omar, M. Martinez-Caoamero, and A. Galvez. 2006. Production of antimicrobial substances by bacteria isolated from fermented table olives. *World Journal of Microbiology and Biotechnology* 22(7): 765–768.

Saavedra, J. M. 2007. Use of probiotics in pediatrics: Rationale, mechanisms of action, and practical aspects. *Nutrition in Clinical Practice* 22: 351–365.

Saavedra, J. M., N. A. Bauman, I. Oung, J. A. Perman, and R. H. Yolken. 1994. Feeding of *Bifidobacterium bifidum* and *Streptococcus thermophilus* to infants in hospital for prevention of diarrhoea and shedding of rotavirus. *The Lancet* 344: 1046–1049.

Saito, T. 2004. Selection of useful lactic acid bacteria from *Lactobacillus acidophilus* group and their applications to functional foods. *Animal Science Journal* 75: 1–13.

Salminen, E., E. Elomaa, J. Minkkinen, H. Vapaatalo, and S. Salminen. 1988. Preservation of intestinal integrity during radiotherapy using live *Lactobacillus acidophilus* cultures. *Clinical Radiology* 39: 435–437.

Sartor, R. B. and S. K. Mazmanian. 2012. Intestinal microbes in inflammatory bowel disease. *American Journal of Gastroenterology Supplements* 1: 15–21.

Sarkar, P. K., B. Hasenack, and M. J. Nout. 2002. Diversity and functionality of *Bacillus* and related genera isolated from spontaneously fermented soybeans (Indian kinema) and locust beans (African soumbala). *International Journal of Food Microbiology* 25: 175–186.

Satish, K. R., P. Kanmani, N. Yuvaraj, K. A. Paari, V. Pattukumar, and V. Arul. 2011. *Lactobacillus plantarum* AS1 binds to cultured human intestinal cell line HT-29 and inhibits cell attachment by enterovirulent bacterium *Vibrio parahaemolyticus*. *Letters in Applied Microbiology* 53(4): 481–487.

Satish, K. R., V. D. Raghu, P. Kanmani, N. Yuvaraj, K. A. Paari, V. Pattukumar, and V. Arul. 2010. Isolation, characterization and identification of a potential probiont from south Indian fermented foods (kallappam, koozh and mor kuzhambu) and its use as biopreservative. *Probiotics and Antimicrobial Proteins* 2: 145–151.

Sato, K., H. Saito, H. Tomioka, and T. Yokokura. 1988. Enhancement of host resistance against *Listeria* infection by *Lactobacillus casei*: Efficacy of cell wall preparation of *Lactobacillus casei*. *Microbiology and Immunology* 32: 1189–1200.

Savadogo, A., C. A. T. Ouattara, I. H. N. Bassole, and S. A. Traore. 2006. Bacteriocins and lactic acid bacteria—A mini review. *African Journal of Biotechnology* 5(9): 678–683.

Sekine, K., T. Toida, M. Saito, M. Kuboyama, T. Kawashima, and Y. Hashimoto. 1985. A new morphologically characterized cell wall preparation (whole peptidoglycan) from *Bifidobacterium infantis* with a higher efficacy on the regression of an established tumour in mice. *Cancer Research* 45: 1300–1307.

Shahani, K. M., B. A. Friend, and P. J. Bailey. 1983. Antitumor activity of fermented colostrum and milk. *Journal of Food Protection* 46: 385–386.

Sharma, A., G. K. Rath, S. P. Chaudhary, A. Thakar, B. K. Mohanti, and S. Bahadur. 2012. *Lactobacillus brevis* CD2 lozenges reduce radiation- and chemotherapy-induced mucositis in patients with head and neck cancer: A randomized double-blind placebo-controlled study. *European Journal of Cancer* 48:875–881.

Shigwedha, N. and L. Jia. 2013. Bifidobacterium in Human GI Tract: Screening, isolation, survival and growth kinetics in simulated gastrointestinal conditions. In *Lactic Acid Bacteria- R and D for Food, Health and Livestock Purposes*, ed. M. Kongo, 281–308, Croatia: InTech.

Singh, A. 2009. Soy whey: A potent functional food adjunct. MTech thesis, IIT Kharagpur, India.

Singh, A., R. K. Singh, and A. K. Sureja. 2007. Cultural significance and diversities of ethnic foods of Northeast India. *Indian Journal of Traditional Knowledge* 6(1): 79–94.

Sinha, P. R. and R. N. Sinha. 2000. Importance of good quality dahi in food. *Indian Dairyman* 52: 45–47.

Songisepp, E., J. Kals, T. Kullisaar, R. Mandar, P. Hutt, M. Zilmer, and M. Mikelsaar. 2005. Evaluation of the functional efficacy of an antioxidative probiotic in healthy volunteers. *Nutrition Journal* 4: 22. doi:10.1186/1475–2891–4–22.

Songisepp, E., T. Kullisaar, P. Hutt, P. Elias, T. Brilene, M. Zilmer, and M. Mikelsaar. 2004. A new probiotic cheese with antioxidative and antimicrobial activity. *Journal of Dairy Science* 87: 2017–2023.

Spanhaak, S., R. Havenaar, and G. Schaafsma. 1998. The effect of consumption of milk fermented by *Lactobacillus casei* strain Shirota on the intestinal microflora and immune parameters in humans. *European Journal of Clinical Nutrition* 52: 1–9.

Stiles, M. E. 1996. Biopreservation by lactic acid bacteria. *Antonie van Leuwenhoek* 70: 331–345.

Swennen, K., C. M. Courtin, and J. A. Delcour. 2006. Non-digestible oligosaccharides with prebiotic properties. *Clinical Reviews in Food Science and Nutrition* 46: 459–471.

Tamang, J. P. and S. Nikkuni. 1996. Selection of starter cultures for the production of kinema a fermented soybean food of the Himalaya. *World Journal of Microbiology and Biotechnology* 12: 629–635.

Tamang, B. and J. P. Tamang. 2009. Lactic acid bacteria isolated from indigenous fermented bamboo products of Arunachal Pradesh in India and their functionality. *Food Biotechnology* 23: 133–147.

Tamang, B., J. P. Tamang, U. Schillinger, C. M. A. P. Franz, M. Gores, and W. H. Holzapfel. 2008. Phenotypic and genotypic identification of lactic acid bacteria isolated from ethnic fermented tender bamboo shoots of North East India. *International Journal of Food Microbiology* 121: 35–40.

Tamang, J. P., B. Tamang, U. Schillinger, C. M. A. P. Franz, M. Gores, and W. H. Holzapfel. 2005. Identification of predominant lactic acid bacteria isolated from traditional fermented vegetable products of the Eastern Himalayas. *International Journal of Food Microbiology* 105(3): 347–356.

Tamang, J. P., N. Tamang, S. Thapa, S. Dewan, B. M. Tamang, H. Yonzan, , A. K. Rai, R. Chettri, J. Chakrabarty, and N. Kharel. 2012. Microorganisms and nutritional value of ethnic fermented foods and alcoholic beverages of North East India. *Indian Journal of Traditional Knowledge* 11(1): 7–25.

Tewary, H. K. and H. G. Muller. 1992. The fate of some oligosaccharides during the preparation of wari and Indian fermented food. *Food Chemistry* 43(2): 107–111.

Thapa, N., J. Pal, and J. P. Tamang. 2004. Microbial diversity in ngari, hentak and tungtap, fermented fish products of North-East India. *World Journal of Microbiology and Biotechnology* 20(6): 599–607.

Thapa, N., J. Pal, and J. P. Tamang. 2006. Phenotypic identification and technological properties of lactic acid bacteria isolated from traditionally processed fish products of the Eastern Himalayas. *International Journal of Food Microbiology* 107(1): 33–38.

Thokchom, S. and S. R. Joshi. 2012. Antibiotic resistance and probiotic properties of dominant lactic microflora from tungrymbai, an ethnic fermented soybean food of India. *Journal of Microbiology* 50(3): 535–539.

Todorov, S., B. Onno, O. Sorokine, J. M Chobert, Ivanova, I., and X. Dousset. 1999. Detection and characterization of a novel antibacterial substance produced by *Lactobacillus plantarum* ST31 isolated from sourdough. *International Journal of Food Microbiology* 48: 167–177.

Tolonen, M., S. Rajaniemi, J. M. Pihlava, T. Johansson, P. E. J. Saris, and E. L. Ryhanen. 2004. Formation of nisin, plant-derived biomolecules and antimicrobial activity in starter culture fermentations of sauerkraut. *Food Microbiology* 21: 167–179.

Tyopponen, S., E. Petaja, and T. Mattila-Sandholm. 2003. Bioprotectives and probiotics for dry sausages. *International Journal of Food Microbiology* 83: 233–244.

Uhlman, L., U. Schillinger, J. R. Rupnow, and W. H. Holzapfel. 1992. Identification and characterization of two bacteriocin-producing strains of *Lactococcus lactis* isolated from vegetables. *International Journal of Food Microbiology* 16: 141–151.

Vasiljevic, T. and N. P. Shah. 2008. Probiotics-From Metchnikoff to bioactives. *International Dairy Journal* 18: 714–728.

Veer, P. V., J. M. Dekker, J. W. J. Lamers, F. J. Kok, E. J. Schouten, Brants, F. Sturmans, and R. J. J. Hermus. 1989. Consumption of fermented milk products and breast cancer: A case–control study in the Netherlands. *Cancer Research* 49(14): 4020–4023.

Vinderola, C. G., M. Medici, and G. Perdigon. 2004. Relationship between interaction sites in the gut, hydrophobicity, mucosal immunomodulation capacities and cell wall protein profiles in indigenous and exogenous bacteria. *Journal of Applied Microbiology* 96: 230–243.

Watanabe, T., K. Hamada, A. Tategaki, H. Kishida, H. Tanaka, M. Kitano, and T. Miyamoto. 2009. Oral administration of lactic acid bacteria isolated from traditional south Asian fermented milk 'Dahi' inhibits the development of Atopic Dermatitis in NC/Nga mice. *Journal of Nutritional Science and Vitaminology* 55: 271–278.

Wollowski, I., G. Rechkemmer, and B. L. Pool-Zobel. 2001. Protective role of probiotics and prebiotics in colon cancer. *The American Journal of Clinical Nutrition* 73: 451S–455S.

Wylie, J. G. and A. Henderson. 1969. Identity and glycogen-fermenting ability of lactobacilli isolated from the vagina of pregnant women. *Journal of Medical Microbiology* 2: 363–366.

Yadav, H., S. Jain, and P. R. Sinha. 2007. Antidiabetic effect of probiotic dahi containing *Lactobacillus acidophilus* and *Lactobacillus casei* in high fructose fed rats. *Nutrition* 23: 62–68.

Yateem, A., M. T. Balba, T. Al-Surrayai, B. Al-Mutairi, and R. Al-Daher. 2008. Isolation of lactic acid bacteria with probiotic potential from camel milk. *International Journal of Dairy Science* 3: 194–199.

Yuan, L., K. Wen, F. Liu, and G. Li. 2013. Dose effects of lab on modulation of rotavirus vaccine induced immune responses. In *Lactic Acid Bacteria—R and D for Food, Health and Livestock Purposes*, ed. J. M. Kongo, Croatia: InTech.

Chapter 4

Diet, Microbiome, and Human Health

Ashfaque Hossain, Saeed Akhter, and Yearul Kabir

Contents

4.1 Introduction

The influence of microorganisms residing in the intestine (gut microbiota) on human health and disease is an area of intense research as health and well-being is of primary concern to us. The gut microbiome (gut microbiota and its collective genomes) plays a key role in homeostasis in humans and a strong relationship exists between diet, microbiota, and our health (Nicholson et al. 2012, Martin et al. 2014). Dietary components and dietary metabolites have roles beyond basic nutrition, and the modulation of the gut microbiome composition by the alteration of food habits has potentialities in health improvement and even disease prevention (Holmes et al. 2012, Guzman et al. 2013). Understanding the complex interaction between diet and the composition and function of human gut microbiota is critical in advancing our knowledge in the formulation of ways of manipulation of microbiota to prevent various health conditions and to improve our health. A growing body of evidence suggests that reprogramming the gut microbiome or its function has beneficial effects on the host metabolism (de Vos and de Vos 2012, Goldsmith and Sartor 2014). The current knowledge of the complex and bidirectional interaction between the gut microbiome and dietary components in relation to human health and disease is reviewed in this chapter.

Virtually every surface of the human body is colonized by microorganisms. The human intestine is the habitat of many species of bacteria along with viruses, unicellular eukaryotes, and other organisms which have evolved and adapted to live, colonize, and grow there, forming a huge ecosystem, the gut microbiota (Bäckhed et al. 2005, Holmes et al. 2011). With an average length of 1.50 m and diameter of 6.4 cm, the human large intestine (colon) represents one of the largest interfaces where host–microbe interactions occur (Cummings and Macfarlane 1991). The intestine is home to an estimated 10^{14} microbial cells (Lepage et al. 2012). The microbes that we carry outnumber us 10:1 in terms of total human body cell (somatic and germ cells) counts. The combined number of genes in the microbiota genome is 150 times larger than the human genome (Neish 2009, Musso et al. 2010, Lepage et al. 2012). Taken together, the information reveals that the human gut microbiome is an ecosystem of the highest complexity. The vast majority of the microbial cells present in the human intestine are bacteria; the other members are viruses (5.8%; estimated 1200 viral genotypes are present; Breitbart et al. 2003), archaea (0.8%), and eukaryotes (0.5%) (Arumugam et al. 2011). Various factors influence the structure and function of gut microbiota. These include the availability of nutrients and antimicrobial compounds, temperature, pH, redox potential, degree of anaerobiosis, and presence of bacteriophages (Kinross et al. 2008). The metabolic activity of the human gut microbes is as robust as that of the liver and it has been suggested to function as an auxiliary, virtual organ (O'Hara and Shanahan 2006, DiBaise et al. 2012). A single layer of epithelial cells separates the gut microbiota from the internal milieu, and the structure and composition of the gut flora reflect the evolution and adaptation at both microbial and host levels promoting extensive, multiple levels of host–microbial interactions (McFall-Ngai et al. 2013). To maintain an intact and functional epithelial barrier is essential as the prevention of an unregulated uptake/translocation of the microbiome or its metabolites is required for the maintenance of host homeostasis (Guzman et al. 2013).

It is increasingly becoming clear that health and disease states can be explained at the individual level, at least in part, by the host–bacterial relationship. Directed manipulation of the microbiome offers a promising avenue for therapeutic applications as studies have shown that the transfer of donor microbiota induces a variety of donor phenotypes into the recipients (Jia et al. 2008). In addition, such practice has also resulted in the accelerated recovery of sick recipients (Prakash et al. 2011, McFall-Ngai et al. 2013).

4.2 Gut Microbiota

Although it is generally accepted that the intestine of a newborn infant is sterile and is rapidly colonized by different microorganisms during and after birth, thus developing the gut microbiota (Mackie et al. 1999), recent evidence shows that colonization of the gut is initiated before birth following ingestion of microbe-containing amniotic fluid by the fetus (Mshvildadze and Neu 2010). The human placenta, although considered sterile, has recently been found to possess a unique microbiome. A population-based cohort of placental specimens collected under sterile conditions from 320 subjects following culture-independent metagenomic analysis showed that the placenta harbors a variety of microbes and the placental microbiome most closely resembles the oral microbiome (Aagaard et al. 2014).

How a child is born (natural delivery or caesarean section) and how that child is fed (breast feeding or bottle feeding) strongly influences the development of gut microbiota (Penders et al. 2006). Hygiene levels and medication are also important in determining the structure of the gut microbiota of infants. The gut microbiota is usually considered fully developed by the age of 4. Each person possesses a unique microbiota and it is stable over time in healthy adults(Vanhoutte et al. 2004, Vrieze et al. 2010). Pioneer bacteria involved in the initial colonization in newborn babies are important in determining the final composition of the microbiota in adults (Guarner and Malagelada 2003).

Metagenomic studies have brought to light the enormous richness and diversity of human gut microbiota compositions. Microorganisms colonize different parts of the gastrointestinal tract (GIT) and bacterial population density varies along the GIT (Guarner and Malagelada 2003, Tappenden and Deutsch 2007, Romano-Keeler et al. 2014). There is a qualitative and quantitative increase in complexity in the bacterial population from the stomach to the colon (Table 4.1). In addition, there is variation in the composition of the flora along the GIT in terms of surface adherent and luminal bacteria. Although the ratio of anaerobes to aerobes is lower at the mucosal surface than in the lumen, the anaerobes outnumber aerobes and facultative anaerobes by two to three orders of magnitude in the overall count (Sekirov et al. 2010).

4.2.1 Diversity of Microbes in Gut Microbiota

The GIT is one of the most complex ecosystems on earth; organisms from all the kingdoms of life such as bacteria, archaea (e.g., methanogens), and eukarea (fungi, helminths, and protozoa) as well as viruses are present in gut microbiota (Norman et al. 2014). Development of culture-independent methods such as 16S ribosomal RNA survey and direct sequencing vastly advanced our knowledge of gut microbiota. Such studies have shown that bacteria living in the human gut achieve the highest cell densities recorded for any ecosystem which is a complex community of the diverse array of bacterial species. Culture-independent metagenomic studies have also revealed that cultivable fecal bacteria represent a fraction of the total bacteria present in the GIT, with the proportion of undescribed species varying from 30% to 90% (Blaut and Clavel 2007, Lagier et al. 2012). In healthy adults, 80% of the identified fecal microbiota belong to four dominant phyla: the Gram-negative *Bacteroidetes* and *Proteobacteria* and the Gram-positive *Actinobacteria* and

Table 4.1 The Number and Type of Bacteria Present in Different Anatomic Sites of the Human Intestine

Anatomic Site	*pH*	*Number of Bacteria*	*Type of Bacteria*
Stomach	2.0	1–10^2	*Lactobacillus* *Streptococcus* *Helicobacter* *Peptostreptococcus*
Duodenum		10^1–10^3	
Jejunum	↑ 4.0–5.0 ↓	10^3–10^4	↑ *Streptococcus* *Lactobacillus*
Ileum		10^7–10^9	*Bacteroides* *Clostridium* *Streptococcus* *Actinomycinaea*
Colon		10^{11}–10^{12}	*Bacteroides* *Clostridium* *Bifidobacterium* *Enterobacteriaceae* *Akkermansia* *Prevotella* *Ruminococcus*

Source: Adapted from Guarner, F. and J. R. Malagelada. 2003. *The Lancet* 360: 512–519; Sekirov, I. et al. 2010. *Physiological Reviews* 90: 859–904.

Note: The pH and functions of the different parts are also listed.

Firmicutes. These include at least 17 families, corresponding to no less than 1250 different species of bacteria (Schuijt et al. 2013). A striking feature of the gut microflora is that the majority of gut bacteria (~65%) are Gram-positive bacteria, virtually all of which are obligate anaerobes; Gram-negative anaerobes account for another 20%–30% of the total gut bacterial population (Bäckhed et al. 2005). In a large-scale culture-independent study Frank et al. (2007) put a much higher number to the bacterial genus and species present in the human gut microbiome. According to this study the human gut microbiome consists of at least 1800 genera and 15,000–36,000 species of bacteria demonstrating that a staggering level of microbial diversity remains to be characterized within the human microbiome.

The firmicutes are with a low G + C content, bacteroidetes and actinobacteria are with a high G + C content (de Vos and de Vos 2012, Schuijt et al. 2013). Gut microbiota exists in a relatively stable condition within the host and takes part in wide ranging metabolic processes (Tremaroli and Bäckhed 2012) but there is substantial variation in the species composition between individuals (Diamant et al. 2011, Flint 2012). Microbiota of each individual has a conserved fraction (core microbiota) which is shared between individuals and which may be needed for correct functioning of the gut and a variable fraction (variable microbiota) (Booijink et al. 2010, Tremaroli and Bäckhed 2012). A core microbiota that comprises 50–100 bacterial species when the frequency of abundance at the phylotype level is not considered, and a core microbiome harboring more than 6000 functional gene groups is present in the majority of human guts surveyed (Zhu et al. 2010).

4.3 Diet Influences Gut Microbiota

The important factors which influence human health are genetics, environment, and diet. Food has a role beyond serving as nutrients. Dietary impacts on health are one of the oldest concepts in medicine (Goldsmith and Sartor 2014). The importance of food in health was acknowledged more than 2500 years ago by Hippocrates by his sayings "death sits in the bowels," "bad digestion is the root of all evil" and his "food as medicine" philosophy (Hawrelak and Myers 2004). The influence of the gut microbiome and its interaction with the host is pivotal to understand nutrition and metabolism (Sekirov et al. 2010, Chen et al. 2014). Diet can influence the composition of gut microbiota and gut microbiota has wide ranging health effects; both positive and negative (Laparra and Sanz 2010, Tremaroli and Bäckhed 2012, Scott et al. 2013). Several lines of evidence suggest that dietary factors might profoundly influence the structure and function of gut microbiota, rapidly and reproducibly (David et al. 2014). These include studies using the mouse model, human clinical studies, epidemiological studies, and metagenomic investigations in humans (Bäckhed et al. 2005, McFall-Ngai et al. 2013). Diet is one of the major determinants for the persistence of a particular bacterium in the gut because the diet provides nutrients not only for the host but also for the bacteria residing there (Blaut and Clavel 2007).

Dietary composition and caloric intake appear to swiftly regulate intestinal microbial composition and function. The relative proportion of the three main macronutrients (carbohydrates, proteins, and fats) influence gut transit time and pH, in addition to the composition of gut microbiota (Scott et al. 2013, Shen et al. 2014). The diet-induced alteration of gut microbiota may change the relative proportion of protective/beneficial bacteria making the host susceptible to disease and/or reducing its efficiency of food utilization (Walker et al. 2011).

Compelling evidence to support the notion that diet modulates the structure and function of gut microbiota came from the studies with resistin-like molecule knockout mice (which are resistant to diet-induced obesity). A high-fat diet resulted in a decrease in *Bacteroidetes* and an increase in *Firmicutes* and *Proteobacteria* in control mice (which became obese) and also in resistin-like molecule knockout mice (which did not become obese) (Hildebrandt et al. 2009). Also transplantation of microbiota from lean or obese humans to germ-free mice established the corresponding phenotypes. The structure of microbiota also shifted accordingly following high-fat or low-fat diets in these microbiologically humanized mice (Turnbaugh et al. 2008) clearly demonstrating that diet influences gut microbiota in a profound way and adiposity is transferrable by fecal transplantation which responds to dietary changes (Petrof and Khoruts, 2014).

Analyses of large metagenome datasets have indicated that the microbial composition of individuals can be described within a few distinctive enterotypes (classification of the human gut microbiome according to the dominant microorganism present) which are independent of age, gender, and nationality and respond differently to diet and drugs (Arumugam et al. 2011). Enterotype *Bacteroides* (type-1) is associated with the consumption of a diet rich in protein and animal fat, while those who ate more fiber and carbohydrates and less animal fat and protein had *Prevotella* enterotype (type-2). Enterotype *Ruminococcus* (type-3) is not so distinct and is partly merged with the Bacteroides enterotype (Wu et al. 2011, Tremaroli and Bäckhed 2012). The enterotypes are stable and a long-term change in dietary habits are probably needed to induce a shift of one enterotype to another, as a 10-day dietary intervention failed to result in the alteration of the enterotype (Wu et al. 2011).

An interesting study by Filippo et al. (2010) showed how diet can impact the shaping of gut microbiota by comparing European children on a Western diet with rural African children who had a fiber-rich diet. Children from a rural African village in Burkina Faso showed a significant enrichment in *Bacteroidetes* with abundance of bacteria from the genus *Prevotella* and *Xylanibacter* and a depletion of *Firmicutes*. *Prevotella* and *Xylanibacter* encode enzymes enabling hydrolysis of cellulose and xylan. These African children indeed demonstrated a higher content of short-chain fatty acids (SCFAs) revealing that the gut microbiota in rural Africa may allow individuals to maximize energy intake from fibers while affording protection from inflammation and infection. In addition, these children showed depletion of *Firmicutes* which are usually abundant in people on a high-protein, high-fat diet (Filippo et al. 2010).

Studies with adult human volunteers have shown that changing the amount and type of carbohydrate consumed over periods of 4 weeks induced a significant change in the composition of the gut microbiota and its metabolic products (Brinkworth et al. 2009, Walker et al. 2011). Difference in gastrointestinal flora between breast-fed and formula milk-fed babies is another example of diet-induced changes in gut microbiota. Several studies have shown that although Bifidobacteria are the most prevalent bacteria in the GIT flora of both feeding groups, the amount is significantly higher in breast-fed than in formula-fed infants (Harmsen et al. 2000). Babies fed breast milk vs. formula milk display very large difference in inflammation and susceptibility to disease. Formula milk also causes a dramatic shift in gut flora from a simple flora dominated by *Bifidobacteria* to a complex adult gut flora; the number of *Escherichia coli* and Bacteroides was significantly higher in formula milk-fed than in breast-fed infants (Vandenplas et al. 2011).

Diet also influences the composition of gut microbiota in the elderly. Bacteroidetes are the dominant member of the gut microbiota and the relative abundance of various groups within the Firmicutes phylotype in the elderly differs from that of young adults (Claesson et al. 2012). Overall, the bacterial diversity of gut microbiota tends to decrease with age (Claesson et al. 2011). Diet not only influences the structure of gut microbiota, it may also induce change in the expression of bacterial cell surface constituents. Gut bacteria *Bacteroides thetaiotaomicron* exhibit changes in the capsular polysaccharide depending on the availability of nutrients (Bäckhed et al. 2005).

4.4 Influence of Gut Microbiota on Metabolism of Diet

A diverse population of bacterial species in the human gut performs important metabolic and immune functions that eventually delineate the nutritional and health status of the host (Selma et al. 2009, Martin et al. 2014). The association of gut microbiota with the host is based on molecular interactions that predominantly affect nutrition, immunity, and metabolism. These complex, site-specific, microbial communities contribute in vitamin synthesis, energy uptake, and the development of immunity in the host (Bik 2009). External environmental factors such as diet, pathogens, or antibiotic treatment and genetic predepositions may disturb the microbial ecosystem leading to "dysbiosis" and impaired activity that can render a negative health effect (Hawrelak and Myers 2004).

The impact of gut microbiota on the nutritional and health status of the host is determined by the modulation of immune and metabolic functions. Enzymatic activities involving transformation of various dietary compounds is also attributed to the microbiome (Laparra and Sanz 2010). Intestinal microbiota is responsible for the fermentation of nondigestible dietary residue in addition to endogenous mucus of the epithelia (Roberfroid et al. 1995).

Several reports elucidate the role of certain specific bacterial species such as Bacteroidetes in the degradation of carbohydrates on account of their ability to possess a large numbers of genes encoding carbohydrate active enzymes and their ability to shift to the specific energy sources available in the gut. The genomic sequencing of gut symbiont *Bacteroides thetaiotaomicron* has shown to encode for 400 enzymes including transport, binding, and digestion of complex carbohydrates (Xu et al. 2003). Similarly, Firmicutes, Actinobacteria, and Verrucomicrobium phyla constitute a group of bacteria that would initiate the degradation of complex substrates including plant cell walls, starch particles, and mucin in the gut. Bacteroidetes and actinobacteria (Bacteroides enterotype) have been shown to associate with saturated fat and animal protein whereas carbohydrates and simple sugars (glucose and fructose) are linked with *Firmicutes* and *Proteobacteria* (Prevotella enterotype). Microbial diversity in the gut is greatly influenced by the type of nutrient as fat and protein are reported to decrease and carbohydrates increase the diversity of human gut microbiome (Delzenne et al. 2011a,b). The emerging concept of prebiotics and their impact on human health requires explorative studies to highlight the complex relationship between diet composition, gut microbiota, and metabolic outputs (Wu et al. 2011, Flint 2012).

Host metabolism is linked with the products of microbial metabolism through signaling mechanisms thereby directly affecting intestinal function, the liver, the brain, and adipose and muscle tissues leading to a rise in the level of obesity and the associated morbidities. Transformation of indigestible food components into molecules by gut microbiota, and providing energy to the host has been linked with obesity pathogenesis due to an excess energy intake (Bäckhed et al. 2007, Tremaroli and Bäckhed 2012).

Dietary bioactive compounds such as prebiotics, polyunsaturated fatty acids (PUFAs), and phytochemicals influence the composition of the gut microbiota and their ability to generate fermentation products. PUFAs including ω-3 and ω-6 fatty acids are associated with various aspects of immunity and metabolism (Laparra and Sanz 2010). The interactions between PUFAs and components of gut microbiota greatly alter their role in metabolism. A growing body of evidence shows that dietary factors can dramatically alter the gut microbiome in ways that contribute to metabolic disturbance and progression of obesity (Cani et al. 2009b). Dietary fat composition can both reshape the gut microbiota and alter host adipose tissue inflammatory/lipogenic profiles. In addition, there exists the interdependency of dietary fat source, commensal gut microbiota, and the inflammatory profile of mesenteric fat that can collectively affect the host metabolic state (Huang et al. 2013).

In a study published recently, a team of researchers found that in mice, just one of species of bacteria, *Akkermansia muciniphila* plays a major part in controlling obesity and metabolic disorders such as type 2 diabetes (Everard et al. 2013). It is the dominant bacterial species in the human gut, representing 3%–5% of the microbial community (Belzer and de Vos 2012). The abundance of this bacterium inversely correlates with body weight in rodents and humans. Interestingly, prebiotic feeding normalized *A. muciniphila* abundance, which correlated with an improved metabolic profile, reversed high-fat diet-induced metabolic disorders including fat-mass gain, metabolic endotoxemia, adipose tissue inflammation, and insulin resistance (Karlsson et al. 2012). In addition, prebiotic feeding of *A. muciniphila* increased the intestinal levels of endocannabinoids that control inflammation, the gut barrier, and gut peptide secretion (Everard et al. 2013).

4.5 Gut Microbial Activity in Health and Diseases

The enormous gene pool of the microbiome provides various enzymes of diverse metabolic pathways which communicate with and affect the host in numerous ways, both beneficial and harmful, acting locally and systemically (Tables 4.2 and 4.3). The adaptable and renewable activity of the microbiome is normally a health asset but certain members of the microbiota can become a liability in genetically susceptible and immunocompromised individuals (Lepage et al. 2012, McDermott and Huffnagle 2014).

4.5.1 Gut Microbial Activity Beneficial to Human

The primary role of the gut bacteria beneficial to the host is the fermentation of non-digestible carbohydrates such as cellulose, hemicellulose, pectins, gum, and resistant starches resulting in generation of SCFAs. In addition to serving as an energy source, SCFAs stimulate differentiation and proliferation of epithelial cells (Slavin 2013, Sharma and Devi 2014). Interaction between the gut bacteria and the host is important in the differentiation and proliferation of IEC, a competent immune system and moderate inflammatory responses (Yu et al. 2012). Also, gut bacteria stimulate the intestinal endocrine cells to stimulate hormones, which in turn enter circulation and can modulate the host function (Sekirov et al. 2010). In addition, gut bacteria communicate directly with immune cells of the gut-associated lymphoid tissue (GALT) and terminal of visceral afferent nerves (Diaz-Heijtz et al. 2011). Gut microbiota also play nonimmune, protective roles by directly blocking intestinal pathogenic microbes to IEC and by enhancing mucosal integrity via epithelial cell stimulation. So the gut microbiota may influence many metabolic processes of the host. It is important that the state of homeostasis is maintained between human hosts and their gut microbiota as it dictates the health and disease states of the host depending upon the relative proportion of beneficial bacteria and harmful bacteria (Kaminogawa 2010). In Table 4.2 the major beneficial effects of gut bacteria are listed. For many of the health benefits offered by the gut bacteria, there are multiple mechanisms involved; only the most common mechanism is mentioned here due to limitations of space.

4.5.2 Dysbiosis Leads to Disease States

Human gut microbiota exists in a state of homeostasis with the host for the benefit of the host and the microbes under normal circumstances. The gut microbiota is a complex ecosystem whose diversity is enormous, and under specific conditions when there is a disruption in the state of homeostasis, it is able to overcome protective host responses and exert pathologic effects (Wallace et al. 2011); the intestinal microbiome is linked to a growing number of over 25 diseases and syndromes (de Vos and de Vos 2012). The intestinal mucosal immune system has developed specialized mechanisms for eliminating the pathogenic microbes while at the same time tolerating the beneficial gut microbiota (Schuijt et al. 2013). Altogether, in indirect or associative support in maintaining the state of host–microbe homeostasis, several mechanisms of mucosal immunity are involved. These include strongly developed innate defense mechanisms ensuring appropriate

Table 4.2 Health Benefits of Gut Microbiota

Health Benefit	*Mechanism/Main Finding*	*References*
Energy harvest	Harvest calorie from undigested ingredients of food.	Jumpertz et al. (2011)
Synthesis of B vitamins and vitamin K	Lactic acid bacteria and *Bifidobacteria* can de novo synthesize biotin, thiamine (B_1), riboflavin (B_2), niacin (B_3), pantothenic acid (B_5), pyridoxine (B_6), cobalamine (B_{12}), folic acid, and vitamin K.	LeBlanc et al. (2013)
Absorption of minerals	SCFAs produced by gut bacteria enhance absorption of calcium, copper, iron, magnesium, and manganese.	Scholz-Ahrens et al. (2007)
Development of immune System	Gut immune maturation depends on colonization with a host-specific microbiota. Pathogens-associated molecular patterns (PAMP) of gut bacterial interact with TLRs and other pattern recognition receptors (PRP) of host cells to modulate development and stimulation both innate and adaptive arms of host immune system.	Chung et al. (2012), Ganal et al. (2012)
Neuronal networking	Interaction between the intestinal microbiota, the gut, and the central nervous system (CNS) is recognized as the microbiome–gut–brain axis. Dysbiosis leading dysregulation of microbiome–gut–brain axis leads to a variety of disease conditions.	Collins et al. (2012), De Vadder et al. (2014)
Angiogenesis	Gut microbiota-derived ligands induce proliferation, migration, tube formation and production of proangiogenic factors, from human intestinal microvascular endothelial cells (HIMECs); vessel sprouting and angiogenesis observed in the *ex vivo* and *in vivo* assays.	Schirbel et al. (2013)
Prevention of allergy	Alteration of gut microbiota resulted in elevated serum IgE concentrations, increased steady-state circulating basophil populations and exaggerated basophil-mediated Th2 cell responses and allergic inflammation. Altered microbiota leads to the induction of immune deviation in infancy. High counts of *Bacteroides* prevented clinical manifestation of atopy.	Hill et al. (2012)
Metabolism of xenobiotics	Gut microbiota modulates hepatic gene expression and function by altering its xenobiotic response to drugs without direct contact with the liver.	Björkholm et al. (2009)
Protection against infection	By outcompeting pathogen for attachment sites, by producing bacteriocins, and by limiting nutrients availability for the pathogens.	Guarner and Malagelada (2003), Canny and McCormick (2008)

Table 4.3 Dysiosis Leads to Disease States

Disease	*Mechanism/Main Findings*	*References*
Atherosclerosis	Metabolism by intestinal microbiota of dietary L-carnitine, a trimethylamine abundant in red meat produces trimethylamine N-oxide (TMAO) and accelerates atherosclerosis in murine model.	Koeth et al. (2013)
Type-2 diabetes	Metagenomic studies have shown that patients with type-2 diabetes gut microbial dysbiosis, show decrease in the abundance of some universal butyrate-producing bacteria and an increase in various opportunistic pathogens.	Qin et al. (2012)
Metabolic endotoxemia	High fat diet-induced changes in gut microbiota leads to increased transit of LPS to systemic circulation which contribute to the development of metabolic endotoxemia and ultimately clinical signs of chronic diseases.	Chang and Li (2011)
Eczema	A diverse and adult-type microbiota in early childhood is associated with eczema and it may contribute to the perpetuation of eczema.	Nylund et al. (2013)
Irritable bowel syndrome	Overgrowth of aerobic bacteria in the small intestine using nitrate generated as a by-product of the inflammatory response; reduced number of *Bifidobacteria* in the gut leading to altered floral–mucosal interactions. The enteric nervous system, and brain–gut–brain axis are directly involved in the pathogenesis.	Kinross et al. (2008)
Altered gut permeability	Altered gut microbiota-induced glucagon like peptide-2 (GLP-2)-driven alteration of gut permeability.	Cani et al. (2009a)
Obesity	An obesity-associated gut microbiome with increased capacity for energy harvest.	Diamant (2011) Everard et al. (2013)
Allergy	Reduced biodiversity and altered gut flora composition early in life fails to confer maximum tolerogenic immunomodulatory effects.	Sjögren et al. (2009), Özdemir (2013) Trompette et al. (2014)
CRC	*Clostridium* and *Bacteroides* enhance the potency of DNA-damaging agents, for example, N-nitorso compounds and heterocyclic amines and increase the growth rate of colonic tumor; *Lactobacillus* and *Bifidobacteria* reduce tumorigenesis	Uccello et al. (2012)
Cancer (other types)	Microbiota changes observed. Microbial-induced inflammation contribute to cancer by stimulating production of cytokines that promote cell proliferation and/or inhibit apoptosis.	Bultman (2014)

Table 4.3 (*Continued*) Dysiosis Leads to Disease States

Disease	*Mechanism/Main Findings*	*References*
Autism	Abnormal energy metabolism by altered gut bacteria results in production of acyl-carnitine and altered production of propionic acid which results in alteration in mitochondrial function leading to neurodevelopmental disorder, autism.	Frye et al. (2013)
Asthma	Change in gut flora early in life leading to inappropriate immune tolerance contributes toward the development of asthma.	McLoughlin and Mills (2011)

function of the mucosal barrier, existence of unique types of lymphocytes and secretory immunoglobulin A (sIgA). Studies with germ-free animals have demonstrated that the gut microbiota plays a vital role in the development of an optimally functioning mucosal immune system (Mazmanian et al. 2005, Kostic et al. 2013).

Human gut microbiota converts L-carnitine into trimethylamine which can promote cardiovascular risk in humans (Zhu et al. 2014). Inadequate or excess stimulation of the immune system is a challenge to host microbe homeostasis and subsequent disease states. A number of cellular components [e.g., lipopolysaccharides (LPS), peptidoglycans, teichoic acids, flagella, superantigens, bacterial DNA, heat-shock protein] and the metabolic products of the gut microbiota are able to stimulate both the innate and adaptive components of the host immunity (Holmes et al. 2011, 2012). Chronic immune activation in response to signals from gut microbiota could pose the risk of chronic, low-grade inflammation, which studies have shown as a predisposing factor for a variety of multifactorial, multigenic complex diseases including obesity, diabetes, inflammatory bowel diseases, rheumatoid arthritis, cardiovascular disease, allergy, asthma, autism, colon cancer, and several infections, inflammatory, autoimmune, and neoplastic disease (Chang and Li 2011, Hormannsperger et al. 2012; Table 4.3). Numerous studies have shown that the modulation of structure and function of gut microbiota by probiotics, prebiotics, synbiotics, cobiotics, and immunobiotics offer a realistic therapeutic and preventive option for these diseases.

A recent study showed that gut bacteria enhances infectivity of certain viruses. The virus becomes covered with LPS molecules from natural gut bacteria, then virus–LPS conjugate interact with TLR4 (receptor of LPS molecules on mammalian cells) to make viral infection possible. Mouse mammary tumor virus (MMTV), poliovirus, and a reovirus which impairs bile duct function all have been shown to use the same LPS-dependent strategy. LPS–TLR4 interaction leads to stimulation of IL-10 production, which suppresses the body's antiviral reaction, further enhancing viral infection. The bacterial cell wall component peptidoglycan also promoted viral infectivity (Wilks and Golovkina, 2012).

4.6 Human Colon as a Fermenter

The main theme of the development of various functional foods such probiotics, prebiotis, cobiotics, synbiotics, and immunobiotics is the improvement of the colonic fermentation process which has been shown to exert profound health benefits on the human host (Blaut and Clavel 2007, Villena and Kitazawa 2014). The human colon is a highly active metabolic organ which acts a fermenter where a variety of undigested food ingredients (mostly complex carbohydrates) are fermented for the benefit of both the microbes and the host (Figure 4.1; Valeur and Berstad 2010). With approximately 1.5 kg of bacteria in the colon (Xu and Gordon 2003), and metabolic activity comparable to the liver (Martin et al. 2009, DiBaise et al. 2012), fermentation in the gut thus plays an important role in the digestive physiology and energy metabolism of the host.

Because of the diversity and metabolic potential of the gut microbiota, gut fermentation is a complicated process resulting in a dynamic gut metabolom (total metabolites) where the end product produced by one organism serves as a growth substrate for the other (Vlieg et al. 2011).

The degradation of complex carbohydrates and plant polysaccharides as a source of energy for human and microbial cells is not completely accomplished by human enzymes and these nondigestible carbohydrates including xylans, resistant starch, cellulose, hemicellulose, pectins, gums, and inulin in addition to certain oligosaccharides that escape digestion are fermented by colonic microbiota resulting in the yield of energy and SCFA (acetate, propionate, and butyrate) (Martens et al. 2011, Pokusaeva et al. 2011). A considerable number of these polymers cannot be degraded by the host; however herbivores possess the ability to meet 70% of their energy requirement from microbial breakdown under the concept of mutualism. The gut microbiome is highly enriched with genes for carbohydrate metabolism encoding a large assortment of enzymes for carbohydrate metabolism (>115 families of glycosidic hydrolases and >21 families of polysaccharide lyase); in contrast the human genome has relatively few genes that encode carbohydrate-metabolizing

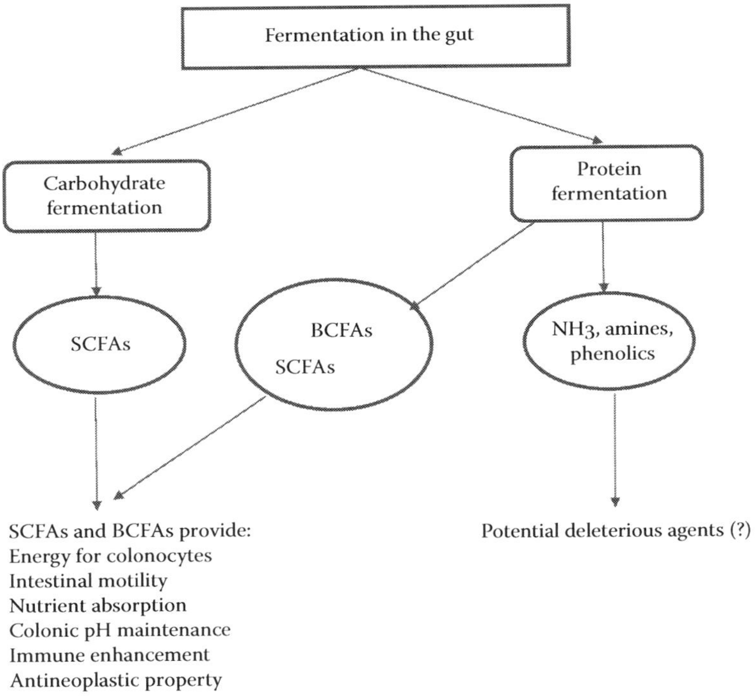

Figure 4.1 Fermentation of carbohydrates and proteins in the gut producing SCFAs, BCFAs, and other products. (From Cummings, J. H. et al. 1987. *Gut* 28: 1221–1227; Macfarlane, G. T. and S. Macfarlane. 2011. *Journal of Clinical Gastroenterology* 45: S120–S127.)

enzymes (Gill et al. 2006, Ley et al. 2006, Flint et al. 2008). During the fermentation process in the colon, the gut microbiota breaks down substances such as resistant starch and dietary fibers which are not completely hydrolyzed in the small intestine by the host enzymes resulting in production of a variety of postbiotics such as SCFAs and gases (e.g., hydrogen, methane, and carbon dioxide) (Topping and Clifton 2001).

A variety of factors influence the fermentation process; the most important factor is the type and amount of complex carbohydrates which pass through the small intestine undigested and reach the colon and its resident microbiota (Tremaroli and Bäckhed 2012, Besten et al. 2013). In addition, the type and amount of various SCFAs produced by fermentation is also influenced by pH, availability of inorganic terminal electron acceptors (e.g., sulfate and nitrate), and large intestine transit time (Macfarlane and Macfarlane 2011).

The microbial population colonizing different parts of the gut influences human health in several ways. Under normal physiological conditions, these microbial communities contribute nutrients and energy to the host through the fermentative process of nondigestible dietary components in the large intestine. Carbohydrates and proteins serve as the main fermentative substrates in the large intestine resulting in the production of a number of products including gases, hydrogen, carbon dioxide, SCFAs, branched chain fatty acids (BCFAs), lactic acid, ethanol, ammonia, amines, phenols, and indoles (Figure 4.1). The human microbiome is also responsible for the maintenance of a balance with the host's metabolism and immune system (MacFarlane and Cummings 1991, Flint et al. 2007, Flint 2012).

4.6.1 Short-Chain Fatty Acids

SCFAs are saturated organic fatty acids with 1–6 carbon atoms and are the principal anions which arise from bacterial fermentation of polysaccharide, oligosaccharide, proteins, peptide, and glycoprotein in the colon (Velázquez et al. 1997, Macfarlane and Macfarlane 2011). The main postbiotic fermentation products of resistant starch and dietary fibers are SCFAs; which includes acetate (C2), propionate (C3), and butyrate (C4)(Figure 4.2).

Various studies demonstrated that SCFA production is in order of acetate > propionate > butyrate in a molar ratio of approximately 3:1:1 mainly in the proximal and transverse colon (Cummings et al. 1987, Cummings and Myers 1991). SCFAs are produced in the range of 150–600 mmol/day (average of 400 mmol/day); more than 95% are immediately absorbed by the colon and the rest excreted in the feces. The SCFAs thus absorbed provide approximately 500 kcals of energy a day; which amounts to 5%–15% of the total caloric needs of an individual on a Western diet (Martin et al. 2014). Absorption of SCFAs by the colonic mucosa is an energy-independent process and the rate of absorption of different SCFAs are same, irrespective of their chain length. In addition to SCFAs, small amounts of isobutyrate, valerate, and isovalerate are also produced (Beyer-Sehlmeyer et al. 2003). The absorbed SCFAs are used as an energy source by the colonocytes (butyrate being the preferred substrate) and also by the other tissues including

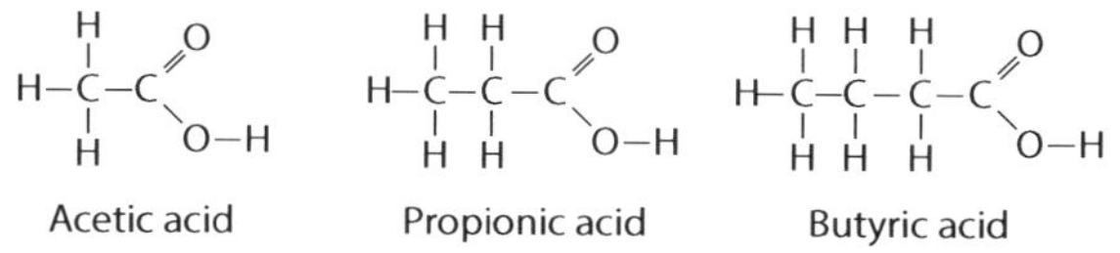

Figure 4.2 Short-chain fatty acids.

the liver and the muscles. In addition to serving as energy, SCFAs also have other important functions (Macfarlane and Macfarlane 2011).

4.6.2 SCFAs and Their Physiologic Effects

By facilitating the uptake of electrolytes and water, SCFAs reduce the osmotic effect of unabsorbed carbohydrate molecules and thus act as an antidiarrheal agent; an individual may suffer from diarrhea (antibiotic associated diarrhea) when the gut microbiota is disrupted resulting in impaired colonic fermentation (Binder 2010). Microbial fermentation products influence gastrointestinal motility and sensitivity and may play a role in the pathogenesis of irritable bowel syndrome. Research data indicate that inadequate β-oxidation of SCFAs as a pathogenic mechanism for ulcerative colitis (Bergman 1990, Cummings et al. 1996, Flint et al. 2007). Brighenti et al. (1995) demonstrated a significant role of acetate and propionate as modulators of glucose metabolism thus resulting in lower glycemic responses to oral glucose owing to the absorption of these SCFAs. Proliferation and differentiation of the IEC is modulated by SCFAs and thus contribute toward the creation of a protective barrier against pathogens (Hooper et al. 2012). SCFAs decrease colonic pH and increase colonic water absorption and thus maintain colonic health. Other health-promoting properties of SCFAs include laxation and vasodilation; SCFAs also play roles in gut motility and gut wound healing (Flint et al. 2007, Tan et al. 2014). SCFAs are incorporated as basic elements in a variety of biosynthetic processes such as lipogenesis, gluconeogenesis, and protein synthesis. SCFAs activate G protein-coupled receptors, GPR41 and GPR43 (Kim et al. 2013) leading to the activation of several intracellular pathways including transcriptional factors such as activating transcriptional factor-2 (ATF-2) and signal transduction mediators protein kinase C and mitogen-activated protein kinases (MAPKs) (Elamin et al. 2013, Kim et al. 2013).

An important method of regulation of gene expression is through acetylation (carried out by the enzyme histone acetyl transferase, HAT) and deacetylation (carried out by the enzyme histone deacetylase, HDAC) of the DNA-binding protein, histone. Acetylation leads to enhanced gene expression, while deacetylation reverses the process. By exerting a negative effect on HDAC activity (Davie 2003), SCFAs are reported to modulate the expression of a number of key regulatory proteins such as NFAT, NFκB, p53, and MyoD (Vinolo et al. 2011). Recent *in vivo* and *in vitro* studies suggest that SCFAs stimulate gut hormone secretion. Colonic enteroendocrine L cells express receptors for SCFAs (free fatty acid receptor, FFA2 and FFA3). The release of insulinotropic hormone, glucagon-like peptide-1 (GLP-1) and an anorectic hormone, peptide YY by colonic enteroendocrine L cells is mediated by SCFAs (Vinolo et al. 2011, Kaji et al. 2014). In an interesting study, Wichmann et al. (2013) showed that SCFAs, by modulating the secretion of the hormone GLP-1, increase intestinal transit time of food in case of energy insufficiency and thus allow for greater energy harvest and absorption in germ-free and antibiotics-treated mouse models.

Butyrate is produced in minimal amount in comparison to acetate and propionate, but is the most studied and is reported to have a more important role in colonic homeostasis and also in wide array of metabolic processes (Nordgaad 1998). Butyrate serves as the primary energy source for the colonocyte, supplying 70%–90% of its energy requirements. It promotes cell repair, proliferation, and differentiation (Canani et al. 2011). By stimulating the healthy growth of colonic cells, butyrate helps prevent colon cancer. Additional properties of butyrate which contribute to preventing colon cancer includes reduction of DNA damage, reduction of the exposure of the colonic mucosa to ammonia, inhibition of the conversion of primary to secondary bile acids (Kaji et al. 2014). Butyrate enhances villi development and promotes the gut barrier function and reduces epithelial permeability which is achieved by upregulation of mucin-associated genes (MUC1-4) in the intestinal goblet cells. Butyrate also upregulates the expression of tight junction proteins such as zonulin and occludin, enhancing intestinal barrier function (Bordin et al. 2004, Gaudier et al. 2004).

Butyrate exerts a differential effect on healthy colonocytes and tumor cell lines. It activates the expression of genes involved in cell proliferation and differentiation in healthy colonocytes; whereas it activates genes which leads to apoptosis in tumor cells (Canani et al. 2011). Butyrate also possesses antimicrobial properties. It is reported to prevent colonization by *Salmonella enteritidis* in experimental animals. Mechanistic studies revealed that it upregulated host defense protein genes and also downregulated invasion genes in *Salmonella*, thereby reducing the ability of the bacteria to attach and invade host cells of the intestinal epithelium (Immerseel et al. 2006, Sunkara et al. 2012).

4.6.3 SCFAs as Modulators of the Immune System

Research in the field of immunology and gut microbiology has shown that SCFAs exert wide ranging effects on immune and inflammatory responses. SCFAs act as chemotactic factors for neutrophils and thus enhance the recruitment of circulating leukocytes to the inflammatory site. SCFAs modulate the production of these inflammatory mediators by neutrophils and other immune cells. Studies have shown that propionate and butyrate reduce the LPS-stimulated production of cytokine-induced neutrophil chemoattractant-2 (CINC-2), tumor necrosis factor (TNF)-α, and nitric oxide (NO) production by neutrophils (Maslowski and Mackay 2011, Vinolo et al. 2011), which contribute toward controlling the inflammatory process involved in the pathogenesis of various diseases including Crohn's disease (Segain et al. 2000).

As IEC are in direct contact with high concentrations of SCFAs, the effects of these fatty acids on these cells have been a topic of intense investigation. By changing the type or the amount of chemokines produced by intestinal cells, SCFAs may alter the recruitment of leukocytes and the pattern of inflammatory mediators produced in this tissue (Vinolo et al. 2011, Zeng et al. 2014). SCFAs are also involved in T cell differentiation. This is achieved by stimulation of production of prostaglandin E2 (PGE2), which by activating its receptor EP4 facilitates Th1 differentiation and Th17 expansion, two subsets of T helper involved in a variety of immune processes including inflammation (Smith et al. 2013).

Studies have identified various structural components and secreted products of gut microorganisms with direct roles in modulating the immune system. Flagellin from the probiotic strain *E. coli* Nissle is reported to induce β-defensin, an antimicrobial peptide implicated in the resistance of epithelial surfaces to microbial colonization (Schlee et al. 2007). A soluble protein p40, derived from probiotic bacteria *Lactobacillus rhamnosus* GG prevented cytokine-induced apoptosis in IEC through the activation of epidermal growth factor receptor (EGFR). Delivery of p40 to the colon prevented and treated colon epithelial cell injury and inflammation and ameliorated colitis in an EGFR-dependent manner (Yan et al. 2011). Butyrate exerts an anti-inflammatory effect by inhibition of NF-kB activation. Studies have shown that it downregulates production of TNF-α in human peripheral monocytes and in macrophage-like synoviocytes in rheumatoid arthritis patients by regulating mRNA degradation (Fukae et al. 2005).

4.6.4 Fermentation of Fat

The interaction of gut microbiota with dietary fat is more complex. Lipid metabolism by gastrointestinal microbes generates multiple fatty acid species that can affect host health. Metabolism of linoleic acid has been associated with several human colonic *Roseburia* species that form either vaccenic acid or a hydroxy-18:1 fatty acid. They may also act as precursors of conjugated linoleic acid (CLA) *cis*-9, *trans*-11-18:2-, the health-promoting compound (Devillard et al. 2007). In a study with germ-free mice it has been found that representative gut bacteria *Lactobacillus plantarum* carry out the metabolism of PUFAs and generates oxo, hydroxyl, and conjugated fatty acids and partially saturated *trans*-fatty acids. These fatty acid intermediates, especially hydroxyl fatty acids, were detected in host organs. The evidence for the fact that the source of these hydroxy fatty acids is the bacterial metabolism of fatty acids came from the observation that the levels of hydroxy fatty acids were much higher in specific pathogen-free mice than in germ-free mice. These findings suggest that lipid metabolism by gastrointestinal microorganisms affect host lipid composition, which in turn may provide new ways for host health improvement by altering lipid metabolism related to the onset of metabolic syndrome (Kishino et al. 2013).

4.6.5 Fermentation of Protein

The dietary proteins which escape digestion in the small intestine, as well as proteins from mucous, enzymes, sloughed epithelial cells, dead host, and bacterial cells are fermented in the colon. Fermentation of proteins leads to the production of SFAs, BCFAs, and amines. In addition, protein fermentation also generates ammonia, phenols, indoles, and sulfurs (Figure 4.1; Macfarlane and Cummings 1991). In contrast to carbohydrate fermentation which takes place in the proximal and transverse colon, protein fermentation mainly occurs in the distal colon, when carbohydrates get depleted. It is generally accepted that protein fermentation is considered detrimental to the host's health; for example, colorectal cancer (CRC) and ulcerative colitis appear most often in the distal colon, which is the primary site of protein fermentation. Some of the proteolytic fermentation products, however, are used by gut microbiota as nitrogenous growth factors. Mucin contains a substantial amount of nitrogen in the form of amino sugars. Fermentation of these sugars releases ammonia which is absorbed from the colon by mucosal cells and contributes to the host's nitrogen balance (Windey et al. 2012).

4.6.6 Bacteria Involved in Gut Fermentation

Bacteroides are the most numerous and most versatile polysaccharide fermenting bacteria of the gut microbiota; other gut fermenters belong to the genera *Bifidobacterium, Ruminococcus, Lactobacillus,* and *Clostridium* (Guarner and Malagelada 2003). In addition to saccharolytic and proteolytic bacteria, methanogens and other bacteria that utilize intermediate fermentation products such as hydrogen, ethanol, lactate, and succinate are also present in large number (Guarner and Malagelada 2003, Nakamura et al. 2010). Gram-positive Firmicutes are the human colonic butyrate producers comprising the two most abundant groups related to *Eubacteriumrectale/Roseburia* spp. and *Faecalibacterium prausnitzii.* Mechanisms proposed in non-gut *Clostridium* spp. whereby butyrate synthesis leads to the energy generation through substrate-level phosphorylation and proton gradients has also been found to be true in majority of gut bacterial species involved in butyrate production (Louis and Flint 2009).

4.7 Concept of Probiotics, Prebiotics, Synbiotics, Cobiotics, and Immunobiotics: Mechanism of Action and Health Claims

Advances in knowledge about gut microbiota through recent studies with functional metagenomics has opened the possibilities of applying this knowledge for rational remodeling for human benefit (Holmes et al. 2012, Guzman et al. 2013). Owing to the inherent plasticity of gut microbiota, the various physiologic features that can be targeted are relative susceptibilities to infections, metabolic syndromes, bioavailability of nutrients, development of innate and adaptive immunity, immune tolerance, development and functioning of the nervous system, and the intestinal barrier function (Delzenne et al. 2011a,b, Martin et al. 2014). Various gut microbiota modifying agents such as probiotics, prebiotics, synbiotics , cobiotics, and immunobiotics can be used to achieve a measurable benefit to the host.

Antibiotics can be used to eliminate or suppress undesirable bacteria from the human host, probiotics can introduce missing or suppressed beneficial bacteria in the gut microbiota, prebiotics can enhance the proliferation of beneficial microbes, synbiotics can synergistically enhance the potency of both probiotics and prebiotics to maximize sustainable changes in the human microbiome (Roberfroid 1998, Lourens-Hattingh and Viljoen 2001, Gibson et al. 2004, Takahashi et al. 2013). Cobiotics, on the other hand, can be beneficial both to the host and to gut microbiota in a targeted health effect, and immunobiotics can promote health through modulation of mucosal immune mechanisms (Greenway et al. 2013, Tomosada et al. 2013). Through strategic use of these gut microbiota modifying processes, either singly or in combination, remodeling of the gut microbiome to suit individual therapeutic needs can be considered (Preidis and Versalovic 2009, Goldsmith and Sartor 2014).

4.7.1 Probiotics

The main theme of probiotic action is its capacity to remodel gut microbiota, which results in subsequent health benefits. Lilley and Stillwell (1965) used this term for the first time describing it as a microbial substance that stimulated the growth of other microorganisms, followed by Sperty (1971) who narrated probiotics as tissue extracts that promoted microbial growth. Parker (1974) used the expression, probiotic as animal supplements containing organisms and substances that would contribute to create a balance of the intestinal flora. Similarly, Fuller (1989) defined probiotics as food supplements with live microorganisms to promote host health by balancing the intestinal flora. Subsequently, Fooks et al. (1999) stated the word probiotic to comprise of two Greek words meaning "for life." Despite a number of other definitions of the term probiotic, the currently prevailing and the most widely accepted one is that "probiotics are live microorganisms, administrated in certain quantities that confer health benefits to the host" (FAO/WHO 2001). Numerous lactic acid bacterial strains are considered as probiotics; however, all of them do not meet the required standard because of their sensitivity to the critical level of acidity and bile salts in the human GIT (Hekmat and Reid 2006). Probiotics are consumed by humans either as a live dietary supplement or as live microflora in fermented foods. The most well-known probiotic-containing food product is *yogurt* (Lourens-Hattingh and Viljoen 2001). Other fermented foods that contain probiotics are some juices and soy drinks, buttermilk, fermented and unfermented milk, some soft cheeses, *sauerkraut*, *miso*, *tempeh*, *kefir*, kimchi, pickles, and *kombucha* tea (Collins and Gibson 1999, Anuradha and Rajeshwari 2005, Shah, 2007, Soccol et al. 2010).

Another significant aspect of probiotics is strain specificity that may create a challenge in research on probiotics or probiotic-containing food products to establish the effectiveness of one strain relative to the other (Canani et al. 2007). Species of *Lactobacillus* and *Bifidobacterium* have been considered the most popular for use in a majority of probiotic products available in the market (FAO/WHO 2001). Rational yoghurts, frozen yogurts, and desserts are the reservoirs of *Lactobacillus bulgaricus* and *Streptococcus thermophilus*, in many parts of the world (Senok 2009). Although these species have been associated with improved lactose digestion and immune enhancement, all of these do not meet the criteria for a probiotic microorganism on account of their sensitivity to the conditions in the GIT where they do not survive in very high numbers. Moreover, other genera, such as *Escherichia* and *Enterococcus* are now marketed as probiotics; however, their safety as probiotics remains a concern for consumers (Eaton and Gasson 2001, Ishibashi and Yamazaki 2001, Senok et al. 2005).

Some of the fundamental properties of probiotic strains that would benefit human health include resistance to acid and bile, attachment to the human gut epithelial cells, colonization in the human intestine, and production of antimicrobial substances (Parvez et al. 2006). Additionally, probiotics would present a characteristic of not being pathogenic, toxic, mutagenic, or carcinogenic in the host organism and should be generally regarded as GRAS (generally recognized as safe) (Mattia and Merker 2008). Moreover, they must be viable during processing and storage, and should offer resistance to the physicochemical processing of the food and must be able to survive the digestion process. They must also possess the ability to adhere and colonize the gut mucosa and promote immunostimulation without an inflammatory effect (Saarela et al. 2000, Prado et al. 2008).

Abundant literature is available to elucidate the multiple health benefits of ingesting probiotic containing foods. Numerous studies explicated the role of probiotics as antimicrobial and antimutagenic (Lourens-Hattingh and Viljoen 2001), anticarcinogenic (Marteau et al. 2001), and antihypertensive (Liong et al. 2009) in humans. Probiotic bacteria not only promote the endogenous host defense mechanisms and the nonimmunologic gut defense (Salminen et al. 1998), but also generate increased humoral immune responses on ingestion thereby promoting the intestine's immunologic barrier (Kaila et al. 1992, Marschan et al. 2008).

Probiotics have demonstrated protection against allergic sensitization and allergic diseases as several studies reported an attenuating effect in allergic symptoms after probiotic treatment (Dotterud et al. 2010) suggesting these syndromes to be mediated by the induction of regulatory mechanisms, such as generation, proliferation, and activity of tolerogenic dendritic cells (DCs) and T cells (Rautava et al. 2006, Lyons et al. 2010). Speculation prevails whether probiotic bacteria imparted such an effect directly or whether it is yielded through probiotic-mediated stabilization of the intestinal microbiota (Bernardo et al. 2012). Probiotics have also been reported to positively impact mineral metabolism, especially bone stability (Arunachalam 1999), attenuation of symptoms of bowel disease, and Crohn's syndrome (Marteau et al. 2004).

More complex and increased beneficial effects of probiotics in humans entail stimulating nonspecific host resistance to microbial pathogens (Perdigon et al. 1986, 1988) and modulating the host's immune responses to deleterious antigens leading to downregulation of hypersensitivity reactions. Enhanced recovery from infection, and antimicrobial functions have been reported as some *Lactobacillus* strains exhibited suppression of pathogenic microorganisms including *Sal. enteritidis*, *E. coli*, *Shigella sonnei*, and *Serratia marcescens* (Drago et al. 1997). Granato et al. (2010) reported a series of physiological benefits of probiotic strains that include regulation of the intestinal flow, control of diarrhea, reduced cholesterol levels, improved lactose tolerance, better absorption of micronutrients, improved immunological system, better urogenital health, prevention of cancer, reduced catabolic products of the kidney and liver, and prevention of arteriosclerosis. The authors further emphasized the potential health outcomes of probiotic ingestion reporting reduced rate of onset of osteoporosis, better development, and improved bioavailability of nutrients. Other clinical studies explained the role of probiotics in improving the mucosal barrier function, increasing allergen-specific IgA levels, and more importantly affecting a range of other immune-modulatory properties (Marschan et al. 2008, West et al. 2009).

Probiotics have been used to treat diseases of the GIT with impressive success. Consumption of yoghurt (a ready source of probiotics) eliminated symptoms of lactose intolerance and improved digestion in people who cannot efficiently absorb lactose (Guarner and Malagelada 2003). A recent study on 3758 children aged 1–5 years revealed that daily intake of a probiotic strain, *Lactobacillus casei* strain Shirota played an important role in the prevention of acute diarrhea in young children in a community setting during a 24-week period (Sur et al. 2011).

Saccharomyces boulardii has been shown to be a highly effective probiotic agent used in preventing gastroenteritis caused by *Shigella flexneri* in a murine model (Zbar et al. 2013). *E. coli* strain Nissle 1917 (EcN) is a less commonly used probiotic. In a study, this strain was found to be safe and well-tolerated and significantly reduced stool frequency in infants and toddlers suffering from acute diarrhea (Henker et al. 2007).

Impressive data are also available on the use of probiotics to boost immune response. Studies with various formulations of probiotics, either alone or in combination, were carried out to determine their effects on immune parameters, infectious outcomes, and inflammatory conditions in humans. These studies revealed that mucosal IgA production (especially in children), phagocytosis, and natural killer cell activity can be enhanced by some probiotic bacteria (Lomax and Clader 2009, Dong et al. 2010). Enteric bacteria induce local immune response in the gut in addition to systemic response. Probiotics have been used to enhance both humoral- and cell-mediated immune response against gastrointestinal pathogens. The specific IgA response was enhanced following probiotic administration in children infected with the rotavirus and in adults undergoing vaccination with an attenuated *Salmonella typhi* strain; enhanced phagocytic of circulating leukocytes was also noted (Majamaa et al. 1995, Schiffrin et al. 1995).

Application of probiotics offers great promise in the treatment of necrotizing enterocolitis (NEC) in premature babies. NEC, an extensive intestinal inflammatory disease of premature infants, is caused, in part, by an excessive inflammatory response to initial bacterial colonization due to the inappropriate expression of innate immune response genes. In a randomized placebo-controlled clinical trial, it was shown that probiotics (*Bifidobacterium infantis* and *Lactobacillus acidophilus)* significantly reduced the incidence of NEC. Probiotics were demonstrated to prevent NEC by modulating enterocyte genes that regulate innate immune-mediated inflammation (Ganguli et al. 2013). Bifidobacteria, the classic probiotic bacteria, exhibit beneficial effects through the modulation of host defense responses and protection against infectious diseases. The inhibitory effect of bifidobacteria can in part be attributed to the increased production of acetate which inhibits translocation of the Shiga-like toxin produced by *E. coli* O157:H7 from the gut lumen to the blood; indicating that acetate produced by protective bifidobacteria improves the intestinal defense mediated by epithelial cells and thereby protects the host against lethal infection (Fukuda et al. 2011).

4.7.2 Prebiotics

A prebiotic is defined by the FAO as "a nonviable food component that confers a health benefit on the host associated with modulation of the microbiota." Prebiotics are non-digestible food ingredients which upon ingestion function by promoting the growth and activity of certain specific colonic microbiota (Gibson and Roberfroid 1995, Roberfroid 2007). Primarily, these indigestible materials are nonviable food components benefitting the host through modulation of the microbiota (Gibson et al. 2004, Pineiro et al. 2008). There have been several criteria to define a prebiotic, however, a prebiotic would indicate resistance to gastric acidity, be fermentable by gut microbiota, and possess the ability to support the growth and/or activity of beneficial gut microflora (Schrezenmeir and de Vrese 2001, Roberfroid 2007).

The majority of prebiotics are dietary fibers such as oligosaccharides, although a variety of food ingredients can function as prebiotics. The proper functioning of prebiotics is related to their metabolism by the probiotics (Gourbeyre et al. 2011). In the absence of dietary fibers in the colon, anaerobic bacteria derive energy from protein fermentation which leads to the generation of toxic and potentially carcinogenic compounds such as phenolic and ammoniac compounds (Kolida et al. 2002, Manning and Gibson 2004). Common prebiotic oligosaccharides are inulin (polymers composed mainly of fructose units, and typically with a terminal glucose), fructose oligosaccharides (FOS), galactooligosaccharides (GOS), sucrose oligosaccharide (SOC), *trans*-galacto-oligosaccharides (TOS), xylooligosaccharides (XOS), pyrodextrins, soy oligosaccharides, and isomaltose-oligosaccharides (Macfarlane et al. 2008). Different members of the gut microbiota have preferential prebiotic substrates; for example, growth of Bifidobacteria is more efficient on fructans in comparison to Clostridia and *Bacteroides* sp. (Prakash et al. 2011, Gourbeyre et al. 2011). GOS being derived from lactose usually consist of chains of galactose monomers (Scholtens et al. 2006), are versatile food ingredients, and possess prebiotic characteristics. However, utilization of GOS by bifidobacteria is still hard to analyze as no precise analytical methods for it exists. Selectivity in consuming several types of GOS by different bifidobacteria denotes targeting prebiotics to focus upon certain bifidobacterial species (Barboza et al. 2009).

4.7.2.1 Inulin and FOS

Inulin and FOS are the most widely consumed prebiotic materials by humans worldwide. These are fructans (polymers of fructose attached by β 1-2 linkage with a terminal glucose residue (Macfarlane et al. 2006). Inulins have a degree of polymerization (DP) of <200 (usually 2–60), whereas a FOS has a DP of <10. These are non-digestible carbohydrates and are transferred to colon and fermented almost quantitatively (ca. 100%; Roberfroid 2007). Inulin possess 25%–35% of food energy of starch and approximately 10% of sweetness of sugar/sucrose making it a versatile food ingredient in many processed foods (Roberfroid 1999). Numerous major dietary sources of prebiotics cover fructans such as inulin, oligofructose, and short-chain FOS. A "high performance" (HP) type of inulin is also available in the market. HP inulin has an average DP of 25 with the residual sugars as well as the oligomers removed. This product provides almost twice the fat mimetic characteristics of standard inulin with no sweetness contribution (Niness 1999). The energy obtained from the fermentation of inulin and FOS is mostly due to production of SCFA and lactate which contribute to 1.5 kcal/g of energy for both inulin and FOS. There is also increasing evidence from human and animal studies that such prebiotics can enhance satiety and decrease energy intake leading to improved control of body weight (Cani et al. 2009a).

Inulin, naturally occurring in onions in high concentration has been shown to possess fructose monomers in high number (10–60) while oligofructose derivatives, found in asparagus, wheat, and artichoke, exist in low number (3–7) of fructose monomers (Gibson et al. 1994). Improved conditions in bowel inflammation, reduction in the production of pro-inflammatory biomarkers on using long-chain inulin along with an increase in intestinal bifidobacteria and lactobacilli have been reported in the literature (Lindsay et al. 2006, Leenen and Dieleman 2007).

4.7.2.2 Health Benefits of Prebiotics

Prebiotics while in the GIT have been reported to deliver beneficial effects in various ways. Prebiotics influence intestinal transit time and normally determine bowel habits. Prebiotics stimulate the growth of a variety of intestinal microbiota including bifidobacteria. Studies have demonstrated the implication of prebiotics in reducing atherosclerosis, osteoporosis, obesity, type-2 diabetes, cancer, infections, and allergies risk in humans (Scholtens et al. 2006, Roberfroid 2007). Human milk oligosaccharides (HMO) are reported to have a range of biological activities beyond providing nutrition to the infant (Barile and Rastall 2013). In addition to the selective stimulation of beneficial bacteria, which is a common property of all prebiotics, certain prebiotics such as GOS can competitively block adhesion of pathogens to IEC. Evidence exists that fructans-type prebiotics such as inulin and FOS can reduce serum cholesterol levels and increase HDL/LDL ratio (Ooi and Liong 2010). Gut microbiota fermentation of prebiotics increases satietogenic and incretin gut peptide production with consequences for appetite reduction and glucose response after a meal (Cani et al. 2009b). In summary, prebiotic food ingredients are vital to support the growth and survival of probiotic organisms in the human intestine. So, beneficial probiotic bacteria need to be constantly introduced in the diet and supplied with proper fibrous diet (prebiotics) to sustain them in the gut so that a healthy microbe–host relationship is maintained.

4.7.3 Synbiotics

As probiotics and prebiotics offer health benefits to humans, it was hypothesized that by combining probiotics and prebiotics, it should be possible to achieve not only the combined effect, but also a synergistic effect. The term synbiotics was proposed by Roberfroid (1998) to describe such a combination of a probiotic and a prebiotic which was more potent than either of these ingredients. In addition to probiotics and prebiotics, studies are conducted to explore various combinations of synbiotics aiming at the modification of gut flora for health benefits. Synbiotics (*Bifidobacterium breve* Yakult and *Lb. casei* Shirota as probiotics, and GOS as a prebiotic) was used to treat D-lactate acidosis. It allowed the reduction in colonic absorption of D-lactate by both prevention of D-lactate-producing bacterial overgrowth and stimulation of intestinal motility, leading to the remission of D-lactate acidosis (Takahashi et al. 2013). Another recent study also showed the usefulness of synbiotics. Phenol and *p*-cresol, as metabolites of aromatic amino acids produced by gut bacteria, are regarded as bioactive toxins and serum biomarkers of a disturbed gut environment. A double-blind placebo-controlled trial on consumption of synbiotics (*Bif. breve* strain Yakult as probiotic and prebiotic GOS as prebiotic) demonstrated reduced serum total phenol levels and prevented skin dryness and disruption of keratinization in healthy adult women providing evidence of health benefits to the skin as well as the gut (Miyazaki et al. 2013). A synbiotic combination of inulin (prebiotic) and *Bifidobacterium longum* (probiotic) was found to be more potent in inhibiting azoxymethane (AOM)-induced aberrant crypt foci in rats in comparison to either inulin or the probiotic alone (Rowland et al. 1998).

4.7.4 Cobiotics

Cobiotics is a newly coined term to describe substances which are utilized by probiotics and also by the host. In contrast, prebiotics are only utilized by probiotics, but not by the host (Greenway et al. 2013). Certain enzymes react with food materials and release nutrients which are stimulatory to the probiotics. Enzymes protease and amylase when incorporated as a cobiotic combination, function as lactogenic factor (stimulate the growth of lactobacilli). Enzymes cellulose and hemicellulose, on the other hand function as a bifidogenic, that is, stimulate the growth of bifidobacteria. In a recent study, the effectiveness of cobiotics has been highlighted. A cobiotic consisting of prebiotic purified inulin, sugar-free blueberry pomace extract, and an oat preparation of purified beta-glucan was used to repair gastrointestinal dysbiosis and found to be highly effective in augmenting glucose control in a type-2 diabetic patient (Greenway et al. 2013).

4.7.5 Immunobiotics

The term "immunobiotics" was coined to identify bacteria that promote health through driving mucosal immune mechanisms, compared to those with strictly local effects (Podleski 2011, Tomosada et al. 2013). Immunobiotics are demonstrably beneficial for treating a variety of mucosal disorders, including inflammatory diseases. Immunobiotic microorganism *Lactobacillus jensenii* TL2937 has been found to interact with IEC and immune cells in experimental models through the modulation of Toll-like receptors (TLRs) to maintain a fine balance between tolerance and inflammation (Villena et al. 2013, Villena and Kitazawa 2014). Interestingly, immunobiotic bacteria has been found to stimulate the immune system at sites beyond the intestinal tract; consumption of *Lb. rhamnosus* CRL1505 (Lr1505) and *Lb. casei* CRL431 (Lc431) resulted in the stimulation of the immune system in the respiratory tract as demonstrated by increased activity of macrophages at those sites (Marranzino et al. 2012). Nasal administration *Lb. rhamnosus* strains have been reported to differentially modulate respiratory antiviral immune responses and induce protection against respiratory syncytial virus infection (Tomosada et al. 2013).

In an attempt to modulate virus-induced inflammation–coagulation interactions to treat acute respiratory virus infections, immunobiotic strain *Lb. rhamnosus* CRL1505 strain was used. The immunobiotic strain triggered activation of TLR-3 by modulating the production of proinflammatory and anti-inflammatory cytokines as well as the expression of tissue factor and thrombomodulin in the lung (Zelaya et al. 2014). The preventive treatment with the immunobiotic bacteria beneficially modulated the finely tuned balance between clearing respiratory viruses (respiratory syncytial virus and influenza virus) and controlling immune-coagulative responses in the lung, allowing normal lung function to be maintained in the face of a viral attack. These findings demonstrate that immunobiotic functional food offers novel preventive and therapeutic approaches to better control virus-inflammatory lung damage (Zelaya et al. 2014).

4.8 Microbiome Metabolites: Effects on Health

Abundant literature confirms the role of microbial metabolites of dietary components in disease prevention and disease risk (Qin et al. 2012, Goldsmith and Sartor 2014). The undigested nutrients including polysaccharides, lipids, and peptides that reach the large intestine unabsorbed positively impact the growth of gut microbiota (Bazzocco et al. 2008, Sekirov et al. 2010). Short SCFAs (acetate, propionate, and butyrate) that are formed as a result of microbial metabolism of dietary carbohydrates are directly linked to the proportion and composition of gut microbiota thereby affecting host health. Similarly, SCFAs are also produced by anaerobic microbial metabolism of peptides and proteins along with several toxic compounds such as ammonia, amines, phenols, thiols, and indols which are potentially harmful to human health (Cummings et al. 1996, Scott et al. 2013).

Phytochemicals, generally regarded as bioactive nonnutrient plant compounds, possess antioxidant, antiestrogenic, anti-inflammatory, immunomodulatory, and anticarcinogenic properties. The currently existing 25,000 phytochemicals exhibit either positive and deleterious effects on human health, for example, vegetables, the major source of nitrates in the human diet, may exert a damaging effect by interacting with several compounds forming nitrosamines, nitrosamides, and nitrosoguanidine that cause DNA damage. Contrarily, a plethora of literature confirms the positive role of dietary bioactive phytochemicals with potential benefit to human health. Nevertheless, components of the gut microbiota are associated with the fermentation, transformation, and bioavailability of these phytochemicals (Scalbert et al. 2002, Qin et al. 2012).

Laparra and Sanz (2010) elucidated the role of phytochemicals and their metabolic products as antimicrobial inhibiting pathogenic bacteria and stimulating the growth of beneficial bacteria in the gut. Moreover, phytochemicals and their derived products potentially affect colonic microbiota, as a part of them remains unabsorbed in the gut and this unabsorbed portion is subsequently metabolized in the liver. These metabolites are excreted through the bile in the form of glucuronides which eventually accumulate in the ileal and colorectal lumen (Bazzocco et al. 2008, Tzonuis et al. 2008).

The metabolism of dietary phenolic compounds results in different types of metabolites in the colon before absorption (Selma et al. 2009). Unabsorbed dietary phenolics and their metabolites possess the ability to act as antimicrobial or bacteriostatic agents. These metabolites inhibit the growth of selective pathogens and promote the growth of commensal bacteria, including some recognized probiotics (Lee et al. 2006, Laparra and Sanz 2010). The rapidly advancing field of medical sciences warrants recognition and understanding of how gut microbiota can beneficially interact with diet and modulate metabolism for improved long-term health status.

4.9 Perspectives

Research on the human microbiome, especially on the interplay between food and gut microbiota leading to health and disease conditions has become one of the most exciting fields in biology; generating fascinating insights into the relations of microbes and man as modulated by diet and the effects of the microbes on our health and well-being. The bidirectional interaction between host and microbe, which appears to influence the host at multiple levels, is crucial for our evolution, development, metabolism, immune function, and susceptibility to infectious and noncommunicable diseases. The influence of diet on gut microbiota is astounding; metagenomic analysis of gut microbial ecology is generating useful information regarding the functional contribution of gut microbiota to its host as modulated by diet and its relationship to health and disease states. It is anticipated that newer methodologies such as metaproteomics, the function-based approach relying on microbial protein expression; metabolomics, the functional analysis of complex microbial populations through analysis of their complete metabolite profiles; metatranscriptomics, which enables community-wide gene expression analysis of gut microbiota, will allow more thorough research leading to varied ways of harnessing the beneficial effects of the modulation of gut microbiota by diet as therapeutic, and even preventive options in future (Lozupone et al. 2012, David et al. 2014).

4.10 Conclusion

The human gut is a natural habitat for a large and dynamic bacterial community. The microbiome (genes and genomes of all the bacteria inhabiting the gut) of each person is distinct and variable but each individual possesses a shared core microbiome which is required for proper maintaining of cross species homeostasis between the gut bacteria and the host. The recent interest in the structure and function of the gut microbiome, its dynamic evolution throughout an individual's life in a host specific manner and how it is modified by diets, has resulted in a series of exciting findings. The advent of culture-independent techniques to study the microbiome has enabled scientists to decipher the dynamics of the complex bidirectional interactions between diet and the microbiome in relation to human health and diseases. Although details of the complex interactions between diet, the microbiome and host health is an emerging area of science, existing knowledge is being used in leveraging the microbiome to develop dietary interventions to counterbalance dysbiosis and to increase overall well-being. However, it is essential to assess the efficacy of the pro/prebiotics to molecular detail and the long-term safety of probiotics, as the impact of prolonged perturbation of the microbiome is largely unknown. Collectively, the research findings reviewed here suggest that more integrative studies will provide all-encompassing knowledge of the complex, multi-level interactions between diet, the microbiome, and host health, which can be utilized to design microbiome-based biomarkers for those at risk of various infectious and metabolic diseases and formulate diet-driven microbiota alteration strategies to improve human health.

References

Aagaard, K., J. Ma, K. M. Antony, R. Ganu, and J. Versalovic. 2014. The placenta harbors a unique microbiome. *Science Translational Medicine* 6: 1–10. DOI: 10.1126/scitranslmed.3008599.

Anuradha, S. and K. Rajeshwari. 2005. Probiotics in health and disease. *Journal of Indian Association of Clinical Medicine* 6: 67–72.

Arumugam, M, J. Raes, E. Pelletier, D. Le Paslier, T. Yamada, D. R. Mende et al. 2011. Enterotypes of the human gut microbiome. *Nature* 473: 174–180.

Arunachalam, K. D. 1999. Role of Bifidobacteria in nutrition, medicine and technology. *Nutrition Research* 19: 1559–1597.

Bäckhed, F., R. E. Ley, J. L. Sonnenburg, D. A. Peterson, and J. I. Gordon. 2005. Host-bacterial mutualism in the human intestine. *Science* 307: 1915–1920.

Bäckhed, F., J. K. Manchester, C. F. Semenkovich, and J. I. Gordon. 2007. Mechanisms underlying the resistance to diet-induced obesity in germ-free mice. *Proceedings of the National Academy of Sciences, USA* 104: 979–984.

Barboza, M., D. A. Sela, C. Prim, R. G. Locascio, S. L. Freeman, J. B. German, D. A. Mills, and C. B. Lebrilla. 2009. Glycoprofiling bifidobacterial consumption of galacto-oligosaccharides by mass spectrometry reveals strain-specific, preferential consumption of glycans. *Applied and Environmental Microbiology* 75: 7319–7325.

Barile, D. and R. A. Rastall. 2013. Human milk and related oligosaccharides as prebiotics. *Current Opinions in Biotechnology* 24: 214–219.

Bazzocco, S., I. Mattila , S. C. Guyot, C. Renard, and A. M. Aura. 2008. Factors affecting the conversion of apple polyphenols to phenolic acids and fruit matrix to short-chain fatty acids by human faecal microbiota in vitro. *European Journal of Nutrition* 47: 442–452.

Belzer, C. and W. M. de Vos. 2012. Microbes inside—From diversity to function: The case of *Akkermansia*. *International Society of Microbial Ecology Journal* 6: 1449–1458.

Bergman, E. N. 1990. Energy contributions of volatile fatty acids from the gastrointestinal tract in various species. *Physiological Review* 70: 567–590.

Bernardo, D., B. Sánchez, H. O. Al-Hassi, E. R. Mann, M. C. Urdaci, S. C. Knight, and A. Margolles. 2012. Microbiota/host crosstalk biomarkers: Regulatory response of human intestinal dendritic cells exposed to *Lactobacillus* extracellular encrypted peptide. *PLoS ONE* 7: e36262.

Besten, G. D., K. V. Eunen, A. K. Groen, K. Venema, D. Reijngoud, and B. M. Bakker. 2013. The role of short-chain fatty acids in the interplay between diet, gut microbiota, and host energy metabolism. *Journal of Lipid Research* 54: 2325–2340.

Beyer-Sehlmeyer, G., M. Glei, and E. Hartmann. 2003. Butyrate is only one of several growth inhibitors produced during gut flora-mediated fermentation of dietary fibre sources. *British Journal of Nutrition* 90: 1057–1070.

Bik, E. M. 2009. Composition and function of the human-associated microbiota. *Nutrition Reviews* 67: S164–S171.

Binder , H. J. 2010. Role of colonic short-chain fatty acid transport in diarrhea. *Annual Review of Physiology* 72 : 297–313.

Björkholm, B., C. M. Bok, A. Lundin, J. Rafter, M. L. Hibberd, and S. Pattersson. 2009. Intestinal microbiota regulate xenobiotic metabolism in the liver. *PLoS ONE* 4:e6958. DOI:10.1371/ journal.pone.0006958.

Blaut, M. and T. Clavel. 2007. Metabolic diversity of the intestinal microbiota; implications for health and disease. *Journal of Nutrition* 137: 7515–7555.

Booijink, C. C., S. El-Aidy, M. Rajilić-Stojanović, H. G. Heilig, F. J. Troost, H. Smidt, M. Kleerebezem, W. M. De Vos, and E. G. Zoetendal. 2010. High temporal and inter-individual variation detected in the human ileal microbiota. *Environmental Microbiology* 12: 3213–3227.

Bordin, M., F. Datri, L. Guillemot, and S. Citi. 2004. Histone deacetylase inhibitors up-regulate the expression of tight junction proteins. *Molecular Cancer Research* 2: 692–701.

Breitbart, M., I. Hewson, B. Felts, J. M. Mahaffy, J. Nulton, P. Salamon, and F. Rohwer. 2003. Metagenomic analysis of an uncultured viral community from human feces. *Journal of Bacteriology* 185: 6220–6223.

Brighenti, F., G. Castellani, L. Benini, M. C. Casiraghi, E. Leopardi, R. Crovetti, and G. Testolin. 1995. Effect of neutralized and native vinegar on blood glucose and acetate responses to a mixed meal in healthy subjects. *European Journal of Clinical Nutrition* 49: 242–247.

Brinkworth, G. D., M. Noakes, P. M. Clifton, and A. R. Bird. 2009. Comparative effects of very low-carbohydrate, high-fat and high-carbohydrate, low-fat weight-loss diets on bowel habit and faecal short-chain fatty acids and bacterial populations. *British Journal of Nutrition* 101: 1493–1502.

Bultman, S. J. 2014. Emerging roles of the microbiome in cancer. *Carcinogenesis* 35: 249–255.

Canani, R. B., P. Cirillo, G. Terrin, L. Cesarano, M. I. Spagnuolo, A. De Vincenzo et al. 2007. Probiotics for treatment of acute diarrhoea in children: Randomised clinical trial of five different preparations. *British Medical Journal* 335: 340–342.

Canani, R. B., M. D. Costanzo, L. Leone, M. Pedata, R. Meli, and E. A. Calignano. 2011. Potential beneficial effects of butyrate in intestinal and extraintestinal diseases. *World Journal of Gastroenterology* 17: 1519–1528.

Cani, P. D., E. Lecourt, M. E. Dewulf, F. M. Sohet, B. D. Pachikian, D. Naslain, F. De Backer, A. M. Neyrinck, and N. M. Delzenne 2009a. Gut microbiota fermentation of prebiotics increases satietogenic and incretin gut peptide production with consequences for appetite sensation and glucose response after a meal. *American Journal Clinical Nutritio*n 90:1236–1243.

Cani, P. D., S. Possemiers, T. Van de Wiele, Y. Guiot, A. Everard, O. Rottier et al. 2009b. Changes in gut microbiota control inflammation in obese mice through a mechanism involving GLP-2-driven improvement of gut permeability. Gut 58: 1091–1103.

Canny, G. O. and B. A. McCormick, 2008. Bacteria in the intestine, helpful residents or the enemies within? *Infection and Immunity* 76 : 3360–3373.

Chang, S. and L. Li. 2011. Metabolic endotoxemia: A novel concept in chronic disease pathology. *Journal of Medical Sciences* 31: 191–209.

Chen J, X. He, and J. Huang. 2014. Diet effects in gut microbiome and obesity. *Journal of Food Sciences* 79: R442-R451.

Chung, H., S. J. Pamap, J. A. Hill, N. K. Surana, S. M. Edelman, E. B. Troy et al. 2012. Gut immune maturation depends on colonization with a host-specific microbiota. *Cell* 149: 1578–1593.

Claesson, M. J., S. Cusack, O. Siobhán, R. O'Sullivan, H. Greene-Diniz, E. de Weerd et al. 2011. Composition, variability, and temporal stability of the intestinal microbiota of the elderly. *Proceedings of the National Academy of Sciences, USA* 108: 4586–4591.

Claesson, M, J., I. B. Jeffery, S. Conde, S. E. Power, E. M. O'Connor, S. Cusack et al. 2012. Gut microbiota composition correlates with diet and health in the elderly. *Nature* 78: 178–184.

Collins, M. D. and G. R.Gibson. 1999. Probiotics, prebiotics, and synbiotics: Approaches for modulating the microbial ecology of the gut. *American Journal of Clinical Nutrition* 69: 1052S–1057S.

Collins, S. M., M. Surette, and P. Bercik. 2012. The interplay between the intestinal microbiota and the brain. *Nature Reviews in Microbiology* 10: 735–742.

Cummings, J. H., E. R. Beatty, S. M. Kingman, S. A. Bingham, and H. N. Englyst. 1996. Digestion and physiological properties of resistant starch in the human large bowel. *British Journal of Nutrition* 75: 733–747.

Cummings, J. H. and G. T. Macfarlane. 1991. The control and consequences of bacterial fermentation in the human colon. *Journal of Applied Bacteriology* 70: 443–459.

Cummings, J. H., E. W. Pomare, W. J. Branch, C. P. Naylor, and G. T. Macfarlane. 1987. Short chain fatty acids in human large intestine, portal, hepatic and venous blood. *Gut* 28: 1221–1227.
David, L. A., C. F. Mauricel, R. N. Carmody, D. B. Gootenberg, J. E. Button, B. E. Wolfe et al. 2014. Diet rapidly and reproducibly alter the human gut microbiome. *Nature* 505: 559–563.
Davie, J. R. Inhibition of histone deacetylase activity by butyrate. 2003. *Journal of Nutrition* 133: 2485S–2493S.
De Vadder, F. D., P. Kovatcheva-Datchary, D. Goncalves, J. Vinera, C. Zitoun, A. Duchampt, F. Bäckhed, and G. Mithieux. 2014. Microbiota-generated metabolites promote metabolic benefits via gut-brain neural circuits. *Cell* 156 : 84–96.
de Vos, W. M. and E. A. de Vos. 2012. Role of the intestinal microbiome in health and disease: From correlation to causation. *Nature Reviews* 70: S45–S56.
Delzenne, N. M., A. M. Neyrinck, and P. D. Cani. 2011a. Modulation of the gut microbiota by nutrients with prebiotic properties: Consequences for host health in the context of obesity and metabolic syndrome. *Microbial Cell Factories* 10: 1–11.
Delzenne, N. M., A. M. Neyrinck, F. Bäckhed, and P. D. Cani. 2011b. Targeting gut microbiota in obesity: Effects of prebiotics and probiotics. *Nature Reviews Endocrinology* 7: 639–646.
Devillard, E., F. McIntosh, S. H. Duncan, and R. J. Wallace. 2007. Metabolism of linoleic acid by human gut bacteria: Different routes for biosynthesis of conjugated linoleic acid. *Journal of Bacteriology* 189: 2566–2570.
Diamant, M., E. E. Blaak, and W. M. de Vos. 2011. Do nutrient–gut–microbiota interactions play a role in human obesity, insulin resistance and type 2 diabetes? *Obesity Reviews* 12: 272–281.
DiBaise, J. K., D. N. Frank, and R. Mathur. 2012. Impact of the gut microbiota on the development of obesity: current concepts. *American Journal of Gastroenterology Supplements*1: 22–27.
Diaz-Heijtz, R., S. Wang, F. Anuar, Y. Qian, B. Björkholm, A. Samuelsson, M. L. Hibberd, H. Forssberg, and S. Pettersson. 2011. Normal gut microbiota modulates brain development and behavior. *Proceedings of the National Academy of Sciences, USA* 108: 3047–3052.
Dong, H., I. Rowland, K. M. Tuohy, L. V. Thomas, and P. Yaqoob. 2010. Selective effects of *Lactobacillus casei* Shirota on T cell activation, natural killer cell activity and cytokine production. *Clinical and Experimental Immunology* 161: 378–388.
Dotterud, C. K., O. Storrø, R. Johnsen, and T. Oien. 2010. Probiotics in pregnant women to prevent allergic disease: A randomized, double-blind trial. *British Journal of Dermatology* 163: 616–623.
Drago, L., M. R. Gismondo, A. Lombardi, C. Haen, and L. Gozzoni. 1997. Inhibition of enteropathogens by new *Lactobacillus* isolates of human intestinal origin. *FEMS Microbiology Letters* 153: 455–463.
Eaton, T. J. and M. J. Gasson. 2001. Molecular screening of *Enterococcus* virulence determinants and potential for genetic exchange between food and medical isolates. *Applied and Environmental Microbiology* 67: 1628–1635.
Elamin, E. E., A. A. Masclee, J. Dekker, H. J. Pieters, and D. M. Jonkers. 2013. Short-chain fatty acids activate AMP-activated protein kinase and ameliorate ethanol-induced intestinal barrier dysfunction in Caco-2 cell monolayers. *Journal of Nutrition* 143: 1872–1881.
Everard, A., C. Belzer, L. Geurts, J. P. Ouwerkerk, C. Druart, L. B. Bindels, Y. Guiot et al. 2013. Cross-talk between *Akkermansia muciniphila* and intestinal epithelium controls diet-induced obesity. *Proceedings of the National Academy of Sciences, USA* 110: 9066–9071.
FAO/WHO. 2001. Joint expert consultation on health and nutritional properties of probiotics in food including powder milk with live lactic acid bacteria. pp. 1–30, Cordoba, Argentina. DOI: fao.org/docrep/fao/009/a0512e00.pdf
Filippo, C. D., D. Cavalieri, M. D. Paola, M. Ramazzotti, J. B. Poullet, S. Massart, S. Collini, G. Pieraccini, and P. Lionetti. 2010. Impact of diet in shaping gut microbiota revealed by a comparative study in children from Europe and rural Africa. *Proceedings of the National Academy of Sciences, USA* 107: 14691–14696.
Flint, H. J. 2012. The impact of nutrition on the human microbiome. *Nutrition Reviews* 70: S10–S13.
Flint, H. J., E. A. Bayer, M. T. Rincon, R. Lamed, and B. A. White. 2008. Polysaccharide utilization by gut bacteria: Potential for new insights from genomic analysis. *Nature Reviews Microbiology* 6: 121–131.
Flint, H. J., S. H. Duncan, K. P. Scott, and Louis, P. 2007. Interactions and competition within the microbial community of the human colon: links between diet and health. *Environmental Microbiology* 9: 1101–1111.

Fooks, L. J., R. Fuller, and G. R. Gibson. 1999. Prebiotics, probiotics and human gut microbiology. *International Dairy Journal* 9: 53–61.

Frank, D. N., A. L. Amand, R. A. Feldman, E. C. Boedeker, N. Harpaz, and N. R. Pace. 2007. Molecular-phylogenetic characterization of microbial community imbalances in human inflammatory bowel diseases. *Proceedings of the National Academy of Sciences, USA* 104: 13780–13785.

Frye, R. E., S. Melnyk, and D. F. MacFabe. 2013. Unique acyl-carnitine profiles are potential biomarkers for acquired mitochondrial disease in autism spectrum disorder. *Translational Psychiatry* 3: e220. DOI:10.1038/tp.2012.143.

Fukae, J., Y. Amasaki, Y. Yamishita, T. Bohgaki, S. Yasuda, S. Jodo, T. Atsumi, and T. Koike. 2005. Butyrate suppresses tumour necrosis factor alpha production by regulatory specific messenger RNA degradation mediated through a CIS-acting AU-rich element. *Arthritis and Rheumatology* 52: 2697–2707.

Fukuda, S., H. Toh, and K. Hase. 2011. Bifidobacteria can protect from enteropathogenic infection through production of acetate. *Nature* 469: 543–547.

Fuller, R. 1989. Probiotics in man and animals. *Journal of Applied Bacteriology* 66: 365–378.

Ganal, S. C., S. L. Sanos, C. Kallfass, K. Oberle, C. Johner, C. Kirschning et al. 2012. Priming of natural killer cells by nonmucosal mononuclear phagocytes requires instructive signals from commensal microbiota. *Immunity* 37: 171–186.

Ganguli, K., D. Meng, S. Rautava, L. Lu, W. A. Walker, and N. Nanthakumar. 2013. Probiotics prevent necrotizing enterocolitis by modulating enterocyte genes that regulate innate immune-mediated inflammation. American Journal of Physiology Gastrointestinal and Liver Physiology 304: G132–G141. DOI: 10.1152/ajpgi.00142.2012.

Gibson, G. R., H. M. Probert, J. V. Loo, R. A. Rastall, and M. B. Roberfroid. 2004. Dietary modulation of the human colonic microbiota: Updating the concept of prebiotics. *Nutrition Research Reviews* 17: 259–275.

Gibson, G. R. and M. B. Roberfroid. 1995. Dietary modulation of the human colonic microbiota: Introducing the concept of prebiotics. *Journal of Nutrition* 125: 1401–1412.

Gibson, G. R, C. L. Wills, and J. Van Loo. 1994. Non-digestible oligosaccharides and bifidobacteria—Implication for health. *International Sugar Journal* 96: 381–387.

Gill, S. R., M. Pop, R. T. DeBoy, P. B. Eckburg, P. J. Turnbaug, B. S. Samuel et al. 2006. Metagenomic analysis of the human distal gut microbiome. *Science* 312: 1355–1359.

Goldsmith, J. R. and R. B. Sartor. 2014. The role of diet on intestinal microbiota metabolism: Downstream impacts on host immune function and health, and therapeutic implications. *Journal of Gastroenterology* 49: 785–798.

Gourbeyre, P., S. Denery, and M. Bodinier. 2011. Probiotics, prebiotics, and synbiotics: Impact on the gut immune system and allergic reactions. *Journal of Leukocyte Biology* 89: 85–695.

Granato, D., G. F. Branco, A. Gomes, C. J. de Assis, F. Faria, and N. P. Shah. 2010. Probiotic dairy products as functional foods. *Comprehensive Reviews in Food Science and Food Safety* 9: 455–470.

Greenway, F., S. Wang, and M. Heiman. 2013. A novel cobiotic containing a prebiotic and an antioxidant augments glucose control and gastrointestinal tolerability of metformin: A case study. *Beneficial Microbes* 17: 1–4.

Gaudier, E., A. Jarry, H. M. Blottiere, P. de Coppet, M. P. Buisine, J. P. Aubert, C. Laboisse, C. Cherbut, and C. Hoebler. 2004. Butyrate specifically modulates MUC gene expression in intestinal epithelial goblet cells deprived of glucose. *American Journal of Physiology Gastrointestinal and Liver Physiology* 287: G1168–G1174.

Guarner, F and J. R. Malagelada. 2003. Gut flora in health and disease. *The Lancet* 360: 512–519.

Guzman, J. R., V. S. Conlin, and C. Jobin. 2013. Diet, microbiome, and the intestinal epithelium: An essential triumvirate? *Biomedical Research International* 2013: 1–12. Article ID 425146.

Harmsen, H. J., A. C. Wildeboer-Veloo, G. C. Raangs, A. Wagendorp, N. Klijn, J. G. Bindels, and G. W. Welling. 2000. Analysis of intestinal flora development in breast-fed and formula-fed infants by using molecular identification and detection methods. *Journal of Pediatric Gastroenterology and Nutrition* 30: 61–67.

Hawrelak, J. A. and S. P. Myers. 2004. The causes of intestinal dysbiosis: A review. *Alternative Medicine Review* 9: 180–197.

Hekmat, S. and G. Reid. 2006. Sensory properties of probiotic yogurt is comparable to standard yogurt. *Nutrition Research* 26: 163–166.

Henker, J., M. Laas, B. M. Blokhin, Y. K. Bolbot, V. G. Maydannik, M. Elze, C. Wolff, and J. Schulze. 2007. The probiotic *Escherichia coli* strain Nissle 1917 (EcN) stops acute diarrhoea in infants and toddlers. *European Journal of Pediatrics* 166: 311–318.

Hill, D. A., M. C. Siracusa, M. C. Abt, B. S. Kim, D. Kobuley, M. Kubo et al. 2012. Commensal bacteria-derived signals regulate basophil hematopoiesis and allergic inflammation. *Nature Medicine* 18: 538–546.

Hildebrandt, M. A, C. Hoffman, S. A. Sherrill-Mix, S. A. Keilbaugh, M. Hamady, Y. Y. Chen, R. Knight, R. S. Ahima, F. Bushman, and G. D. Wu. 2009. High fat diet determines the composition of the murine gut microbiome independently of obesity. *Gastroenterology* 137: 1716–1724.

Holmes, E., J. V. Li, T. Athanasiou, H. Ashrafian, and J. K. Nicholson. 2011. Understanding the role of gut microbiome–host metabolic signal disruption in health and disease. *Trends in Microbiology* 19: 349–359.

Holmes, E., J. Kinross, G. R. Gibson, R. Burcelin, W. Jia, S. Pettersson, and J. K. Nicholson. 2012. Therapeutic modulation of microbiota-host metabolic interactions. *Science Translational Medicine* 4: 1–11. DOI: 10.1126/scitranslmed.3004244.

Hooper, L. V., D. R. Littman, and A. J. Macpherson. 2012. Interactions between the microbiota and the immune system. *Science* 336: 1268–1273.

Hormannsperger, G., T. Clavel, and D. Haller. 2012. Gut matters: Microbe–host interactions in allergic diseases. *Journal of Allergy and Clinical Immunology* 129: 1452–1459.

Huang, E. Y., V. A. Leone, S. Devkota, Y. Wang, M. J. Brady, and E. B. Chang. 2013. Composition of dietary fat source shapes gut microbiota architecture and alters host inflammatory mediators in mouse adipose tissue. *Journal of Parenteral and Internal Nutrition* 37: 746–754.

Immerseel, F. V., J. B. Russell, M. D. Flythe, I. Gantois, L. Timbermont, F. Pasmans, F. Haesebrouck, and R. Ducatelle. 2006. The use of organic acids to combat *Salmonella* in poultry: A mechanistic explanation of the efficacy. *Avian Pathology* 35: 182–188.

Ishibashi, N. and S.Yamazaki. 2001. Probiotics and safety. *American Journal of Clinical Nutrition* 73: 465–470.

Jia, W., H. Li, L. Zhao, and J. K. Nicholson. 2008. Gut microbiota: A potential new territory for drug targeting. *Nature Review Drug Discovery* 7: 123–129.

Jumpertz, R., D. S. Le, P. J. Turnbaugh, C. Trinidad, C. Bogardus, J. I. Gordon, and J. Krakoff. 2011. Energy-balance studies reveal associations between gut microbes, caloric load, and nutrient absorption in humans. *American Journal of Clinical Nutrition* 94: 58–65.

Kaila, M., E. Isolauri, E. Soppi, E. Virtanen, S. Laine, and H. Arvilommi. 1992. Enhancement of the circulating antibody secreting cell response in human diarrhea by a human *Lactobacillus* strain. *Pediatric Research* 32: 141–144.

Kaji, I, S. Karaki, and A. Kuwahara. 2014. Short-chain fatty acid receptor and its contribution to glucagon-like peptide-1 release. *Digestion* 89: 31–36.

Kaminogawa, S. 2010. Effects of food components on intestinal flora, intestinal immune system and their mutualism. *Bioscience Microflora* 29: 69–82.

Karlsson, C. L., J. Onnerfalt, J. Xu, G. Molin, S. Ahrne, and K. Thorngrem-Jerneck, 2012. The microbiota of the gut in preschool children with normal and excessive body weight. *Obesity* 20: 2257–2261.

Kim M. H., S. G. Kang, J. H. Park, M. Yanagisawa, and C. H. Kim. 2013. Short-chain fatty acids activate GPR41 and GPR43 on intestinal epithelial cells to promote inflammatory responses in mice. *Gastroenterology* 145: 396–406.

Kinross, J. M., A. C. von Roon, E. Holmes, A. Darzi, and J. K. Nicholson. 2008. The human gut microbiome: Implications for future health care. *Current Gastroenterology Report* 10: 396–403.

Kishino, S., M. Takeuchi, S. Park, A. Hirata, N. Kitamura, J. Kunisawa et al. 2013. Polyunsaturated fatty acid saturation by gut lactic acid bacteria affecting host lipid composition. *Proceedings of the National Academy of Sciences, USA* 110: 17808–17813.

Koeth, R. A., Z. Wang, B. S. Levison, J. A Buffa, E. Org, B.T. Sheehy et al. E. B. Britt, X. Fu, Y. Wu, L. Li. et al. 2013. Intestinal microbiota metabolism of L-carnitine, a nutrient in red meat, promotes atherosclerosis. *Nature Medicine*19: 576–585.

Kolida, S., K. Tuohy, and G. R. Gibson. 2002. Prebiotic effects of inulin and oligofructose. *British Journal of Nutrition* 87: S193–S197.

Kostic, A. D., M. R. Howitt, and W. S. Garrett. 2013. Exploring host–microbiota interactions in animal models and humans. *Genes & Development* 27: 701–718.

Lagier, J. C., M. Million, P. Hugon, F. Armougom, and D. Raoult. 2012. Human gut microbiota: Repertoire and variations. *Frontiers in Cellular and Infection Microbiology* 2: 1–19.

Laparra, J. M. and Y. Sanz. 2010. Interactions of gut microbiota with functional food components and nutraceuticals. *Pharmacology Research* 61: 219–225.

LeBlanc, J. G., C. Milani, G. S. de Giori, F. Sesma, D. van Sinderen, and M. Ventura. 2013. Bacteria as vitamin supplier to their host: A gut microbiota perspective. *Current Opinions in Biotechnology* 24: 160–168.

Lee, H. C., A. M. Jenner, C. S. Low, and Y. K. Lee. 2006. Effect of tea phenolics and their aromatic fecal bacterial metabolites on intestinal microbiota. *Research in Microbiology* 157: 876–884.

Leenen, C. H. M and L. Dieleman. 2007. Inulin and oligofructose in chronic inflammatory bowel disease. *Journal of Nutrition* 137: 2572S–2575S.

Lepage, P., M. C. Leclerc, M. Joossens, S. Mondot, H. M. Blottière, J. Raes, D. Ehrlich, and J. Doré. 2012. A metagenomic insight into our gut's microbiome. *Gut* 62: 146–158. DOI:10.1136/gutjnl-2011-301805.

Ley R.E, P. J. Turnbaugh, S. Klein, and J. I. Gordon. 2006. Microbial ecology: Human gut microbes associated with obesity. *Nature* 444: 1022–1023.

Lilley, D. M. and R. H. Stillwell. 1965. Probiotics: growth promoting factors produced by microorganisms. *Science* 147: 747–748.

Lindsay, J. O., K. Whelan, A. J. Stagg, J. O. Lindsay, K. Whelan, A. J. Stagg et al. 2006. Clinical, microbiological, and immunological effects of fructo-oligosaccharide in patients with Crohn's disease. *Gut* 55: 348–355.

Liong, M. T., W. Y. Fung, J. A. Ewe, C. Y. Kuan, and H. S. Lye. 2009. The improvement of hypertension by probiotics: Effects on cholesterol, diabetes, renin, and phytoestrogens. *International Journal Molecular Science* 10: 3755–3775.

Lomax, A. R. and P. C. Calder. 2009. Probiotics, immune function, infection and inflammation: A review of the evidence from studies conducted in humans. *Current Pharmaceutical Design* 15: 1428–1458.

Louis, P. and H. J. Flint. 2009. Diversity, metabolism and microbial ecology of butyrate-producing bacteria from the human large intestine. *FEMS Microbiology Letter* 294: 1–8.

Lourens-Hattingh, A. and B. Viljoen. 2001. Yogurt as probiotic carrier food. *International Dairy Journal* 11: 1–17.

Lozupone, C. A., J. I. Stombaugh, J. I. Gordon, J. K. Jansson, and R. Knight. 2012. Diversity, stability and resilience of the human gut microbiota. *Nature* 489: 220–230.

Lyons, A., D. O'Mahony, F. O'Brien, J. MacSharry, B. Sheil, M. Ceddia et al. 2010. Bacterial strain-specific induction of Foxp31 T regulatory cells is protective in murine allergy models. *Clinical and Experimental Allergy* 40: 811–819.

Macfarlane, G. T. and J. H. Cummings. 1991. The colonic flora, fermentation and large bowel digestive function. In S. F. Phillips, J. H. Pemberton and R. G. Shorter (Eds.), *The Large Intestine: Physiology, Pathophysiology and Disease*. New York: Raven Press Ltd, pp. 51–92.

Macfarlane, S., G. T. Macfarlane, and J. H. Cummings. 2006. Prebiotics in the gastrointestinal tract. *Alimentary Pharmacology and Therapeutics* 24: 701–713.

Macfarlane, G. T. and S. Macfarlane. 2011. Fermentation in the human large intestine its physiologic consequences and the potential contribution. *Journal of Clinical Gastroenterology* 45: S120–S127.

Macfarlane, G. T., H. Steed, and S. Macfarlane.2008. Bacterial metabolism and health-related effects of galacto-oligosaccharides and other prebiotics. *Journal of Applied Microbiology* 104: 305–344.

Mackie, R. I., A. Sghir, and H. R. Gaskins.1999. Developmental microbial ecology of the neonatal gastrointestinal tract. *American Journal of Clinical Nutrition* 69: 1035S–1045S.

Majamaa, H., F. Isolauri, M. Saxelin, and T. Vesikari. 1995. Lactic acid bacteria in the treatment of acute rotavirus gastroenteritis. *Journal of Pediatric Gastroenterology and Nutrition* 20: 333–338.

Manning, T. S. and Gibson, G. R. 2004. Microbial-gut interactions in health and disease: Prebiotics. *Best Practice and Research in Clinical Gastroenterology* 18: 287–298.

Marranzino, G., J. Villena, S. Salva, and S. Alvarez. 2012. Stimulation of macrophages by immunobiotic *Lactobacillus* strains: Influence beyond intestinal tract. *Microbiology and Immunology* 56: 771–781.

Marschan, E., M. Kuitunen, K. Kukkonen, T. Poussa, A. Sarnesto, T. Haahtela, R. Korpela, E. Savilahti, and O. Vaarala. 2008. Probiotics in infancy induce protective immune profiles that are characteristic for chronic low-grade inflammation. *Clinical and Experimental Allergy* 38: 611–618.

Marteau, P. R., M. Vrese, C. J. Cellier, and J. Schrezenmeir. 2001. Protection from gastrointestinal diseases with the use of probiotics. *American Journal of Clinical Nutrition* 73: 430–436.

Marteau, P., P. Lepage, I. Mangin, A. Suau, J. Doré, P. Pochart, and P. Seksik. 2004. Gut flora and inflammatory bowel disease. *Alimentary Pharmacology and Therapeutics* 20: 18–23.

Martens, E. C., Lowe, E. C. Chiang, H. N. A. Pudlo, M. Wu, N. P. McNulty, D. W. Abbott et al. 2011. Recognition and degradation of plant cell wall polysaccharides by two human gut symbionts. *PLoS Biology* 9: e1001221.

Martin, R., S. Miguel, J. Ulmer, P. Langella, and L. G. Bermudez-Humaran. 2014. Gut ecosystem: how microbes help us. *Beneficial Microbes* 28: 1–15.

Martin, F. P., N. Sprenger, I. K. Yap, Y. Wang, R. Bibiloni, F. Rochat et al. 2009. Pan-organismal gut microbiome-host metabolic crosstalk. *Journal of Proteome Research* 8: 2090–2105.

Maslowski, K. M. and C. R. Mackay. 2011. Diet, gut microbiota and immune responses. *Nature Immunology* 12: 5–9.

Mattia, A. and R. Merker. 2008. Regulation of probiotic substances as ingredients in foods: Premarket approval or "generally recognized as safe" notification. *Clinical Infectious Disease* 2: S115–S118.

Mazmanian, S. K., C. H. Liu, A. O. Tzianabos, and D. L. Kasper. 2005. An immunomodulatory molecule of symbiotic bacteria directs maturation of the host immune system. *Cell* 122: 107–118.

McDermott, A. J. and G. B. Huffnagle. 2014. The microbiome and regulation of mucosal immunity. *Immunology* 142: 24–31.

McFall-Ngai, M., M. G. Hadfield, T. C. G. Bosch, H. V. Carey, T. Domazet-Lošo, A. E. Douglas et al. 2013. Animals in a bacterial world, a new imperative for the life sciences. *Proceedings of the National Academy of Sciences, USA* 110: 3229–3236.

McLoughlin, R. M. and K. H. G. Mills. 2011. Influence of gastrointestinal commensal bacteria on the immune responses that mediate allergy and asthma. *Journal of Allergy and Clinical Immunology* 127: 1097–1107.

Miyazaki, K., N. Masuoka, M. Kano, and R. Iizuka. 2013. *Bifidobacterium* fermented milk and galacto-oligosaccharides lead to improved skin health by decreasing phenols production by gut microbiota. *Beneficial Microbes* 17: 1–8.

Mshvildadze, M. and J. Neu. 2010. The infant intestinal microbiome: Friend or foe? *Early Human Development* 86: 67–71.

Musso, G., R. Gambino, and M. Cassader. 2010. Obesity, diabetes and gut microbiota: The hygiene hypothesis expanded? *Diabetes Care* 33: 2277–2284.

Nakamura, N., H. Lin, C. McSweeney, R. Mackie, and H. Gaskins. 2010. Mechanisms of microbial hydrogen disposal in the human colon and implications for health and disease. *Annual Reviews in Food Science and Technology* 1: 363–395.

Neish, A.S. 2009. Microbes in gastrointestinal health and disease. *Gastroenterology* 136: 65–80.

Nicholson, J. K., E. Holmes, and J. Kinross. 2012. Host-gut microbiota metabolic interactions. *Science* 336: 1262–1267.

Niness, K. R. 1999. Nutritional and health benefits of inulin and oligofructose. *Journal of Nutrition* 129: 1402S–1406S.

Nordgaard, I. 1998. Colon as a digestive organ: the importance of colonic support for energy absorption as small bowel failure proceeds. *Danish Medical Bulletin* 45: 135–156.

Norman, J. M., S. A. Handley, and W. Virgin. 2014. Kingdom-agnostic metagenomics and the importance of complete characterization of enteric microbial communities. *Gastroenterology* 146: 1459–1469. DOI: 10.1053/j.gastro.2014.02.001.

Nylund, L., R. Satokari, J. Nikkilä, M. Rajilić-Stojanović, M. Kalliomäki, E. Isolauri, S. Salminen, and W. M. de Vos. 2013. Microarray analysis reveals marked intestinal microbiota aberrancy in infants having eczema compared to healthy children in at-risk for atopic disease. *BMC Microbiology* 13: 12 DOI:10.1186/1471-2180-13-12.

O'Hara, A. M. and F. Shanahan. 2006. The gut flora as a forgotten organ. *EMBO Report* 27: 688–693.

Ooi, L., and M. Liong. 2010. Cholesterol-lowering effects of probiotics and prebiotics: A review of *in vivo* and *in vitro* findings. *International Journal of Molecular Sciences* 11: 2499–2522.

Özdemir, O. 2013. Preventative and therapeutic role of probiotics in various allergic and autoimmune disorders. *Journal of Evidence Based Complementary and Alternative Medicine* 18: 121–151.

Parker, R. B. 1974. Probiotics, the other half of the antibiotic story. *Animal Nutrition and Health* 29: 4–8.

Parvez, S., K. A. Malik, S. A. Kang, and H. Y. Kim. 2006. Probiotics and their fermented food products are beneficial for health. *Journal of Applied Bacteriology* 100: 1171–1185.

Penders, J., C. Thijs, C. Vink, F. F. Stelma, B. Snijders, I. Kummeling, P. A. van den Brandt, and E. E. Stobberingh. 2006. Factors influencing the composition of the intestinal microbiota in early infancy. *Pediatrics* 118: 511–521.

Perdigon, G., M. E. de Macıas, S. Alvarez, G. Oliver, and A. A. de Ruiz-Holgado. 1986. Effect of per orally administered lactobacilli on macrophage activation in mice. *Infection and Immunity* 53: 404–410.

Perdigon, G., M. E. de Macıas, S. Alvarez, G. Oliver, and A. P. de Ruiz Holgado. 1988. Systemic augmentation of the immune response in mice by feeding fermented milks with *Lactobacillus casei* and *Lactobacillus acidophilus*. *Immunology* 63: 17–23.

Petrof, E. O. and A. Khoruts. 2014. From stool transplants to next-generation microbiota therapeutics. *Gastroenterology* 146: 1573–1582.

Pineiro, M., N. G. Asp, G. Reid, S. Macfarlane, L. Morelli, O. Brunser, and K. Tuohy. 2008. FAO Technical meeting on prebiotics. *Journal of Clinical Gastroenterology* 42: S156–S159.

Podleski, W. K. 2011. Dietary prevention, control, and protection toward allergic disorders: A word in favor of immunobiotics. *Annals of Allergy Asthma and Immunology* 106: 177. DOI:10.1016/j.anai.

Pokusaeva, K., G. F. Fitzgerald, and D. Sinderen. 2011. Carbohydrate metabolism in Bifidobacteria. *Genes and Nutrition* 6: 285–306.

Prado, F. C., J. L. Parada, A. Pandey, and C. R. Soccol. 2008. Trends in non-dairy probiotic beverages. *Food Research International* 41: 111–123.

Prakash, S., L. Rodes, M. Coussa-Charley, and C. Tomaro-Duchesneau. 2011. Gut microbiota: Next frontier in understanding human health and development of biotherapeutics. *Biologics* 5: 71–86.

Preidis, G. A. and Versalovic, J. 2009. Targeting the human microbiome with antibiotics, probiotics, and prebiotics: Gastroenterology enters the metagenomics era. *Gastroenterology*136: 2015–2031.

Qin, J., Y. Li, Z. Cai, S. Li, J. Zhu, F. Zhang et al. 2012. A metagenome-wide association study of gut microbiota in type 2 diabetes. *Nature* 490: 55–60.

Romano-Keeler, J., D. J. Moore, C. Wang, R. M. Brucker, C. Fonnesbeck, J. C. Slaughter et al. 2014. Early life establishment of site-specific microbial communities in the gut. *Gut Microbes* 5: 192–201.

Rautava, S., H. Arvilommi, and E. Isolauri. 2006. Specific probiotics in enhancing maturation of IgA responses in formula-fed infants. *Pediatric Research* 60: 221–224.

Roberfroid, M. B. 2007. Prebiotics: the concept revisited. *Journal of Nutrition* 137: 830S–837S.

Roberfroid, M. B. 1998. Prebiotics and synbiotics: concepts and nutritional properties. *British Journal of Nutrition* 80: S197-S200.

Roberfroid, M. B. 1999. Caloric value of inulin and oligofructose. *Journal of Nutrition* 129: 1436S–1437S.

Roberfroid, M. B., F. Bornet, C. Bouley, and J. H. Cummings. 1995. Colonic microflora: Nutrition and health: Summary and conclusions of an International Life Sciences Institute (ILSI) (Europe)] workshop held in Barcelona, Spain. *Nutrition Reviews* 53: 127–130.

Rowland, I. R., C. J. Rumney, J. T. Coutts, and L. C. Lievense. 1998. Effect of *Bifidobacterium longum* and inulin on gut bacterial metabolism and carcinogen-induced aberrant crypt foci in rats. *Carcinogenesis.*19: 281–285.

Saarela, M., G. Mogensen, R. Fonden, J. Matto, and T. Mattila-Sandholm. 2000. Probiotic bacteria: Safety, functional and technological properties. *Journal of Biotechnology* 84: 197–215.

Salminen, S., C. Bouley, and M. C. Boutron-Ruault. 1998. Functional food science and gastrointestinal physiology and function. *British Journal of Nutrition* 80: 147–171.

Scalbert, A., C. Morand, C. Manach, and C. Remesy. 2002. Absorption and metabolism of polyphenols in the gut and impact on health. *Biomedicine and Pharmacotherapy* 56: 276–282.

Schiffrin, E., F. Rochat, H. Link-Amster, J. Aeschlimann, and A. Donnet-Hugues. 1995. Immunomodulation of blood cells following the ingestion of lactic acid bacteria. *Journal of Dairy Sciences* 78: 491–497.

Schirbel, A., S. Kessler, F. Rieder, G. West, N. Rebert, K. Asosingh, C. McDonald, and C. Fiocchi. 2013. Pro-angiogenic activity of TLRs and NLRs: a novel link between gut microbiota and intestinal angiogenesis. *Gastroenterology* 144: 613–629.

Schlee, M., J. Wehkamp, A. Altenhoefer, T. A. Oelschlaeger, E. F. Stange, and K. Fellermann. 2007. Induction of human β-Defensin 2 by the probiotic *Escherichia coli* Nissle 1917 is mediated through flagellin. *Infection and Immunity* 75: 2399–2407.

Scholtens, P. A., M. S. Alles, J. G. Bindels, E. G. van der Linde, J. J. Tolboom, and J. Knol. 2006. Bifidogenic effects of solid weaning foods with added prebiotic oligosaccharides: A randomised controlled clinical trial. *Journal of Pediatric Gastroenterology and Nutrition* 42: 553–559.

Scholz-Ahrens, K. E., P. Ade, B. Marten, P. Weber, W. Timm, Y. Açil, C. Glüer, and J. Schrezenmeir. 2007. Prebiotics, probiotics, and synbiotics affect mineral absorption, bone mineral content, and bone structure. *Journal of Nutrition* 137: 838S–846S.

Schrezenmeir, J. and M. de Vrese. 2001. Probiotics, prebiotics, and synbiotics—Approaching a definition. *American Journal of Clinical Nutrition* 73: 361S–364S.

Schuijt, T. J., T. Poll, W. M. de Vos, and W. J. Wiersinga. 2013. Human microbiome: The intestinal microbiota and host immune interactions in the critically ill. *Trends in Microbiology* 21: 221–229.

Scott, K. P., S. W. Gratz, P. O. Sheridan, H. J. Flint, and S. H. Duncan. 2013. The influence of diet on the gut microbiota. *Pharmacology Research* 69: 52–60.

Segain, J. P., D. B. Raingeard, and A. Bourreille. 2000. Butyrate inhibits inflammatory responses through NFkappaB inhibition: implications for Crohn's disease. *Gut* 47: 397–403.

Sekirov, I., S. L. Russell, C. M. Antunes, and B. B. Finlay. 2010. Gut microbiota in health and disease. *Physiological Reviews* 90: 859–904.

Selma, M. V., J. C. Espin, and F. A. Tomas-Barberan. 2009. Interaction between phenolics and gut microbiota: Role in human health. *Journal of Agricultural and Food Chemistry* 57: 6485–6501.

Senok, A. C. 2009. Probiotics in the Arabian Gulf region. *Food and Nutrition Research* 1: 1–6.

Senok, A. C., A. Y. Ismaeel, and G. A. Botta. 2005. Probiotics: Facts and myths. *Clinical Microbiology and Infection* 11: 958–966.

Shah, N. P. 2007. Functional cultures and health benefits. *International Dairy Journal* 17: 1262–1277.

Sharma, M and M. Devi. 2014. Probiotics: A comprehensive approach toward health foods *Critical Reviews in Food Sciences and Nutrition* 54: 537–552.

Shen, W., H. R. Gaskins, and M. K. McIntosh. 2014. Influence of dietary fat on intestinal microbes, inflammation, barrier function and metabolic outcomes. *Journal of Nutritional Biochemistry* 25: 270–280.

Sjögren, Y. M., M. C. Jenmalm, M. Fagerås-Böttcher, B. Björkstén, and E. Sverremark-Ekström. 2009. Altered early infant gut flora in children developing allergy up to five years of age. *Clinical and Experimental Allergy* 39: 518–526.

Slavin, J. 2013. Fiber and prebotics: Mechanisms and health benefits. *Nutrients* 5: 1417–1436.

Smith, P. M., M. R. Howitt, and N. Panikov. 2013. The microbial metabolites, short-chain fatty acids, regulate colonic T_{reg} cell homeostasis. *Science* 341: 569–573.

Soccol, C. R., L. P. D. S. Vandenberghe, and M. R. Spier. 2010. The potential of probiotics. *Food Technology and Biotechnology* 48: 413–434.

Sperty, G. S. 1977. *Probiotics*. West Point, CT: AVI Publishing, 200pp.

Sunkara, L. T., W. Jiang and G. Zhang. 2012. Modulation of antimicrobial host defense peptide gene expression by free fatty acids. *PLoS ONE* 7: e49558. DOI:10.1371/journal.pone.0049558.

Sur, D., B. Manna, and S. K. Niyogi. 2011. Role of probiotic in preventing acute diarrhoea in children: A community based, randomized, double-blind placebo-controlled field trial in an urban slum. *Epidemiology and Infection* 139: 919–926.

Takahashi, K., H. Terashima, K. Kohno, and N. Ohkohchi. 2013. A stand-alone synbiotic treatment for the prevention of D-lactic acidosis in short bowel syndrome. *International Surgery* 98: 110–113.

Tan J., McKenzie, C., Potamitis, M, Thorburn, A. N., Mackay, C. R., and Macia, L. 2014. The role of short-chain fatty acids in health and disease. *Advances in Immunology* 121: 91–119.

Tappenden, K. A. and A. S. Deutsch. 2007. The physiological relevance of the intestinal microbiota—Contributions to human health. *Journal of American College of Nutrition* 26: 679S–683S.

Tomosada, Y., E. Chiba, H. Zelaya, T. Takahashi, K. Tsukida, H. Kitazawa, S. Alvarez, and J. Villena. 2013. Nasally administered *Lactobacillus rhamnosus* strains differentially modulate respiratory antiviral immune responses and induce protection against respiratory syncytial virus infection. *BMC Immunology* 14: 40. DOI:10.1186/1471-2172-14-40.

Topping, D. L. and P. M. Clifton. 2001. Short chain fatty acids and human colonic function: Roles of resistant starch and nonstarch polysaccharides. *Physiological Reviews* 81: 1031–1064.

Tremaroli, V. and F. Bäckhed, F. 2012. Functional interactions between the gut microbiota and the host metabolism. *Nature* 489: 242–249.

Trompette, A., E. S. Gollwitzer, and K. Yadava. 2014. Gut microbiota metabolism of dietary fiber influences allergic airway disease and hematopoiesis. *Nature Medicine* 20: 159–166.

Turnbaugh, P. J., F. Bäckhed, L. Fulton, and J. I. Gordon. 2008. Diet-induced obesity is linked to marked but reversible alterations in the mouse distal gut microbiome. *Cell Host and Microbe* 3: 213–223.

Tzonuis, X., J. Vulevic, G. G. Kuhnle, T. George, J. Leonczak, G. R. Gibson, C. Kwik-Uribe, and J. P. Spencer. 2008. Flavanol monomer-induced changes to the human faecal microflora. *British Journal of Nutrition* 99: 782–792.

Uccello, M., G. Malaguarnera, F. Basile, V. D'agata, M. Malaguarnera, G. Bertino, M. Vacante, F. Drago, and A. Biondi. 2012. Potential role of probiotics on colorectal cancer prevention. *BMC Surgery* 12: S35. DOI:10.1186/1471-2482-12-S1-S35

Valeur, J and A. Berstad. 2010. Colonic fermentation: A neglected topic in human physiology education. *Advances in Physiology Education* 34: 22. DOI:10.1152/advan.00103.2009.

Vandenplas, Y., G. Veereman-Wauters, E. De Greef, S. Peeters, A. Casteels, T. Mahler, T. Devreker, and B. Hauser. 2011. Probiotics and prebiotics in prevention and treatment of diseases in infants and children. *Journal of Pediatrics* 87: 292–300.

Vanhoutte, T., G. Huys, E. Brandt, and J. Swings. 2004. Temporal stability analysis of the microbiota in human feces by denaturing gradient gel electrophoresis using universal and group-specific 16S rRNA gene primers. *FEMS Microbiology Ecology* 48: 437–446.

Velázquez, O. C, H. M. Lederer, and J. L. Rombeau. 1997. Butyrate and the colonocyte. *Advances in Experimental Medicine and Biology* 427: 123–134.

Villena, J., S. Salva, N. Barbieri, and S. Alvarez. 2013. Immunobiotics for the prevention of bacterial and viral respiratory infections. In: H. Kitazawa, J. Villena, and S. Alvarez (Eds.), *Probiotics: Immunobiotics and Immunogenics*. Boca Raton, FL: CRC Press, pp. 128–168.

Villena, J. and H. Kitazawa. 2014. Modulation of Intestinal TLR4-Inflammatory Signaling pathways by probiotic microorganisms: Lessons learned from *Lactobacillus jensenii* TL2937. *Frontiers in Immunology* 4: 1–12. DOI: 10.3389/fimmu.2013.00512.

Vinolo, M. A. R., H. G. Rodrigues, R. T. Nachbar, and R. Curi. 2011. Regulation of inflammation by short chain fatty acids. *Nutrients* 3: 858–876.

Vlieg, E. T. V, P. Veiga, C. Zhang, M. Derrien, and L. Zhao. 2011. Impact of microbial transformation of food on health-from fermented foods to fermentation in the gastro-intestinal tract. *Current Opinions in Biotechnology* 22: 1–9.

Vrieze, A., F. Holleman, E. G. Zoetendal, W. M. de Vos, J. B. Hoekstra, and M. Nieuwdorp. 2010. The environment within: How gut microbiota may influence metabolism and body composition. *Diabetologia* 53: 606–613.

Walker, A.W., J. Ince, S. H. Duncan, L. M. Webster, G. Holtrop, X. Ze et al. 2011. Dominant and diet-responsive groups of bacteria within the human colonic microbiota. *International Society for Microbial Ecology Journal* 5: 220–230.

Wallace, T. C., F. Guarner, K. Madsen, M. D. Cabana, G. Gibson, E. Hentges, and M. I. Sanders. 2011. Human gut microbiota and its relationship to health and disease. *Nutrition Reviews* 69: 392–403.

West, C. E., M. L. Hammarstrom, and O. Hernell. 2009. Probiotics during weaning reduce the incidence of eczema. *Pediatric Allergy and Immunology* 20: 430–437.

Wichmann, A., A. Allahyar, T. U. Greiner, H. Plovier, G. O. Lundén, T. Larsson, D. J. Drucker, N. M. Delzenne, P. D. Cani, and F. Bäckhed. 2013. Microbial modulation of energy availability in the colon regulates intestinal transit. *Cell Host Microbe* 14: 582–590.

Windey, K., V. D. Preter, and K. Verbeke. 2012. Relevance of protein fermentation to gut health. *Molecular Nutrition and Food Research* 56: 184–196.

Wu, G. D., J. Chen, C. Hoffmann, K. Bittinger, Y. Chen, S. A. Keilbaugh et al. 2011. Linking long-term dietary patterns with gut microbial enterotypes. *Science* 334: 105–108.

Wilks, J. and T. Golovkina. 2012. Influence of microbiota on viral infections. *PLoS Pathogens* 8: e1002681. DOI:10.1371/journal.ppat.1002681.

Xu, J., M. K. Bjursell, J. Himrod, S. Deng, L. K. Carmichael, H. C. Chiang, L. V. Hooper, and J. I. Gordon 2003. A genomic view of the human-*Bacteroides thetaiotaomicron* symbiosis. *Science* 299: 2074–2076.

Xu, J. and J. I. Gordon. 2003.Honor thy symbionts. *Proceedings of the National Academy of Sciences, USA* 100: 10452–10459.

Yan, F., H. Cao, T. L. Cover, M. K. Washington, Y. Shi, L. Liu, R. Chaturvedi, R. M. Jr. Peek, K. T. Wilson, and D. B. Polk. 2011. Colon-specific delivery of a probiotic-derived soluble protein ameliorates intestinal inflammation in mice through an EGFR-dependent mechanism. *Journal of Clinical Investigation* 121: 2241–2253.

Yu, L. C., J. Wang, S. Wei, and Y. Ni. 2012. Host–microbial interactions and regulation of intestinal epithelial barrier function: From physiology to pathology. *World Journal of Gastrointestinal Pathophysiology* 15: 27–43.

Zbar, N. S., L. F. Nashi, and S. M. Saleh. 2013. *Saccharomyces boulardii* as effective probiotic against *Shigella flexneri* in mice. *International Journal of Materials, Methods and Technology* 1: 17–21.

Zelaya, H., K. Tsukida, E. Chiba, G. Marranzino, S. Alvarez, S. H. Kitazawa, G. Agüero, and J. Villena. 2014. Immunobiotic lactobacilli reduce viral-associated pulmonary damage through the modulation of inflammation-coagulation interactions. *International Immunopharmacology* 19: 161–173.

Zeng, H., D. L. Lazarova, and M. Bordonaro. 2014. Mechanisms linking dietary fiber, gut microbiota and colon cancer prevention. *World Journal of Gastrointestinal Oncology* 6: 41–51.

Zhu, Y., E. Jameson, M. Crosatt, H. Schäfer, K, Rajakumar, T. D. Bugg, and Y. Chen. 2014. Carnitine metabolism to trimethylamine by an unusual Rieske-type oxygenase from human microbiota. *Proceedings of the National Academy of Sciences, USA* 111: 4268–4273.

Zhu, B., X. Wang and L Li. 2010. Human gut microbiome: The second genome of human body. *Protein Cell* 1: 718–725.

Chapter 5

Health Benefits of Fermented Dairy Products

Baltasar Mayo and Leocadio Alonso

Contents

5.1 Introduction

Although the region in which milking was first practiced remains unknown, direct evidence for dairying in the seventh millennium BC in northwestern Anatolia has been recently reported (Evershed et al. 2008). Organic (lipid) residues preserved in archaeological pottery have provided further evidence for the use of processed (fermented) milk in the sixth millennium BC in Eastern Europe, and in the fourth millennium BC in Britain (Copley et al. 2006). Therefore, fermentation is without any doubt among the oldest techniques of food preservation. It is also an easy way to derive new products. Indeed, milk can be transformed into a vast array of fermented products (Table 5.1), which are important from both nutritive and economical points of view (Kosikowski and Mistry 1997, Tamime 2002, de Ramesh et al. 2006, Robinson and Tamime 2006). More than 400 generic names are applied to traditional and industrialized fermented milk beverages (Robinson and Tamime 2006), and 500–1000 different cheese types have been proposed (Kosikowski and Mistry 1997) (Figures 5.1 through 5.3). Although the list of presentation still continues to be increasing, the real number of different varieties is thought to be much shorter.

5.2 Milk Fermentation and Lactic Acid Bacteria

The natural (spontaneous) fermentation of milk is due to the development of several species of lactic acid bacteria (LAB) (Wouters et al. 2002), a diverse group of bacteria producing lactic acid as the major end product from carbohydrate utilization. LAB are non-sporeformer, anaerobic, aerotolerant microorganisms presenting limited biosynthetic capabilities, thus requiring a rich medium to grow and a series of growth factors such as amino acids, vitamins, purines, and pyrimidines (Carr et al. 2002). Typical LAB members belong to the genera *Lactococcus, Lactobacillus, Leuconostoc,* and *Pediococcus.* Nowadays, although phylogenetically unrelated, *Propionibacterium* and *Bifidobacterium* species are also considered among the LAB, because they are frequently found in the same ecological niches and used for similar industrial applications (Parente and Cogan 2004). LAB species form part of human diet from immemorial times through various fermented products, including dairy commodities. This and the fact that they do not normally produce

Table 5.1 Principal Categories and Relevant Microbial Characteristics of Fermented Milk Products

Milk or Cheese	*Type*	*Starter*	*Starter Function*	*Relevant Microorganisms*								
				Lcl	*Lcc*	*Ln*	*Ec*	*St*	*Lb*	*Ll*	*Lh*	*Other Microbial Types*
Fermented Milks												
Lactic fermentation												
NFMs												
Noninoculated		NoS	LA, AR	++	++							Lactobacilli
Inoculated		BS	LA, AR	++	++							Lactobacilli
Yogurt, Dahi, Zabady		DS	LA, AR, TX					++	++			
Probiotic milks												
Acidophilus milk		DS	LA, AR									*Lb. acidophilus*
Yakult		DS	LA, AR									*Lb. casei*
Other		DS	LA, AR					++	++			*Lb. rhamnosus/ Lb. johnsonii*
Yeast/lactic fermentation												
Kefir		KG	LA, AR, G, TX	+	+	+	+	+	++	++	+	Yeasts
Koumiss		BS	LA, AR, G, TX	+	+	+	+		++	++		Yeasts
Viili, långfil		BS	LA, AR, TX	++	++							*G. candidum*

(*Continued*)

Table 5.1 (*Continued*) Principal Categories and Relevant Microbial Characteristics of Fermented Milk Products

Milk or Cheese	*Type*	*Starter*	*Starter Function*	*Relevant Microorganisms*								
				Lcl	*Lcc*	*Ln*	*Ec*	*St*	*Lb*	*Ll*	*Lh*	*Other Microbial Types*
Acidophilus yeast milk		DS	LA, AR, G, TX									*Lb. acidophilus/ Saccharomyces boulardii*
Cheeses												
Acid curd	Cottage, Quark	MS, DS	LA, D	++	++	+						
Enzymatic curd												
Bacterial ripened												
"Pasta Filata"	Mozzarella	NS, MS	LA, AR				+	++	+	+	+	
High salt content	Feta	MS	LA	++	+		++					Lactobacilli
Cheese with eyes	Edam, Gouda	MS	LA, G, P	++	++	+	+					Propionibacteria
	Emmental	MS	LA, G, P, PAG	++	++	+	+	++	+	+	+	*Propionibacterium freudenreichii/ P. shermanii/P. thoenii*
Semihard	Caerphilly	MS, NoS	LA, D	++			+					Lactobacilli
Hard	Cheddar, Manchego	DS, MS, NoS	LA,P, D, AR	++	+	+	++		-			Lactobacilli/yeasts

Extra-hard	Grana Padano, Parmesano	NoS, MC, WC	LA, P, AR, PAG				++	++	++	++	++	lactobacilli/yeasts
Smear ripened	Brick, Limburger, Munster	MS	LA, AR, TX	++	++	+	++					*Brevibacterium linens/ Kokuria* spp./ *Micrococcus* spp.
Mold ripened												
Internal molds (blue cheese)	Roquefort, Gorgonzola, Stilton	MS, DS	LA, G, P, L	++		+	++					*Penicillium roqueforti/* lactobacilli/yeasts
External molds (moldy cheese)	Brie, Camembert	MS, DS	LA, P, L	++	++	+	+					*Penicillium camemberti/ G. candidum/* lactobacilli
Whey cheese	Ricotta, Requesón	NoS										

Source: Compiled from Kosikowski, F. V. and V. V. Mistry. 1997. *Cheese and Fermented Milk Foods*, 3rd edn., Connecticut: LLC Westport.; Fox, P. F. et al. 2000. *Fundamentals of Cheese Science*. Gaithersburg: AN Aspen Publication; Reprinted from *Cheese: Chemistry, Physics and Microbiology. Major Cheese Groups*, 3rd ed. San Diego. Fox, P. F. et al., Copyright 2004, with permission from Elsevier.

Key of abbreviations: NoS, no starter; DS, defined starter; BS, backslopping; KG, kefir grain; MS, mixed starter; MC, milk cultures; WC, whey cultures. LA, lactic acid; D, diacetyl; AR, other aroma compounds; G, gas (CO_2); P, proteolysis; L, lipolysis; PAG, propionic acid and gas; TX, texture. Lcl, *Lactococcus lactis* subsp. *lactis;* Lcc: *Lactococcus lactis* subsp. *cremoris;* Ln, *Leuconostoc mesenteroides;* Ec, *Enterococcus faecium* and/or *E. faecalis;* St, *Streptococcus thermophilus;* Lb, *Lactobacillus delbrueckii* subsp. *bulgaricus;* Ll, *Lactobacillus delbrueckii* subsp. *lactis;* Lh, *Lactobacilus helveticus.* ++ , dominant species; +, minority or occasional species.

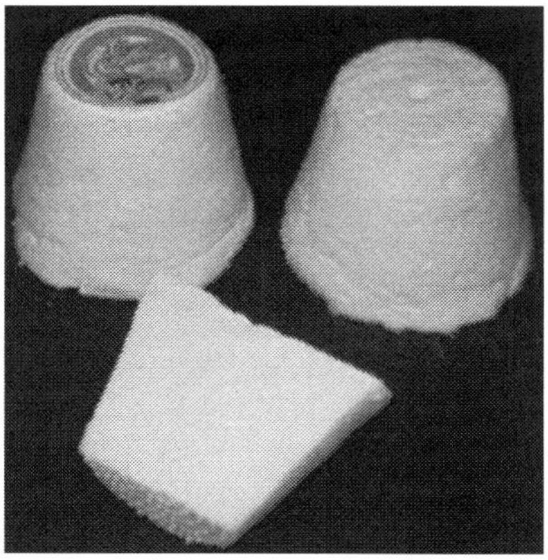

Figure 5.1 Aguega´l Pitu cheese, an acid-coagulated, Spanish traditional cheese.

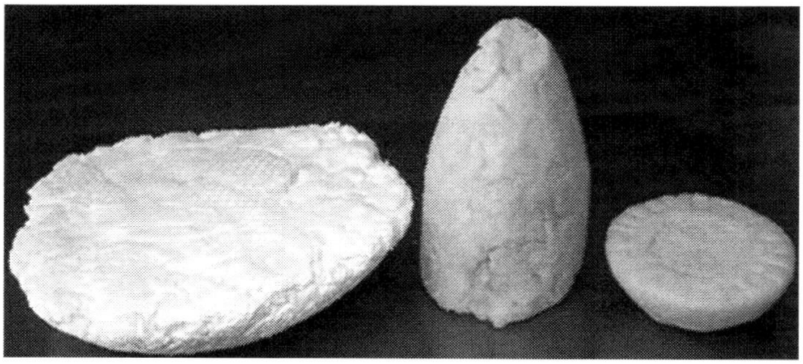

Figure 5.2 Different production stages of Casín cheese (*torta*, *gorollo*, and ripened cheese), a kneaded, crust-free, and lipolyzed cheese.

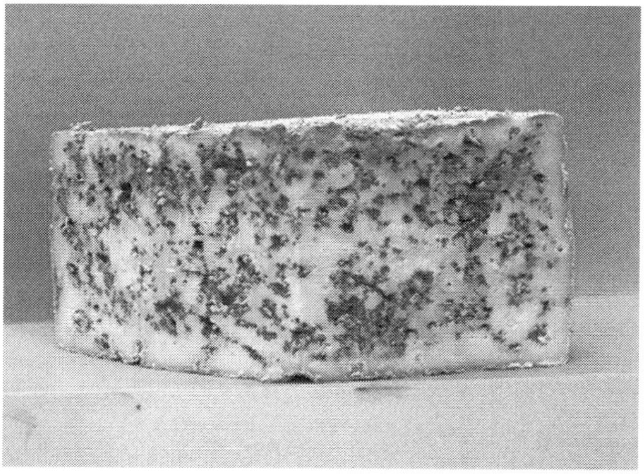

Figure 5.3 Cabrales, the star of the Spanish traditional, blue-veined cheeses. Ripening of this cheese takes place in natural caves where the *Penicillium roqueforti* develops.

infections have endowed LAB with a generally regarded as safe (GRAS) status. The growth of these bacteria in milk causes a rapid drop in pH (acidification) due to the production of lactic acid from the utilization of lactose (Mayo et al. 2010a). LAB development also plays a role in predigestion of other nutrients of milk, thus increasing their bioavailability. Furthermore, during growth in milk, LAB produce new metabolites that enhance the organoleptic and sensorial (taste and flavor) properties of fermented milk products (Smit et al. 2005, Smid and Kleerebezem 2014). The acidification further inhibits or kills many pathogenic and spoilage microorganisms, which assures the microbial stabilization of the fermented products as compared with milk. Beyond lactic acid production, inhibition of undesirable microorganisms is enhanced by some other bacterial metabolites (acetic acid, H_2O_2, diacetyl, bacteriocins) (Dalié et al. 2010), which further improve the stability and safety of fermented milk products.

Acidification also creates appropriate conditions for the subsequent chemical and biochemical pathways occurring during the ripening of fermented dairy foods (Smit et al. 2005). In modern industry, spontaneous fermentations have been replaced by the addition of well-characterized LAB strains (starters), which bring about fermentations in a more reliable way (Mills et al. 2010). Besides starters, other microorganisms (adjunct and/or maturing cultures) can be added to milk for the purpose of health, aspect and for the formation of flavor and taste compounds. More recently, probiotic, nonpathogenic microorganisms that have an influence on the consumer's health are often incorporated into traditional and/or new fermented milk products (Fontana et al. 2013). The binomial LAB-health was already reinforced in the early last century with Metchnikoff's postulates, which proposed a key role for the LAB species present in yogurt for the maintenance of intestinal microbial balance necessary for health (Metchnikoff 1907). Indeed, health benefits associated with the consumption of fermented dairy products are mostly mediated by the LAB species, which bring about the fermentation and are still alive in the final product or by the metabolites they produce during fermentation and/or ripening.

5.2.1 Dairy Products and Probiotics

Although nonviable bacteria and bacterial components (e.g., DNA) have also been reported to produce some beneficial effects (Jijon et al. 2004, Rachmilewitz et al. 2004), probiotics have been defined as "live microorganisms which, when administered in adequate amounts, confer a health benefit to the host" (FAO/WHO 2002). Recently, the FAO/WHO definition of probiotic has been reinforced as relevant and sufficient to accommodate current and anticipated future applications (Hill et al. 2014). Probiotic microorganisms are thought to contribute to health maintenance by enhancing beneficial metabolic (production of organic acids, vitamins), protective (inhibition or exclusion of harmful bacteria, antitoxin, and anticarcinogenic activity) and trophic activities (Guarner and Malagelada 2003).

Since the early twentieth century (Rettger et al. 1935), species of LAB and bifidobacteria, have been used in various "ready-to-use preparations" to restore the intestinal microbial balance when it is disturbed (fever, infections, antibiotic treatments, etc) (Guarner and Malagelada 2003). Although LAB and bifidobacteria remain as the common species, many microbial types are used at present as probiotics (Table 5.2). Fundamental knowledge relating to the mechanisms by which probiotics contribute to host health and well-being is still scarce. Such knowledge is essential to scientifically support their purported health benefits and their subsequent inclusion in functional foods (Klaenhammer and Kullen 1999). The probiotic definition not only embraces the microorganisms added to feed and foods for a health benefit (Table 5.2), but also food products, food supplements, and other presentations containing such microorganisms.

Table 5.2 Representative LAB Strains Used as Probiotics and Some of Their Claimed Health Effects

Species	*Strain*	*Commercial Product/s*	*Health Effect/s*
Bifidobacterium breve	UCC2003	–	Reduces symptoms of chronic IBD
Bifidobacterium animalis subsp. *lactis*	Bb12	Probiotic yogurt, dairy products	Alleviates allergy, reduces rotavirus infection, reduces travelers' diarrhea, improves oral vaccination
Enterococcus faecalis	Symbioflor 1	Food supplements	–
Enterococcus faecium	SF68	Food supplements	–
Lactobacillus acidophilus	La5	Probiotic yogurt, acidophilus milk, cheese	Reduces antibiotic-associated diarrhoea, improves intestinal microbial balance
Lactobacillus acidophilus	NCFO 1748	Food supplements	Reduces harmful enzymatic activities in faeces, prevents post-radiation diarrhoea, alleviates constipation
Lactobacillus delbrueckii subsp. *bulgaricus*	Many	Yogurt, cheese	Improves intestinal microbial balance; reduces antibiotic-associated diarrhoea, alleviates lactose intolerance
Lactobacillus casei	Shirota	Acidified milk	Shortens rotavirus diarrhoea, stimulates immune response, reduces recurrent bladder cancer
Lactobacillus johnsonii	La1	Probiotic yogurt, acidified milk	Improves response to oral vaccination, reduces colonization by *Helicobacter pylori*, alleviates inflammation
Lactobacillus plantarum	299v	Fruit beverages, fermented cereals, food supplements	Alleviates IBS syndrome, reduces LDL cholesterol levels
Lactobacillus reuteri	SD2112	Food supplements	Shortens rotavirus diarrhoea
Lactobacillus rhamnosus	GG	Probiotic yogurt, acidified milk, cheese	Shortens rotavirus diarrhoea, stimulates immune response, alleviates chronic inflammation of intestine, prevents and treat allergy

Table 5.2 (*Continued*) Representative LAB Strains Used as Probiotics and Some of Their Claimed Health Effects

Species	*Strain*	*Commercial Product/s*	*Health Effect/s*
Lactobacillus salivarius	UCC118	–	Reduces symptoms of chronic inflammatory diseases
Propionibacterium freudenreichii	JS	Food supplements	–
Streptococcus thermophilus	Many	Yogurt, cheese	Improves intestinal microbial balance, reduces antibiotic-associated diarrhoea, alleviates lactose intolerance

Source: Compiled from Ouwehand, A. C., S. Salminen, and E. Isolauri. 2002. *Antonie van Leeuwenhoek* 82: 279–289; de Vrese, M. and J. Schrezenmeir. 2008. *Advances in Biochemistry, Engineering and Biotechnology* 111: 1–66; Kiwaki, M. and K. Nomoto. *Handbook of Probiotics and Prebiotics*, 2nd edn., Hoboken. pp. 449–457. 2009. Copyright Wiley-VCH Verlag GmbH & Co. KGaA. Reproduced with permission.

Dairy products continued to be the principal vehicles for the administration and consumption of probiotics (Stanton et al. 2005).

5.3 Traditional and New Dairy Products

The diversity of fermented dairy products is large as it is influenced by the use of milk from different animal species and a variety of mixtures. Technologies of manufacturing and ripening have multiplied the panoply of fermented dairy products (Table 5.1). Manufacturing technologies affect the physical, chemical, and thus the sensory properties of the products. In addition, milk origin and dairy technologies pose a strong selection pressure on the microorganisms than can survive technological processes and develop in each fermentation. Addition of sugar, fruits, condiments, grains, herbs, and the application of preservation methods, such as concentration, drying, or freezing, can further enlarge the number of varieties.

5.3.1 Natural Fermented Milk

The origin of natural fermented milk (NFM) can be assumed to have started soon after the first human populations settled themselves some 15,000 years ago around the Middle East (Mayo et al. 2010b). From those ancient times up to now, production of NFM spread through the entire world, using in each region the available type of milk. Evidence of such products can still be found in large areas of Africa, Middle East, Asia, and even in Europe (Figure 5.4). Products such as *ergo* from Ethiopia, *rayeb, lben, laban, kad, zabady, zeer* from Morocco and Northern African and Middle East countries, *roub* from Sudan, *amasi* (*hodzeko, mukaka wakakora*) from Zimbabwe, *filmjölk* and *långfil* from Sweden, *chhurpi, mohi, shoyu, philu, somar* from the Himalayas, and many others (Mayo et al. 2010b, Tamang et al. 2012).

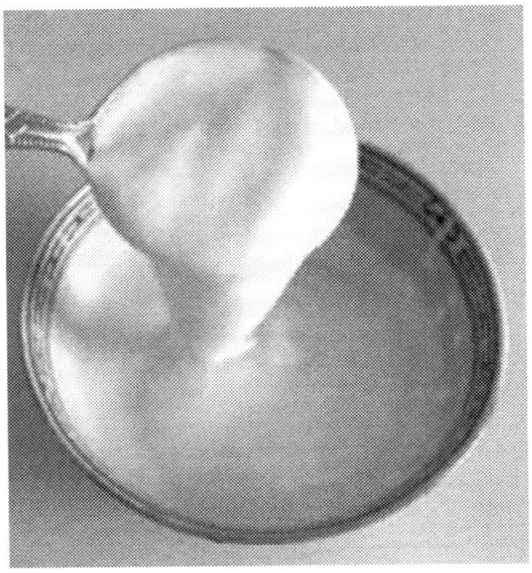

Figure 5.4 Texture appearance of a, yogurt-like, naturally fermented milk (NFM).

A common feature of NFM is the development of mesophilic LAB species, which are responsible for lowering of the pH and for the production of the most typical flavor and aroma compounds (Smid and Kleerebezem 2014). Two basically different NFM subclasses can be distinguished, inoculated and noninoculated NFM. The latter type is made by leaving plain milk at room temperature until enough acidity is formed and the coagulum appears. Depending on the preferences, it can be stored for days or weeks, during which stronger flavors develop. In contrast, traditional inoculated NFM are usually manufactured by backslopping (inoculation with a portion of previous batch) techniques (Robinson and Tamime 2006).

NFM is also the basis for more processed commodities, such as butter and its byproduct buttermilk, cottage cheese, cheeses, and whey, as the manufacturing process of all these products starts by an initial acidification of milk. Some of these products are partially dried (*leben zeer, than*), preserved in oil (*labneh anbaris, shanklish*), added with spices (*shanklish, mish*), mixed with wheat products (*kishk*), and so on. Butter is made by churning fat-enriched milk or cream, in a process that separates the fat fraction of the milk from the whey.

5.3.2 Yogurt

Yogurt is defined by the Codex Alimentarius of 1992 as a coagulated milk product that results from lactic fermentation of milk by *Lactobacillus delbrueckii* subsp. *bulgaricus* and *Streptococcus thermophilus* (FAO/WHO 2003). Production and consumption of yogurt was confined to communities in Eastern Europe, the Balkans, Middle East, and India until recently (Kosikowski and Mistry 1997). However, a general perception of the beneficial health effects associated with its consumption increased production in the developed world since 1960. Today, yogurt is the major commercial fermented milk around the world. Among the factors contributing to the great success of this fermented milk, image of a natural product, attractive organoleptic characteristics (fresh, acidulated taste, and pleasant flavor), nutritional value, prophylactic and therapeutic properties, and moderate cost (due to the high productivity of the production lines) can all be mentioned (Tamime and Robinson 2007). Yogurt can be produced from the milk of cow, buffalo, goat, sheep, yak, and other mammals; although cow's milk is predominant. Varieties of yogurt available include plain (set), fruit-flavored, whipped, drinking type (stirred), smoked, dried, strained, and frozen (Tamime and Robinson 2007).

In some countries the term yogurt is restrained to the fermented milk made by using exclusively these two bacterial types, while in others incorporation of probiotic cultures is also allowed. In this last case, *Lactobacillus acidophilus, Bifidobacterium* spp., *Lactobacillus casei, Lactobacillus rhamnosus, Lactobacillus gasseri*, and *Lactobacillus johnsonii* are among the commonest adjunct cultures (Guarner et al. 2005).

5.3.2.1 Yogurt-Related Traditional Products

Fermented milk products manufactured by thermophilic bacteria include not only yogurt but also other fermented milks, such as Bulgarian buttermilk, *zabady*, and *dahi* (Kosikowski and Mistry 1997, Robinson and Tamime 2006, Shiby and Mishra 2013). Bulgarian buttermilk is a type of cultured buttermilk fermented with *Lb. bulgaricus*. Yogurt made domestically in Egypt is called *zabady* (El-Baradei et al. 2008). *Dahi* or *Indian yogurt* is a lesser known ethnic fermented milk product consumed in India and neighboring countries (Tamang 2010). It is made from yak's or cow's milk by essentially the same technology as *zabady*.

5.3.3 Kefir, Koumiss, and Related Products

Fermented milk products that are manufactured using starter cultures containing yeasts include *acidophilus-yeast milk, kefir, koumiss*, and *viili* (Kosikowski and Mistry 1997, de Ramesh et al. 2006). Of these, *kefir* is the most popular. It originates in the Balkan region; though nowadays is widely produced throughout the world. *Kefir* is a viscous, acidic, and mildly alcoholic milk beverage produced by fermentation of milk with a kefir grain as the starter culture (FAO/WHO 2003). The kefir grain is an inert polysaccharide matrix in which a relatively stable and specific microbial community composed of different LAB, acetic acid bacteria, and yeast species coexists in a complex symbiotic relationship (Farnworth 2005). After the fermentation, the grain is recovered and can be reused to inoculate a new fermentation, in a way similar to the backslopping practice. This product is manufactured under a variety of names in different geographical areas of the Balkan-Caucasian region, including *kephir, kiaphur, kefer, knapon, kepi*, and *kippi*.

Koumiss is a natural fermented dairy product from the Caucasian area. It is also produced under other names such as *kumis, kumys*, or *kymys*. Furthermore, similar products are produced in Central Asia (Mongolia and China), where they are called *chigee* and *airag* (Kosikowski and Mistry 1997, Tamang 2010). *Koumiss* is defined by the use in its production of mare's milk, which contains less casein and fatty matter than cow's milk. *Koumiss* presents a dispersed coagulum giving the product a smoother taste as compared with kefir. The traditional manufacture of *koumiss* involves storing of mare's milk in animal skin bags, where a natural or induced (inoculated) acidification process takes place. Dry *koumiss* is usually kept from season to season and the distinctive starters are transferred from one generation to another within the families for backslopping. In the modern production of *koumiss*, cow's milk tends to replace mare's milk as the starting material, for which cow's milk has to be adapted by dilution for mimicking mare's milk (Kücükcetin et al. 2003).

5.3.4 Viili

Viili is a traditional Finnish fermented milk product originally made in the summertime as a way to preserve an excess of milk. It is also known as *viilia*; and similar and related products are *piima, pitkapiima,* and *viilipiima* from Finland; *långfil* and *tatmjolk* from Sweden; *taette* from Norway, *ymer* from Denmark, and *skyr* from Iceland (Tamime 2002). Most of these products share a thick and sticky consistency, with some degree of stretchiness plus a subtle sweet taste.

Viili is produced by fermenting milk with special strains of *Lactococcus lactis* subsp. *lactis* and *Lc. lactis* subsp. *cremoris* producing extracellular polysaccharides (EPS) (Macura and Townsley 1984). Typical of *viili* is the presence of the fungus *Geotrichum candidum* that develops on the product surface forming a velvety layer similar to that in Camembert and Brie cheeses. *G. candidum* consumes lactate, lowering the acidity of the product, and produces the characteristic moldy aroma of *viili* (Kahala et al. 2008). The EPS act as food stabilizers, preventing syneresis and graininess, and provide the product with a natural ropiness (Macura and Townsley 1984). Beyond their rheological role, EPS have recently been claimed to promote the development of beneficial populations in the gut after consumption (Ruas-Madiedo et al. 2006).

5.3.5 Probiotic Fermented Milks

5.3.5.1 Acidophilus Milk

Acidophilus milk was one of the first probiotic milks derived from Metchnikoff's observations. It is produced by a *Lb. acidophilus* strain isolated from the feces of a breast-feeding infant. *Lb. acidophilus* strains are considered to fulfill most of the basic criteria of probiotics: survive gastrointestinal transit, bile and acid tolerance, and antimicrobial production. In the past, the *acidophilus milk* was marketed by fermenting sterilized milk with *Lb. acidophilus* strains (Kosikowski and Mistry 1997). Today, nonfermented (sweet) *acidophilus milk* is preferred. Manufacturing of *sweet acidophilus milk* involves incorporation of a concentrate culture of *Lb. acidophilus* into sterilized low-fat milk (de Ramesh et al. 2006). Furthermore, addition of probiotic microorganisms, for example, bifidobacteria, is a common practice.

5.3.5.2 Acidophilus-Yeast Milk

Acidophilus-yeast milk is made by joining *Lb. acidophilus* with a special type of *Saccharomyces cerevisiae, Saccharomyces boulardii* (Czerucka et al. 2007). This tropical yeast was first isolated from lychees and mangosteensin in 1923 by Henri Boulard. *Sacch. boulardii* has been shown to be nonpathogenic, nonsystemic (remaining in the gastrointestinal tract rather than spreading elsewhere in the body), and to grow well at the unusually high temperature of 37°C (Kotowska et al. 2005).

5.3.5.3 Yakult

Yakult is a Japanese probiotic milk product made by fermenting a mixture of skimmed milk with a special strain (Shirota) of the bacterium *Lb. casei*. The claimed benefits of yakult are supported by an array of scientific studies (reviewed recently by Kiwaki and Nomoto 2009), ranging from maintenance of gut flora, modulation of the immune system, regulation of bowel habits, and alleviation of constipation. It also seems to be effective in curing various gastrointestinal infections.

5.3.5.4 Other Commercial Fermented Milks

More recently, a large array of probiotic fermented milks are sold in the market. These include some of the most successful probiotic strains (Table 5.2), such as *Lb. casei* DN114001 (*Actimel*®, Danone), *Lb. johnsonii* La1 (*LC1*®, Nestlé), *Lb. rhamnosus* ®GG (*LGG*®, Valio), *Lb. plantarum* 299v (*ProViva*®, Skåne Dairy), and *Bifidobacterium animalis* subsp. *lactis* Bb12 (Chr. Hansen, bifidobacterium-containing yogurt).

5.3.6 Cheese

In terms of production and global consumption, cheese is the most important milk-derived product. It is estimated that world production of cheese is around 20 million tons per year (FIL-IDF 2012). Cheese is the generic name of a group of fermented-milk-based food products produced worldwide in a great variety and diversity of forms, textures, and flavors (Figures 5.1 through 5.3 and 5.5). This is a reflection of the great variety of technologies practiced that include the type of milk (cow's, sheep's, goats', buffalo's), the mode of coagulation (acidic, enzymatic), the type of the coagulant (rennet, vegetable, microbial), and the manufacturing and ripening conditions (Kosikowski and Mistry 1997, Law 1999).

Acid-induced milk gels are very stable if left undisturbed, but if they are accidentally or intentionally broken, curd and whey separates. Removing of whey gives rise to a product that can be consumed fresh or stored for long periods if properly salted and/or dehydrated. Today, acid-coagulated cheeses (*Cottage cheese, Cream cheese, Quarg, Fromage frais, Queso blanco*) may still represent 25% of the total cheese production, and in some countries are the principal varieties (Kosikowski and Mistry 1997). Enzymatic milk gels are more stable than those obtained by acidification. These are formed by treatment of cheese milk with proteolytic enzymes disturbing the equilibrium of casein micelles primarily by digestion of the κ-casein component. Enzymatic curds can be heavily processed by cutting, stirring, washing, heating, pressing, and so on to various extents giving rise to a huge diversity of cheese families (Fox et al. 2000). Mixed acid and enzymatic coagulations are rather common, thus enlarging the cheese type within each family. On the basis of the principal ripening agent and/or

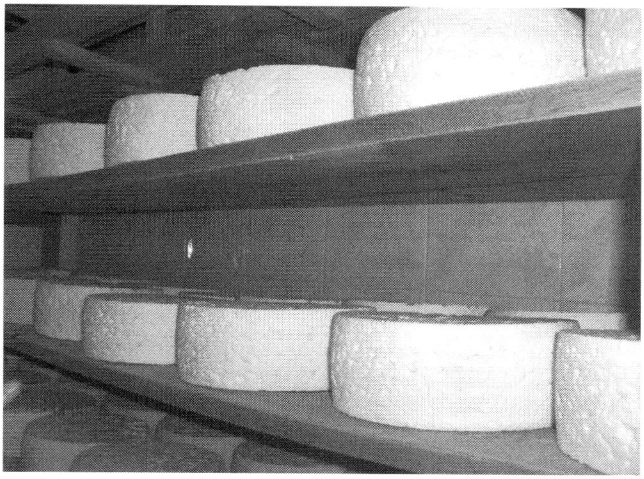

Figure 5.5 Cheese shelves of Cabrales cheese.

their characteristic technology, cheeses can be classified into three different super families: internal bacterially ripened, mold-ripened, and surface-ripened (Law 1999, Fox et al. 2000). Internal bacterially ripened include cheese groups of very hard (*Grana Padano, Parmesan*), hard (*Cheddar, Ras*), semihard (*Caerphilly, Mahón*), cheeses with eyes (such as the Swiss-types, *Emmental* and *Gruyère*, and Dutch-types, *Edam* and *Gouda*), heavily salted cheeses (*Feta, Domiati*), and "pasta filata" varieties (*Mozzarella, Provolone*). Mold-ripened (*Penicillium* spp.) varieties would include those with mold in the surface (*Brie, Camembert*) and those with internal molds (*Roquefort, Gorgonzola, Stilton, Danablue, Cabrales*) (Figure 5.3). The surface-ripened cheese super-family groups a large number of varieties, including *Limburger, Munster, Taleggio,* and *Tilsit*, among others.

As in other dairy products, particular manufacturing and ripening conditions are thought to select for the typical microbial groups present in cheese milk (Beresford et al. 2001, Wouters et al. 2002), which develop within the cheese matrix and generate or influence the final sensory properties of the mature cheese. These microorganisms include not only LAB species (all cheese types), but also bacteria from some other groups such as propionibacteria (*Emmental, Gruyère*), brevibacteria, and corynebacteria (surface-ripened cheeses), and so on. Beyond bacteria, variable numbers of yeasts are also present in most cheese varieties (Wouters et al. 2002).

5.3.6.1 Probiotic Cheese

Cheese is one of the most versatile food products, which offers many marketing opportunities for using it as a probiotic carrier. Though LAB strains from traditional cheeses may have functional properties of probiosis similar or higher than those from intestinal sources (Wu et al. 2009, Sabir et al. 2010, Meira et al. 2012, Papanikolaou et al. 2012), the supplementation of cheese with recognized probiotic bacteria would increase further the added value of these products (Gomes da Cruz et al. 2008). Within the cheese matrix, entrapped bacteria are protected by protein and fat constituents during storage and gastric transit (protection against gastric juice, bile salts, and digestive enzymes), which would increase delivery of viable probiotics to the gastrointestinal tract (GIT) (de Vrese and Schrezenmeir 2008). In addition, probiotic bacteria and particularly acid-susceptible bifidobacteria may result in a better protection from acid due to the cheese buffering capacity. However, added probiotic bacteria may antagonize starter cultures or have a direct effect on composition, texture, and/or sensory properties of the cheeses (Stanton et al. 1998, de Vrese and Schrezenmeir 2008). Therefore, a careful selection of the functional strain/s to be included in each cheese type would be required.

5.4 Health Benefits of Fermented Dairy Products

5.4.1 Nutritional Value of Dairy Products as Compared with Milk

The nutrient composition of fermented dairy products derives from the nutrient composition of milk. Milk itself is a source of important functional components, such as calcium, phosphorous, vitamins, lactoferrin, and so on (Jenkins and McGuire 2006). Species, breed, feed, stage of lactation, age, and environmental factors all affect the nutritional composition of milk. Variables such as temperature and storage conditions, type and duration of treatments (homogenization, pasteurization, temperature and length of fermentation and ripening) during processing do also affect the nutritional value of the milk and its functional components. The final nutritional composition of fermented foods is also affected by the microbial types involved in fermentation and ripening (Beermann and Hartung 2013). Fermented products are a source of the beneficial bacteria involved in manufacturing, as well as a source of functional metabolites produced during growth (organic acids, folic acid, bioactive peptides), which further increase the health value of fermented dairy products (Table 5.3).

5.4.1.1 Vitamins-B

LAB species require several vitamins but some cultures are capable of synthesizing B vitamins such as folates (B-9, B-11) and B-12 (LeBlanc et al. 2011). Judicious selection of both primary and secondary lactic cultures and fermentation conditions has been shown to increase vitamin concentrations in fermented foods (Wouters et al. 2002, Leblanc et al. 2011).

5.4.1.2 Lactose

A large part of the world's population shows low levels of the enzyme β-galactosidase (lactase) in the mucosa of the small intestine (de Vrese et al. 2001). These individuals suffer intolerance symptoms when lactose-containing milk is present in their diet. There is good scientific evidence for the alleviation of lactose intolerance symptoms by the consumption of yogurt containing live *Streptococcus thermophilus* and *Lb. bulgaricus* (Pelletier et al. 2001) and other dairy products such as *kefir* (Hertzler and Clancy 2003). During fermentation, the bacterial β-galactosidase activities increase the enzymatic conversion of lactose to its absorbable monosaccharide components, glucose, and galactose. However, other factors seem to play a role, as the same total amount of lactose is better tolerated in yogurt than in milk by lactose maldigesters (Labayen et al. 2001).

5.4.1.3 Protein

Milk proteins from fermented dairy products are thought to be more easily digested than those of milk. In addition to protein degradation by the coagulant agent, bacterial predigestion of milk proteins and rennet-derived peptides may also occur. In fact, the activity of LAB proteases and peptidases is preserved throughout the shelf life of the fermented products. Consequently, content of peptides and free amino acids increases as ripening and storage progress (Ash and Wilbey 2010). However, the proteolytic system components of different LAB species and strains do not have the same activity, which contributes to a large variation in the type and levels of peptides and free amino acids in different dairy products (Liu et al. 2010). A major part of the aroma and taste components of most dairy products come from the catabolism of amino acids (Smit et al. 2005, Smid and Kleerebezem 2014).

In addition to a role in nutrition, proteins may have further health benefits due to the release by proteolysis of encrypted bioactive peptides (López-Expósito et al. 2012). According to their physiological activity, bioactive peptides can exert antihypertensive, antimicrobial, antioxidant, anticarcinogenic properties (López-Expósito et al. 2012). Milk proteins are considered the most important source of bioactive peptides and an increasing number of bioactive peptides have been identified in milk protein hydrolysates and fermented dairy products (Gómez-Ruiz et al. 2004, Madureira et al. 2010).

5.4.1.4 Lipids

Lipids contribute little to the attribute of most dairy products (Smit et al. 2005). Except in mold-ripened cheeses, minor amounts of fatty acids (FA) are released as a result of lipase activity

Table 5.3 Bioactive Chemical Components from Milk and Fermented Dairy Products and Their Health-Related Functionality

Bioactive Component	*Function or Process Affected*
Minerals	
Calcium	Bone health, heart health
Phosphorous	
Vitamins	
Vitamin A	Metabolism, growth promoter, bone health vision, reduced risk of colon cancer
Vitamin D	
Vitamin B	
Proteins	
Whey proteins	Weight management, immune system enhancer, antimicrobial, binding toxic substances
Lactoperoxidase	
Lactoferrin	
Immunoglobulins	
Peptides and Amino Acids	
Glycomacropeptides	Antiproliferative, immunomodulation, muscle tone, dental health, hypertension, cognition, mood, stress
Bioactive peptides	
Gamma-aminobutyric acid	
Lipids and Fatty Acids	
Conjugated linoleic acid (CLA)	Anti-inflammatory, lipid-lowering, heart disease prevention, inhibit atherosclerosis, cognition, mood, stress, inhibition of cancer, cell growth
Phospholipids	
Milk fat globule membrane	
α-Linoleic acid	
Mono- and polyunsaturated acids	
Sphingolipids	
Carbohydrates	
Lactose	Anticariogenic, digestive health, bifidogenic
Lactulose Lactic acid	
Galacto-oligosaccharides (GOS)	

Table 5.3 (*Continued*) Bioactive Chemical Components from Milk and Fermented Dairy Products and Their Health-Related Functionality

Bioactive Component	*Function or Process Affected*
Acids	
Lactic acid	Antimicrobial, gut health
Acetic acid	
Propionic acid	

Source: Compiled from Korhonen, H. J. 2009. *Bioactive Components in Milk and Dairy Products*, Oxford: Wiley-Blackwell, 15–38; Wijesinha-Bettoni, R. and B. Burlingame. 2013. *Milk and Dairy Products in Human Nutrition*, Roma: Food and Agriculture Organization, 41–102.

(Collins et al. 2003). FA in milk fat is primarily saturated (SFA) (63.7%) and monounsaturated (MUFA) (29.1%), with minor amounts of polyunsaturates (PUFA) (4.1%). Although not all FA have the same biological effects, high intake of saturated fat is generally perceived to be unhealthy, largely because it elevates blood total and low-density lipoprotein (LDL) cholesterol levels, which are risk factors for cardiovascular diseases (German and Dillard 2006). Epidemiological data suggest that MUFA (oleic acid-18:1c9) and PUFA (linoleic-18:2-omega-6 and alpha-linolenic-18:3-omega-3 acids) are favorable for health (Gebauer et al. 2011). Vaccenic acid (VA) and the naturally occurring isomer of conjugated linoleic acid (CLA), cis-9, trans-11 (c9, t11-CLA) are dietary trans fatty acids formed by biohydrogenation of vegetable oils in ruminants, which have been associated with health (Bhardwaj et al. 2011, Gebauer et al. 2011). Different LAB strains have been reported to produce CLA (Alonso et al. 2003, Macouzet et al. 2009). Such strains can be utilized to enhance CLA content in dairy products. Traditional cheeses (Schirone et al. 2011) and yogurt (Serafeimidou et al. 2012) have also been reported to contain variable levels of c9, t11-CLA. *In-vitro* studies and experimental models suggest that VA and CLA may beneficially affect risk of cardiovascular diseases and cancer (Beppu et al. 2006, Coakley et al. 2006). However, current clinical studies, which have been conducted with insufficient statistical power, produced inconclusive results. Therefore, further research is needed to determine the effects of these compounds in humans, as current clinical data do not consistently support the findings from experimental studies.

The consumption of milk fat globule membrane (MFGM) alone as a nutraceutical or as a dietary food supplement, or the consumption of food products enforced by MFGM is thought to be beneficial due to the presence of biologically active phospholipids, such as sphingomyelin, phosphatidylcholine, and phosphatidylethanolamine (Alonso et al. 2009). Phospholipids are currently considered to influence numerous cell functions including growth and development, molecular transport, absorption, and stress response. These processes might modulate myelination in the central nervous system affecting memory and development of Alzheimer's disease (Horrocks and Farooqui 2004).

5.4.2 Prevention and Treatment of Gut Disorders

A large list of pathologies and intestinal disorders have been related to an unbalanced gut microbiota (Guarner and Malagelada 2003). Dairy products, particularly yogurt, and probiotic strains belonging to different LAB species have been shown to prevent and/or alleviate a variety of gastrointestinal diseases and dysfunctions (Ouwehand et al. 2002, Ceapa et al. 2013). In some cases, restoration of the microbial balance by the use of probiotics has a clear beneficial health effect in the treatment and/or prevention of such diseases.

5.4.2.1 Travelers' Diarrhea

Travelers' diarrhea continues to be a significant health problem among tourists visiting developing countries. The two most common etiologic agents of the disease are enterotoxigenic and enteroaggregative *Escherichia coli*. Less frequently, other invasive enteropathogens such as *Shigella*, *Campylobacter jejuni*, *Salmonella* spp., and invasive *E. coli* may cause watery diarrhea and dysentery. The gut-associated lymphoid tissue (GALT) plays a key role as a first line of defense against ingested pathogens. The secretory immunoglobulin A (sIgA) is the main effector of the mucosal adaptive immune system. IgA concentration in the gut has been shown to be modulated by LAB species (Puri et al. 1996). Consequently, many studies have been conducted on the value of probiotic LAB preparations for reducing the risk of travelers' diarrhea. However, inconsistent results have frequently been reported with unexplained geographic differences in protection rates (Koo and DuPont 2006). The use of diverse probiotic strains, administration vehicles, and dosage schedules may contribute to the heterogeneity of the results, together with a different etiological agent (McFarland 2007).

5.4.2.2 Viral Diarrhea

Rotaviruses are responsible for about one-third of the cases of severe diarrhea in children in both developed and developing countries (Parashar et al. 2006). Rotaviruses invade the mature enterocytes of the villi in the jejunum and ileum, where they replicate causing partial disruption of the intestinal mucosa and impairing sodium and chloride transport. Yogurt feeding in children with acute watery diarrhea decreased stool frequency and shortened the duration of diarrheal episodes (Boudraa et al. 2001). Recent meta-analysis of randomized, controlled studies found that yogurt seems to prevent and treat successfully acute viral diarrhea in children (van Neil et al. 2002). Probiotic strains may have a beneficial effect via a different mechanism, avoiding the absorption of the virus by improving the barrier effect of mucus, glycocalyx, and intercellular junctions. Furthermore, probiotics can hinder virus-induced pathology by stimulating innate and/or adaptive immunity, such as increase in the number of IgA-secreting cells (Colbère-Garapin et al. 2007).

5.4.2.3 Antibiotic-Associated Diarrhea by Clostridium difficile

Antimicrobial therapy disturbs the endogenous gut microbiota, frequently resulting in diarrhea. In the majority of cases, diarrhea is due to the overgrowth of *C. difficile*, a Gram-positive, spore-forming anaerobe, present in low numbers in the intestine (Thompson 2008). Many clinical studies have investigated the efficacy of probiotics in the protection and relapse of *C. difficile* diarrhea. However, probiotics cannot be considered as a group, instead studies should focus on specific strains. By using this approach, several works and meta-analysis studies have proved that both *Lb. rhamnosus* GG and other probiotic strains are effective in the treatment of acute diarrhea (McFarland 2006; Szajewska et al. 2007).

5.4.2.4 Infections by Helicobacter pylori

Helicobacter pylori is an infectious agent, spread worldwide and causing gastritis, peptic ulcers, and gastric cancer. It colonizes and occasionally invades the epithelial cells of the stomach. *In-vitro* studies have demonstrated the ability of various *Lactobacillus* strains to attenuate growth and inhibit the adhesion of *H. pylori* to the gastric mucosa (Coconnier et al. 1998). Animal and human studies have also shown the ability of probiotic lactobacilli to significantly decrease gastritis activity and *H. pylori* density (Wang et al. 2004). It has also been shown that pretreatment with *Lactobacillus*- and *Bifidobacterium*-containing yogurt can improve the efficacy of the triple and quadruple antimicrobial therapy in the eradication of residual *H. pylori* (Wang et al. 2004). Probiotics may further have a significant role in the settings of *H. pylori* therapy by preventing the side effects associated with antibiotic treatment (Cremonini et al. 2002).

5.4.2.5 Constipation

Constipation is a disorder of the motor activity of the large bowel and its main symptom is straining on defecation. Constipation is associated with striking changes in the fecal microbiota, intestinal permeability, and systemic immune response (Khalif et al. 2005). Low levels of *Bifidobacterium* and *Lactobacillus* populations have frequently been found in constipated patients (Khalif et al. 2005). Therefore, the use of LAB-containing fermented products is a first approach of treatment, which has a long history of success (Salminen et al. 1998).

5.4.2.6 Inflammatory Bowel Diseases (IBD)

IBD includes Crohn's disease, ulcerative colitis (UC), and pouchitis, which are characterized by deregulation of the immune system leading to inflammation of the GIT. The interaction of LAB with the mucosal epithelial cells and the cells of GALT has been suggested as the most important mechanism by which these bacteria enhance a proper gut immune function. Thus, benefits of dairy products containing live bacteria may account by their immunomodulation capacity (Granier et al. 2013). Indeed, yogurt consumption has seemed to enhance the immune response in immunocompromised populations such as the elderly (Meydani and Ha 2000). Several reports also indicate that consumption of yogurt or intake of some LAB strains modulates the production of cytokines, which are primarily immune system effectors (Solis-Pereyra et al. 1997, Borruel et al. 2002).

5.4.2.7 Irritable Bowel Syndrome (IBS)

Ten to fifteen percent of the western population suffers, to a varying degree, from IBS in the lower GIT. IBS is characterized by abdominal discomfort or pain and an altered bowel function. Inflammation and immune dysfunction are thought to play an important role in IBS (Chadwick et al. 2002). Though studies differed in the definition of IBS, probiotic strains used, trial design, and primary and secondary outcomes scored, promising results have been reported regarding the relief of IBS symptoms by the use of specific probiotics (O'Mahony et al. 2005).

5.4.3 Allergy

It is estimated that 20% of the population in industrialized areas suffers from some form of allergy (atopic eczema, allergic rhinitis, and asthma). The current aims of intervention are to avert deviant microbiota development, strengthen the GIT barrier function, and alleviate abnormal immune responsiveness (Isolauri et al. 2008). During maturation of the immune system, probiotics may provide alternative microbial stimulation (Isolauri et al. 2000). Feeding *Lb. rhamnosus* GG to 159 pregnant women with a family history of atopic disease and their newborn infants during the first months of life, Kalliomäki et al. (2001) showed a significant reduction in the prevalence of atopic dermatitis in infants. The protective effect was also seen in a four-year follow-up study (Kalliomäki et al. 2003). This strongly suggests that LGG seems to be effective not only for treatment but also for prevention of allergies. These data are in good agreement with the results of a very recent meta-analysis (Lee et al. 2008), indicating prevention of atopic dermatitis by probiotics.

Cow's milk protein allergy (CMPA) is an immunological reaction to one or more milk proteins affecting 2%–7.5% of children (Solinas et al. 2010). Persistence of the condition into adulthood is low as tolerance is developed within 2–4 years of age. Preliminary digestion of caseins during maturation or storage of dairy products has been shown to facilitate loss of allergenic reactivity during gut digestion, thus increasing tolerance (Alessandri et al. 2012).

5.4.4 Cancer

Owing to the difficulty of carrying out such studies in humans, evidence for the potential use of fermented dairy products in cancer treatment and prevention comes currently from *in-vitro* and animal studies. On the basis of a systematic review of epidemiological studies, the World Cancer Research Fund and American Institute for Cancer Research report concluded that there is a probable association between milk intake and lower risk of colorectal cancer, a probable association between diets high in calcium and increased risk of prostate cancer, and limited evidence of an association between milk intake and lower risk of bladder cancer (Lampe 2011). The mechanisms by which fermented dairy products and probiotics may inhibit the development and/or proliferation of cancer are not yet fully understood. However, there is evidence of a decrease in intestinal inflammation, enhanced immune function, suppression of intestinal bacteria involved in pro-carcinogenic and mutagenic pathways, binding of potential food carcinogens, and production of antitumorigenic substances (Rachid et al. 2002, Geier et al. 2006). Furthermore, the antitumor activity of dairy products might be due to their antioxidative properties (Güven et al. 2003). Related to these functions, the ability of LAB bacteria to bind toxins (mycotoxins, cyanobacterial toxins, heavy metals) from foods, water, and diet (El-Nezami et al. 2002, Halttunen et al. 2007) may prove a further way of cancer prevention.

In addition to bacteria, fungal metabolites may also be involved in the progression of cancer and/or in the efficacy of anticancer treatments. In this respect, andrastin A, a secondary metabolite produced by *Penicillium roqueforti* in blue cheese (Figure 5.3) under ripening condition (Nielsen et al. 2005, Fernández-Bodega et al. 2009), has been shown to inhibit the efflux of anticancer drugs in multidrug-resistant cancer cells.

5.4.5 Prevention of Dental Caries and Oral Health

Milk has been shown to be minimally cariogenic in animal studies and "tooth friendly" in animal trials (Schachtele and Jensen 1984). Among fermented dairy products, cheese is known as a cariostatic food due to its ability in stimulating salivary flow, increasing rate of sugar clearance, inhibition of plaque bacteria, delivery of high amounts of calcium and inorganic phosphate to plaque, and increasing the pH (Kashket and DePaola 2002). Most of these effects have been shown to be mediated by micellar casein (Guggenheim et al. 1999). However, inhibition of cariogenic-proactive microorganisms, such as *Streptococcus mutans* and *Candida* species has also been shown to be protective. A combination of *Lactobacillus rhamnosus* GG and bifidobacteria using cheese as a vehicle resulted in a reduction in dental caries, which correlated with reduced counts of *S. mutans* and yeasts in saliva (Ahola et al. 2002). Reduced prevalence of oral *Candida* and prevention of hyposalivation in the elderly have been proposed as the major effect of probiotic cheese with *Lb. rhamnosus* GG (Hatakka et al. 2007).

5.5 Future Prospects in Functional Dairy Products

Although health-related properties of traditional and new fermented products should be scientifically demonstrated, attempts to increase the functionality of dairy products are necessary to maintain or enhance their beneficial status. Some of these are briefly discussed in the following paragraphs.

5.5.1 Reduction in Lactose and Fat and Intervention on the Fatty Acid Profile

Milk and dairy products contain animal fat composed mainly of triglycerides (>95%), of which mostly are SFA (63.7%). High intake of saturated fat has been shown to lead to weight gain and obesity, and contribute to the development of heart diseases (Micha and Mozaffarian 2010). Association between consumption of milk and milk products has been further associated with high total serum cholesterol levels (Astrup et al. 2011). Thus, reduction in the SFA and cholesterol contents should produce healthier dairy products. In fact, yogurt with a reduced fat content is currently the rule and not the exception (Adolfsson et al. 2004). More difficulties have been encountered in reducing fat content in cheese. Reduced cheddar cheese resulted in a completely different ripening biochemistry, which lead to an imbalance of many flavor-contributing compounds (Drake et al. 2010). Sixty-five to ninety-five percent reduction of cholesterol has recently been achieved in nonhomogenized milk by beta-cyclodextrin (Alonso et al. 2009). Reduced-cholesterol cheese has been reported to produce much higher levels of bitter amino acids than the control cheese (Kwak et al. 2002). Further, as shown by sensory analysis, the texture score of cholesterol-reduced cheese decreased dramatically with ripening time. Supplementing ruminant animal diets with fat of different origins has been investigated as a means to alter fatty acid composition of food products, including milk and milk-derived products (Hess et al. 2008). Enhancing the CLA content of milk through nutritional manipulation is one of the most pursued effects (Jenkins and McGuire 2006, Fontecha et al. 2011).

5.5.2 Dairy Products Containing Probiotics, Prebiotics, or Both (Synbiotics)

Fermented dairy products are currently the principal vehicle of bacterial probiotics (Ouwehand et al. 2002, Stanton et al. 2005). Probiotic strains may also be incorporated into traditional dairy products, including cheese (Gomes da Cruz et al. 2008; Table 5.2). Survival at low pH, however, is a property limiting the application of many commercial probiotic strains into fermented products. New probiotic strains more resistant to acidity are being fostered among isolates from traditional dairy products (Gueimonde and Salminen 2006). In addition to better survival, these new strains can grow into the dairy products during manufacturing and ripening, while maintaining good technological properties (Wu et al. 2009, Sabir et al. 2010, Papanikolaou et al. 2012).

The addition of prebiotics, nonassimilable food components that can be utilized by the endogenous beneficial populations, could increase the actual levels of such bacteria and their activities in the GIT (de Vrese and Schrezenmeir 2008), thus enhancing the production of active metabolites. After consumption, prebiotics can additionally favor the development of probiotic strains (Oliveira et al. 2009). Combination of both probiotics and prebiotics in a single product (synbiotic) may be better suited for enhanced survival of the probiotic strains in fermented milks and/or may have stronger beneficial effects after consumption (de Vrese and Schrezenmeir 2008, Kolida and Gibson 2011, Ceapa et al. 2013).

5.5.3 Dairy Products Containing Bioactive Compounds

γ-Aminobutyric acid (GABA), a nonprotein amino acid, possesses well-known physiological functions such as neurotransmission, induction of hypotension, and diuretic and tranquilizer effects (Wong et al. 2003). GABA is synthesized by glutamate decarboxylase, a widely distributed enzyme among eukaryotic and prokaryotic organisms, including strains of LAB species (Siragusa et al. 2007). Selected producers could be employed as starter and/or adjunct cultures for the development of health-promoting dairy products enriched with GABA (Inoue et al. 2003).

5.5.4 Recombinant LAB: Vaccines and Nutraceuticals

During the last 25 years, a vast array of genetic tools and engineering techniques had been developing for *Lactococcus lactis* and some lactobacilli species (de Vos and Hugenholtz 2004). Owing to their GRAS status, LAB species are receiving increased attention for the expression of therapeutic proteins, such as human interleukin-10 and interferon-gamma (Steidler and Rottiers 2007), and for the presentation of antigens for mucosal immunization (Oliveira et al. 2006). Administration of therapeutic molecules via mucosal routes through consumption of a dairy product offers important advantages over systemic delivery such as reduction of secondary effects, easy administration, and the possibility to modulate both systemic and mucosal immune responses (Bermúdez-Humarán et al. 2011). The production of therapeuticals and vaccines through fermentation by functional starters in an inexpensive medium (milk) would further enforce their clinical use.

5.6 Conclusion

Fermented milk foods form a vast family of products having improved nutritional value and sensory properties as compared with the milk source. They have traditionally been considered not only as nutritive foods, but also as ancient medical remedies. The beneficial effects on human health of the consumption of certain traditional and new fermented dairy products are now well established. In fact, it has been recently hypothesized that cheese and other dairy products might be the missing link to the French paradox, the epidemiological phenomenon of low rates of cardiovascular mortality despite high saturated fat consumption (Petyaev and Bashmakov 2012). However, fundamental knowledge relating to the mechanisms by which these products contribute to consumers' health and well-being are still scarce. Such knowledge is essential to scientifically support their purported health benefits, enhancing the positive effectors (microbial populations, metabolites) and counteracting, whenever possible, detrimental undesirable components.

Acknowledgments

The work at the author's laboratory has been supported by projects from the Spanish Ministry of Economy and Competitiveness (AGL2007-61869 and AGL2011-24300).

References

Adolfsson, O., S. N. Meydani, and R. M. Russell. 2004. Yogurt and gut function. *American Journal of Clinical Nutrition* 80: 245–256.

Ahola, A. J., H. Yli-Knuuttila, T. Suomalainen, T. Poussa, A. Ahlstrom, J. H. Meurman, and R. Korpela. 2002. Short-term consumption of probiotic-containing cheese and its effect on dental caries risk factors. *Archives of Oral Biology* 47: 799–804.

Alessandri, C., S. Sforza, P. Palazzo, F. Lambertini, S. Paolella, D. Zennaro, C. Rafaiani et al. 2012. Tolerability of a fully maturated cheese in cow's milk allergic children: Biochemical, immunochemical, and clinical aspects. *PLoS One* 7: e40945.

Alonso, L., P. Cuesta, and S. E. Gilliland. 2003. Production of free conjugated linoleic acid by *Lactobacillus acidophilus* and *Lactobacillus casei* of human intestinal origin. *Journal of Dairy Science* 86: 1941–1946.

Alonso, L., P. Cuesta, J. Fontecha, M. Juárez, and S. E. Gilliland. 2009. Use of beta-cyclodextrin to decrease the level of cholesterol in milk fat. *Journal of Dairy Science* 92: 863–869.

Ash, A. and A. Wilbey. 2010. The nutritional significance of cheese in the UK diet. *International Journal of Dairy Technology* 63: 305–319.

Astrup, A., J. Dyerberg, P. Elwood, K. Hermansen, F. B. Hu, M. U. Jakobsen, F. J. Kok et al. 2011. The role of reducing intakes of saturated fat in the prevention of cardiovascular disease: Where does the evidence stand in 2010. *American Journal of Clinical Nutrition* 93: 684–688.

Beppu, F., M. Hosokawa, L. Tanaka, H. Kohno, T. Tanaka, and K. Miyashita. 2006. Potent inhibitory effect of trans9, trans11 isomer of conjugated linoleic acid on the growth of human colon cancer cells. Journal of Nutritional Biochemistry 17: 830–836.

Beresford, T. P., N. A. Fitzsimons, N. L. Brennan, and T. M. Cogan. 2001. Recent advances in cheese microbiology. *International Dairy Journal* 11: 259–274.

Bermúdez-Humarán, L. G., P. Kharrat, J. M. Chatel, and P. Langella. 2011. Lactococci and lactobacilli as mucosal delivery vectors for therapeutic proteins and DNA vaccines. *Microbial Cell Factory* 10 (Supp. 1): S4.

Bhardwaj, S., S. J. Passi, and A. Misra. 2011. Overview of trans fatty acids: Biochemistry and health effects. *Diabetes and Metabolic Syndrome: Clinical Research and Reviews* 5: 161–164.

Beermann, C. and J. Hartung. 2013. Physiological properties of milk ingredients released by fermentation. *Food Functionality* 4: 185–199.

Borruel, N., M. Carol, F. Casellas, M., Antolín, F. de Lara, E. Espín, J. Naval, F. Guarner, and J. R. Malagelada. 2002. Increased mucosal tumor necrosis factor alpha production in Crohn's disease can be downregulated ex vivo by probiotic bacteria. *Gut* 51: 659–664.

Boudraa, G., M. Benbouabdellah, W. Hachelaf, M. Boisset, J. F. Desjeux, and M. Touhami. 2001. Effect of feeding yogurt versus milk in children with acute diarrhoea and carbohydrate malabsorption. *Journal of Pediatric Gastroenterology and Nutrition* 33: 307–313.

Carr, F. J., D. Chill, and N. Maida. 2002. The lactic acid bacteria: A literature survey. *Critical Reviews in Microbiology* 28: 281–370.

Ceapa, C., H. Wopereis, L. Rezaïki, M. Kleerebezem, J. Knol, and R. Oozeer. 2013. Influence of fermented milk products, prebiotics and probiotics on microbiota composition and health. *Best Practices in Research Clinical Gastroenterology* 27: 139–155.

Chadwick, V. S., W. Chen, D. Shu, B. Paulus, P. Bethwaite, A. Tie, and I. Wilson. 2002. Activation of the mucosal immune system in irritable bowel syndrome. *Gastroenterology* 122: 1778–1783.

Coakley, M., M. C. Johnson, E. McGrath, S. Rahman, R. P. Ross, G. F. Fitzgerald, R. Devery, and C. Stanton. 2006. Intestinal bifidobacteria that produce trans-9, trans-11 CLA: A fatty acid with anti-proliferative activity against SW480 and HT-29 colon cancer cells. *Nutrition and Cancer* 56: 95–102.

Coconnier, M. H., V. Lievin, E. Hemery, and A. L. Servin. 1998. Antagonistic activity against *Helicobacter* infection *in vitro* and *in vivo* by the human *Lactobacillus acidophilus* strain LB. *Applied and Environmental Microbiology* 64: 4573–4580.

Colbère-Garapin, F., S. Martin-Latil, B. Blondel, L. Mousson, I. Pelletier, A. Autret, A. François, V. Niborski, G. Grompone, G. Catonnet, and A. van de Moer. 2007. Prevention and treatment of enteric viral infections: Possible benefits of probiotic bacteria. *Microbes and Infection* 9: 1623–1631.

Collins, Y. F., P. L. H. McSweeney, and M. G. Wilkinson. 2003. Lipolysis and free fatty acid catabolism in cheese: A review of current knowledge. *International Dairy Journal* 13: 841–866.

Copley, M. S., R. Berstan, S. N. Dudd, G. Docherty, A. J. Mukherjee, V. Straker, S. Payne, and R. P. Evershed. 2006. Direct chemical evidence for widespread dairying in prehistoric Britain. *Proceedings of the Natural Academy of Science USA* 100: 1524–1529.

Cremonini, F., S. Di Carlo, M. Covino, A. Armuzzi, M. Gabrielli, L. Santarelli, E. C. Nista, G. Cammarota, G. Gasbarrini, and A. Gasbarrini. 2002. Effect of different probiotic preparations on anti-*Helicobacter pylori* therapy-related side effects: A parallel group, triple blind, placebo-controlled study. *The American Journal of Gastroenterology* 97: 2744–2749.

Czerucka, D., T. Piche, and P. Rampal. 2007. Review article: Yeast as probiotics. *Saccharomyces boulardii. Alimentary and Pharmacological Therapy* 26: 767–78.

Dalié, D. K. D., A. M. Deschamps, and F. Richard-Forget. 2010. Lactic acid bacteria—potential for control of mould growth and mycotoxins: A review. *Food Control* 21: 370–380.

de Ramesh, C. C., C. H. White, A. Kilara, and Y. H. Hui. 2006. *Manufacturing Yogurt and Fermented Milks.* Oxford: Blackwell Publishing.

de Vos, W. M., and J. Hugenholtz. 2004. Engineering metabolic highways in lactococci and other lactic acid bacteria. *Trends in Biotechnology* 22: 72–79.

de Vrese, M., A. Stegelmann, B. Richter, S. Fenselau, C. Laue, and J. Schrezenmeir. 2001. Probiotics: Compensation for lactase insufficiency. *The American Journal of Clinical Nutrition* 73–2: S421–S429.

de Vrese, M. and J. Schrezenmeir. 2008. Probiotics, prebiotis, and synbiotics. *Advances in Biochemistry, Engineering and Biotechnology* 111: 1–66.

Drake, M. A., R. E. Miracle, and D. J. McMahon. 2010. Impact of fat reduction on flavor and flavor chemistry of Cheddar cheeses. *Journal of Dairy Science* 93: 5069–5081.

El-Baradei, G., A. Delacroix-Buchet, and J.-C. Ogier. 2008. Bacterial biodiversity of traditional Zabady fermented milk. *International Journal of Food Microbiology* 121: 295–301.

El-Nezami, H., N. Polychronaki, S. Salminen, and H. Mykkanen. 2002. Binding rather than metabolism may explain the interaction of two food-Grade *Lactobacillus* strains with zearalenone and its derivative alpha-zearalenol. *Applied and Environmental Microbiology* 68: 3545–3549.

Evershed, R. P., S. Payne, A. G. Sherratt, M. S. Copley, J. Coolidge, D. Urem-Kotsu, K. Kotsakis et al. 2008. Earliest date for milk use in the Near East and southeastern Europe linked to cattle herding. *Nature* 455: 528–531.

FAO/WHO. 2002. Report of a Joint FAO/WHO Working Group on Drafting Guidelines for the Evaluation of Probiotics in Food. London, Ontario, Canada, April 30 and May 1, 2002. ftp://ftp.fao.org/es/esn/food/wgreport2.pdf.

FAO/WHO. 2003. CODEX Standard for Fermented Milks. Codex Stan 243–2003. Reviewed 2008. http://www.codexalimentarius.net/download/standards/400/CXS_243e.pdf.

Farnworth, E. R. 2005. Kefir-a complex probiotic. *Food Science and Technology Bulletin: Functional Foods* 2: 1–17.

Fernández-Bodega, M. A., E. Mauriz, A. Gómez, and J. F. Martín. 2009. Proteolytic activity, mycotoxins and andrastin A in *Penicillium roqueforti* strains isolated from Cabrales, Valdeón and Bejes-Tresviso local varieties of blue-veined cheese. *International Journal of Food Microbiology* 136: 18–25.

FIL-IDF. 2012. The World Dairy Situation 2012. *FIL-IDF Bulletin* 458/2012.

Fontana, L., M. Bermúdez-Brito, J. Plaza-Díaz, S. Muñoz-Quezada, and A. Gil. 2013. Sources, isolation, characterisation and evaluation of probiotics. *British Journal of Nutrition* 109: S35–S50.

Fontecha, J., L. M. Rodríguez-Alcalá, M. V. Calvo, and M. Juárez. 2011. Bioactive milk lipids. *Current Nutrition in Food Science* 7: 155–159.

Fox, P. F., T. P. Guinee, T. M. Cogan, and P. L. H. McSweeney. 2000. *Fundamentals of Cheese Science.* Gaithersburg: AN Aspen Publication.

Fox, P. F., P. L. H. McSweeney, T. M. Cogan, and T. P. Guinee. 2004. *Cheese: Chemistry, Physics and Microbiology. Major Cheese Groups*, 3rd ed. San Diego: Elsevier Academic Press.

Gebauer, S. K., J. M. Chardigny, M. U. Jakobsen, B. Lamarche, A. L. Lock, S. D. Proctor, and D. J. Baer. 2011. Effects of ruminant trans fatty acids on cardiovascular disease and cancer: A comprehensive review of epidemiological, clinical, and mechanistic studies. *Advances in Nutrition* 2: 332–354.

Geier, M. S., R. N. Butler, and G. S. Howarth. 2006. Probiotics, Prebiotics and Synbiotics, a role in chemoprevention for colorectal cancer? *Cancer Biology and Therapy* 5: 1265–1269.

German, J. B. and C. J. Dillard. 2006. Composition, structure and absorption of milk lipids: A source of energy, fat soluble nutrients and bioactive molecules. *Critical Reviews in Food Science and Nutrition* 46: 57–92.

Gomes da Cruz, A., F. C. Alonso Buriti, C. H. Batista de Souza, J. A. Fonseca Faria, and S. M. Isay Saad. 2008. Probiotic cheese: Health benefits, technological and stability aspects. *Trends in Food Science and Technology* 20: 344–354.

Gómez-Ruiz J. A., M. Ramos, and I. Recio. 2004. Angiotensin converting enzyme-inhibitory activity of peptides isolated from Manchego cheese: Stability under simulated gastrointestinal digestion. *International Dairy Journal* 14: 1075–1080.

Granier, A., O. Goulet, , and C. Hoarau. 2013. Fermentation products: Immunological effects on human and animal models. *Pediatric Research* 74: 238–244.

Guarner, F. and J. R. Malagelada. 2003. Gut flora in health and disease. *Lancet* 360: 512–9.

Guarner, F., G. Perdigon, G. Corthier, S. Salminen, B. Koletzko, and L. Morelli. 2005. Should yoghurt cultures be considered probiotic? *British Journal of Nutrition* 93: 783–786.

Gueimonde, M. and S. Salminen. 2006. New methods for selecting and evaluating probiotics. *Digestive and Liver Disease* 38–2: S242–S247.

Guggenheim, B., R. Schmid, and J.-M. Aeschlimann. 1999. Powdered milk micellar casein prevents oral colonization by *Streptococcus sobrinus* and dental caries in rats: A basis for the caries-protective effect of dairy products. *Caries Research* 33: 446–454.

Güven, A., A. Güven, and M. Gülmez. 2003. The effect of kefir on the activities of GSH-Px, GST, CAT, GSH and LPO levels in carbon tetrachloride-induced mice tissues. *Journal of Veterinary Medicine* Series B 50: 412–416.

Halttunen, T., S. Salminen, and R. Tahvonen. 2007. Rapid removal of lead and cadmium from water by specific lactic acid bacteria. *International Journal of Food Microbiology* 114: 30–35.

Hatakka, K., A. Ahola, H. Yli-Knuuttila, M. Richardson, T. Poussa, J. H. Meurman, and R. Korpela. 2007. Probiotics reduce the prevalence of oral candida in the elderly-a randomized controlled trial. *Journal of Dental Research* 86: 125–130.

Hertzler, S. R. and S. M. Clancy. 2003. Kefir improves lactose digestion and tolerance in adults with lactose maldigestion. *Journal of American Diet Association* 103: 582–587.

Hess, B. W., G. E. Moss, and D. C. Rule. 2008. A decade of developments in the area of fat supplementation research with beef cattle and sheep. *Journal of Animal Science* 86: E188–E204.

Hill, C., F. Guarner, G. Reid, G. R. Gibson, D. J. Merenstein, B. Pot, L. Morelli et al. 2014. The International Scientific Association for Probiotics and Prebiotics consensus statement on the scope and appropriate use of the term probiotic. *Nature Reviews on Gastroenterology and Hepatology* 11: 506–514.

Horrocks, L. A. and A. A. Farooqui. 2004. Docosahexaenoic acid in the diets: Its importance in main and restoration of neural membrane function. *Prostaglandins, Leukotrienes and Essential Fatty Acids* 70: 361–372.

Inoue, K., T. Shirai, H. Ochiai, M. Kasao, K. Hayakawa, M. Kimura, and H. Sansawa. 2003. Blood-pressure-lowering effect of a novel fermented milk containing gamma-aminobutyric acid (GABA) in mild hypertensives. *European Journal of Clinical Nutrition* 57: 490–495.

Isolauri, E., T. Arvola, Y. Sutas, E. Moilanen, and S. Salminen. 2000. Probiotics in the management of atopic eczema. *Clinical and Experimental Allergy* 30: 1605–1610.

Isolauri, E. and S. Salminen, Nutrition, Allergy, Mucosal Immunology, and Intestinal Microbiota (NAMI) Research Group Report. 2008. Probiotics: Use in allergic disorders: A Nutrition, Allergy, Mucosal Immunology, and Intestinal Microbiota (NAMI) Research Group Report. *Journal of Clinical Gastroenterology* 42–2: S91–S96.

Jenkins, T. C. and M. A. McGuire. 2006. Major advances in nutrition: Impact on milk composition. *Journal of Dairy Science* 89: 1302–1310.

Jijon, H., J. Backer, H. Diaz, H. Yeung, D. Thiel, C. McKaigney, C. de Simone, and K. Madsen. 2004. DNA from probiotic bacteria modulates murine and human epithelial and immune function. *Gastroenterology* 126: 1358–1373.

Kahala, M., M. Mäki, A. Lehtovaara, J. M. Tapanainen, R. Katiska, M. Juuruskorpi, J. Juhola, and V. Joutsjoki. 2008. Characterization of starter lactic acid bacteria from the Finnish fermented milk product viili. *Journal of Applied Microbiology* 105: 1929–1938.

Kalliomäki, M., S. Salminen, H. Arvilommi, P. Kero, P. Koskinen, and E. Isolauri. 2001. Probiotics in primary prevention of atopic disease: A randomized placebo-controlled trial. *Lancet* 357: 1076–1079.

Kalliomäki, M., S. Salminen, T. Poussa, H. Arvilommi, and E. Isolauri. 2003. Probiotics and prevention of atopic disease: 4-year follow-up of a randomized placebo-controlled trial. *Lancet* 361: 1869–1871.

Kashket, S. and D. P. DePaola. 2002. Cheese consumption and the development and progression of dental caries. *Nutrition Reviews* 60: 97–103.

Khalif, I. L., E. M. Quigley, E. A. Konovitch, and I. D. Maximova. 2005. Alterations in the colonic flora and intestinal permeability and evidence of immune activation in chronic constipation. *Digestive and Liver Diseases* 37: 838–849.

Kiwaki, M. and K. Nomoto. 2009. *Lactobacillus casei* Shirota. In: *Handbook of Probiotics and Prebiotics*, 2nd edn., eds. Y. K. Lee, and S. Salminen, Hoboken: Wiley, pp. 449–457.

Klaenhammer, T. R. and M. J. Kullen. 1999. Selection and design of probiotics. *International Journal of Food Microbiology* 45: 45–57.

Kolida, S. and G. R. Gibson. 2011. Synbiotics in health and disease. *Annual Reviews in Food Science and Technology* 2: 373–393.

Koo, H. L. and H. L. DuPont. 2006. Current and future developments in travelers' diarrhoea therapy. *Expert Review of Anti-infective Therapy* 4: 417–427.

Korhonen, H. J. 2009. Bioactive Components in bovine milk. In: *Bioactive Components in Milk and Dairy Products*, ed. Y. W. Park, Oxford: Wiley-Blackwell, 15–38.

Kosikowski, F. V. and V. V. Mistry. 1997. *Cheese and Fermented Milk Foods*, 3rd edn., ed. F. V. Kosikowski. Connecticut: LLC Westport.

Kotowska, M., P. Albrecht, and H. Szajewska. 2005. *Saccharomyces boulardii* in the prevention of antibiotic-associated diarrhoea in children: A randomized double-blind placebo-controlled trial. *Alimentary and Pharmacology Therapy* 21: 583–590.

Kücükcetin, A., H. Yaygin, J. Hinrichs, and U. Kulozik. 2003. Adaptation of bovine milk towards mares' milk composition by means of membrane technology for Koumiss manufacture. *International Dairy Journal* 13: 945–951.

Kwak, H. S., C. S. Jung, S. Y. Shim, and J. Ahn. 2002. Removal of cholesterol from Cheddar cheese by beta-cyclodextrin. *Journal of Agriculture and Food Chemistry* 50: 7293–7298.

Labayen, I., L. Forga, A. González, I. Lenoir, and A. J. Martínez. 2001. Relationship between lactose digestion, gastrointestinal transit time and symptoms in lactose malabsorbers after dairy consumption. *Alimentary and Pharmacological Therapy* 15: 543–549.

Lampe, J. W. 2011. Dairy products and cancer. *Journal of American College Nutrition* 30–1: S464–S470.

Law, B. A. 1999. *Technology of Cheesemaking. Sheffield Food Technology*. Boca Raton: CRC Press LLC.

LeBlanc, J. G., J. E. Laiño, M. J. del Valle, V. Vannini, D. van Sinderen, M. P. Taranto, G. F. de Valdez, G. S. de Giori, and F. Sesma. 2011. B-group vitamin production by lactic acid bacteria-current knowledge and potential applications. *Journal of Applied Microbiology* 111: 1297–1309.

Lee, J., D. Seto, and L. Bielory. 2008. Meta-analysis of clinical trials of probiotics for prevention and treatment of pediatric atopic dermatitis. *Journal of Allergy and Clinical Immunology* 121: 116–121.

Liu, M., J. R. Bayjanov, B. Renckens, A. Nauta, and R. J. Siezen. 2010. The proteolytic system of lactic acid bacteria revisited: A genomic comparison. *BMC Genomics* 11: 36.

López-Expósito I., L. Amigo, and I. Recio. 2012. A mini-review on health and nutritional aspects of cheese with a focus on bioactive peptides. *Dairy Science and Technology* 92: 419–438.

Macouzet, M., B. H. Lee, and N. Robert. 2009. Production of conjugated linoleic acid by probiotic *Lactobacillus acidophilus* La-5. *Journal of Applied Microbiology* 106: 1886–1891.

Macura, D. and P. M. Townsley. 1984. Scandinavian ropy milk—Identification and characterization of endogenous ropy lactic streptococci and their extracellular excretion. *Journal of Dairy Science* 67: 735–744.

Madureira, A. R., T. Tavares, A. M. P. Gomes, M. E. Pintado, and F. X. Malcata. 2010. Physiological properties of bioactive peptides obtained from whey proteins. *Journal of Dairy Science* 93: 437–455.

Mayo, B., T. Aleksandrzak-Piekarczyk, M. Fernández, M. Kowalczyk, P. Álvarez-Martín, and J. Bardowski. 2010a. Updates in the metabolism of lactic acid bacteria. In: *Biotechnology of Lactic Acid Bacteria. Novel Applications*, eds. F. Mozzi, R. Raya, and G. Vignolo, Hoboken: Wiley-Blackwell, pp. 3–33.

Mayo, B., M. S. Ammor, S. Delgado, and A. Alegría. 2010b. Fermented milk products. In *Fermented Foods and Beverages of the World*, eds J. P. Tamang, and K. Kailasapathy, New York: CRC Press, pp. 263–288.

McFarland, L. V. 2006. Meta-analysis of probiotics for the prevention of antibiotic associated diarrhoea and the treatment of *Clostridium difficile* disease. *American Journal of Gastroenterology* 101: 812–822.

McFarland, L. V. 2007. Meta-analysis of probiotics for the prevention of traveller's diarrhoea. *Travel Medicine and Infectious Disease* 5: 97–105.

Meira, S. M., V. E. Helfer, R. V. Velho, F. C. Lopes, and A. Brandelli. 2012. Probiotic potential of *Lactobacillus* spp. isolated from Brazilian regional ovine cheese. *Journal of Dairy Research* 79: 119–127.

Metchnikoff, E. 1907. *The Prolongation of Life*. London: Heinemann.

Meydani, S. N., and W. K. Ha. 2000. Immunologic effects of yogurt. *American Journal of Clinical Nutrition* 71: 861–872.

Micha, R. and D. Mozaffarian. 2010. Saturated fat and cardiometabolic risk factors, coronary heart disease, stroke, and diabetes: A fresh look at the evidence. *Lipids* 45: 893–905.

Mills, S., O. O'Sullivan, C. Hill, G. Fitzgerald, and R. P. Ross. 2010. The changing face of dairy starter cultures: From genomics to economics. *International Journal of Dairy Technology* 63: 149–170.

Nielsen, K. F., P. W. Dalsgaard, J. Smedsgaard, and T. O. Larsen. 2005. Andrastin A-D, *Penicillium roqueforti* metabolites consistently produced in blue-mold-ripened cheese. *Journal of Agricultural and Food Chemistry* 53: 2908–2913.

O'Mahony, L., J. McCarthy, P. Kelly, G. Hurley, F. Luo, K. Chen, G. C. O'Sullivan, B. Kiely, J. K. Collins, F. Shanahan, and E. M. Quigley. 2005. *Lactobacillus* and *Bifidobacterium* in irritable bowel syndrome: Symptom responses and relationship to cytokine profiles. *Gastroenterology* 128: 541–451.

Oliveira, M. L., A. P. Arêas, I. B. Campos, V. Monedero, G. Pérez-Martínez, E. N. Miyaji, L. C. Leite, K. A. Aires, and H. P. Lee. 2006. Induction of systemic and mucosal immune response and decrease in *Streptococcus pneumoniae* colonization by nasal inoculation of mice with recombinant lactic acid bacteria expressing pneumococcal surface antigen A. *Microbes and Infection* 8: 1016–1024.

Oliveira, R. P. S., A. C. R. Florence, R. C. Silva, P. Perego, A. Converti, L. A. Gioielli, and M. N. Oliveira. 2009. Effect of different prebiotics on the fermentation kinetics, probiotic survival and fatty acids profiles in nonfat symbiotic fermented milk. *International Journal of Food Microbiology* 128: 467–472.

Ouwehand, A. C., S. Salminen, and E. Isolauri. 2002. Probiotics: An overview of beneficial effects. *Antonie van Leeuwenhoek* 82: 279–289.

Papanikolaou, Z., M. Hatzikamari, P. Georgakopoulos, M. Yiangou, E. Litopoulou-Tzanetaki, and N. Tzanetakis. 2012. Selection of dominant NSLAB from mature traditional cheese according to their technological properties and *in vitro* intestinal challenges. *Journal of Food Science* 77: M298–M306.

Parashar, U. D., C. J. Gibson, J. S. Bresse, and R. I. Glass. 2006. Rotavirus and severe childhood diarrhoea, *Emerging Infectious Diseases* 12: 304–306.

Parente, E. and T. M. Cogan. 2004. Starter cultures: General aspects. In *Cheese: Chemistry, Physics and Microbiology, vol 1: General Aspects,* 3rd edn., eds. P. F. Fox, P. L. H. McSweeney, T. M. Cogan, and T. P. Guinee, London: Elsevier Academic Press, pp. 123–147.

Pelletier, X., S. Laure-Boussuge, and Y. Donazzolo. 2001. Hydrogen excretion upon ingestion of dairy products in lactose-intolerant male subjects: Importance of the live flora. *European Journal of Clinical Nutrition* 55: 509–512.

Petyaev, I. M. and Y. K. Bashmakov. 2012. Could cheese be the missing piece in the French paradox puzzle? *Medical Hypotheses* 79: 746–749.

Puri, P., A. Rattan, R. L. Bijlani, S. C. Mahapatra, and I. Nath. 1996. Splenic and intestinal lymphocyte proliferation response in mice fed milk or yogurt and challenged with *Salmonella typhimurium*. *International Journal of Food Science and Nutrition* 47: 391–398.

Rachid, M. M., N. M. Gobbato, J. C. Valdéz, H. H. Vitalone, and G. Perdigón. 2002. Effect of yogurt on the inhibition of an intestinal carcinoma by increasing cellular apoptosis. *International Journal of Immunopathology and Pharmacology* 15: 209–216.

Rachmilewitz, D., K. Katakura, F. Karmeli, T. Hayashi, C. Reinus, B. Rudensky, S. Akira, K. Takeda, J. Lee, K. Takabayashi, and E. Raz. 2004. Toll-like receptor 9 signalling mediates the anti-inflammatory effects of probiotics in murine experimental colitis. *Gastroenterology* 126: 520–528.

Rettger, L. F., M. N. Levy, L. Weinstein, and J. E. Weiss. 1935. *Lactobacillus acidophilus and its Therapeutic Applications.* New Haven: Yale University Press.

Robinson, R. K. and A. Y. Tamime. 2006. Types of Fermented Milks. In: *Fermented Milks*, ed. A. Y. Tamime, Hoboken: Wiley, pp. 1–10.

Ruas-Madiedo P., M. Gueimonde, A. Margolles, C. G. de los Reyes-Gavilán, and S. Salminen. 2006. Short communication: Effect of exopolysaccharide isolated from "viili" on the adhesion of probiotics and pathogens to intestinal mucus. *Journal of Dairy Science* 89: 2355–2358.

Sabir, F., Y. Beyatli, C. Cokmus, and D. Onal-Darilmaz. 2010. Assessment of potential probiotic properties of *Lactobacillus* spp., *Lactococcus* spp., and *Pediococcus* spp. strains isolated from kefir. *Journal of Food Science* 75: M568–M573.

Salminen, S., A. C. Ouwehand, and E. Isolauri. 1998. Clinical applications of probiotic bacteria. *International Dairy Journal* 8: 563–572.

Schachtele, C. F. and M. E. Jensen. 1984. Can foods be ranked according to their cariogenic potential. In: *Cariology Today*, ed. B. Guggenheim, Basel: Karger, pp. 136–146.

Schirone, M., R. Tofalo, G. Mazzone, A. Corsetti, and G. Suzzi. 2011. Biogenic amine content and microbiological profile of Pecorino di Firandola cheese. *Food Microbiology* 28: 128–136.

Serafeimidou, A., S. Zlatanos, K. Laskaridis, and A. Segredos. 2012. Chemical characteristics, fatty acid composition and conjugated linoleic acid (CLA) content of traditional Greek yogurts. *Food Chemistry* 134: 1839–1846.

Shiby, V. K. and H. N. Mishra. 2013. Fermented milks and milk products as functional foods—a review. *Critical Reviews in Food Science and Nutrition* 53: 482–496.

Siragusa, S., M. De Angelis, R. Di Cagno, C. G. Rizzello, R. Coda, and M. Gobbetti. 2007. Synthesis of gamma-aminobutyric acid by lactic acid bacteria isolated from a variety of Italian cheeses. *Applied and Environmental Microbiology* 73: 7283–7290.

Smid, E. J. and M. Kleerebezem. 2014. Production of aroma compounds in lactic fermentations. *Annual Reviews of Food Science and Technology* 5: 313–326.

Smit, G., B. A. Smit, and E. J. Engels. 2005. Flavour formation by lactic acid bacteria and biochemical flavour profiling of cheese products. *FEMS Microbiology Reviews* 29: 591–610.

Solinas, C., M. Corpino, R. Maccioni, and U. Pelosi. 2010. Cow's milk protein allergy. *Journal of Maternal, Fetal and Neonatal Medicine* 23–3: S76–S79.

Solis-Pereyra, B., N. Aattouri, and D. Lemonnier. 1997. Role of food in the stimulation of cytokine production. *American Journal of Clinical Nutrition* 66: S521–S525.

Stanton, C., G. Gardiner, P. B. Lynch, J. K. Collins, G. F. Fitzgerald, and R. P. Ross. 1998. Probiotic Cheese. *International Dairy Journal* 8: 491–496.

Stanton, C., R. P. Ross, G. F. Fitzgerald, and D. van Sinderen. 2005. Fermented functional foods based on probiotics and their biogenic metabolites. *Current Opinion in Biotechnology* 16: 198–203.

Steidler, L. and P. Rottiers, P. 2007. Therapeutic drug delivery by genetically modified *Lactococcus lactis. Annals of New York Academy of Science* 1072: 176–186.

Szajewska, H., A. Skorka, M. Ruszczynski, and D. Gieruszczak-bialek. 2007. Meta-analysis: *Lactobacillus* GG for treating acute diarrhoea in children. *Alimentary Pharmacology and Therapeutics* 25: 871–881.

Tamang, J. P. 2010. *Himalayan Fermented Foods: Microbiology, Nutrition and Ethnic Values.* Boca Raton: CRC Press.

Tamang, J. P., N. Tamang, S. Thapa, S. Dewan, B. M. Tamang, H. Yonzan, A. K. Rai, R. Chettri, J. Chakrabarty, and N. Kharel. 2012. Microorganisms and nutritional value of ethnic fermented foods and alcoholic beverages of North East India. *Indian Journal of Traditional Knowledge* 11: 7–25.

Tamime, A. Y. 2002. Fermented milks: A historical food with modern applications-a review. *European Journal of Clinical Nutrition* 56–4: S2–S15.

Tamime, A. Y. and R. K. Robinson. 2007. *Yoghurt Science and Technology*. Cambridge: Woodhead Publishing.
Thompson, I. 2008. *Clostridium difficile*-associated disease: Update and focus on non-antibiotic strategies. *Age and Ageing* 37: 14–18.
van Niel, C. W., C. Feudtner, M. M. Garrison, and D. A. Christakis. 2002. *Lactobacillus* therapy for acute infectious diarrhoea in children: A metaanalysis. *Pediatrics* 109: 1046–1049.
Wang, K. Y., S. N. Li, C. S. Liu, D. S. Perng, Y. C. Su, D. C. Wu, C. M. Jan, C. H. Lai, T. N. Wang, and W. M. Wang. 2004. Effects of ingesting *Lactobacillus*-and *Bifidobacterium*-containing yogurt in subjects with colonized *Helicobacter pylori*. *The American Journal of Clinical Nutrition* 80: 737–741.
Wijesinha-Bettoni, R. and B. Burlingame. 2013. Milk and dairy products composition. In *Milk and Dairy Products in Human Nutrition*, eds. E. Muehlhoff, A. Bennett, and D. McMahon, Roma: Food and Agriculture Organization, 41–102.
Wong, C. G., T. Bottiglieri, and O. C. Snead III. 2003. GABA, γ-hydroxybutyric acid, and neurological disease. *Annual of Neurology* 54–6: S3–S12.
Wouters, J. T. M, E. H. E Ayad, J. Hugenholtz, and G. Smit. 2002. Microbes from raw milk for fermented dairy products. *International Dairy Journal* 12: 91–109.
Wu, R., L. Wang, J. Wang, H. Li, B. Menghe, J. Wu, M. Guo, and H. Zhang. 2009. Isolation and preliminary probiotic selection of lactobacilli from Koumiss in Inner Mongolia. *Journal of Basic Microbiology* 49: 318–326.

Chapter 6

Functional Properties of Fermented Milks

Nagendra P. Shah

Contents

6.1 Introduction

Fermentation is one of the oldest techniques employed by humans to preserve milk. It is believed that fermented milk originated in the Middle East before the Phoenician era. *Laban* or *labneh*, the traditional Egyptian fermented milk, is reported to have been consumed around 7000 BC (Kosikowski and Mistry 1997). It is reported that according to the Persian tradition, the long life of Abraham was due to the consumption of fermented milk. It is believed that the Tartars and Mongols spread the practice of drinking fermented milk in Asia. Fermented milk still remains very popular in South East Asia, Iraq, Syria, and Turkey. It also plays an important role in the diets of Europeans. Today, fermented milks are manufactured in many countries around the world and play an important role in human nutrition. Fermented milk provides both the nutritional function and the physiological function. The nutritional function is due to the nutrients present in milk and the physiological function refers to the therapeutic functions beyond the nutritional function (Shah 2001).

6.1.1 Nutritional Attributes of Fermented Milk

To understand the nutritional attributes of fermented milk, one needs to appreciate the nutritional values of milk. The macronutrients such as carbohydrates, proteins, and lipids found in milk differ from one species to other (Jensen 1995). Milk is a complete food for newborn mammals and contains approximately 5% lactose, 3.3% protein, 4% fat, and 0.7% minerals used for the growth and development of mammals (McJarrow et al. 2009) and for their immunity. Nutritionally fermented milk has a similar composition to that of the unfermented counterpart from which it is made. However, bacterial fermentation results in the lowering of lactose and increasing the level of lactic acid in fermented milk. Milk is also a good source of micronutrients including calcium, phosphorus, magnesium, and zinc. Milk proteins have a high nutritive value due to the favorable balance of essential amino acids. Human milk contains low protein, low minerals, and a high lactose level compared with cow's milk. Following sections discuss the nutritional attributes of milk constituents.

6.1.1.1 Lactose

During fermentation, lactic acid bacteria (LAB) convert 20%–30% of the lactose into lactic acid. Consequently, the lactose level in fermented milk or yoghurt can be lower than that of milk. Lactose is considered as excellent food for babies and has a favorable effect in the intestinal tract. Generally, yoghurt is supplemented with 2%–4% skim milk powder, so the protein and sugar contents are usually higher than that of cow's milk. Yoghurts with lower lactose content may be better tolerated by lactose-intolerant individuals. Yoghurts fortified with skim milk powder and containing higher levels of lactose are also better tolerated by lactose malabsorbers.

Lactose stimulates gastrointestinal activity. It increases the capacity of the body to utilize phosphorus and calcium. Lactose has beneficial effects on the absorption of calcium. Polysaccharides such as cellulose are generally added to the yoghurt mix as a stabilizer and many of these polysaccharides are considered as the "bifidus factor" and may prevent constipation by providing bulk. Lactic acid acts as a preservative by reducing pH, which inhibits the growth of potential harmful spoilage bacteria. Lactic acid also influences the physical properties of casein curd to induce a finer suspension, which seems to promote digestibility.

6.1.1.2 Milk Proteins

Milk protein is considered to be of high nutritional value in terms of its biological value (BV), net protein utilization (NPU) and protein efficiency ratio (PER). Caseins and whey proteins contain high levels of essential amino acids; hence, proteins in milk are of excellent quality. Fermented milk and yoghurt making involves heat treatment and the use of starter bacteria, which increase the levels of soluble proteins, nonprotein nitrogen, and free amino acids. Feeding of fermented milk and yoghurt is reported to result in increased weight gains and increased feeding efficiency in rats compared to that of the milk from which it was prepared.

Milk is heat treated (typically 85°C for 30 min) for making fermented milk or yoghurt. This results in denaturation of whey proteins and produces a soft curd when milk proteins are coagulated by acid produced by LAB. Such soft curd shows characteristics more like human milk and is easily digestible as a substitute for mother's milk than harder curd. The soft curd is also better digested by children without causing any discomfort. Because of heat treatment and denaturation of whey proteins and aggregation with casein, a more open structure of casein aggregates is formed which allows proteolytic enzymes of the gastrointestinal tract freer access during digestion.

The digestibility of milk protein is the highest (>90%) among proteins. Additionally, proteins in fermented milk including yoghurt have been found to be better digestible than those in milk (Vass et al. 1984). This is possibly due to the decrease in protein particle size and an increase in soluble nitrogen, nonprotein nitrogen, and free amino acids during the heat processing of milk and proteolysis by starter bacteria. This favorable protein utilization and improvement in body mass were found in animals kept on fermented milk diets (Vass et al. 1984).

6.1.1.3 Milk Fat

Milk contains approximately 4% fat. Milk fat has the highest value as an energy source with each gram of fat providing 9 kcal (Kurmann and Rasic 1988). Starter bacteria in fermented milk do not alter the level of fat during fermentation. Milk fat is highly digestible. Lactic acid resulting from milk fermentation has been found to promote peristaltic movement, which improves the overall digestion and absorption of food. Milk fat improves consistency and mouthfeel of the product. Milk fat supplies essential fatty acids including linoleic and linolenic acid and fat-soluble vitamins such as vitamin A, carotene, vitamin D, E, and K. Choline, a constituent of phospholipid, promotes the oxidation of lipids in the liver and acts to maintain equilibrium in cholesterol concentration. Fermented milk including yoghurt is reported to lower cholesterol levels in human volunteers. The subjects consumed 240 mL of yoghurt three times per day.

6.1.1.4 Vitamins and Minerals

The level of fat-soluble vitamins (particularly vitamin A and D) is dependent on the fat content of the product made from milk. The vitamin content of fermented milk in general is higher as starter bacteria synthesize certain B group vitamins during fermentation. Fermented milk is an excellent source of vitamins B_1, B_2, B_6, B_{12}, and pantothenic acid and vitamin C. However, the majority of vitamin C is lost by heat treatment and vitamin B_{12} is undetectable after storage for 5 days (Kurmann and Rasic 1988). Levels of some B vitamins, particularly vitamin B_{12}, are reduced due to the requirement of some LAB for this vitamin. Some lactic bacteria are able to synthesize the B vitamin folic acid.

The mineral content is not altered during fermentation; however, reports suggest that the utilization of Ca, P, and iron in the body is better for fermented milk than for cow's milk. The utilization of Ca and P in the body is better in the presence of lactose and vitamin D. Calcium is required for bone metabolism and the prevention of osteoporosis. Yoghurts contain appreciable quantity of sodium and potassium and thus may not be suitable for feeding babies less than 6 months, unless these minerals are reduced prior to manufacturing of fermented milk or yoghurt.

6.1.2 Health Properties of Fermented Milk

Fermented milk provides additional health benefits than those provided by milk including the improvement in lactose digestion, antimicrobial activity, and anticancer effect (Table 6.1).

6.1.2.1 Improved Lactose Digestion

A large number of people in the world are unable to digest and absorb lactose and are classified as lactose malabsorbers. In such people, lactosein milk is not completely hydrolyzed into monosaccharides, glucose, and galactose with the help of the β-D-galactosidase (or lactase) enzyme (Savaiano et al. 1984, Shah 1993, 1994, Shah and Jelen 1991, Shah et al. 1992). This group of people often complains of "gastric distress" after consuming unfermented milk (Onwulata et al. 1989). The unabsorbed lactose reaches colon, where it is fermented by colonic flora to volatile fatty acids, lactic acid, CO_2, H_2, and CH_4. The unhydrolyzed lactose withdraws water and electrolytes from the duodenum and jejunum. This leads to bloating, flatulence, abdominal pain, and diarrhea in lactose malabsorbers, depending on the amount of lactose consumed (Savaiano et al. 1984, 1987, Shah et al. 1992, Madry et al. 2011).

Fermented milk or yoghurt appears to be well tolerated by lactose malabsorbers. The traditional cultures used in making yoghurt (*Lactobacillus delbrueckii* ssp. *bulgaricus* and *Streptococcus thermophilus*) contain substantial quantities of β-D-galactosidase, and it has been suggested that the consumption of fermented milk or yoghurt may assist in alleviating the symptoms of lactose malabsorption. Several studies have reported that yoghurt is tolerated well by lactose malabsorbers. The lactase enzyme elaborated by these bacteria and the oro-cecal transit time in viscous products such as yogurt (Shah et al. 1992) are responsible for the better tolerance of lactose or digestion of lactose in fermented milk. Starter bacteria can convert on an average 25%–30% of lactose into lactic acid; hence, the lactose content in fermented milk is lower than that in milk (Shah et al. 1992).

6.1.2.2 Antimicrobial Activity

Starter bacteria in fermented dairy foods produce antimicrobial substances such as lactic acid and hydrogen peroxide. Lactic acid can lower pH in the gut and has a bactericidal or bacteriostatic effect. The low pH resulting from the production of lactic acid during fermentation creates an undesirable environment for the growth of spoilage microorganisms. Starter bacterium such as

Table 6.1 Properties of Fermented Milk

No.	*Therapeutic Properties*	*Possible Causes and Mechanisms*
1	Improved digestibility	Partial breakdown of protein and improved bioavailability of nutrients.
2	Lactose tolerance	Reduced lactose in the product and further availability of bacterial lactase enzyme in the intestine for lactose hydrolysis.
3	Anticarcinogenic effect	Inhibition of carcinogens and enzymes involved in converting procarcinogens to carcinogens.
4	Increased vitamin contents	Synthesis of group B vitamins during fermentation.

Source: From Buttriss J. 1997. *International Journal of Dairy Technology* 50(1): 21–27; Panesar, P.S. 2011. *Food and Nutrition Sciences* 2: 47–51.

Lb.delbrueckii ssp. *bulgaricus* produces bacteriocin like antimicrobial substances such as bulgarin, which has an antimicrobial effect. Two types of lactic acid, L (+) and D (−) are produced during fermentation by LAB. Some species of bacteria such as *Lb. delbrueckii* ssp. *bulgaricus* and *Lactococcus lactis* produce only D (−) lactic acid.

6.1.2.3 Anticancer Effect

Fermented milk has been found to suppress the multiplication of cancer cells in mice (Kumar et al. 2012). The antiproliferative effect of fermented milk on the growth of the human breast cancer line has been demonstrated. Only live starter bacteria appear to have an anticancer effect. Similarly, antimutagenic effects of starter bacteria have been reported. The antitumor actions of fermented milk are claimed to be due to the stimulation of the immune functions of the body as well as the improvement in the intestinal microflora population. Fermented milk has been found to reduce the levels of fecal enzymatic activities such as β-glucuronidase, azoreductase, and nitroreductase, which catalyze conversion of procarcinogens to carcinogens.

The therapeutic properties of fermented milk containing probiotic organisms are shown in Table 6.2.

Table 6.2 Therapeutic Properties of Fermented Milk Containing Probiotic Organisms

Therapeutic Properties	*Possible Causes and Mechanisms*	*References*
Colonization of gut and inhibition of pathogenic organisms	Survive gastric acid, tolerate bile concentration, and adhere to intestinal surface and production of inhibitory compounds against pathogens.	Alakomi et al. (2000)
Lactose tolerance	Reduced lactose in the product and further availability of bacterial lactase enzyme in the intestine for lactose hydrolysis.	Vesa et al. (1996) Montalto et al. (2005) Hertzler and Clancy (2003)
Hypocholesterolaemic effect	Production of inhibitors of cholesterol synthesis, deconjugation of biles, and assimilation of cholesterol.	Mann and Spoerry (1974), Liong and Shah (2005), Begley et al. (2006)
Anticarcinogenic effect	Inhibition of carcinogens and enzymes involved in converting procarcinogens to carcinogens.	Rafter (2002)
Stimulation of the host immunological system	Enhancement of macrophage formation, stimulation of suppressor cells and production of interferon.	Anderson (2000), Pasare and Medzhitov (2005), Granucci and Ricciardi-Castagnoli (2003)
Control of vaginal infections	Improvement of therapeutic outcome in women with bacterial vaginosis by probiotic strains in dairy product.	Falagas et al. (2007)
Antimutagenic effect	Antimutagenic activity produced by probiotic bacteria against mutagens and promutagens such as 2-nitrofluourene, alfatoxin-B, and 2-amino-3methyl-3H-imidazoquinoline.	Lankaputhra and Shah (1998a,b)

A recent trend has been to add probiotic organisms to fermented milk, hence, this fermented milk can provide additional benefits beyond what milk and fermented milk can provide. A number of health benefits are claimed for probiotic organisms, *Lactobacillus acidophilus*, *Bifidobacterium* spp., and *Lactobacillus casei*, and therefore for products containing probiotic organisms (Shah 2000). The health benefits of probiotic bacteria include improvement in lactose metabolism, antimicrobial properties, antimutagenic and anticarcinogenic properties, reduction in serum cholesterol, antidiarrhea properties, immune system stimulation, and improvement in inflammatory bowel disease. There is some evidence to support the view that the oral administration of probiotic organisms is able to restore the normal balance of microbial populations in the intestine (Armuzzi et al. 2001, Cats et al. 2003). The dominance of probiotic organisms prevents colonization by undesirable microorganisms such as *Escherichia coli* or yeasts (e.g., *Candida* spp.) and the suppression of the growth of putrefactive bacteria. This may prevent the liberation of carcinogenic compounds by these organisms in the colon. Antibiotic treatment affects the population of probiotic organisms, which can be restored through the consumption of fermented milk containing *Lactobacillus* and *Bifidobacterium*.

6.1.2.4 Antimicrobial Properties

Probiotic bacteria produce organic acids such as lactic and acetic acids, hydrogen peroxide, and bacteriocins. Acetic and lactic acids are the main organic acids produced. Other acids produced in small quantities include citric acid, hippuric acid, orotic acid, and uric acid (Lankaputhra and Shah 1998a). Lactic and acetic acids account for over 90% of the acids produced. Lowering of pH due to lactic acid or acetic acid produced by these bacteria in the gut has a bactericidal or bacteriostatic effect (Alakomi et al. 2000).

The antimicrobial substances are produced to suppress the multiplication of pathogenic and putrefying bacteria. Because of these virtues, probiotic bacteria show strong antimicrobial properties against Gram-positive bacteria such as *Staphylococcus aureus*, *Clostridium perfringens* rather than against Gram-negative bacteria such as *Salmonella typhimurium* and *E. coli*. Hydrogen peroxide in the presence of organic acids such as lactic acid is inhibitory to bacteria (Lankaputhra and Shah 1998b). *Lb. acidophilus* is reported to produce acidophilin, lactobacillin, and lactodin, which show antimicrobial activity against *E. coli*, *Salmonella*, *Shigella*, and *Pseudomonas*. Hence, *Lb. acidophilus* can suppress putrefactive bacteria in the gut.

Some health-promoting roles of fermented milk containing *Lb. acidophilus*, *Bifidobacterium* spp., and *Lb. casei* are shown in Table 6.3.

Two types of lactic acid L (+) and D (–) are produced during fermentation by LAB. Some species of bacteria such as *Lb. delbrueckii* ssp. *bulgaricus* and *Lc. lactis* produce only D (–) lactic acid, whereas some lactic streptococci and *L. casei* produce L (+) lactic acid. *Lactobacillus helveticus* and *Lb. acidophilus* produce a racemic mixture of L (+) and D (–) lactic acid (Table 6.3). D (–) lactic acid is not metabolized to pyruvic acid in the body due to a lack of the D2-hydroxy acid dehydrogenase and this results in acidosis in neonatal infants. L (+) isomer is completely harmless. Bifidobacteria and *Lb. casei* produce L (+) lactic acid. Thus, the lactic acid produced by bifidobacteria and *Lb. casei* is easily metabolized, while providing antimicrobial properties (Shah 1999). Several researchers/investigators reported that *Lactobacillus* spp. showed a broad inhibitory spectrum against *E. coli* and *Staph. aureus* (Erdourul and Erbilir 2006, Ronka et al., 2003, Ryan et al. 2008). Ashraf et al (2009) concluded that all lactobacilli tested (except *Lb. delbruckii*) restrained the growth of *E. coli* and *Staph. aureus*. Also the most recent group of researchers (Ali et al. 2013) evaluated the probiotic potential of *Lactobacillus* spp., *Bifidobacterium* spp., and *Streptococcus* spp.

Table 6.3 Types of Lactic Acid Produced by Probiotic Bacteria

Bacteria	*D* (−)	*L* (+)
Bifidobacteria	−	+
Lb. casei	−	+
Lb. helveticus	+	+
Lb. acidophilus	+	+

Source: From Shah, N.P. 1999. *Probiotica* 6: 1–3.

isolated from dairy sources and found that Lactobacillus spp. could possibly be used as a novel strain against *E. coli* and *Staph. Aureus* pathogens

6.1.2.5 Anticarcinogenic Properties

LAB and fermented products made from LAB have potential anticarcinogenic activity (Mitsuoka, 2014). *Bifidobacterium longum* and *Bifidobacterium infantis* are effective antitumor agents. Their mode of action may be by the suppression of bacterial enzymes, by activation of the host immune system, and the reduction of intestinal pH. The antitumor effect of *Lb. acidophilus* was reported by Goldin and Gorbach (1977, 1984). Oral dietary supplements containing viable cells of *Lb. acidophilus* decreased the bacterial enzymes, β-glucuronidase, azoreductase, and nitroreductase. These enzymes catalyze conversion of procarcinogens to carcinogens. The anticarcinogenic effects of *Lb. acidophilus* or bifidobacteria may possibly be due to the direct removal of procarcinogens, and the activation of the body's immune system. It has been reported that short-chain fatty acids produced by *Lb. acidophilus* and *Bifidobacterium, Lactobacillus plantarum* and *Lactobacillus rhamnosus* were found to inhibit the generation of carcinogenic products by reducing enzyme activities (Cenci et al. 2002). However, some strains of *Lb. acidophilus* and *Bifidobacterium* spp. reduce the levels of enzymes such as β-glucuronidase, azoreductase, and nitroreductase responsible for activation of procarcinogens and reduce the risk of tumor development (Yoon et al. 2000). The effect is particularly due to *Lb. acidophilus, Lactobacillus* GG, and *Bifidobacterium* spp. Starter bacteria such as *S. thermophilus* and *Lb. delbrueckii* ssp. *bulgaricus* did not have any effect on fecal enzyme activities.

Direct removal of procarcinogens by probiotic bacteria might involve a reduction in the rate at which nitrosamines are produced. Probiotic bacteria may remove the sources of procarcinogens or the enzymes that lead to the formation of carcinogens. It has been shown that probiotic bacteria can greatly reduce the mutagenicity of nitrosamines. This may be due to the fact that certain species of probiotic bacteria, such as *Bifidobacterium breve*, have high absorbing properties for carcinogens, such as those produced upon charring of meat products (Mitsuoka 2014). A reduction in excreted carcinogens and in bacterial procarcinogenic enzymes has been observed in mice fed with *B. breve* and fructooligosaccharides. It has been found that probiotic microorganisms reduce colon cancer risks by inhibiting carcinogen-induced DNA damage in the gut of rats (Wollowski et al. 1999) but similar data in humans is lacking. Therefore, to enhance the knowledge of effects of probiotics in humans, fecal water genotoxicity was investigated. The human data reviewed by Pool-Zobel (2005) show that inulin-type fructans containing diets reduces the colon cancer risks by reducing the exposure to genotoxic carcinogens in the gut.

Other investigators (Lee et al. 2007) studied the probiotic properties of *Bacillus polyfermenticus* SCD and found that this strain had strong adherence properties in the human colon and anticarcinogenic properties *in vitro* and *in vivo*.

Probiotics may play a role in decreasing cancer evidence. The studies have shown that certain numbers of *Lactobacillus* and *Bifdobacterium* spp. reduce the production of carcinogenic enzymes from colonic flora and also reduce the production of antimutagenic organic acids and enhance the host's immune system (Hirayama and Rafter 1999, Kumar et al. 2010). The recent review (Shida and Namoto 2013) summarizes the possible immunomodulatory concept by which *Lb. casei* strain Shirota (LcS) strain, one of the most popular probiotics, exerts anticancer activity.

In the presence of probiotic bacteria, the proliferation of tumors is reported to decrease considerably. Tumor suppression via the body's immune response system has been reported. The injection of cell wall fractions into growing tumors caused regression of the tumors and activation of the immune response. The cell wall fractions of *B. infantis* are claimed to contain active antitumor constituents. The enhancement in the body's defenses may be due to the increased production of IgA antibodies by probiotic bacteria. The presence of *B. longum* in the gut of gnotobiotic C3H/He male mice has been found to reduce the incidence of liver tumors. The effect is claimed to be due to the stimulation of the immune response of the host or to decreasing the activity of some fecal bacterial enzymes by bifidobacteria. However, further research is needed in this area and more evidence is required to verify these claims. Finally, some investigators extensively looked into the anticarcinogenic effects of probiotic bacteria. They found very promising results and showed that purified lipoteichoic acid from *Lb. rhamnosus* GG acts as an oral photoprotective agent against UV-induced carcinogenesis (Weill et al. 2013).

6.1.2.6 Antimutagenic Properties

Studies have shown a negative correlation between the incidences of certain cancers and consumption of fermented milk products (Orrhage et al. 1994). Antimutagenic activity of fermented milk has been demonstrated *in vitro* against a large spectrum of mutagens including 4-nitroquinoline-N′-oxide, 2-nitrofluorene, and benzopyrene. The antimutagenic effect of fermented milks has been detected against a range of mutagens and promutagens in various test systems based on microbial and mammalian cells (Ayebo et al. 1982). Although there is no direct evidence regarding antimutagenic or anticarcinogenic properties of bifidobacteria in human subjects, studies conducted using human cell lines have shown that certain strains have positive effects that could lead to the prevention of cancer. As most of the probiotic organisms produce various short-chain fatty acids such as acetic and butyric acids, these acids may be responsible for the antimutagenic effect observed in bifidobacteria. The mechanism of antimutagenicity of probiotic bacteria has not been understood or identified so far and remains speculative. It has been suggested that microbial binding of mutagens could be the possible mechanism of antimutagenicity (Orrhage et al. 1994).

Lankaputhra and Shah (1998b) studied the levels of acetic, butyric, lactic, and pyruvic acids produced by probiotic bacteria (*Lb. acidophilus* and bifidobacteria) as determined by high-performance liquid chromatography (HPLC). All strains produced acetic, lactic, pyruvic, and butyric acids. Other acids produced in small quantities were citric, hippuric, orotic, and uric acid. Lankaputhra and Shah (1998b) studied the antimutagenic activity of these acids produced by probiotic bacteria against eight mutagens and promutagens including 2-nitroflourene (NF), aflatoxin-B (AFTB), and 2-amino-3-methyl-3H-imidazoquinoline (AMIQ). AFTB is a diet-related potent mutagen produced by a fungal strain of *Aspergillus flavus*, which is a major food-contaminant species prevalent in most Asian countries. The AMIQ is a heterocyclic amine mutagen. This is a major mutagen formed in heat-processed beef in Western diets (Lankaputhra and Shah, 1998a,b). The TA-100 mutant of *S. typhimurium* (His^-) strain is used as a mutagenicity indicator organism. The mutagenicity test is carried out using the Ames Salmonella test (Lankaputhra and Shah 1998b). While acetic acid showed higher antimutagenic activity than lactic or pyruvic acids, butyric acid showed a broad-spectrum antimutagenic activity against all mutagens or promutagens studied. Butyric acid is claimed to prevent carcinogenic effects at molecular (DNA) level (Smith 1995).

Lankaputhra and Shah (1998b) also reported that live bacterial cells showed higher antimutagenicity than killed cells against the mutagens studied. This suggests that live bacterial cells may metabolize or bind the mutagens. The inhibition of mutagens and promutagens by probiotic bacteria appeared to be permanent for live cells and temporary for killer cells. Killed cells released mutagens and promutagens when extracted with dimethyl sulfoxide. The results emphasized the importance of consuming live probiotic bacteria and of maintaining their viability in the intestine in order to provide the efficient inhibition of mutagens. It has been reported that unfermented milk exerted lower antimutagenic activity, whereas fermented milk showed a higher antimutagenic activity (Hsieh and Chou 2006). They also found that soymilk fermented with both *S. thermophilus* and *Bif. infants* exhibited the highest antimutagenicity of 85.07% and 85.78%, respectively, against 4-nitroquinoline-N-oxide (4-NQO) and 2-dimethyl-4-amino-biphenyl (DMAB). Recent research has paid attention to the effects of probiotics on the antimutagenic activities of crude peptide extracted from yoghurt (Sah et al. 2014) and found that *Lb. acidophilus*, *Lb.casei*, and *Lactobacillus paracasei* subsp. *paracasei* liberated from yoghurt showed strong antimutagenicity (26.35%).

6.1.2.7 Reduction in Serum Cholesterol

Studies have shown that consuming certain cultured dairy products can help reduce the serum cholesterol level. The feeding of fermented milks containing very large numbers of probiotic bacteria (~10^9 bacteria/g) to hypercholesterolemic human subjects has resulted in lowering cholesterol from 3.0 to 1.5 g/L (Homma 1988). The role of bifidobacteria in reducing serum cholesterol is not completely understood. Mann and Spoerry (1974) suggested that consumption of fermented dairy products could help lower serum cholesterol. They observed a decrease in serum cholesterol levels in men fed with large quantities of milk fermented with *Lactobacillus*. This may have been due to the production of hydroxymethylglutarate by LAB, which inhibits hydroxymethylglutaryl-CoA reductases required for the synthesis of cholesterol. Rao et al. (1981) reported that metabolites from orotic acid formed during the fermentation of dairy products may help lower cholesterol level. According to Jaspers et al. (1984), uric acid inhibits cholesterol synthesis and orotic acid and hydroxymethylglutamic acid reduce serum cholesterol. However, the role of bifidobacteria in lowering cholesterol is still debated. Klaver and Meer (1993) reported that removal of cholesterol from the culture medium by *Lb. acidophilus* and other species is not due to the bacterial uptake of cholesterol, but results from bacterial bile salt deconjugating activity. The deconjugation of bile acid by the intestinal flora may influence the serum cholesterol level. The deconjugated bile acid does not absorb lipids as readily as the conjugated counterpart, leading to a reduction in cholesterol level.

Lb. acidophilus and bifidobacteria actively assimilated cholesterol and other organic acids. Reports by Gilliland et al. (1985) show that *Lb. acidophilus* itself may take up cholesterol during growth in the small intestine and make it unavailable for absorption into the blood stream. Anderson and Gilliland (1999) also reported that *Lb. acidophilus* reduces the serum cholesterol level significantly by the consumption of yoghurt and due to the direct breakdown of cholesterol and the deconjugation of bile salt. The effects of LAB on cholesterol levels are therefore inconsistent and range from a significant reduction to no reduction. The exact mechanism remains unknown. However, it has been reported that human isolates of *Lactobacillus fermentum* KC5b was represented as a novel/candidate probiotic and was also able to remove a maximum of 14.8 mg of cholesterol per gram (dry weight) of cells from the culture medium (Pereira and Gibson 2002). Recently, many researchers have increased their interest/attention in treating hypercholesterolemia in humans using bile salt deconjugation by LAB (Jones et al. 2004, Lim et al. 2004). Other promising investigations screened 11 strains of Lactobacilli and analyzed bile salt deconjugation ability, bile salt hydrolase (BSH) activity, and coprecipitation of cholesterol with deconjugated bile (Liong and Shah 2005) and found that *Lb. acidophilus* strains had higher deconjugation ability than *Lb. casei* strains. Bifidobacteria can actively assimilate cholesterol and other organic acids. The organisms themselves may take up cholesterol during their growth in the small intestine and make it unavailable for absorption into the blood stream. Lavanya and coworkers (2011) finally proved that the probiotic microorganisms isolated from fermented milk reduces the cholesterol level in the presence of 0.3% bile salt ranging from 28% to 83%. The most recent reviewers highlighted the ability of all these probiotics as a novel alternative to chemical drugs to reduce blood cholesterol level (Anandharaj et al. 2014).

6.1.2.8 Immune System Stimulation

Immunomodulation by *Lb. acidophilus* and bifidobacteria has been observed (Schiffrin et al. 1995). The mechanism for immunomodulation is not clearly understood. The translocation of a small number of ingested bacteria via M cells to the Payer's patches of the gut-associated lymphoid tissue in the small intestine is claimed to be responsible for enhancing immunity. The ingestion of probiotic yoghurt has been reported to stimulate cytokine production in blood cells (Solis-Pereira and Lemonnier 1996) and enhance the activities of macrophages (Marteau et al. 1997).

6.1.3 Prebiotics and Synbiotics

The beneficial effects of the presence of bifidobacteria in the gastrointestinal tract are dependent on their viability and metabolic activity. The growth of bifidobacteria is dependent on the presence of a complex carbohydrate known as oligosaccharides. To maximize effectiveness of bifidus products, prebiotics are used in probiotic foods. Prebiotics are "non-digestible food that beneficially affects the host by selectively stimulating the growth and/or activity of one or a limited number of bacteria in the colon" (Gibson and Roberfroid 1995).

Some oligosaccharides, due to their chemical structure, are resistant to digestive enzymes and therefore pass into the large intestine where they become available for fermentation by saccharolytic bacteria. Compounds which are either partially degraded or not degraded by the host and are preferentially utilized by bifidobacteria as carbon and energy sources are referred to as "bifidogenic factors." Some bifidogenic factors that are of commercial significance include fructooligosaccharides, lactose derivatives such as lactulose, lactitol, galactooligosaccharides, and soybean oligosaccharides (O'Sullivan 1996). Resistant starch and non-starch oligosaccharides are classified as colonic foods, but not as prebiotics because they are not metabolized by certain beneficial bacteria (O'Sullivan 1996). Djouzi and Andrieux (1997) studied the effects of three oligosaccharides on the metabolism of intestinal microflora in germ-free rats inoculated with human fecal flora. Fructooligosaccharides and galacto-oligosaccharides increased the bifidobacteria number by 2 log cycles.

Products that contain both prebiotics and probiotics are referred to as "synbiotics." Synbiotics are a combination of the effects of probiotics and prebiotics to produce health-enhancing functional food ingredients. Japan is the world leader in probiotic and prebiotic products. The majority of yoghurts marketed in recent years in Australia, the United States, and Europe contain probiotic bacteria and some form of prebiotics. Liong and Shah (2006) evaluated the effectiveness of three synbiotic diets [(a) LF diet, (b) LMdiet, (c) LFM diet] to minimize serum cholesterol in male rats. They found that the symbiotic (LFM) diet that contained *L. casei* ASCC 292, fructooligosaccharide, and maltodextrin significantly reduced cholesterol levels.

6.2 Conclusions

Probiotic foods are a good example of functional foods, that are becoming increasingly popular. Several health benefits have been claimed for probiotic bacteria; however, not all probiotic bacteria are effective in providing health benefits. Proper strain selection should be carried out in order to incorporate the strains that provide the claimed health benefits. The combination of prebiotics along with probiotic bacteria to modify gastrointestinal flora have the potential to provide a complete food for maximum health benefits.

References

Alakomi, H.L., Skytta, E., Saarela, M., Mattila-Sandholm, T., Latva-Kala, K., and Helander, I.M. 2000. Lactic acid permeabilizes Gram-negative bacteria by disrupting the outer membrane. *Applied and Environmental Microbiology* 66: 2001–2005.

Ali, F.S., Saad, O.A.O., and Hussain, S.A. 2013. Antimicrobial activity of probiotic bacteria. *Egyptian Academic Journal of Biological Sciences* 5(2): 21–34.

Anandharaj, M., Sivasankari, B., and Rani, R.P. 2014. Effects of probiotics, prebiotics, and synbiotics on hypercholesterolemia: A review. *Chinese Journal of Biology* 2014:1–7.

Anderson, K.V. 2000. Toll-like receptors: Critical proteins linking innate and acquired immunity. *Current Opinion in Immunology* 12: 13–19.

Anderson, K.V. and Gilliland, S.E. 1999. Effect of fermented milk (yogurt) containing *Lactobacillus acidophilus* L1 on serum cholesterol in hypercholesterolemic humans. *Journal of the American College of Nutrition* 18(1): 43–50.

Armuzzi, A., Cremonini, F., Bartolozzi, F., Canducci, F., Candelli, M., Ojetti, V., Cammaroto, G. et al. 2001. The effect of oral administration of *Lactobacillus GG* on antibiotic-associated gastrointestinal side-effects during *Helicobacter pylori* eradication therapy. *Alimentary Pharmacology and Therapeutics* 15:163–169.

Ashraf, M., Arshad, M., Siddique, M., and Muhammad, G. 2009. *In vitro* screening of locally isolated Lactobacillus species for probiotic properties. *Pakistan Veterinary Journal* 29(4):186–190.

Ayebo, A.D., Shahani, K.M., Dam, R., and Friend, B.A. 1982. Ion exchange separation of the antitumor component(s) of yogurt dialysate. *Journal of Dairy Science* 65(2): 2388–2390.

Begley, M., Hill, C., and Gahan, C.G.M. 2006. Bile salt hydrolase activity in probiotics. *Applied and Environmental Microbiology* 72: 1729–1738.

Buttriss, J. 1997. Nutritional properties of fermented milk products. *International Journal of Dairy Technology* 50(1):21–27.

Cats, A., Kulpers, E.J., Bosschaert, M.A., Pot, R.G., Vandenbroucke-Gauls, C.M., and Kusters, J.G. 2003. Effect of frequent consumption of *Lactobacillus casei* – containing milk drink in *Helicobacter pylor*-colonised subjects. *Alimentary Pharmacology Therapeutics* 17(3):429–435.

Cenci, G., Rossi, J., Throtta, F., and Caldini, G. 2002. Lactic acid bacteria isolated from dairy products inhibit genotoxic effect of 4-nitroquinoline-1-oxide in SOS-chromotest. *Systematic and Applied Microbiology* 25 (4):483–90.

Djouzi, Z. and Andrieux, C. 1997. Compared effects of three oligosaccharides on metabolism of intestinal microflora in rats inoculated with a human faecal flora. *British Journal of Nutrition* 78(2): 313–24.

Erdourul, O. and Erbilir, F. 2006. Isolation and characterization of *Lactobacillus bulgaricus* and *Lactobacillus casei* from various foods. *Turkish Journal of Biology* 30:39–44.

Falagas, M.E., Betsi, G.I., and Athanasiou, S. 2007. Probiotics for the treatment of women with bacterial vaginosis. *Clinical Microbiology and Infection* 13(7): 657–664.

Gibson, G.R. and Roberfroid, M.B. 1995. Dietary modulation of the human colonic microbiota: introducing the concept of prebiotics. *Journal of Nutrition* 125: 1401–1412.

Gilliland, S.E., Nelson, C.R., and Maxwell, C. 1985. Assimilation of cholesterol by *Lactobacillus acidophilus*. *Appliedand Environmental Microbiology* 49(2): 377–381.

Goldin, B.R. and Gorbach, S.L. 1977. Alterations in faecalmicroflora enzymes related to diet, age, lactobacillus supplement and dimethyl hydrazine. *Cancer* 40: 2421–2426.

Goldin, B.R. and Gorbach, S.L. 1984. The effect of milk and *Lactobacillus* feeding on human intestinal bacterial enzyme activity. *American Journal of Clinical Nutrition* 39:756–761.

Granucci, F. and Ricciardi-Castagnoli, P. 2003. Interactions of bacterial pathogens with dendritic cells during invasion of mucosal surfaces. *Current Opinion in Microbiology* 6:72–76.

Hertzler, S.R. and Clancy, S.M. 2003. Kefir improves lactose digestion and tolerance in adults with lactose maldigestion. *Journal of the American Dietetic Association* 103: 582–587.

Hirayama, K. and Rafter, J. 1999. The role of lactic acid bacteria in colon cancer prevention: mechanistic considerations. *Antonie van Leeuwenhoek* 76(1): 391–394.

Homma, N. 1988. Bifidobacteria as a resistance factor in human beings. *Bifidobacteria Microflora* 7: 35–43.

Hsieh, M.L. and Chou, C.C. 2006. Mutagenicity and antimutagenic effect of soymilk fermented with lactic acid bacteria and bifidobacteria. *International Journal of Food Microbiology* 111: 43–47.

Jaspers, D.A., Massey, L.K. and Leudecke, L.O. 1984. Effect of consuming yoghurts prepared with three culture strains on human serum lipoproteins. *Journal of Food Science* 49:1178–1181.

Jensen, R. G. 1995. *Handbook of milk composition*. San Diego: Academic Press, pp. 1–3.

Jones, M. L., Chen, H., Ouyang, W., Metz, T., and Prakash, S. 2004. Microencapsulated genetically engineered *Lactobacillus Pantarum* 80 (pCBH1) for bile acid deconjugation and its implication in lowering cholesterol. *Journal of Biomedicine and Biotechnology* 2004(1): 61–69.

Klaver, F.A.M. and Meer, R.V.D. 1993. The assumed assimilation of cholesterol by lactobacilli and *Bifidobacteriumbifidum* is due to their bile salt deconjugating activity. *Applied and Environmental Microbiology* 59(4):1120–1124.

Kosikowski, F. and Mistry, V.V. 1997. Fermented milk foods—Origins and principles, Vol. 1. Wesport, CT, USA: F.V. Kosikowski-L.L.C., pp. 87–108.

Kumar, M., Kumar, A., and Nagpal, R. 2010. Cancer preventing attributes of probiotics: An update. *International Journal of Food Sciences and Nutrition* 61(5): 473–496.

Kumar, M., Verma, V., Nagpal, R., Kumar, A., Behare, P.V., and Agarwal, P.K. 2012. Anticarcinogenic effect of probiotic fermented milk and chlorophyllin on aflatoxin-B?-induced liver carcinogenesis in rats. *British Journal of Nutrition* 107(7): 1006–1016.

Kurmann, J.A. and Rasic, J.L. 1988. Technology of fermented special products. Fermented milks: Science and technology. *International Dairy Federation* Bulletin No. 277. Brussels: IDF, pp. 101–109.

Lankaputhra, W.E.V. and Shah, N.P. 1998a. Adherence of probiotic bacteria to human colonic cells. *Bioscience and Microflora* 17:105–113.

Lankaputhra, W.E.V. and Shah, N.P. 1998b. Antimutagenic properties of probiotic bacteria and of organic acids. *Mutation Research* 397:169–182.

Lavanya, B., Sowmiya, S., Balaji, S., and Muthuvelan, B. 2011. Plasmid profiling and curing of Lactobacillus strains isolated from fermented milk for probiotic applications. *Advance Journal of Food Science and Technology* 3(2): 95–101.

Lee, N.K., Park, J.S., Park, E., and Paik, H.D. 2007. Adherence and anticarcinogenic effects of *Bacillus polyfermenticus* SCD in the large intestine. *Letters in Applied Microbiology* 44: 274–278.

Lim, H.J., Kim, S.Y., and Lee, W.K. 2004. Isolation of cholesterol-lowering lactic acid bacteria from human intestine for probiotic use. *Journal of Veterinary Science* 5(4):391–395.

Liong, M.T. and Shah, N.P. 2005. Acid and bile tolerance and cholesterol removal ability of lactobacilli strains. *Journal of Dairy Science* 88(1): 55–66.

Liong, M.T. and Shah, N.P. 2006. Effects of *Lactobacillus caseisynbiotic* on serum lipoprotein, intestinal microflora and organic acids in rats. *Journal Dairy Science* 89(5): 1390–1399.

Mądry, E., Krasińska, B., Woźniewicz, M. G., Drzymała-Czyż, S.A., Bobkowski, W., Torlińska, T., and Walkowiak, J.A. 2011. Tolerance of different dairy products in subjects with symptomatic lactose malabsorption due to adult type hypolactasia. *Gastroenterology Review* 5: 310.

McJarrow, P., Schnell, N., Jumpsen, J., and Clandinin, T. 2009. Influence of dietary gangliosides on neonatal brain development. *Nutrition reviews* 67(8):451–463.

Mann, G.V. and Spoerry, A. 1974. Studies of a surfactant and cholesterolemia in the Massai. *American Journal of Clinical Nutrition* 27:464–469.

Marteau, P., Vaerman, J.P., Dehennin, J.P., Bord, S., Brassart, D., Pochart, P., Desjeux, J.F., and Rambaud, J.C. 1997. Effects of intrajejunal perfusion and chronic ingestion of *Lactobacillus johnsonii*strain La1 on serum concentrations and jejunal secretions of immunoglobulins and serum proteins in healthy humans. *Gastroentérologiecliniqueetbiologique* 21(4): 293–298.

Mitsuoka, T. 2014. Development of Functional Foods. *Bioscience of Microbiota, Food and Health* 33(3): 117–128.

Montalto, M., Nucera, G., Santoro, L., Curigliano, V., Vastola, M., Covino, M., Cuoco, L., Manna, R., Gasbarrini, A., and Gasbarrini, G. 2005. Effect of exogenous beta-galactosidase in patients with lactose malabsorption and intolerance: a crossover double-blind placebo-controlled study. *European Journal of Clinical Nutrition* 59: 489–493.

O'Sullivan, M.G. 1996. Metabolism of bifidogenic factors by gut flora–An overview. *International Dairy Federation* Bulletin, No. 313: 23, Brussels: IDF.

Onwulata, C.I., Ramkishan Rao, D., and Vankineni, P. 1989. Relative efficiency of yogurt, sweet acidophilus milk, hydrolysed-lactose milk, and a commercial lactase tablet in alleviating lactose maldigestion. *American Journal of Clinical Nutrition* 49: 1233–1237.

Orrhage, K., Sillerstrom, E., Gustafsson, J.A., Nord, C.E., and Rafter, J. 1994. Binding of mutagenic heterocyclic amines by intestinal and lactic acid bacteria. *Mutation Research* 311: 239–248.

Panesar, P.S. 2011. Fermented dairy products: Starter cultures and potential nutritional benefits. *Food and Nutrition Sciences* 2: 47–51.

Pasare, C. and Medzhitov, R. 2005. Toll-like receptors: Linking innate and adaptive immunity. *Advances in Experimental Medicine and Biology* 560: 11–18.

Pereira, D.I.A. and Gibson, G.R. 2002. Cholesterol assimilation by lactic acid bacteria and bifidobacteria isolated from the human gut. *Applied and Environmental Microbiology* 68: 4689–4693.

Pool-Zobel, B.L. 2005. Inulin-type fructans and reduction in colon cancer risk: Review of experimental and human data. *British Journal of Nutrition* 93(1): S73–S90.

Rafter, J. 2002. Lactic acid bacteria and cancer: Mechanistic perspective. *British Journal of Nutrition* 88(supl.): S89–S94.

Rao, D.R., Chawan, C.B., and Pulusani, S.R. 1981. Influence of milk and thermophilus milk on plasma cholesterol levels and hepatic cholesterogenesis in rats. *Journal of Food Science* 46(5): 1339–1341.

Ronka, E., Malinena, E., Saarelab, M., Rinta-Koskic, M., Aarnikunnasa, J., and Palva, A., 2003. Probiotic and milk technological properties of *Lactobacillus brevis*. *International Journal of Food Microbiology* 83: 63–74.

Ryan, K.A., Jayaraman, T., Daly, P., Canchaya, C., Curran, S., Fang, F., Quigley, E. M., and O'Toole, P.W. 2008. Isolation of Lactobacilli with probiotic properties from the human stomach. *Letters in Applied Microbiology* 47(4): 269–274.

Sah, B.N., Vasilijevic, T., McKechnic, S., and Donkor, O.N. 2014. Effect of probiotics on antioxidant and antimutagenic activities of crude peptides extracted from yoghurt. *Food Chemistry* 156: 264–270.

Savaiano, D.A., ElAnouar, A.A., Smith, D.J., Levitt, M.D. 1984. Lactose malabsorption from yogurt, pasteurized yogurt, sweet acidophilus milk, and cultured milk in lactase-deficient individuals. *American Journal of Clinical Nutrition* 40: 1219.

Savaiano, D. A. and Levitt, M.D. 1987. Milk intolerance and microbe-containing dairy foods. *Journal of Dairy Science* 70(2): 397–406.

Schiffrin, E.J., Rochat, F., Link-Amster, H., Aeschlimann, J.M., and Donnet-Hughes, A. 1995. Immunomodulation of human blood cells following the ingestion of lactic acid bacteria. *Journal of Dairy Science* 78(3): 491–197.

Shah, N.P. 1993. Effectiveness of dairy products in alleviation of lactose intolerance. *Food Australia* 45:268–271.

Shah, N.P. 1994. *Lactobacillus acidophilus* and lactose intolerance: a review. *Asean Food Journal* 9(2): 47–54.

Shah, N.P. 1999. Probiotic bacteria: antimicrobial and antimutagenic properties. *Probiotica* 6: 1–3.

Shah, N.P. 2000. Probiotic bacteria: Selective enumeration and survival in dairy foods. *Journal of Dairy Science* 83: 894–907.

Shah, N.P. 2001. Functional foods, probiotics and prebiotics. *Food Technology* 55(11): 46–53.

Shah, N.P., and Jelen, P. 1991. Lactose absorption by post-weanling rats from yoghurt, quarg, and quarg whey. *Journal of Dairy Science* 74:1512–1520.

Shah, N.P., Fedorak, R.N., and Jelen, P. 1992. Food consistency effects of quarg in lactose absorption by lactose intolerant individuals. *International Dairy Journal* 2:257–269.

Shida, K. and Nomoto, K. 2013. Probiotics as efficient immunopotentiators: Translational role in cancer prevention. *The Indian Journal of Medical Research* 138(5): 808–814.

Smith, J.G. 1995. Molecular and genetic effects of dietary derived butyric acid. *Food Technology* 49:87–90.

Solis-Pereira, B. and Lemonnier, D. 1996. Induction of human cytokines by bacteria used in dairyfoods. *Nutrition Research* 13:1127–1140.

Vass, A., Szakaly, S., and Schmidt, P. 1984. Experimental study of the nutritional biological characters of fermented milks. *Acta Medica Hungarica* 41(2-3): 157–161.

Vesa, T.H., Marteau, P., Zidi, S., Briet, F., Pochart, P., and Rambaud, J.C. 1996. Digestion and tolerance of lactose from yoghurt and different semi-solid fermented dairy products containing *Lactobacillus acidophilus* and bifidobacteria in lactose maldigesters—Is bacterial lactase important? *European Journal of Clinical Nutrition* 50: 730–733.

Weill, F.S., Cela, E.M., Paz, M.L., Ferrari, A., Leoni, J., and Gonzalez Maglio, D.H. 2013. Lipoteichoic acid from *Lactobacillus rhamnosus GG* as an oral photoprotective agent against UV-induced carcinogenesis. *British Journal of Nutrition* 109: 457–466.

Wollowski, I., Bakalinsky, A.T., Neudecker, C., and Pool-Zobel, B.L. 1999. Bacteria used for the production of yoghurt inactive carcinogens and prevent DNA damage in the colon of rats. *Journal of Nutrition* 129: 77–82.

Yoon, H., Benamouzig, R., Little, J., Francois-Collange, M., and Tome, D. 2000. Systematic review of epidemiological studies on meat, dairy products and egg consumption and risk of colorectal adenomas. *European Journal of Cancer Prevention* 9: 151–164.

Chapter 7

Health Benefits of Yogurt

Ramesh C. Chandan

Contents

7.1 Introduction

Recent knowledge supports the hypothesis that diet may play a beneficial role in some diseases because the main role of diet is to provide sufficient nutrients to meet metabolic requirements while giving the consumer a feeling of satisfaction and well-being (Granato et al. 2010). The diet-health link is now an integral part of a healthy life style. The role of diet and specific foods for the

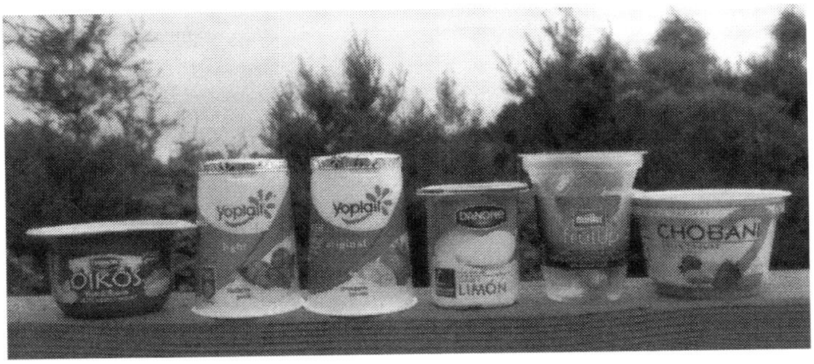

Figure 7.1 Commercial yogurt samples.

prevention and treatment of disease and improvement of body functions is now being recognized. Currently, an interactive discipline of nutrition and food science has produced an array of food products that represent a vibrant, dynamic, and emerging segment of the food industry. Such foods in the diet furnish traditionally recognized nutrients and additionally provide specific health benefits. The objective of consuming these foods is to rectify or manage certain disease states, reduce the risk of disease, or maintain good health. Yogurt has been a part of the human diet for several thousands of years and constitutes a notable example of such functional foods.

This chapter presents an overview of the benefits of consuming yogurt. The components of milk, the starting material of yogurt, furnish vital nutrients to the consumers of yogurt. In addition, the yogurt culture (*Lactobacillus delbrueckii* subsp. *bulgaricus* and *Streptococcus thermophilus*) and its fermentation products provide tangible health benefits. Most yogurts now do contain supplemental probiotic organisms (lactobacilli and bifidobacteria) which confer additional health benefits. Accordingly, probiotics are also discussed briefly to discuss additional overall benefits attributed to yogurt intake.

Some international brands of commercial yogurt are shown in Figure 7.1.

7.2 Basics of Yogurt Science and Technology

7.2.1 Definition of Yogurt

Yogurt is defined by the US Food and Drug Administration (FDA CFR 2011) as the food produced by culturing a standardized yogurt mix (defined below) with a characterizing bacterial culture that contains the lactic acid-producing bacteria *Lb. delbrueckii* subsp. *bulgaricus* and *Strep. thermophilus*. The dairy ingredients permitted in the yogurt mix are cream, milk, partially skimmed milk, or skim milk, used alone or in combination. One or more of the other optional ingredients are also allowed to increase the nonfat solids of the food provided that the ratio of protein to nonfat solids and the protein efficiency ratio of all the protein present in the mix shall not be decreased as a result of adding such ingredients. These optional ingredients include concentrated skim milk, nonfat dry milk, buttermilk, whey, lactose, lactalbumins, lactoglobulins, or whey modified by partial or complete removal of lactose, and or minerals, to increase the nonfat solids of the food. Yogurt, before the addition of bulky flavors, contains not less than 3.25% milk fat and not less than 8.25% milk solids not fat (SNF), and has a titratable acidity of not less than 0.9%, expressed as lactic acid (Hui 2012). The food may be homogenized and shall be pasteurized or ultrapasteurized prior to the addition of the bacterial culture. Flavoring ingredients may be added after pasteurization or ultrapasteurization. To extend the shelf life of the food, yogurt may be heat-treated after culturing is completed, to destroy viable microorganisms. However, the parenthetical phrase "heat-treated after culturing" shall follow the name of the food (yogurt) on the label.

Optional ingredients are also defined in the regulations.

1. Vitamins A and D. If added, vitamin A shall be present in such quantity that each 946 mL (quart) of the food contains not less than 2000 International Units (IU) thereof, within limits of current good manufacturing practice. If added, vitamin D shall be present in such quantity that each 946 mL (quart) of the food contains 400 IU thereof, within limits of current good manufacturing practice (Hui 2012)
2. Nutritive carbohydrate sweeteners: sugar (sucrose), beet or cane; invert sugar (in paste or syrup form); brown sugar; refiner's syrup; molasses (other than blackstrap); high fructose corn syrup; fructose; fructose syrup; maltose; maltose syrup, dried maltose syrup; malt extract, dried malt extract; malt syrup, dried malt syrup; honey; maple sugar, except table syrup
3. Flavoring ingredients
4. Color additives
5. Stabilizers

7.2.2 Low-Fat Yogurt

Low-fat yogurt has a similar description as given earlier for yogurt, except the milk fat of the product before addition of bulky flavors is not less than 0.5% and not more than 2% (Hui 2012). The minimum SNF content is the same (8.25%) as in yogurt.

7.2.3 Nonfat Yogurt

Nonfat yogurt is the product as per the previous description of yogurt, except the milk fat content before the addition of bulky flavors is less than 0.5% (Hui 2012). The minimum SNF content is the same (8.25%) as in yogurt.

7.2.4 National Yogurt Association Criteria for Live and Active Culture Yogurt

According to the National Yogurt Association (NYA) (1996), *live and active culture yogurt* is the food produced by culturing permitted dairy ingredients with a characterizing culture in accordance with the FDA standards of identity for yogurt. In addition to the use of *Lb. delbrueckii* subsp. *bulgaricus* and *Strep. thermophilus*, live and active culture yogurt may contain other safe and suitable food-grade bacterial cultures. Heat treatment of live and active yogurt, with the description of yogurt, with the intent to kill the culture is not consistent with the maintenance of live and active cultures in the product. Producers of live and active culture yogurt should ensure proper practices of distribution, code dates, and product handling conducive to the maintenance and activity of the culture in the product. Live and active culture yogurt must satisfy the following requirements:

The product must be fermented with both *Lb. delbrueckii* subsp. *bulgaricus* and *Strep. thermophilus*. The cultures must be active at the end of the stated shelf life as determined by the activity test described below. Compliance with this requirement shall be determined by conducting an activity test on a representative sample of yogurt that has been stored at temperatures between 0 and 7°C (32 and 45°F) for refrigerated cup yogurt. The activity test is carried out by pasteurizing 12% solids nonfat dry milk (NFDM) at 92°C (198°F) for 7 min, cooling to 43°C (110°F), adding 3% inoculum of the material under test, and fermenting at 43°C (110°F) for 4 h. The total organisms are to be enumerated in the test material both before and after fermentation by official standard methodology. The activity test is met if there is an increase of 1 log or more during fermentation. In the case of refrigerated cup yogurt, the total population of organisms in live and active culture yogurt must be at least 10^8 cfu/g at the time of manufacture. It is anticipated that if proper distribution practices and handling instructions are followed, the total organisms in refrigerated cup of live and active culture yogurt at the time of consumption will be at least 10^7 cfu/g.

7.2.5 Frozen Yogurt

Frozen yogurt resembles ice cream in its physical state. Both soft-serve and hard-frozen yogurts are popular. These are available in nonfat and low-fat varieties. Frozen yogurt is generally a low acidity product. The industry standards require a minimum titratable acidity of 0.30%, with a minimum contribution of 0.15% as a consequence of fermentation by yogurt bacteria (Chandan 2013).

7.2.6 Yogurt Processing

Details for yogurt science and technology are given elsewhere (Chandan and Nauth 2012, Chandan and Kilara 2013, Chandan 2013, 2014). For yogurt fermentation, the bulk starter is prepared from skim milk with total solids raised from 8.8% to 10%–12% by fortifying with nonfat dry milk. The fortified skim milk is heated to 93–96°C (200–205°F) for 10 min and cooled to 43°C (110°F). It is inoculated with frozen or freeze-dried yogurt culture, stirred for 5 min and incubated quiescently at 43°C (110°F) for 6–8 h to reach 0.9% titratable acidity. The starter is cooled to 4°C (40°F).

Yogurt is a Grade A product (USDHHS 2011). Raw milk and all the dairy ingredients of yogurt must conform to Grade A ordinance. The yogurt mix is prepared from whole milk, partially skimmed milk, condensed skim, nonfat dry milk, whey protein concentrate, and cream. Sucrose is also added at this point for fruit-flavored yogurt. Stabilizers may also be added to prevent the surface appearance of whey and to improve and maintain body, texture, viscosity, and mouthfeel. Whey protein, gelatin, starch, modified starch, and tapioca-based starches may be used without affecting the flavor of yogurt. The mix is heat treated at 85–95°C (185–203°F) and then held for 10–40 min, followed by homogenization treatment carried in two stages; first stage is at 10–20 mega Pascal and the second stage is at 3.5. The mix is then cooled to 43°C (110°F) and inoculated with the yogurt starter. It is then incubated at 43–45°C (109–113°F) until it reaches a pH of 4.7–4.8. Yogurt is cooled quickly to 4°C (40°F).

Greek-style yogurt is prepared by the straining/centrifugation of yogurt made from skim milk. Acid whey is generated in its production. The solids recovered are then used as plain Greek style yogurt or they may be blended with cream, sugar, fruit base, and flavor to produce different varieties. Greek yogurt has grown to occupy 50% of the total yogurt market in the United States. It has twice as much protein as regular yogurt. It resembles *shrikhand* in India and *quark* in Europe.

7.3 Health Aspects of Yogurt

7.3.1 Nutrient-Based Health Attributes

Milk is the main ingredient of yogurt. Fermented milks are enhanced functional foods due to the fact that they contain nutrients of milk as well products of metabolic activities of starter microorganisms in the product. Furthermore, they contain live and active cultures in significant numbers to effect physiological benefits to the consumer (Chandan 2011, 2014, Shah et al. 2013). Generally, yogurt has a higher nutrient density related to 13%–15% milk solids compared with milk at 12.3%. Accordingly, yogurt contains more protein, calcium, and other nutrients than milk, reflecting the extra solids-not-fat content. Greek-style yogurt contains twice as much protein as compared to conventional yogurt. Bacterial mass content and the products of the lactic fermentation further distinguish yogurt from milk. Fat content is standardized to meet consumer demand for low-fat to fat-free foods.

Milk has been described as nature's nearly perfect food as it provides vital nutrients including proteins, essential fatty acids, minerals, and lactose in balanced proportions (Chandan and Kilara 2008, 2013). Milk is composed of a unique set of constituents. These constituents perform a nutritional function as well as physiological functions. They act independently and synergistically with each other. The role of major and minor constituents in human nutrition is intertwined with newly discovered physiological benefits. We will briefly highlight both nutritional and physiological benefits of consuming yogurt and fermented milks.

Leading nutrition experts recognize milk and milk products as important constituents of a well-balanced and nutritionally adequate diet. In this regard, yogurt and milk products complement and supplement nutrients available from grains, legumes, vegetables, fruits, meat, seafood, and poultry. The typical nutritional profile of yogurt is shown in Table 7.1.

Various milk constituents as well as products of yogurt fermentation contribute physiological effects (Table 7.2).

Major milk constituents contributing to nutritional value (Chandan and Kilara 2008) of yogurt are discussed below.

7.3.1.1 Milk Proteins

The major proteins of milk are casein and whey proteins in the ratio of 80 to 20. Casein further consists of various fractions including α_{S1} and α_{S2} -casein, β-casein, and κ-casein (Table 7.3). Also shown are the major whey proteins of milk.

The nutritional value of milk proteins has been recognized for many years. Compared to plant proteins, dairy proteins provide the highest quality and absorption characteristics (Chandan and Kilara 2008, 2013). In other words, to achieve the requisite amino acids, our requirement for protein is much lower when milk proteins are included in our diet.

Both caseins and whey proteins of milk possess biological and physiological properties. The biological properties of milk proteins are summarized in Table 7.4.

In studies with mice, it has been shown that whey proteins enhance humoral immune response (Chandan and Kilara 2008). The sulfhydryl containing amino acids, cysteine and glutathione, are related to immune response. Whey proteins are rich in cysteine. β-Lactoglobulin contains 33 mg of cysteine per gram protein, while α-lactalbumin and bovine serum albumin contain 68 and 69 mg cysteine per gram protein, respectively (Chandan and Kilara 2008). The –SH compounds are also involved in quenching toxic free-radicals.

Table 7.1 Typical Nutritional Profile of Yogurt

Type of Yogurt	*Plain*			*Vanilla*	*Fruit-Flavored*	
	Whole Milk	*Low Fat*	*Nonfat*	*Low Fat*	*Low Fat*	
					#1	*#2*
Nutrient (per 100 g)						
Moisture	87.9	85.07	85.23	79.00	74.48	75.30
Calories (kcal)	61	63	56	85	102	99
Protein (g)	3.47	5.25	5.73	4.93	4.37	3.98
Total fat (g)	3.25	1.55	0.18	1.25	1.08	1.15
Saturated fatty acids (g)	2.096	1.00	0.116	0.806	0.697	0.742
Monounsaturated fatty acids (g)	0.893	0.426	0.049	0.343	0.297	0.316
Polyunsaturated fatty acids (g)	0.092	0.044	0.005	0.036	0.031	0.033
Cholesterol (mg)	13	6	2	5	4	5
Carbohydrates (g)	4.66	7.04	7.68	13.80	19.05	18.64
Total dietary fiber (g)	0	0	0	0	0	0
Sugars, total (g)	4.66	7.04	7.68	13.80	19.05	18.64
Calcium (mg)	121	183	199	171	152	138
Iron (mg)	0.05	0.08	0.09	0.07	0.07	0.06
Magnesium (mg)	12	17	19	16	15	13
Phosphorus (mg)	95	144	157	135	119	109
Potassium (mg)	155	234	255	219	195	177
Sodium (mg)	46	70	77	66	58	53
Zinc (mg)	0.59	0.89	0.97	0.83	0.74	0.67
Ascorbic acid (mg)	0.5	0.8	0.9	0.8	0.7	0.6
Thiamin (mg)	0.029	0.044	0.048	0.042	0.037	0.034
Riboflavin (g)	0.142	0.214	0.234	0.201	0.178	0.162
Niacin (mg)	0.075	0.114	0.124	0.107	0.095	0.086
Vitamin B-6 (mg)	0.032	0.049	0.053	0.045	0.040	0.037
Folate (DFE) (μg)	7	11	12	11	9	9
Vitamin B-12 (μg)	0.37	0.56	0.61	0.53	0.47	0.43
Vitamin A (RAE) (μg)	27	14	2	12	10	11
Vitamin A (IU)	99	51	7	43	36	40

Table 7.1 (*Continued*) Typical Nutritional Profile of Yogurt

Type of Yogurt	*Plain*			*Vanilla*	*Fruit- flavored*	
	Whole Milk	*Low Fat*	*Nonfat*	*Low Fat*	*Low Fat*	
					#1	*#2*
Vitamin E (α-tocopherol) (mg)	0.06	0.03	0.00	0.02	0.02	0.02
Vitamin D (D2 + D3) μg	0.1	0.0	0.0	0.0	0.0	0.0
Vitamin D (IU))	2.0	1.0	0	1	1	1
Vitamin K (phylloquinone)	0.2	0.2	0.2	0.1	0.1	0.1

Source: From Chandan, R.C. Chapter 16 in *Dairy Ingredients for Food Processing*. pp. 387–419. 2011. Copyright Wiley-VCH Verlag GmbH & Co. KGaA. Reproduced with permission; U.S. Department of Agriculture (USDA), June 20, 2014. National Nutrient Data base for Standard Reference Release 26. Basic Reports 01116 to 01121. USDA, Washington, DC.

TABLE 7.2 Milk Constituents with Putative Physiological Effects

Component	*Health Effect*
Butyric acid CLA	Reduce colon cancer risk. Modulate immune function, reduce risk of cancer (stomach, colon, breast, and prostate)
Sphingolipids	May reduce risk of colon cancer
Stearic acid	May modulate blood lipids to reduce risk of cardiovascular and heart disease
Triglycerides	May enhance long-chain fatty acid and calcium absorption
Whey proteins	May modulate immune system, reduce risk of heart disease and cancer, lower blood pressure
Glycomacropeptide	Prevent dental caries, gingivitis, antiviral, antibacterial, bifidogenic
Immunoglobulins	Antibodies against diarrhea and GI tract disturbances
Lactoferrin	Toxin binding, antibacterial, immune modulating, anticarcinogenic, antioxidant, iron absorption
Lactoperoxidase	Antimicrobial
Lysozyme	Antimicrobial, synergistic with immunoglobulins and lactoferrin
Lactose	Calcium absorption
Calcium	Prevent osteoporosis and cancer, control hypertension

Source: From Chandan, R.C. 1999. *Journal of Dairy Science* 82: 2245–2256; Chandan, R.C. Chapter 16 in *Dairy Ingredients for Food Processing*. pp. 387–419. 2011. Copyright Wiley-VCH Verlag GmbH & Co. KGaA. Reproduced with permission.

Table 7.3 Fractions of Casein and Whey Proteins of Cow's Milk

	Concentration (g/L)
Casein Fractions	
α-$_{s1}$-Casein	10.3
α-$_{s2}$-Casein	2.7
β-Casein	9.7
κ-Casein	3.5
C-terminal β-Casein fragments	0.8
Whey Proteins Fractions	
N-terminal β-casein fragments	0.8
β-Lactoglobulin	3.4
α-Lactalbumin	1.3
Immunoglobulins	0.8
Bovine serum albumin	0.4
Lactoferrin	0.02–0.20
Lactoperoxidase	0.03
Lysozyme	130 μg/L

Source: From Chandan, R.C. 1999. *Journal of Dairy Science* 82: 2245–2256; Chandan, R.C. Nutritive and health attributes of dairy ingredients. Chapter 16 in *Dairy Ingredients for Food Processing*. 2011. pp. 387–419; Korhonen, J.J. and Marnila, P. Chapter 8 in *Milk and Dairy Products in Human Nutrition: Production, Composition and Health*. 2013. pp. 148–171; Kukovics, S. and Nemeth, T. Chapter 5 in *Milk and Dairy Products in Human Nutrition: Production, Composition and Health*. 2013. pp. 80–110. Copyright Wiley-VCH Verlag GmbH & Co. KGaA. Reproduced with permission.

α-Lactalbumin is a calcium binding protein and thereby enhances calcium absorption. It is an excellent source of essential amino acids such as tryptophan and cysteine (Chandan 2011). Tryptophan regulates appetite, sleep-waking rhythm, and pain perception. Cysteine is important in functions of –SH compounds. α-Lactalbumin interacts with galactosyltransferase enzyme to promote transfer of galactose from UDP-galactose to glucose to form lactose in the mammary gland.

The immunoglobulins of milk are important for imparting immune defense to the host. IgG1 is a major component (Chandan 2011). Milk contains 0.6 g/L, whereas colostrum contains a substantially higher level of 48 g/L. Other fractions are IgG2, IgA, IgM, all of which provide passive immunity. Lactoferrin has a role in the nonspecific defense of the host against invading pathogens. It is active against several Gram-positive and Gram-negative bacteria, yeasts, fungi, and viruses. Its iron-binding characteristic aids in enhancing iron absorption (Chandan and Shah 2013). Lactoferrin stimulates and protects cells involved in the host defense mechanism. Furthermore, it controls cytokine response.

7.3.1.1.1 Bioactive Peptides

Functional peptides are generated during digestive processes in the body and during the fermentation processes used in fermented dairy foods. They arise from casein as well as from whey proteins (Table 7.4). These peptides are inactive in the native proteins but assume activity after they are released from them. They contain 3–64 amino acids and display a largely hydrophobic character and are resistant to hydrolysis in the gastrointestinal tract (Chandan 2011). They can be absorbed in intact form to exert various physiological effects locally in the gut or may have a systemic effect after entry into the circulatory system. Casomorphins and lactophorins derived from milk proteins are known to be opioid agonists while lactoferroxins and casooxins act as opioid antagonists. The opioids have analgesic properties similar to aspirin. Casokinins are

Table 7.4 Some Functional Properties of Major Milk Proteins and Bioactive Peptides Derived from Them

Protein	*Function*
Caseins	Precursors of bioactive peptides, iron carriers (Ca, Fe, Zn, Cu)
Casomorphins from α- and β-caseins	Opioid agonists
Casoxins from κ-casein	Opioid agonists
Casokinins from α- and β-caseins	Antihypertensive
Casoplatelins from κ-casein and transferring	Antithrombotic
Casecidin from α- and β-caseins	Antimicrobial
Isracidin from α-casein	Antimicrobial
Immunopeptides from α- and β-caseins	Immunostimulants
Phosphopeptides from α- and β-caseins	Mineral carriers
Glycomacropeptide from κ-casein	Antistress effects
α-Lactalbumin	Ca carrier
α -Lactorphin	Lactose synthesis in mammary glands, anticarcinogenic and immunomodulatory effects. Opioid agonists
β-Lactoglobulin	Possible antioxidant, retinol carrier, fatty acid binding
β-Lactorphin	Opioid agonists
Immunoglobulins A, M and G	Protectection of immune system, provide antibodies
Lactoferricin from lactoferrin	Opioid agonists

Source: From Park 2009; Chandan, R.C. Chapter 16 in *Dairy Ingredients for Food Processing*. pp. 387–419. 2011; Korhonen, J.J. and Marnila, P. Chapter 8 in *Milk and Dairy Products in Human Nutrition: Production, Composition and Health*. 148–171. 2013; Kukovics, S. and Nemeth, T. Chapter 5 in *Milk and Dairy Products in Human Nutrition: Production, Composition and Health*. pp. 80–110. 2013. Copyright Wiley-VCH Verlag GmbH & Co. KGaA. Reproduced with permission.

antihypertensive (lower blood pressure), casoplatelins are antithrombotic (reduce blood clotting), immunopeptides are immunostimulants (enhance immune properties), and phosphopeptides are mineral carriers.

Casein phosphopeptides may aid in the bioavailability of calcium, phosphorus, and magnesium for optimum bone health (Chandan 2011, Park 2009). They may also be helpful in preventing dental caries. They may also have a role in secretion of entero-hormones and immune enhancement. The role of casein peptides in the regulation of blood pressure is showing promise. The conversion of angiotensin-I into angiotensin-II is inhibited by certain hydrolyzates of casein and whey proteins (Chandan and Kilara 2008). Since angiotensin-II raises blood pressure by constricting blood vessels, its inhibition causes the lowering of blood pressure. This ACE inhibitory activity would therefore make yogurt and dairy foods a natural functional food for controlling hypertension (Chandan 2011). A commercial ingredient derived by the hydrolysis of milk protein has an anxiolytic bioactive peptide with antistress effects. Psychometric tests and measurement of specific hormonal markers have displayed an antistress effect.

The glycomacropeptide released from κ-casein as result of proteolysis may be involved in regulating digestion as well as in modulating platelet function and thrombosis in a beneficial way. It is reported to suppress appetite by stimulating the CCK hormone. Consequently, it may be a significant ingredient of satiety diets designed for weight reduction. Furthermore, this peptide may inhibit binding of toxins in the gastrointestinal tract. Some miscellaneous bioactive factors are being discovered. Specific proteins for binding vitamin B_{12}, folic acid, and riboflavin may assist in enhancing the bioavailability from milk and other foods. The fat globule membrane protein called butyrophilin is a part of the immune system. Other growth factors in milk may help gut repair after radiation or chemotherapy.

7.3.1.2 Lactose

Lactose, the milk sugar, stimulates the absorption of calcium and magnesium. It has a relatively low glycemic index compared with glucose or sucrose, and hence is suitable for diabetics. It is less cariogenic than other sugars (Chandan 2011). Lactose stimulates bifidobacteria in the colon and thereby prevents infection and improves intestinal health.

Heated milk contains up to 0.2% lactulose, a lactose derivative. Since lactulose is not a digestible ingredient, it acts somewhat like a soluble fiber. Lactulose is generally used for treatment of constipation and chronic encephalopathy. Some recent data indicates that lactulose may enhance calcium absorption in the intestine.

7.3.1.3 Milk Fat

Several positive findings have emerged for the consumption of milk fat. Milk fat exists in an emulsion form in milk making it highly digestible. Also, milk fat contains 10% short- and medium-chain fatty acids. Their 1:3 positions in the glyceride molecule allow gastric lipase with specificity for these positions to predigest them in the stomach itself (Chandan 2011). Butyric acid, a characteristic fatty acid of milk fat, is absorbed in the stomach and small intestine and provides energy similar to carbohydrates. Medium chain fatty acids are transported to the liver for a rapid source of energy. The fatty acids lower the pH facilitating protein digestion. At the same time the acid barrier for pathogenic activity is enhanced. Free fatty acids and monoglycerides are surface tension lowering agents, thereby exerting an anti-infective effect.

Milk fat is a concentrated form of energy. Fat protects the organs and insulates the body from environmental temperature effects. It carries vitamins A, D, E, and K and supplies essential fatty acids including arachidonic acid, linolenic acid, omega 3-linoleic, eicosopentaenoic acid, and docosahexaenoic acid (Chandan 2011). The essential fatty acids cannot be synthesized by the body and must be supplied by the diet.

Conjugated linoleic acids (CLA) are a class of fatty acids found in animal products such as milk and yogurt (Chandan 2011). Rumen flora synthesizes CLA, which have been demonstrated to exhibit potent physiological properties. CLA are strong antioxidant constituents of milk fat and may prevent colon cancer and breast cancer. CLA's has been shown to enhance immune response. Prostaglandin PGE-2 promotes inflammation, artery constriction, and blood clotting. CLA may reduce risk of heart disease by reducing levels of prostaglandin PGE-2. Studies have indicated that CLA may increase bone density, reduce chronic inflammation, and normalize blood glucose levels by increasing insulin sensitivity.

Another constituent of milk fat is sphingolipids. They occur at a level of only 160 μg/kg. Recent studies show that they are hydrolyzed in the gastrointestinal tract to ceramides and sphingoid bases, which help in cell regulation and function. Studies on experimental animals show that sphingolipids inhibit colon cancer, reduce serum cholesterol, and elevate the good cholesterol HDL. They could protect against bacterial toxins as well as against infection.

Butyric acid is liberated from milk fat by lipase in the stomach and small intestine. It may exert beneficial effects on the gastric and intestinal mucosa cells. In the colon, butyric acid is formed by the fermentation of carbohydrates by the resident microbiota. Butyric acid in the colon works as a substrate for colon cells and confers anticancer properties.

7.3.1.4 Minerals and Vitamins

Milk and dairy products are, in general, an excellent source of calcium, phosphorus, and magnesium in the diet. High levels of these minerals are in optimum ratio for bone growth and maintenance. As a food source, milk offers good bioavailability of minerals and vitamins. To prevent osteoporosis, the continued consumption of milk is cited as important by leading experts in nutrition and medical science. Other functions of calcium involve regulation of blood pressure and prevention of colon cancer. Milk is a good source of water-soluble B-vitamins (Chandan 2011). The fat-soluble vitamins A, D, E, and K are well known for their beneficial role in human nutrition.

7.3.2 Health Attributes due to Probiotic and Beneficial Cultures

Probiotics may be defined as a food or supplement containing concentrates of defined strains of living microorganisms that on ingestion in certain doses exert health benefits beyond inherent basic nutrition (Chandan and Kilara 2013). They are believed to contribute to the well-being of the consumer by improving the host's microbial balance in the gastrointestinal tract. This definition stresses the importance of ingestion of several hundred millions of live and active microbial culture. There has been marked proliferation in the number of probiotic products on the market. Probiotics and associated ingredients might add an attractive dimension to cultured dairy foods for effecting special functional attributes. Milk is an excellent medium to carry or generate live and active cultured dairy products. The buffering action of the milk proteins keeps the probiotics active during their transit through the gastrointestinal tract. Some other carriers are fruit juices, candies, ice cream, and cheese.

7.3.2.1 Beneficial Microflora

Cultures associated with health benefits are yogurt bacteria (*Strep. thermophilus* and *Lb. delbrueckii* spp. *bulgaricus*), other lactobacilli and bifidobacteria (Chandan 1999). Table 7.5 gives a list of various probiotics being used in commercial fermented milks.

Yogurt organisms possess a distinctly high lactase activity, making it easily digestible by individuals with a lactose-maldigestion condition. To bolster probiotic function, most commercial yogurt is now supplemented with *Lactobacillus acidophilus* and *Bifidobacterium* spp. The strains of lactic acid bacteria used in probiotics are mostly intestinal isolates such as *Lb. acidophilus, Lb. casei, Enterococcus faecium, Enterococcus faecalis,* and *Bifidobacterium bifidum*. Yogurt starter bacteria, *Lb. delbrueckii* ssp. *bulgaricus* and *Strep. thermophilus*, are also included in this table because yogurt has been associated with several health benefits in the past (Chandan and Nauth 2012). They are now reported to persist and remain viable throughout the gastrointestinal tract of rats and humans. The necessity for continuous ingestion in such cases is obvious.

7.3.2.2 Major Benefits

In the literature, a number of healthful benefits of yogurt and fermented milks have been assigned against colitis, constipation, various kinds of diarrhea, gastric acidity, gastroenteritis, indigestion, intoxication (bacterial toxins), diabetes, hypercholesteremia, kidney and bladder disorders, lactose intolerance, liver and bile disorders, obesity, skin disorders, tuberculosis, vaginitis and urinary tract infections, cancer prevention, prevention and treatment of *Helicobacter pylori* gastritis, and irritable bowel syndrome (Chandan and Nauth 2012).

It is generally agreed that *Lb. delbrueckii* subsp. *bulgaricus* and *Strep. thermophilus*, the yogurt bacteria do not adhere to the mucosal surfaces of the intestinal tract during their transit through the gut. Feeding trials with Gottingen minipigs appear to indicate that these yogurt organisms do survive the passage to the terminal ileum (Chandan and Nauth 2012). The numbers detected (10^6–10^7 cfu/g of chyme) are considered to be high enough to be considered for a potential probiotic. It is believed that the gut is home to 400–500 species of organisms. The colonic microbial population is 10 times total body cells. Studies have indicated that the total microbiota of each adult individual has a unique pattern reflecting their differences in composition which is partly dependent on the host genotype. Various health benefits of consuming yogurt containing probiotics have been enumerated in many recent articles (Donovan and Shamir 2014). They are summarized in Table 7.6.

Other reports indicate benefits for prevention of HIV infection, management of dyslipidemia, autism, obesity and diabetes, prevention of recurrence of Crohn's disease, and prevention of urinary tract infections. In addition to probiotics, prebiotics also confer benefits to the consumer (Chandan 2011).

Prebiotic is defined as a nondigestible food ingredient that beneficially affects the host by selectively stimulating the growth and/or activity of one or a limited number of bacteria in the colon that can improve the host health (Chandan 2011). The beneficial effects of the presence of bifidobacteria in the gut are dependent on their viability and metabolic activity. Their growth is stimulated by the presence of complex carbohydrates known as oligosaccharides. Fructo-oligosaccharides (FOS) are well-known prebiotics. FOS may contain 2–8 units in a chain. Inulin, a type of FOS, extracted from chicory root has a degree of polymerization (DP) up to 60. FOS and inulin occur naturally in a variety of fruits, vegetables, and grains, especially chicory, Jerusalem artichoke, bananas, onion, garlic, asparagus, barley, wheat, and tomatoes.

Table 7.5 Probiotic and Beneficial Microorganisms in Commercial Products

Lactobacillus acidophilus
Lactobacillus amylovorus
Lactobacillus crispatus
Lactobacillus johnsoni LA1
Lactobacillus gasseri ADH
Lactobacillus casei/paracasei
Lactobacillus casei subsp. *rhamnosus*
Lactobacillus reuteri
Lactobacillus brevis
Lactobacillus delbrueckii subsp. *bulgaricus*
Lactobacillus fermentum
Lactobacillus gallinarum
Lactobacillus gasseri
Lactobacillus helveticus
Lactobacillus plantarum
Lactobacillus rhamnosus
Lactobacillus salivarius
Bifidobacterium adolescentis
Bifidobacterium animalis
Bifidobacterium bifidum
Bifidobacterium breve
Bifidobacterium infantis
Bifidobacterium longum
Streptococcus thermophilus
Enterococcus faecium
Enterococcus faecalis
Pediococcus acidilactici
Saccharomyces cerevisiae (boulardii)
Bacillus cereus var. toyoi

Source: From Granato, D. et al. 2010. *Comprehensive Reviews in Food Science and Food Safety* 9: 455–470; Chandan, R.C. and Nauth, K.R. 2012. Chapter 12 in *Handbook of Animal-Based Fermented Food and Beverages*, CRC Press, Boca Raton, FL. pp. 213–233; Franz, C.M.A.P., Cho G-S., and Holzapfel, W.H. 2013. Chapter 1 in *Probiotic and Prebiotic Foods: Technological, Stability and Benefits to Human Health.* Nova Science Publishers, NY. pp. 1–23.

Table 7.6 A Summary of Health Benefits of Consumption of Yogurt and Probiotics

Benefit	*Remarks*
Alleviation of lactose intolerance symptoms	Lactose malabsorption is caused by sensitivity to milk sugar lactose in persons lacking the intestinal lactase enzyme. The symptoms include bloating, flatulence, and diarrhea. The enzyme lactase present in yogurt culture assists in lactose digestion and provides relief from the symptoms
Improvement of digestive health	Yogurt culture and probiotics promote a healthy digestive tract by restoring balance in the gut organisms in favor of good bacteria. This change leads to regularity and curbs the growth of undesirable organisms causing diarrhea. Probiotics are helpful in conditions such as irritable bowel syndrome, Crohn's disease, and ulcerative colitis. Alleviation of microbial overpopulation in the small intestine. Treatment of antibiotic-related, rotaviral and *Clostridium difficile* diarrhea, and infant gastroenteritis
Suppression of pathogenic organisms	Lactic acid production in the colon decreases pH leading to suppression of pathogens. Reduces yeast infection. Protection and cure of vaginitis in women
Improvement in bone health maintenance	Yogurt nutrients calcium, magnesium, phosphorus, potassium and protein function together to promote strong healthy bones
Blood pressure control	Yogurt minerals calcium, magnesium and potassium help to lower blood pressure
Cardiovascular benefits	Reduction of serum cholesterol and coronary atherosclerosis by probiotics. Reduction in blood pressure is also documented
Weight control and obesity	Treatment of fatty liver
Inhibition of carcinogen production	Reduction of harmful fecal enzymes, biomarkers of cancer initiation. Prevention of bladder and colon cancer. Positive effects on cervical and bladder cancer
Maintenance of intestinal barrier function	Stimulates mucous production
Modulation of systemic immune responses	Alleviation of dermatitis and skin allergies. Prevention of eczema
Modulation of local immune responses	Inhibition of rotavirus
Beauty and cosmetic benefits	Yogurt's high zinc content keeps skin healthy. Topical application of yogurt fights acne and pimples and helps alleviation of skin discoloration

Source: From Chandan, R.C. Chapter 16 in *Dairy Ingredients for Food Processing*. pp. 387–419. 2011. Copyright Wiley-VCH Verlag GmbH & Co. KGaA. Reproduced with permission; Shah, N.P., da Cruz, A.G., and Faria, J.d.A.F. (Editors) 2013. *Probiotics and Probiotic Foods: Technology, Stability and Benefits to Human Health*. Nova Science Publishers, New York; Heath, S.J., Lewis, J.D.N., and Candy, D.C.A. 2013. Chapter 3 in *Probiotics and Probiotic Foods: Technological, Stability and Benefits to Human Health*. Nova Science Publishers, NY. pp. 41–48.

Prebiotic fermentation leads to health benefits such as increased fecal biomass, and increased stool weight and/or frequency. Prebiotics are fermented by bifidobacteria with the production of short-chain fatty acids (SCFA), mainly acetate, propionate, and butyrate, hydrogen, and carbon dioxide. The production of SCFA leads to lower pH in the colon which facilitates absorption of calcium, magnesium, and zinc. Lower pH also restricts pathogenic and other harmful bacteria thus reducing or eliminating precarcinogenic activity.

Synbiotic refers to a product in which a probiotic and prebiotic are combined. The synbiotic effect may be directed toward two different regions, both the large and small intestines. The combination of pre- and probiotic in one product has been shown to confer benefits beyond those of either on its own.

7.3.2.2.1 Role of Intestinal Flora

The belief in the beneficial effects of the probiotic approach is based on the knowledge that the intestinal microflora provides protection against various diseases (Chandan 1999, 2011, Prentice 2014). The human colon contains colonies of many genera of bacteria. Their number exceeds human body cells. It is recognized that approximately 67% of human immune function is located in the colon. Probiotics have been with us for as long as people have eaten fermented milks. It has been shown that germ-free animals are more susceptible to disease than their conventional counterparts who carry a complete gut flora. This difference has been shown for infections caused by *Salmonella enteritidis* and *Clostridium botulinum*. Another source of evidence that supports the protective effect of the gut flora is the finding that antibiotic-treated animals, including humans can become more susceptible to disease (Saavedra 1995). In humans, pseudomembranous colitis, a disease caused by *Clostridium difficile*, is almost always a consequence of antibiotic treatment (Chandan and Shah 2013).

More supporting evidence comes from experiments in which dosing with fecal suspensions has been shown to prevent infection. In humans it has been shown that *C. difficile* infection can be reversed by administering fecal enemas derived from a healthy human adult. Probiotics also deplete the essential nutrients for the pathogenic organisms thus eliminating their growth. Yogurt is helpful in maintaining gut health (Morelli 2014).

7.3.2.2.2 Mode of Health Benefits Ascribed to Yogurt Consumption

Figure 7.2 illustrates how yogurt and cultured dairy products might exert functional benefits to the consumer (Chandan 1999, Chandan and Shah 2013). Potential mechanisms by which probiotics may exert their beneficial effects are: (a) competition with other microflora for nutrients, (b) production of acids inhibitory to certain enteropathogens, (c) production of bacteriocins or inhibitory metabolites, (d) immunomodulation, and (e) competition for adhesion to intestinal mucosa.

Next, some major known health benefits of consuming yogurt as corroborated by human clinical work are discussed below. Yogurt and fermented dairy products have been recommended in global health according to the proceedings of the first global summit on the health effects of yogurt (Donovan and Shamir 2014, German 2014).

7.3.2.2.3 Ameliorating Symptoms of Lactose Intolerance

There is strong clinical evidence in the literature about the improvement of lactose utilization by yogurt in a large proportion of the world's population who are unable to effectively digest lactose

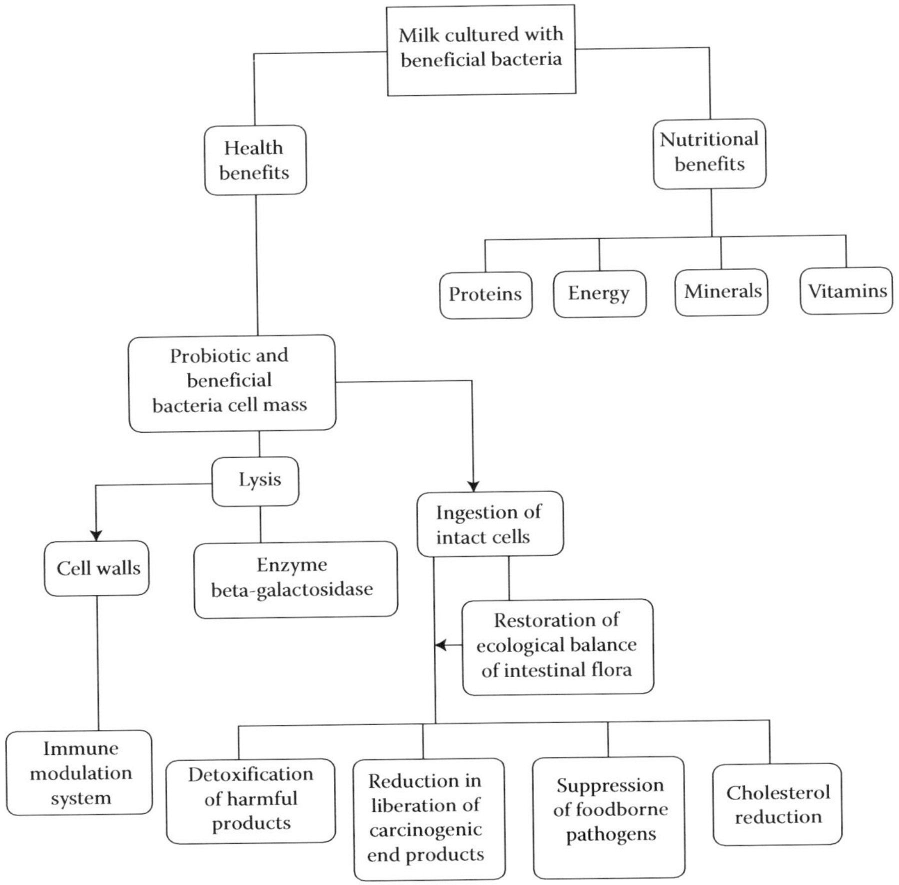

Figure 7.2 Possible mode of health benefits of yogurt and cultured foods. (From Chandan, R. C. 1999. *Journal of Dairy Science* 82: 2245–2256; Chandan, R.C. and Shah, N.P. Chapter 20 in *Manufacturing Yogurt and Fermented Milks*. pp. 413–431. 2013. Copyright Wiley-VCH Verlag GmbH & Co. KGaA. Reproduced with permission.)

(Prentice, 2014, Savaiano 2014). The enzyme lactase responsible for lactose digestion, although present in the suckling infant, disappears after weaning. In areas of the world where milk is not a staple food, the lack of this enzyme causes no problems. Lactose malabsorption refers to incomplete digestion of lactose resulting in a flat or low rise in blood sugar following ingestion of lactose in a clinical lactose intolerance test. The disaccharide lactose is hydrolyzed to glucose and galactose by lactase and subsequently absorbed in the small intestine. Lactase is a constitutive, membrane bound enzyme located in the brush borders of the epithelial cells of the small intestine. The intact residual lactose left over following impaired lactase activity enters the colon where it is fermented by inherent microflora to generate organic acids, carbon dioxide, methane, and hydrogen. The fermentation products together with the osmotically driven excessive water drawn into the colon are primarily responsible for abdominal pain, bloating, cramps, diarrhea, and flatulence. These symptoms are associated with lactose maldigestion when lactose is not fully digested in the small intestine. It has been known for some time that lactose-deficient subjects tolerate lactose in yogurt better than the same amount of lactose in milk. It is possible to show increased lactase activity in the small intestine of humans that have been fed yogurt.

7.3.2.2.4 Bone Health

One of the primary functions of calcium along with protein is to provide strength and structural properties to the bones and teeth. The major sources of dietary calcium are dairy products which are excellent sources of bioavailable calcium. The addition of lactic acid to unfermented yogurt and regular yogurt display improved bone mineralization as compared with unfermented yogurt. It is postulated that the acidic pH due to added lactic acid or naturally contained in fermented yogurt converts colloidal calcium to its ionic form and allows its transport to the mucosal cells of the intestine. Yogurt consumption improves bone health and reduces the risk of fractures in later life (Morelli 2014, Prentice 2014).

7.3.2.2.5 Enhanced Digestion

Yogurt is easier to digest because it assists in lactose and protein digestion. Some of the lactose content is metabolized during fermentation. The remaining intact lactose is broken down to easily absorbable glucose and galactose by the constituent lactase enzyme of the culture (Morelli 2014). In addition, the heating step during yogurt processing denatures whey proteins making them less allergenic. The subsequent fermentation process results in partial digestion of the casein and whey protein by the protein hydrolyzing enzymes of yogurt culture. Compared with milk, the lactic acid content and the vitamin B content of yogurt further assists in overall digestion.

7.3.2.2.6 Reduction in Serum Cholesterol and Cardio-Metabolic Diseases

Research data obtained from clinical studies suggests that yogurt consumption as a part of a healthy diet may be beneficial in the prevention of cardiovascular diseases (Astrup 2014, Marette and Pickard-Deland 2014). Probiotics help to partially reduce cholesterol levels circulating in blood. Some studies have indicated a modest lowering of serum cholesterol in subjects consuming milk fermented with *Lb. acidophilus, Lb. rhamnosus GG* and yogurt cultures. Because of bioavailability of the inherent calcium and potassium, yogurt prevents high blood pressure. Yogurt appears to reduce the risk of metabolic syndrome and related diseases like diabetes.

7.3.2.2.7 Prevention of Diarrhea, Vaginitis, and Dermatitis

Probiotics improve the efficiency of the digestive tract especially when the bowel function is poor. The establishment of probiotics in the gastrointestinal tract may provide prophylactic and therapeutic benefits against intestinal infections. Probiotics may have a role in circumventing traveler's diarrhea. Yogurt supplemented with probiotic organisms reduces the duration of certain types of diarrhea. Yogurt with probiotics has been recommended to replace milk during the treatment of diarrhea because it is tolerated better than milk. A double blind study has shown that only 7% of infants receiving probiotic formula containing *Bif. bifidum* and *Strep. thermophilus* develop diarrhea against 31% incidence in the placebo group (Saavedra et al. 1994). The vaginal microflora changes drastically during bacterial infection. Bacteria of genera *Escherichia, Proteus, Klebsiella* and *Pseudomonas* along with yeast, *Candida albicans* are recognized as etiological agents in urinary tract infection among adult women. It has been shown that the normal urethral, vaginal, and cervical flora of healthy females can competitively block the attachment of uropathogenic bacteria to the surfaces of uroepithelial cells. Lactobacilli strains supplemented in the diet or directly applied are reported to coat the uroepithelial wall and prevent the adherence of uropathogens. Milk fermented with yogurt cultures and *Lb. casei* influenced the intestinal microflora of infants (Guerin-Danan et al. 1998).

7.3.2.2.8 Anticarcinogenesis

Bifidobacteria, and lactobacilli, especially *Lb. acidophilus* have been shown to have powerful anti-carcinogenic features, which are active against certain tumors. An epidemiological study reported a positive correlation between the consumption of probiotics and the prevention of colon cancer. Several reports suggest the prevention of cancer initiation by various probiotics by reducing fecal procarcinogenic enzymes nitroreductase and azoreductase (Lee et al. 1996).

7.3.2.2.9 Immunomodulatory Role

An interesting development in recent years has been the finding that lactobacilli administered by mouth can stimulate macrophage activity against several different species of bacteria (Brassart and Schiffrin 1997, Lee et al. 1996, El-Abbadi et al. 2014). For example, *Lb. casei* given to mice increased phagocytic activity. Lactobacilli injected intravenously are reported to survive in the liver, spleen, and lungs and enhance natural killer cell activity.

7.3.2.2.10 Production of Vitamins and Control of Pathogenic Organisms

Probiotics also produce some of the B-vitamins including niacin, pyridoxine, folic acid, and biotin. In addition, they produce antibacterial substances, which have antimicrobial properties against disease-causing bacteria. Acidophilin produced by *Lb. acidophilus* is reported to inactivate 50% of 27 different disease-causing bacteria. Children with Salmonella poisoning and Shigella infections were cleared of all symptoms using *Lb. acidophilus. Bifidobacterium bifidum* effectively kills or controls *Escherichia coli, Staph. aureus,* and *Shigella*. Acidophilus is also reported to control viruses such as herpes (Chandan and Shah 2013).

7.3.2.2.11 Weight Management

Several studies have been conducted to determine the role of milk and yogurt on human body composition and weight control. This work has suggested that yogurt consumption is associated with a reduced risk of weight gain and obesity (Astrup 2014). Some studies have suggested yogurt may help in reducing or controlling weight and waist circumference in men and women (Jacques and Wang 2014, Kelishadi et al. 2014).

7.3.2.2.12 Reduction of Duration of Common Cold

A recent review supports that consuming yogurt with probiotics decreases the duration of the common cold and upper respiratory tract infections (King et al. 2014). Probiotics have been reported to be useful in the treatment of acne, psoriasis, eczema, allergies, migraine, gout, rheumatic and arthritic conditions, cystitis, candidiasis, colitis and irritable bowel syndrome, and some forms of cancer.

7.3.3 Efficacy Level of Yogurt Cultures

Since the efficacy of yogurt is directly related to the number of live and active cells consumed, it is important to specify potency or colony forming units (CFU) of the culture per unit weight or volume of the product. Many scientists recommend that live and active yogurt should deliver a minimum of 10 million CFU of live and active culture per ml of the product. This level equates to a dose of 100 million CFU of the culture cells when 100 mL of yogurt is consumed (Chandan and Nauth 2012).

7.4 Conclusion

Yogurt has been a part of the human diet for many centuries. Medical research in recent years has corroborated ancient beliefs about the health benefits of yogurt consumption. Milk being the raw material of yogurt and other fermented milks provides nutrients such as vital proteins, milk fat, lactose, minerals, and vitamins. These nutrients have been established to be healthful as a part of the human diet and are strongly associated with adult height and general well-being. More recently, based on clinical and scientific studies, the consumption of milk and dairy products has been advocated as necessary for bone health, weight control and prevention of coronary heart disease, hypertension, and diabetes. Yogurt and fermented milks provide additional health benefits ascribed to the presence of live and active cultures and the metabolic products contained therein. Clinical trials have provided fairly conclusive evidence for the beneficial role of yogurt consumption in gut ecology and in normalizing the composition of beneficial gut bacteria, and for the prevention of gastrointestinal infections. For a certain segment of the human population, the consumption of lactose contained in milk products causes symptoms of bloating, gas, and diarrhea. However, the cultures contained in yogurt provide the enzyme lactase needed for lactose digestion. Thus, lactose-intolerant individuals can safely consume yogurt and derive the full nutritional benefit of dairy products. Similarly, scientific evidence is strong for alleviating the diarrhea associated with travel, antibiotic consumption, and other digestive conditions. There is strong evidence that yogurt consumption boosts the immune system, prevents cancer of the gastrointestinal tract, and certain other organs. More research is needed to ascertain preliminary reports indicating benefits related to *Heliobacter pylori* infection, Crohn's disease, irritable gut syndrome, inflammatory bowel disease, and celiac disease. Similarly, confirmation is needed for antimutagenic effects, antiviral properties, and several other benefits associated with yogurt consumption.

References

Astrup, A. 2014. First global summit on the health benefits of yogurt: Yogurt and dairy product consumption to prevent cardiometabolic diseases: Epidemiologic and experimental studies. *American Journal of Clinical Nutrition* 99: 1235S–1242S.

Brassart, D. E. and Schiffrin, J. 1997. The uses of probiotics to reinforce mucosal defence mechanisms. *Trends in Food Science and Technology* 8: 321–326.

Chandan, R.C. 1999. Enhancing market value of milk by adding cultures. *Journal of Dairy Science* 82: 2245–2256.

Chandan, R.C. 2011. Nutritive and health attributes of dairy ingredients. Chapter 16 in *Dairy Ingredients for Food Processing*. Editors: R.C. Chandan and A. Kilara. Wiley-Blackwell, Ames, Iowa, USA. pp. 387–419.

Chandan, R.C. 2013. History and Consumption Trends. Chapter 1 in *Manufacturing Yogurt and Fermented Milks*. 2nd Edition. Editors: R.C. Chandan and A. Kilara. John Wiley & Sons, Chichester, West Sussex, UK. pp. 3–20.

Chandan, R.C. 2014. Dairy—Fermented Products. Chapter 18 in *Food Processing: Principles and Applications*. 2nd Edition. Editors: S. Clark, S. Jung, and B. P. Lamsal. John Wiley and Sons, Ltd., Chichester, West Sussex, UK. pp. 405–436.

Chandan, R.C. and Kilara, A. 2008. Role of Milk and Dairy Foods in Nutrition and Health. Chapter 18 in *Dairy Processing and Quality Assurance*. Editors: R. C. Chandan, A. Kilara, and N. P. Shah. Wiley-Blackwell, Ames, IA. pp. 411–428.

Chandan, R.C. and Kilara, A. (Editors). 2013. *Manufacturing Yogurt and Fermented Milks*, 2nd. John Wiley & Sons, Chichester, West Sussex, UK. pp. 477.

Chandan, R.C. and Nauth, K.R. 2012. Yogurt. Chapter 12 in *Handbook of Animal-Based Fermented Food and Beverages*, 2nd. Editors: Y.H. Hui, E.O. Evranuz, and R.C. Chandan. CRC Press, Boca Raton, FL. Pages 213–233.

Chandan, R.C. and Shah, N.P. 2013. Functional Foods and Disease Prevention. Chapter 20 in *Manufacturing Yogurt and Fermented Milks*, 2nd. Editors: R.C. Chandan and A. Kilara. John Wiley and Sons, Ltd., Chichester, West Sussex, UK. pp. 413–431.

Donovan, S.M. and Shamir, R. 2014. Introduction to the yogurt in nutrition initiative and the first global summit on the health benefits of yogurt. *American Journal of Clinical Nutrition* 99: 1209S–1211S.

El-Abbadi, N.H., Dao, M.C., and Meydani, S.N. 2014. First global summit on the health benefits of yogurt: Yogurt: Role in healthy and active aging. *American Journal of Clinical Nutrition* 99: 1263S–1270S.

FDA 2011. Code of Federal Regulations 2011: Title 21, Part 131. Milk and Cream 133. Yogurt, Low Fat Yogurt and Nonfat Yogurt. Revised as of April 1, 2011. US Department of Health and Human Services, Food and drug Administration, GMP Publications, Washington, DC. pp. 31–39.

Franz, C.M.A.P., Cho, G-S., and Holzapfel, W.H. 2013. Probiotics: Taxonomy and Technological Features. Chapter 1 in *Probiotic and Prebiotic Foods: Technological, Stability and Benefits to Human Health*. Editors: N.P. Shah, A.G. da Cruz, and J. de A.F. Faria, Nova Science Publishers, NY. pp. 1–23.

German, J.B. 2014. First global summit on the health benefits of yogurt: The future of yogurt: Scientific and regulatory needs. *American Journal of Clinical Nutrition* 99: 1271S–1278S.

Granato, D., Branco, G.F., Cruz, A.G., Faria, J. de A.F., and Shah, N.P. 2010. Probiotic dairy products as functional foods. *Comprehensive Reviews in Food Science and Food Safety* 9: 455–470.

Guerin-Danan, C., Chabanet, C., Pedone, C., Popot, F., Vaissade, P., Bouley, C., Szylit, O., and Andrieux. C. 1998. Milk Fermented with Yogurt Cultures and *Lactobacillus casei* Compared with Yogurt and Gelled Milk: Influence on Intestinal Microflora in Healthy Infants. *American Journal of Clinical Nutrition*, 67: 111–117.

Heath, S.J., Lewis, J.D.N., and Candy, D.C.A. 2013. Mechanisms of Probiotics. Chapter 3 in *Probiotics and Probiotic Foods: Technological, Stability and Benefits to Human Health*. Editors: N.P. Shah, A.G. da Cruz, and J. de A.F. Faria. Nova Science Publishers, NY. pp. 41–48.

Hui, Y.H. 2012. Cottage Cheese and Yogurt: Standards, Grades, and Specifications. Chapter 19 in *Handbook of Animal-Based Fermented Food and Beverages*. 2nd Edition. Editors: Y.H. Hui, E.O. Evranuz, R.C. Chandan. CRC Press, Boca Raton, FL. pp. 319–332.

Jacques, P.F. and Wang, H. 2014. First global summit on the health benefits of yogurt: yogurt and weight management. *American Journal of Clinical Nutrition* 99: 1212S–1216S.

Kelishadi, R., Farajian, S., Safavi, M., Mirlohi, M., and Hashemipour, M. 2014. A randomized triple-masked controlled trial on the effect of synbiotics on inflammation markers in overweight children. *Jornal de Pediatra* 90(2): 161–168.

King, S., Glanville, J., Sanders, M.E., Fitzgerald, A., and Varley, D. 2014. Effectiveness of probiotics on the duration of illness in healthy children and adults who develop common acute respiratory infections: A scientific review and meta-analysis. *British Journal of Nutrition* doi:10.1017/S0007114514000075. pp. 1–14.

Korhonen, J.J. and Marnila, P. 2013. Milk Bioactive Proteins and Peptides. Chapter 8 in *Milk and Dairy Products in Human Nutrition: Production, Composition and Health*. Editors: Y.W. Park and G.F.W. Haenlein. John Wiley and Sons, Ltd., Chichester, West Sussex, UK. pp. 148–171.

Kukovics, S. and Nemeth, T. 2013. Milk major and minor proteins, polymorphisms and non-protein nitrogen. Chapter 5 in *Milk and Dairy Products in Human Nutrition: Production, Composition and Health*.

Editors: Y.W. Park and G.F.W. Haenlein. John Wiley and Sons, Ltd., Chichester, West Sussex, UK. pp. 80–110.

Lee H., Rangavajhyala, N., Gradjean, G., Shahani K.M. 1996. Anticarcinogenic effect of *Lactobacillus acidophilus* on n-nitrosobis (2-oxopropyl) amine induced colon tumor in rats. *Journal of Applied Nutrition* 48: 59–66.

Marette, A., and Pickard-Deland, E. 2014. First global summit on the health benefits of yogurt: Yogurt consumption and impact on health: Focus on children and cardiometabolic risk. *American Journal of Clinical Nutrition* 99: 1243S–1247S.

Morelli, L. 2014. First global summit on the health benefits of yogurt: Yogurt, living cultures, and gut health. *American Journal of Clinical Nutrition* 99: 1248S–1250S.

National Yogurt Association. 1996. Live and Active Culture Program Procedure. McLean, Va.

Park, Y.W. 2009. Overview of Bioactive Components in Milk and Dairy Products. Chapter 1 in *Bioactive Compounds of Milk and Dairy Products*. Editor: Y. W. Park. Wiley Blackwell, Wiley-Blackwell, Ames, Iowa, USA. pp. 3–12.

Prentice, A.M. 2014. First global summit on the health benefits of yogurt. Dairy products in global health. *American Journal of Clinical Nutrition* 99: 1212S–1216S.

Saavedra, J.M. 1995. Microbes to fight microbes: A not so novel approach to controlling diarrheal disease. *Journal of Pediatric Gastroenterology* 21: 125–129.

Saavedra, J.M., Bauman, N.A., Oung, I., Perman, J.A., and Yolken, R.H. 1994. Feeding of *Bifidobacterium bifidum* and *Streptococcus thermophilus* to infants in hospital for prevention of diarrhea and shedding of rotavirus. *Lancet* 344: 1046–1049.

Savaiano, D.A. 2014. First global summit on the health benefits of yogurt: Lactose digestion from yogurt: Mechanism and relevance. *American Journal of Clinical Nutrition* 99: 1251S–1255S.

Shah, N.P., da Cruz, A.G., and Faria, J.d.A.F. (Editors) 2013. *Probiotics and Probiotic Foods: Technology, Stability and Benefits to Human Health*. Nova Science Publishers, New York.

U.S. Department of Agriculture (USDA), June 20, 2014. National Nutrient Data base for Standard Reference Release 26. Basic Reports 01116 to 01121. USDA, Washington, DC.

U.S. Department of Health and Human Services. 2011. Grade "A" Pasteurized Milk Ordinance. 2011 Revision. Department of Public Health, USDHHS, Food and Drug Administration, Washington, DC.

Chapter 8

Health Benefits of Ethnic Indian Milk Products

R. K. Malik and Sheenam Garg

Contents

8.1 Introduction

India is the world's largest milk producer, accounting for more than 16% of the world's milk production. It is also the world's largest consumer of milk and milk products; consuming almost all of the milk it produces (Nargunde 2013). Milk products are the major source of inexpensive, nutritious food available for millions of people in India and the only protein source from animals which is widely accepted by the larger segment of India's vegetarian population, particular among the rural landless, and among small, and marginal farmers and women (Reddy 2010). Production of traditional dairy products in India is estimated at over Rs. 150,000 crores, while the organized sector accounts for Rs. 30,000 crores. These products include curd, *ghee, makkhan, malai, khoa, chhana, paneer, shrikhand,* and a variety of milk sweets, some of which are now increasingly produced by the organized sector in milk plants. These products have great social, religious, cultural, medicinal, and economic significance and have been established over a long period of time with the culinary skills of sweet makers—the *halwais* (Pal and Raju 2007). It is estimated that about 50% of the total milk produced in India is transformed into traditional milk products. Traditional dairy products not only have an established market in India but also have great export potential because of the strong presence of the Indian diaspora in many parts of the world (Rao and Raju 2003).

Dairy foods constitute one of the most important components of the human diet in India as in many other regions of the world. The history of Indian dairy products is perhaps as old as Indian civilization itself. Even as our ancestors began to domesticate milch animals, they found innovative ways to convert highly perishable milk into more stable and longer lasting milk products. It is a part of Indian culture to revere cows. It is a customary practice to grace Indian ceremonies and functions with *ghee, butter, dahi, chhas,* and so on. Traditional milk products represent the most prolific segment of the Indian dairy industry. From time immemorial, traditional Indian foods with their extraordinary variety and richness have served people's need for nutrition and sound health and have also reflected the intimate relationship established with farms and with animals. In ancient India, dairy products had an important bearing on the socio-cultural life of the people. Some dairy products were used for medicinal purposes in ancient Ayurveda as well as in household remedies (Lourens-Hattingh and Viljoen 2001).

Milk is a complete food for newborn mammals characterized by the unique biological secretion of the mammary gland endowed by nature with nutrients to fulfil the nutritional needs of offspring. It is the sole food during the early stages of the development of a child. Milk contains well-balanced macronutrients, including the carbohydrate, fat, and protein required for mammalian growth and development. It is also a good source of micronutrients including calcium, magnesium, and zinc. Milk proteins have a high nutritive value due to the favorable balance of essential amino acids (Buttriss 1997). They are, however, deficient in sulfur-containing amino acids such as cysteine and methionine. Milk also contains antimicrobial substances, which provide protection against infection to neonates. Milk and milk-derived products (Figure 8.1) constitute a significant part of the diet of all ethnic groups of all ages, including a proportion of the food

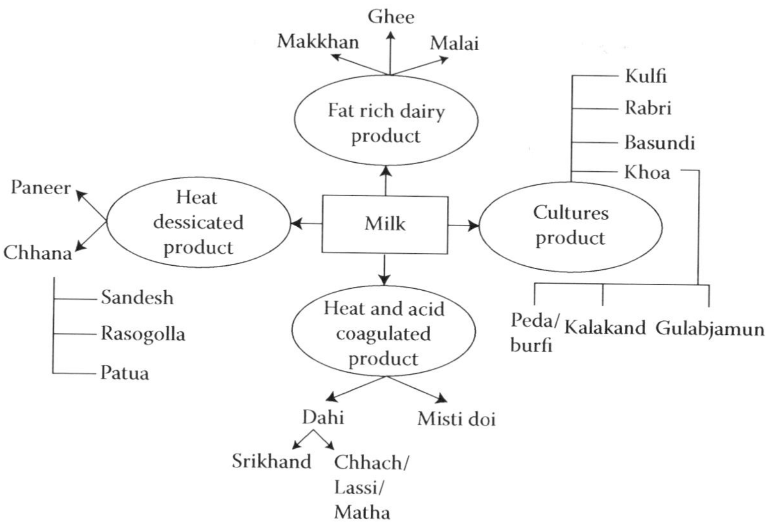

Figure 8.1 Classification of Indian dairy products.

provided to infants. Amongst the several milk products, fermented milks are of great importance worldwide because of their nutritional, organoleptic, and shelf-life properties that are significantly improved in contrast to the raw material that is, milk. Originally fermented milks were developed as a means of preserving the nutrients of milk.

The health benefits of milk and dairy products are well-known to mankind ever since medieval times and may be attributed to the biological active components that are present in milk and milk products (Abdel-Salam 2010). These products contain health benefits providing bioactive peptides, antioxidants, vitamins, specific proteins, oligosaccharides, organic acids, highly absorbable calcium, conjugated linoleic acid (CLA), and probiotic bacteria. These compounds show a wide range of bioactivities, namely, modulation of digestive and gastrointestinal functions, and immune-regulation. Dairy products can potentially be used for improved health or well-being in a range of areas, including antimicrobial function, cardiovascular health, gastrointestinal problems, defense against free radical oxidation and for the enhancement of psychological functions (Bharti et al. 2012). In this chapter, various ethnic Indian dairy products and their health benefits are discussed (Figure 8.1).

8.2 Dahi

The Indian curd known as *dahi* is a well-known fermented milk product consumed by a large section of the population throughout the country, either as a part of daily diet or as a refreshing beverage. The word *dahi* comes from Sanskrit word "dadhi"; there are numerous references to *dahi* in the ancient "vedas" (Yegna Narayan Aiyar 1953). The "Rigveda" mentions curdling of milk with a starter from earlier stock or with pieces of various green leaves, *palasha* bark, and *putika* creeper (Anantakrishnan and Srinivasan 1964). *Dahi* was eaten with barley or rice. The churning of *dahi* to make butter at home and utilizing the refreshing buttermilk with left-over globules of butter in it as a refreshing drink has been practiced for several centuries. According to FSSR

Table 8.1 Average Composition of *Dahi*

Constituent (%)	*Cow Milk*	*Buffalo Milk*	*Skim Milk*
Moisture	85–88	82–85	89–92
Fat	3.5–4.5	6.0–8.0	0.05–0.1
Protein	3.0–3.5	3.5–4.0	3.3–3.5
Lactose	3.8–4.5	4.6–5.2	4.7–5.3
Ash	0.64–0.66	0.7–0.72	–
Lactic acid	0.5–1.0	0.5–1.1	0.5–1.1

Source: Rangappa, K.S. and K.T. Achaya. 1974. *Indian Dairy Products*. Asia Publishing House, Bombay, India, pp. 386.

(2011), *dahi* means the product obtained from pasteurized or boiled milk by souring, natural, or otherwise by harmless bacterial culture. According to the Bureau of Indian Standards (BIS), *dahi* is a product obtained from the lactic fermentation of cow or buffalo or mixed milk through the action of a single or mixed strains of lactic acid bacteria (LAB). This definition does not include milk coagulated by the addition of acids or milk coagulating enzymes. The average composition of *dahi* depends upon the type of milk used (Table 8.1).

Dahi finds a very prominent position in Indian culture, food habits, religious ethos, as also in other South Asian countries (Figure 8.2). In India, *dahi* is traditionally prepared on a small scale in each household using buffalo, cow, or goat milk. Generally, a mixture of cow and buffalo milk is used. Now, the commercial production of *dahi* has become a major activity of the dairy industry in India. It has been estimated that about 50% of the total milk produced in India is converted into traditional fermented milk products (Khurana and Kanawjia 2007) and this sector is showing an annual growth rate of more than 20% (Figure 8.2).

8.2.1 Nutritional Value of Dahi

Dahi is a highly nutritious food containing all the nutrients present in milk (Islam et al. 2010), which is further improved under the influence of the metabolic activity of the starter culture during fermentation. *Dahi* is considered a better food than milk due to its better digestibility. The dietetic value of *dahi* is due to its content of vitamins, proteins, minerals, carbohydrates, and various therapeutic activities (Sarkar 2008). About 20%–30% lactose is hydrolyzed to its absorbable monosaccharide components, glucose and galactose (Bourlioux and Pochart 1988), which makes it suitable for lactose intolerant people. *Dahi* differs from yogurt in its use of mixed starters of mesophilic lactococci. A principal flavor-inducing metabolite is diacetyl, which is appreciated more by people of South Asian origin compared with the acetaldehyde flavor in yogurt (Yadav et al. 2007).

Both heat treatment and acid production result in the finer coagulation of casein, which may also contribute to the greater protein digestibility of *dahi* than that of milk (Adolfsson et al. 2004), making it suitable for children and the elderly. Balasubramanyam et al. (1984) mentioned net protein utilization (NPU), protein efficiency ratio (PER), and biological value (BV) of *dahi* to be 82 ± 0.25, 3.2, 92 ± 1.15, respectively. An improvement in nutritional characteristics is ascribed to improved digestion and absorption of amino acids (Wong et al. 1993) and the presence of easily assimilable proteins resulting from proteolytic activity of starter cultures (Sarkar and Mishra 1998).

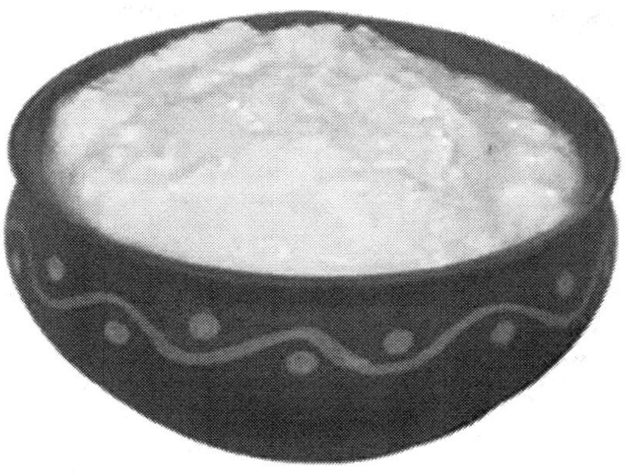

Figure 8.2 Indian dahi.

Dahi has been shown to have a higher concentration of CLA, a long chain bio-hydrogenated derivative of linoleic acid, than the milk from which it has been processed (Shantha et al. 1995). The acidic pH of *dahi* ionizes calcium and thus facilitates intestinal calcium uptake (Bronner and Pansu 1999). During *dahi* manufacture, the maximum increases in folic acid followed by riboflavin and thiamine have been noted (Sharma and Lal 1997), thus making *dahi* a better source of vitamins.

8.2.2 LAB Starter Cultures for Dahi

Specific fermentation under controlled conditions results in a specific fermented product with enhanced organoleptic, nutritional, and therapeutic qualities. The type of starter culture, time, and temperature of incubation used has an impact on the curd formation which in turn affects the sensory and textural qualities of cultured products (Mogra and Choudhry 2008). The amount of inoculum is important for a normal acidification process (Tamime and Robinson 1985). Traditionally, *dahi* or *chhash* of the previous day containing an assorted mixture of LAB is used as the starter culture. Apparently, the microflora depends on the incubation temperature and the time of incubation and storage. Usually, the lactic starter bacteria consist of *Lactococcus lactis* subsp. *lactis, cremoris,* and *diacetylactis, Leuconostoc, Lactobacillus* spp. and *Streptococcus thermophilus. Lactobacillus* spp. dominate in sour *dahi* due to their higher acid tolerance, while lactococci dominate in sweet *dahi* (Aneja et al. 2002). In southern parts of India people consume sour *dahi* wherein lactobacilli and yeast dominate.

A BIS (1980) recommends the use of cultures of *Lactococcus lactis, Lactococcus diacetylactis,* and *Lactococcuscremoris,* singly or in combination with or without *Leuconostoc* species for the preparation of *dahi.* In addition to the above combinations of starter cultures *Lactobacillus delbrueckii* subsp. *bulgaricus, Lactobacillus acidophilus, Lactobacillus casei,* and *Strep. thermophilus* may also be used. Starter cultures not only initiate, but also carry out every change to attain the desired body, texture, and flavor in the cultured dairy product. Furthermore, starters play a preservative role in suppressing spoilage flora, thus increasing shelf-life. Another vital function relates to their protective role in retarding or inhibiting pathogenic flora, and the formation of entero-toxins in the finished cultured dairy product. The starter culture thus determines the shelf-life and the safety of cultured dairy products (Chandan et al. 2006).

8.3 Srikhand

Srikhand is a semisolid sweetish-sour traditional fermented milk product of Indian origin and is very popular in Gujarat, Maharashtra, and certain parts of Karnataka, and Madhya Pradesh (Aneja et al. 2002) (Figure 8.3). *Srikhand* is traditionally produced in the unorganized sector by age old methods. Like *dahi*, it is very refreshing, particularly during the summer months. *Srikhand* is prepared by lactic acid coagulation of milk and expulsion of whey from curd followed by blending of cream, sugar, flavor, color, and spices. Generally, the fermentation of milk is carried out by back-slopping, which contains a mixed type of LAB. The use of the right type of culture is essential for the manufacture of *srikhand.* A mixed culture containing *Lc. lactis* subsp. *lactis*, *Lc. lactis* subsp. *diacetylactis*/*Leuconostoc, Lc.* and *lactis* subsp. *cremoris* in the ratio 1:1:1 is recommended (Aneja et al. 2002). Other recommended cultures are yogurt cultures *Strep. thermophilus* and *Lactobacillusdelbrueckii* subsp. *bulgaricus* in the ratio of 1:1.

According to BIS standards, *srikhand* shall contain not less than 8.5% milk fat (on dry basis not less than 9% protein) and should not contain more than 72.5% sugar on a dry basis. *Srikhand* is prepared by using whole milk as a basic raw material. Usually buffalo milk is preferred as it has a high fat, SNF, and calcium content. In recent years *srikhand* with different flavors such as *kesar, elaichi,* and mango is commercially manufactured in organized dairy sector.

8.4 Chakka

Chakka is obtained by removal of whey from *dahi* and is a base product for *srikhand.* The quality of *srikhand*, the final product is largely governed by the physical and chemical properties of the *chakka*. The yield of the *chakka* depends upon the heat treatment and the total solid contents of the skim milk and the starter culture (Aneja et al. 2002). In the past attempts have been made to prepare *chakka* using direct acidification technology (Sharma and Reuter 1993). *Chakka* prepared from curd using different food grade acids viz., lactic, hydrochloric, and citric acid has been found to be unsatisfactory because of predictable graininess. *Chakka* has better shelf-life than *dahi* due

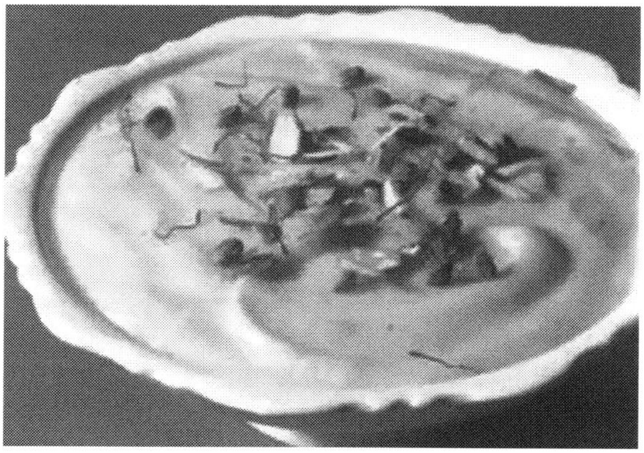

Figure 8.3 Srikhand.

to relatively higher acidity, reduced moisture content (Garg et al. 1983), added sugar (Patel and Chakraborty 1998) and low water activity.

8.5 *Lassi* (Stirred *Dahi*)

Lassi is a refreshing traditional summer beverage of North India, originally from Punjab, prepared by blending *dahi* with water, salt, and spices until frothy. It is estimated that approximately 2144 million liters of *lassi* is produced in India annually. A traditional *lassi* is sometime flavored with sugar, rose water and/or lemon, mango, strawberry, or other fruit juices (Figure 8.4). *Lassi* production has been taken up by the organized sector using different formulations. There are no legal standards or quality standards for this product. Its chemical composition depends on the initial composition of the milk, the degree of concentration of the milk solids, and the quantity of sugar added (Aneja et al. 1989). UHT *lassi* has also been introduced in the market as a long shelf-life product packaged in tetra packs.

8.6 Mattha/Chhach/Chhas

Mattha, chhach, or *chhas* are synonyms for buttermilk which is commonly consumed in all parts of India (Anantakrishnan and Srinivasan 1964). It is a popular refreshing summer beverage. It is a phospholipid-rich fluid fraction obtained as a by-product during the churning of *dahi* while making *makhan* (*desi* fresh butter). It is prepared by churning set *dahi* mixed with water till the butter floats up and is scooped out. The butter is then recovered and the residual watery fluid is consumed as *chhas*. It is a highly flavorful and mildly to highly acidic. The fat retained in *chhas* is comparatively high in low melting constituents of milk fat. The product is also rich in protein and

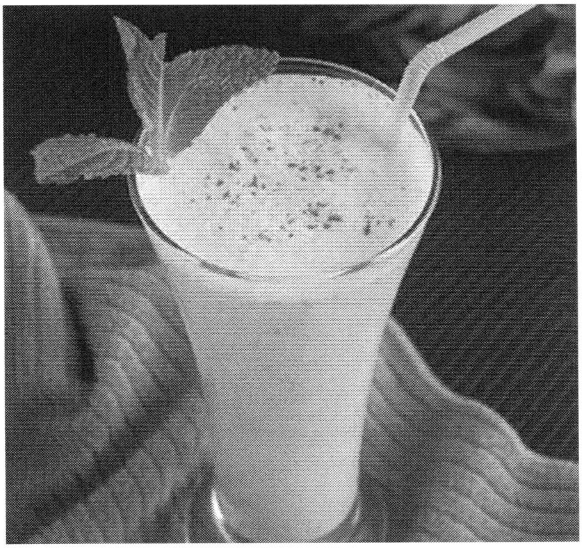

Figure 8.4 Flavored lassi.

lactose (Achaya 1998). The high number of live bacteria present is also thought to provide other healthful and digestive benefits.

8.7 Misti Doi

Misti doi also known as *payodhi* or *lal dahi* is a very popular dessert in the eastern part of India particularly West Bengal, and in Bangladesh (Aneja et al. 2002). It is characterized by a fermented milk product with a light brown color and firm body with a cooked or caramelized flavor (Figure 8.5). Traditionally, *misti doi* is prepared from cow or mixed milk. It contains 2%–9% fat, 10%–14% solids-not-fat, and 17%–19% sugar. The most common sweetener used is cane sugar. In some special varieties of mishit *doi*, fresh palm jaggery is used as a sweetener. The milk is first boiled with the required amount of sugar and partially concentrated by simmering over a low fire, during which it develops a distinctive light cream to light brown caramel color and flavor. It is then cooled to the ambient temperature and cultured with lactic *dahi* culture (1%) and poured into earthen vessels and left undisturbed overnight for fermentation. When a firm body curd has set, it is stored at a low temperature (4°C) and served chilled (De 2002, Aneja et al. 2002, Singh 2007). The most common sweetener used is cane sugar. Due to its pleasant caramel flavor yet sour taste it is liked by all people of all ages. There is now technology available for the industrial manufacture of *misti doi* (Ghosh and Rajoria 1990).

8.8 Makkhan

Makkhan is the traditional unsalted butter made by hand churning whole milk *dahi* (De 1980). Beginning from Vedic times (3000–2000 BC) there is documented proof confirming that *makkhan* was widely used by the early inhabitants of India for both dietary as well as religious purposes. Buffalo milk because of its high fat content and larger fat globules gives higher yields of *makkhan* (FAO 1990). *Makkhan* has a typical soft body and a smooth grainy texture and a distinctive

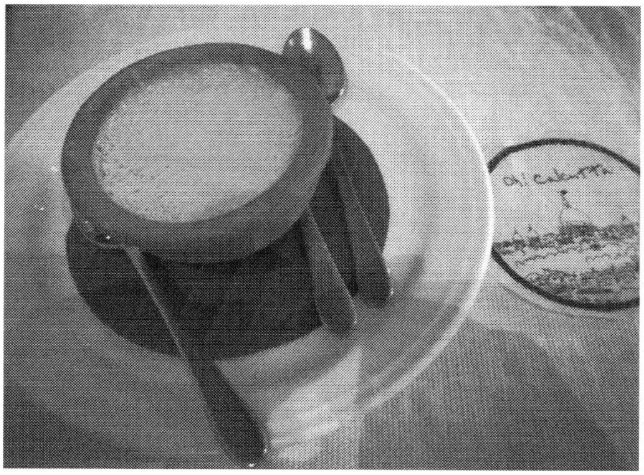

Figure 8.5 Misti doi.

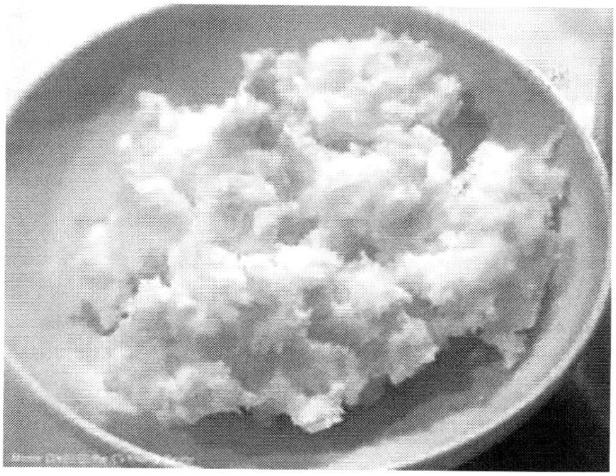

Figure 8.6 Makkhan.

pleasant aroma and flavor derived from the fermented dahi from which it is made. There is no addition of salt or coloring material (Figure 8.6).

Makkhan contains vitamin A, D, E, and K (fat-soluble vitamins) and a small amount of essential fatty acids, arachidonic and linoleic acids. Butter or *makkhan* provides a high calorie value. According to Rujjuta, food that provides high amounts of calories are also more beneficial to the human body, 100 g of butter or *makkhan* provides 750 calories. The molecular structure of butter helps it pass through the layers of tissue that are otherwise impermeable, like that of the brain. It helps the transportation of nutrients to the brain and takes away wastes from it, making the brain function optimally. Butter is packed with the essential mineral selenium, a potent antioxidant along with vitamin E which helps to smoothen the skin and keeps it healthy and elastic. This is what gives that healthy glow to one's skin. In Ayurveda, a number of practitioners prescribe the use of white butter as a remedy for ailments such as ear problems, insomnia, bed wetting, sexual weakness, and even for mental illnesses. It is especially advised for mothers-to-be during their fourth month of pregnancy since it helps nourish the growing child and eases labor. Due to its structure, it helps in the production of compounds that lubricate joints and is especially good for people suffering from arthritis since it increases the lubrication between joints thus helping in reducing the pain associated with the condition. Since butter contains arachidonic acid (AA) that plays an important role in brain function and the maintenance of a healthy cellular structure, it is very good for the proper development of a child's brain. Apart from this, butter has a unique highly absorbable form of vitamin D that is essential for the proper functioning of the synapses (the portion between two nerves that helps the relay of information to and from the brain). Since children's brains are still forming, giving them the right and most essential nourishment is of utmost importance.

8.9 Ghee

Ghee, also known as *ghrita*, has been used in Ayurveda for thousands of years. *Ghee* is mostly prepared by the traditional method used by Indian households or by the direct creamery method at an industry level. Ayurvedic landmarks suggest that *ghrita* made from cow milk is superior

(Joshi 2014). Ancient Sanskrit literature describes *ghee* as a food fit for the gods and a commodity of enormous value. *Ghee* is fairly shelf-stable mainly due to its low moisture content and possible antioxidative properties. *Ghee* contains 99%–99.5% fat and less than 1% moisture, unsaponifiable matter and traces of charred casein, carotene, and fat-soluble vitamins (Srinivasan and Anantakrishnan 1979). The storage stability and quality of *desi ghee* is better than that of direct cream or creamery butter *ghee* because of the presence of phospholipids (Ramamurthy and Narayanan 1971). *Ghee* is one of the four basic elements in Indian cooking. *Ghee*, the Indian name for clarified butterfat is obtained by heat clarification and desiccation of sour cream, cream, or butter at 105–110°C. Heat induced changes in milk proteins/lactose during the clarification process impart a distinctive pleasant cooked flavor to ghee. *Ghee* is the largest indigenous milk product, with an important place in the Indian dietary scenario. The health benefits of the consumption of ghee described in Ayurvedic literature are as follows:

1. *Ghee* increases intelligence, enhances memory power, rejuvenates the skin from inside and increases its glow. It boosts body energy, detoxifies and nourishes the body, normalizes *vata*, (imbalance of *vata* causes diseases), increases clarity of voice, normalizes *pitta*, improves digestion, and increases body fire.
2. *Ghee* increases the quality and quantity of semen, is very effective in eye disorders, and acts as a good *Rasayana* (or rejuvenation, a traditional Ayurvedic therapy to restore the body's vitality to its fullest capacity).
3. *Ghee* is excellent for joint health as it lubricates and oxygenates them.
4. *Ghee* helps you destress, sleep better, and wake up fresher. *Ghee* takes nutrients from your food and delivers them through fat permeable membranes as in the brain.
5. The antioxidants in *ghee* make it a miraculous antiwrinkling and antiageing therapy.
6. *Ghee* is a saturated fat—such a unique structure that actually helps mobilize fats from stubborn fat areas of the body.
7. The SusrutaSamhita claims that *ghee* is good for all parts of the body, and it is the ultimate overall remedy for *pitta* (inflammatory) problems, and is the medium of choice (*anupan*) for mixing medicines for these conditions. Specifically, *ghee* is said to promote memory, intelligence, the quantity and quality of semen, and enhance digestion.

8.10 Fermented Milk Products of North-East India and The Himalayan Region

Yak milk is processed into a number of dairy products such as fermented milk (*kurut*), cheese (*chhurpi), chhur churpen, churkham, chhu, philuk, shyow,* and *maa* (Tamang 2010, Thapa 2002). The chemical composition of yak cheese is around 68.2% of total solids, 49.4% of butterfat on a dry matter basis, and 1.37% of salt. It is largely consumed in the Himalayan highlands and its industrial production has not yet been standardized (Prashant et al. 2009). *Chhurpi* is a white, soft product with a mild to strong flavor and is consumed as a curry mix with wild edible ferns (*Diplazium* spp.), pickles and condiments along with boiled rice in meals (Tamang et al. 2000). In a ripened *chhurpi,* LAB strains except *Leuconostoc mesenteroides* BFE1637 showed high degree of hydrophobicity. This is a significant property of LAB that assists in colonization of epithelial cells. Enzymes such as peptidases and esterase-lipases of LAB strains may play an important role in the improvement of the cheese quality. Similarly, *chhu (sheden)* is a strong flavored traditional cheese-like product in Sikkim, the Darjeeling hills, Arunachal Pradesh, and Ladakh. It is consumed as a curry by cooking it in butter along with onions, tomatoes, and chillies,mixed with beef or yak meat. In a study of the lactic microflora of *chhu*, Dewan and Tamang (2006) observed that LAB were the predominant microflora in this product (8.1–8.8 logCFU/g) and several strains of LAB showed a high degree of hydrophobicity, good acidification and curd forming characteristics, and no production of biogenic amines, thus indicating for their potential use as starter culture.

Shyow is a thick *dahi* (curd) like product, prepared from yak milk, while *mohi* is a refreshing drink prepared by the churning and diluting of *dahi*. *Philu* is a typical indigenous cream-like milk product obtained from cow milk or yak milk and is mostly eaten as a cooked paste delicacy with boiled rice by the Sikkimese (Dewan and Tamang 2007). *Somar* is a soft paste, strongly flavored with a bitter taste, and is consumed as soup along with cooked rice or finger-millet by the Sherpas of Sikkim. The various lactic organisms isolated from these conventional dairy products produce various enzymes such as esterase, phosphatase, leucine-arylamidase, b-galactosidase, and peptidase. These strains inhibited pathogens such as *Enterobacter agglomerans, Enterobacter cloacae,* and *Klebsiella pneumonia*, showed no production of any undesirable biogenic amines and high degree of relative hydrophobicity (0.75%), as judged by the bacterial adherence to hydrocarbon (Dewan and Tamang 2007).

8.11 Beneficial Compounds of Milk Products and Their Health Aspects

Diet and lifestyle are the major factors thought to influence susceptibility to many diseases. Our digestive tract is at the interface of the food we ingest and our metabolism. A high-fat or high-calorie diet associated with exaggerated postprandial spikes in glucose and lipids generate excess free radicals that can trigger a chain of biochemical reactions resulting in chronic, low-grade systemic inflammation (Malik et al. 2014). Concomitantly, the intake of a high-fat diet can also alter gut bacteria and affect intestinal barrier function and favors endotoxemia and inflammation. Thus, a high calorie diet may induce inflammation both at the cellular and systemic level. Inflammation thus induced has been found to play a key role in the pathogenesis of obesity, metabolic syndrome, insulin resistance, type-2 diabetes, coronary heart disease, endothelial dysfunction, prothrombic processes, and Alzheimer's disease. There is strong evidence from gut microbiota studies that alterations in gut bacteria are strongly associated with high circulating endotoxin levels, inflammation, and associated disorders by a mechanism that increases intestinal permeability. The plausible mechanisms include the ability of the microbes to extract energy from the diet, altered fatty acid metabolism within the adipose tissue and liver, and changes in the intestinal barrier integrity.

With this in view, several physical, psychological, pharmaceutical, and dietary therapies have been proposed for the management of these conditions/disorders. However, dietary strategies have been found to be more appropriate without any adverse health effects. The application of ethnic fermented foods as biotherapeutics is the new emerging area in developing dietary strategies and many people are interested in learning the facts behind these health claims. Fermented foods are now well recognized as powerful functional food and dietary ingredients with multiple health promoting functions along with the ability to fight specific diseases (Lourens-Hattingh and Viljoen). They are currently the major focus of attention all over the world to be explored as potential biotherapeutics in the management of several inflammatory metabolic disorders.

8.11.1 Lactulose

Lactulose also called 4-O-β-D-galactopyranosyl-D-fructose is a synthetic disaccharide which is not normally present in raw milk, but is produced due to heat processes. Lactulose is an osmotic laxative, that is, it draws more water into the colon and can thus offer relief in constipation, including chronic constipation within about 24–48 h. Lactulose is not digested in the small intestine as it lacks the specific disaccharidase. It transits unchanged to the colon where it serves as an energy source for the carbohydrate-splitting bacteria, predominantly *Lactobacillus acidophilus* and *Lactobacillus bifidus* (Luzzana et al. 2003). According to Prasad et al. (2007) lactulose exerts significant beneficial effects on the impaired neuronal function and cognitive performance of Portal Systemic Encephalopathy (PSE) patients. There is plenty of anecdotal evidence that lactulose at dosages of up to 60 g per day can kill intruders by inducing a sharp drop of the colonic pH, which makes the survival of *Salmonella* difficult (Schumann 2002). Endotoxins are the "toxic poop" of the bacteria that colonize the gut. In a study Koutelidakis et al. (2003) demonstrated that jaundice patients who had been pretreated with lactulose showed a significantly reduced increase in endotoxins after surgery. These observations were supported by animal experiments that have shown that oral lactulose administration reduced the mortality associated with endotoxin in obstructive jaundice.

Lactulose reduces the baseline ammonia influx from the gut by reducing its production via the acidifying effects of lactulose (Wright et al. 2011). Lactulose also possesses a protective effect on colon carcinogenesis. This type of cancer usually develops in the presence of high amounts of secondary bile salts, which could partially explain the reported lower rate of cancer recurrence in colon cancer patients who were treated with lactulose. Rodent studies also suggested that lactulose has a direct protective effect on the DNA of the colon mucosa of rats. In addition to its (more or less) direct effects, the lactulose induced increase in *Bifidobacteria* may also have cancer protective effects—not just in the colon, but in the mammary glands and liver as well (Reddy and Rivenson 1993). Moreover, lactulose can significantly augment the absorption of calcium, magnesium, zinc, copper, and iron (Seki et al. 2007). It has been revealed that the effects of lactulose are sufficient enough to exert anti-osteoporotic effects in a rodent model (Pometto et al. 2005).

8.11.2 Milk Bioactive Peptides

Milk contains many peptides and proteins, which exhibit bacteriostatic and bactericidal properties in their intact form (Bagnicka et al. 2010). In the current scenario, milk proteins are considered the most important source of bioactive peptides with numerous health benefits which also provide interesting opportunities to the dairy industry. Moreover, these peptides are being incorporated in the form of ingredients in functional foods, dietary supplements, and even pharmaceuticals with the purpose of delivering specific health benefits. Milk protein is considered to be of high nutritional value in terms of its biological value, net protein utilization, and protein-efficiency ratio. The proteins in milk are of excellent quality, as caseins and whey proteins (α-lactalbumin and β-lactoglobulin) contain high levels of essential amino acids.

Bioactive peptides, defined as specific protein fragments (3–20 amino acid sequences) have a positive impact on body functions or conditions and may ultimately influence health (Möller et al. 2008). The functional properties of such peptides are revealed only after the degradation of the native protein structure. This degradation may be a consequence of (a) enzymatic hydrolysis by digestive enzymes, (b) fermentation of milk with proteolytic starter cultures, (c) proteolysis by enzymes derived from microorganisms or plants, and (d) proteolytic action by indigenous proteases present in milk. In many studies a combination of 1 and 2 or 1 and 3, respectively, has proven effective in generating short functional peptides (Korhonen 2009).

Many dairy starter cultures are highly proteolytic and the release of different bioactive peptides from milk proteins through microbial proteolysis is now well documented (Matar et al. 2003, Fitzgerald and Murray 2006, Gobbetti et al. 2007). The type of starter culture used is one of the main factors that influence the synthesis of peptides in fermented milks. It is very challenging to select the right strains or combination of strains with optimum proteolytic activity and lysis tendency at the right time.

Milk fermentation has been described as a strategy to release bioactive peptides from caseins and whey proteins such as antihypertensive, antimicrobial, antioxidative, antithrombotic, immunomodulatory, mineral binding, and opioid (Gobbetti et al. 2004). At present, milk proteins are considered the most promising candidates for various health-promoting functional foods targeted at heart, bone, and digestive system health as well as improving immune defense, mood, and stress control (Korhonen 2009). Native sequences of milk proteins may contain fragments that exert various activities, such as antihypertensive, antithrombotic, opioid, opioid antagonist, immunomodulatory, antibacterial, antifungal, antiviral, antioxidant, binding and transporting metals, preventing amnesia, and causing smooth muscle contractions (Atanasova and Ivanova 2010). In addition, such peptides show a much lower allergenicity than the protein from which they are formed. Figure 8.7 displays the potential health targets of milk-derived bioactive peptides.

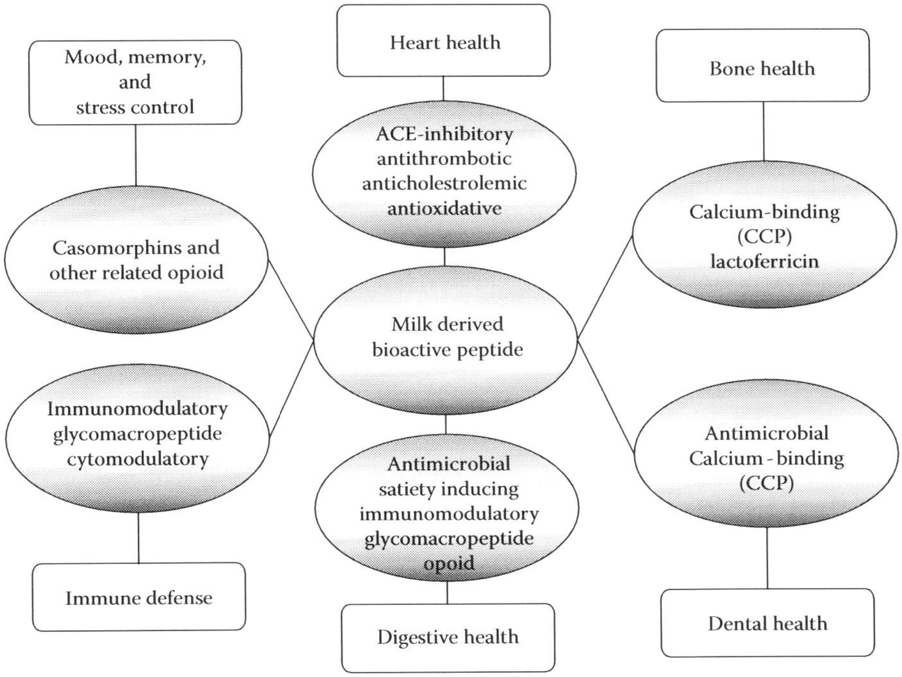

Figure 8.7 Functionality of milk protein-derived bioactive peptides and their potential health targets. (Adapted from Korhonen, H. 2009. *Journal of Functional Foods* 1(2): 177–187.)

8.12 Bioactive Peptides Produced by Lactic Fermentation and Their Potential Health Benefits

Several LAB possess the ability to hydrolyze milk proteins. This is of great advantage as the peptides and amino acids released from milk proteins during fermentation contribute to the typical aroma, flavor, and texture of the product. The proteolytic system of the LAB consists of cell-wall bound proteinases and several intracellular peptidases. In fermented milk products, the longer oligopeptides derived from milk proteins as a result of fermentation can be a source of the liberation of bioactive peptides when further degraded by intracellular peptidases after the lysis of bacterial cells (Meisel and Bockelman 1999). In the gastrointestinal tract, the digestive enzymes may further degrade long oligopeptides, leading to a possible release of bioactive peptides. On release of these bioactive peptides in the intestine they may act locally or pass through the intestinal wall into the blood circulation and end up at the target organ. Further, they may regulate the physiological condition through the modulation of the neural, immune, vascular, or endocrine system. Though no systematic study has been done on the release of bioactive peptides and their physiological effects from ethnic fermented dairy products, there are several reports regarding bioactive peptides released from casein and whey proteins during the fermentation of milk with various cultures. Nakamura et al. (1995a,b) identified two ACE-inhibitory peptides (Val-Pro-Pro, Ile-Pro-Pro) in milk that was fermented with a starter culture composed of *Lactobacillus helveticus* and *Saccharomyces cerevisiae*. This enzyme plays a crucial role in the regulation of blood pressure in mammals. In a study conducted at NDRI on the bio-functional property of traditional Indian *lassi* prepared from buffalo milk (Padghan and Mann 2012) 24 peptides were identified in *lassi* which was prepared using a *dahi* culture. The bioactive peptides found in *lassi* showed partial or complete homology to the milk protein bioactive peptides having ACE inhibitory, immunomodulatory, antioxidant, opioid, and cytomodulatory activities. The formation of bioactive peptides may explain the health promoting properties of milk products containing LAB.

8.12.1 Opioid Peptides

It is a common belief that falling asleep is easier after drinking a glass of *lassi* or *chhach*. Ofcourse, babies often fall asleep after breast or bottle feeding. Now studies provide evidence that there are certain bioactive peptides referred to as opioid peptides that play an active role in the nervous system and can induce sleep. They can have agonistic or antagonistic activity. Recent studies have provided evidence that there are peptides in dairy products which play an active role in the nervous system; these are opioid peptides. The first major opioid peptides discovered were β-casomorphins, fragments of β-casein (Smacchi and Gobbetti 1998). β-casein derived opioid peptides (β-casomorphins) or their precursors have been detected in the duodenal chime of mini-pigs, in the plasma of newborn calves, and in the human small intestine upon oral administration of casein or milk (Fitzgerald and Meisel 2003). These opioid peptides are opioid receptor ligands with agonistic or antagonistic activities which can interact with their endogenous ligands and with exogenous opioids and opioid antagonists. Thus, orally administered opioid peptides may modulate the absorption process in the gut and influence the gastrointestinal function in two ways: first by affecting smooth muscles, which reduces the transit time and second by affecting the intestinal transport of electrolytes, which explain their antisecretory properties. Once absorbed into the blood, these peptides can travel to the brain and various other organs and elicit pharmacological properties similar to opium or morphine (Meisel and Schlimme 1990). Interestingly, an α_s1-casein derived peptide f(91–100) has been demonstrated to possess anxiolytic like stress relieving properties in animal models and human studies (Lefranc 2001).

8.12.2 ACE-Inhibitory Peptides

Many dairy starter cultures are highly proteolytic. The formation of bioactive peptides can, thus, be expected during the manufacture of fermented dairy products like various cheese varieties and fermented milk. Also, LAB have been demonstrated to produce different bioactive peptides possessing ACE-inhibitory activity in milk during fermentation (Donkor et al. 2007). Several studies have demonstrated that *Lb. helveticus* strains, in particular, are capable of releasing antihypertensive peptides, the best known of which are ACE-inhibitory tri-peptides Val-Pro-Pro (VPP) and Ile-Pro-Pro (IPP). The antihypertensive capacity of these peptides has been demonstrated in several rat model and human studies (Hirota et al. 2007).

Biologically, the active peptides derived from fermented food proteins with an affinity to modulate blood pressure have been thoroughly studied. Angiotensin I converting enzyme (ACE; kinases II peptidyldipeptide hydrolase, EC 3.4.15.1) is important for blood pressure regulation. In the event where decreased blood volume or decreased blood flow to the kidneys is sensed, renin acts on angiotensinogen to form angiotensin I. ACE then catalyzes the hydrolysis of the inactive prohormone angiotensin I (decapeptide) to angiotensin II (octapeptide). This results in an increase in blood pressure through vasoconstriction, via increased systemic resistance and stimulated secretion of aldosterone resulting in increased sodium and water absorption in the kidneys. ACE also inactivates the vaso-dilating peptide bradykinin (nonapeptide) and endogenous opioid peptide Met-enkephalin.

Recent scientific evidence indicated that an adequate intake of calcium, potassium, and magnesium helps to reduce blood pressure. Ethnic dairy products are a very useful source of these micronutrients along with the bioactive peptides termed as casokininins or ACE I peptides with a potential to reduce blood pressure due to their ability to inhibit angiotensin I converting enzyme (ACE) and block conversion of angiotensin I to angiotensin II, a potent vasoconstrictor.

8.12.3 Antioxidant Peptides

During normal reactions within the body, free radicals are generated during respiration in aerobic organisms particularly vertebrates and humans. In addition to the physiological production of oxidants and their secondary reactions, there are other sources for production of oxidants. Oxidation of fats and oils during the processing and storage of food products worsen the quality of their lipid content and nutritive values. Consumption of these potentially toxic products can give rise to several diseases. Additionally, UV radiation can stimulate the generation of a variety of oxidants. An excessive amount of reactive radicals can result in damage of proteins and mutation in DNA, oxidation of membrane phospholipids, and modification in low density lipoproteins (LDL) (Alaiz et al. 1994); which in turn, initiates several diseases including atherosclerosis, arthritis, diabetes, and cancer.

Under normal conditions, antioxidant defense systems can remove reactive species through enzymatic antioxidants; such as super oxide dismutase (SOD) and glutathione peroxidase and nonenzymatic antioxidants; and proteins and peptides, antioxidant vitamins, trace elements, coenzymes, and cofactors. On the other hand, antioxidative peptides can also be generated from casein by hydrolysis using digestive enzymes or by the fermentation of milk with proteolytic LAB strains (Korhonen and Pihlanto 2003) which result in the prevention of many lifestyle disorders.

Proteolytic activation of bioactive sequence by LAB has the great advantage of using food grade microorganisms to enrich food with bioactive elements.

8.12.4 Immunomodulatory Action of Bioactive Peptides

Diet has very important role to play in the human body's defense against infections. Recent studies have pointed toward the role of functional peptides in this regard and the two main activities are stimulation of the immune system (imunomodulatory activity) and inhibition of pathogenic bacteria (antimicrobial activity) (Hata et al. 1996, Minkiewicz et al. 2000). The immunomodulatory action of bioactive peptides is related to the stimulation of the proliferation of human lymphocytes and macrophage phagocytic activity (Szwajkowska et al. 2011). Furthermore, many cytochemical studies indicate that peptides can induce apoptosis of cancer cells (López-Expósito and Recio 2008). Numerous studies have focused on the multipotential activity of lactoferricin (Lfcin)—a product of hydrolytic degradation of lactoferrin (LF) under acidic pH (Oo et al. 2010). Lactoferrin itself exhibits a strong bactericidal activity through its ability to bind iron. This peptide shows a considerably higher antimicrobial activity than the native protein. Furthermore, Lfcin has been found effective in the treatment of some cancer varieties, such as leukemia and neuroblastoma (Gifford et al. 2005). Lactoferrampin (Lfampin) is another peptide derived from lactoferrin. It has a wide spectrum of antifungal and antibacterial properties. The peptide exerts antifungal (against *Candida*) activity higher than LF and is also active against various pathogens such as *Clostridium perfringens, Haemophilus influenzae, Helicobacter pylori, Listeria monocytogenes, Staphylococcalenteritis, Staphylococcal aureus, Staph. mutans,* and *Vibrio cholerae* (Van der Kraan et al. 2005). It has been suggested that lactoferrin and its derivatives affect the production of cytokines involved in the immune reactions of the organism (Möller et al. 2008). Moreover, it is also suggested to use them as food preservatives (Haque and Chand 2008).

The whey protein fraction of bovine milk consists mainly of β-lactoglobulin (β-LG) and α-lactalbumin (α-LA). Native α-lactalbumin has immunomodulatory properties, but does not affect microorganisms, whereas products of its degradation by trypsin and chemotrypsin (f1–5, f17–31-SS-f109–114 and f61–68-SS-f75–80) or pepsin exhibit both immunomodulatory and antimicrobial properties against bacteria, viruses, and fungi (Kamau et al. 2010). Biological properties of peptides encoded in the structure of β-LG have been a subject of studies aiming at the inhibition of the human immunodeficiency virus type 1 by use of chemically modified β-LG (3-hydroxyphthaloyl-β–LG) (Taha et al. 2010). Numerous studies are dedicated to the casein fraction, which accounts for 80% of total milk protein and is a rich source of bioactive peptides that stimulate and aid the immune system. Hydrolysis of αs2-casein (by chymosin acting at neutral pH) results in releasing casocidin. This peptide shows antibacterial properties against *Staphylococcus* spp., *Sarcina* spp., *Bacillus subtilis, Diplococcus pneumoniae,* and *Staph. pyogenes* (Silva and Malcata 2005). Caseicins A, B, and C are released from αs1-casein during fermentation of milk by *Lb. acidophilus*. Characteristic of caseicins A (αs1-CN f21-29) and B (αs1-CN f30-37) is their particularly high activity against *Escherichia coli* O157:H7 and *Enterobacter sakazakii* (Hayes et al. 2005). It is also noteworthy that the peptides derived from α-casein promote the growth of probiotic *Lb. acidophilus* while inhibit that of pathogenic bacteria (Srinivas and Prakash 2010) indicating their positive effect on the gastrointestinal tract. The glycomacropepetide (GMP) formed during fermentation by LAB has membranolytic properties, which determine its bactericidal properties (Dashper et al. 2005). The peptide has GMP and its derivatives possess immunomodulatory properties, they also inhibit hemagglutination caused by the influenza virus, binding

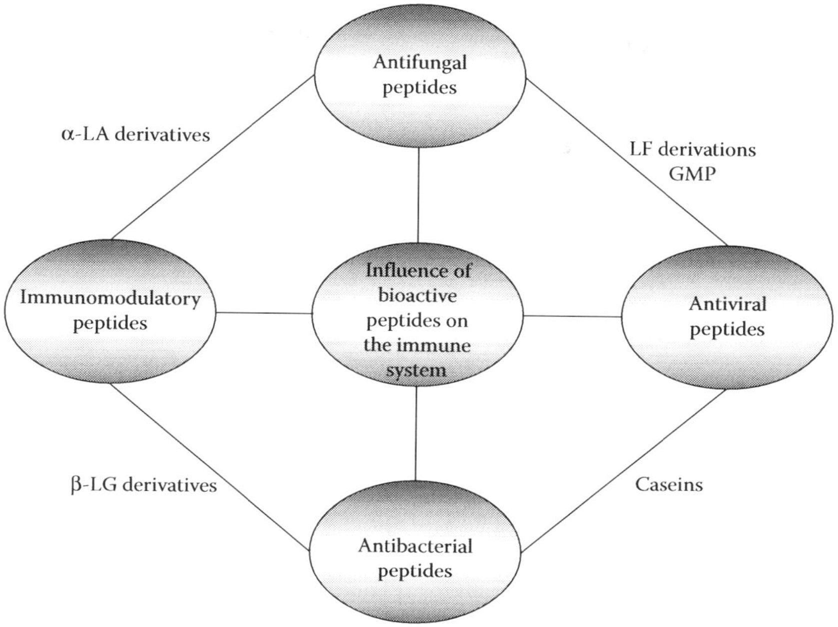

Figure 8.8 Influence of selected peptides from bovine milk on the immune system. (Adapted from Szwajkowska et al. 2011. *Animal Science Paper and Reports* 29: 269–280.)

the toxins of *Vibrio cholerae* bacterium. In addition, these peptides inhibit the adherence of *Staph. mutans*, responsible for caries development. The action of selected biopeptides on the immune system is presented in Figure 8.8.

8.12.5 Caseinophosphopeptides for Bone Formation and Anticariogenic Effect

The potential of fermented dairy products such as *dahi, lassi, chhas, srikhand,* and so on, as a source of functional casein peptides is immense. Specific CPPs can form soluble organophosphate salts and lead to enhanced calcium absorption by limiting the precipitation of calcium in the distal ileum. Reports on the effect of CPPs on mineral solubility or absorption are inconsistent partly due to the diversity of the experimental approaches used (Meisel and Fitzgerald 2003). However, many animal and human studies have reported the presence of CPPs *in vivo* upon ingestion of milk, and fermented dairy products. Since CPPs can bind and solubilize minerals, they have been considered physiologically beneficial in the prevention of osteoporosis, dental caries, hypertension, and anemia. The anticariogenic effect of CPPs has been well documented. CPPs can have an anticariogenic effect by promoting recalcification of tooth enamel. Moreover, glycomacropeptide (GMP) derived from kappa casein seems to contribute to the anti-caries effect by inhibiting the adhesion and growth of plaque forming bacteria on oral mucosa. Another interesting property associated with CPPs is their potential to enhance mucosal immunity. It has been demonstrated that oral administration of a commercial CPP preparation enhanced the intestinal IgA levels of piglets (Otani et al. 2000).

8.13 Health Associated Effects of Bioactive Lipids

Milk fat is known for its high proportion of saturated fatty acids and thus associated with an increased risk of coronary heart disease (CHD). However, only three (lauric, myristic, and palmitic) among the different saturated fatty acids in milk have the property to raise blood cholesterol. At least one third of the fatty acids are unsaturated with the cholesterol lowering tendency (German and Dillard 2006). Moreover, ethnic fermented dairy products prepared by nonspecific (mixed lactic microflora) or defined strains of lactic starters contain components such as CLA, antioxidants, and LAB which have at least a protective if not, a hypocholesterolemic effect (Rogelj 2000). Calcium plays an important role in mediating vascular contraction and vasodilation, muscle contraction, nerve transmission, and glandular secretion. Milk fat components such as CLA, sphingomyelin, butyric acid, β-carotene, and vitamin A and B have anticarcinogenic potential. Milk fat is not only a source of bioactive lipid components in ethnic fermented foods but also serves as an important delivery medium for nutrients including fat soluble vitamins. Butyric acid is found only in the fat of ruminants and is believed to be an important anticarcinogen which, together with etheric lipids, vitamin A, D, E and the CLA, forms a protective barrier mainly against different nontransmissible diseases (German 1999, Parodi 1999, 2004). Caprylic and capric acid may have antiviral activities. Lauric acid may have antiviral and antibacterial functions (Sun et al. 2002, Thormar and Hilmarsson 2007) as well as anticaries and antiplaque activity (Schuster et al. 1980).

CLA has received considerable attention on account of its potent biological properties. CLA is mainly produced through the actions of the anaerobic rumen bacteria when dietary linoleic and linolenic acid are converted to trans-vaccenic acid by the enzyme linoleic acid isomerase, a process called biohydrogenation (Stanton et al. 2003). Intestinal bifidobacteria have also been shown to produce adequate amounts of CLA (Coakley et al. 2006, 2003). CLA has been shown to reduce the risk of heart disease, several types of cancer, and to enhance bone formation and immune function in both human and animal models. Indeed, investigations using animal models have demonstrated that CLA is anticarcinogenic for many types of cancer (Belury 2002, Ip et al. 2002, Whigham et al. 2000). Furthermore, experimental animal studies have indicated that CLA may have beneficial effects on the atherosclerotic process, including reduced LDL cholesterol level, reduced oxidation of LDL cholesterol, slowed development of atherosclerotic lesions, and reduced severity of preexisting lesions (Kritchevsky et al. 2004). The potential anticarcinogenic effect associated with CLA has been demonstrated in a number of *in vitro* and animal studies. Results of these studies suggest that CLA can have a preventative effect on gastrointestinal and colon cancers. These observations have been made based on the ability of CLA to inhibit cell proliferation and induce apoptosis in human cancer cell lines (Kim et al. 2002, Cho et al. 2003, 2005, Soel et al. 2007). The ability of certain strains of bifidobacteria and lactobacilli to produce CLA isomers may also be linked to their health enhancing properties (Coakley et al. 2003, Akalin et al. 2007, Yadav et al. 2007). Other potential health benefits which may be attributed to CLA intake include increased expression of inflammatory response mediators and improvements in bone health (Bhattacharya et al. 2006).

8.14 Health Aspects of Vitamins Produced during Milk Fermentation

Dairy fermentation by LAB can result in the production of a number of vitamins including folate, vitamin B12, riboflavin, and vitamin K, which may impart additional nutritional and or/health value to foods. Folate is an essential vitamin for growth and reproduction in all vertebrates in that it plays a vital role in the biosynthesis of nucleotides and cofactors involved in a number of metabolic reactions within cells. It is reported to play a role in the prevention of several disorders including neural tube defects, some forms of cancer, neuropsychiatric disorders, and coronary heart disease (Ames 1999, Collins 1994, Finglas et al. 2003). Many strains used in ethnic fermented products including strains of *Lactobacillus*, *Streptococcus*, *Lactococcus*, and *Leuconostoc* spp. possess the biosynthetic capability to produce folate in the environment (Lin and Young 2000, Hugenholtz and Smid 2002, Hugenholtz et al. 2002, Crittenden et al. 2003, Sybesma et al. 2004). Moreover, *Strep. thermophilus* used in the manufacture of *dahi* resulted in an increased level of folate being produced.

Vitamin B12 (cobalamin) is an essential cofactor involved in the metabolism of nucleic acids, amino acids, fatty acids, and carbohydrates (Quesada-Chanto et al. 1994, Crittenden et al. 2003). It is primarily found in foods such as red meat and milk as a result of rumen microbial action but a number of intestinal bacteria such as some strains of bifidobacteria, *Lactobacillus*, and propionibacteria are also efficient producers of this vitamin. Vitamin B2 (riboflavin) is a precursor of the coenzymes flavin adenine dinucleotide (FAD) and flavin mononucleotide (FMN) and is therefore required by all flavoproteins. Deficiencies in the vitamin have been associated with inflammation of the skin and mouth, deterioration in vision, loss of hair, and lack of growth. The genetic determinants for riboflavin production have been identified in *Lc. Lactis* (Burgess et al. 2004).

Vitamin K is a generic term for the family of compounds that have a common 2-methyl-1,4-napthoquinone nucleus but differ in the structures of the side chain at 3-position, that are synthesized by plants and bacteria. Vitamin K is a cofactor for the enzyme vitamin K-dependent carboxylase which catalyzes the conversion of glutamic acid to γ-carboxyglutamic acid (Gla). This reaction is essential for optimal Ca^{++} binding and hence the functionality of a range of vitamin K-dependent proteins in blood and bone. Bacteria produce a family of vitamin K_2 forms referred to as menaquinones, including a variety of LAB such as *Lactococcus* and *Leuconostoc* (Morishita et al. 1999).

8.15 Lactose Intolerance

Lactose intolerance (LI), also known as lactose malabsorption is the most common type of carbohydrate malabsorption. It is associated with the inability to digest lactose into its constituents, glucose and galactose, due to low levels of lactase enzyme activity. Symptoms related to LI appear 30 min to 2 h after consumption of food products containing lactose. Related symptoms include: bloating, cramping, flatulence, and loose stools. The highest rates of LI are found in Asians, Native Americans, and African Americans (60%–100%), while the lowest rates are found in people of northern European origin (including northern Americans). The consumption of the lactase enzyme as a food supplement may assist in restoring adequate levels of the enzyme needed for hydrolysis of lactose, especially for patients with low, or nonexistent levels of lactase. On the other hand, lactase products are problematic since not all lactase preparations are of the same concentration. Several lines of evidence show that the appropriate strain of LAB, in adequate amounts, can alleviate symptoms of lactose intolerance. *Strep. thermophilus*, *Lb. bulgaricus*, and other lactobacilli used in fermented milk products deliver enough bacterial lactase to the intestine and stomach where lactose is degraded to prevent symptoms in lactase nonpersistent individuals (Aso and Akazan 1992). Other cultures in fermented milk products that reduce symptoms of lactose intolerance in both children and adults include *Lb. delbrueckii* subsp. *bulgaricus*, *Strep. thermophilus*, and *Bifidobacterium longum* (Martini et al. 1991). The residual amount of lactose after its partial utilization by LAB for the production of lactic acid and other compounds may help in alleviating the adverse effects of lactose intolerance (Ayebo and Shahani 1980). Consumption of ethnic fermented dairy products containing appropriate strains and levels of LAB may thus be a good way to incorporate dairy products and their accompanying nutrients back into the diets of lactose intolerant individuals.

8.16 Control of Blood Cholesterol and Hyperlipidemia

Cholesterol is essential for many functions in the human body. It acts as a precursor to certain hormones and vitamins and is a component of cell membranes and nerve cells. However, elevated levels of total blood cholesterol or other blood lipids are considered risk factors for developing coronary heart disease. Although, humans synthesize cholesterol to maintain minimum levels for biological functioning, diet also is known to play a role in serum cholesterol levels, although the extent of influence varies significantly from person to person. For example, butter or *makkhan* contains lecithin, a substance that helps in the proper assimilation and metabolism of cholesterol and other dietary fats. This helps in break-down and use of fat more efficiently, leading to loss of weight. It satiates any cravings during dieting. Moreover, LAB have been evaluated for their effect on serum cholesterol levels. Clinical studies on the effect of lowering of cholesterol or low-density lipid (LDL) levels in humans have not been conclusive. There have been some human studies that suggest that blood cholesterol levels can be reduced by consumption of probiotic-containing dairy foods. A study revealed that milk decreases cholesterol concentrations and that with greater milk consumption, a greater decrease in cholesterol concentrations occurs. Milk has been proposed to act as an inhibitor of cholesterol synthesis (Mann 1974). Cultured milk products exert their effect on cholesterol by secreting bile salt hydrolase which catalyzes the hydrolysis of glycine or taurine conjugated bile salts. These deconjugated bile salts are less soluble and less efficiently reabsorbed which results in excretion of free bile acids in feces (De Rodas et al. 1996). The cholesterol lowering property of probiotic *dahi* containing selected strains of *Lb. acidophilus* and *Bif. bifidum* was evaluated in rats by Rajpal and Kansal (2009). They found that the cholesterol and plasma triacylglycerol (TAG) contents in the liver were lower in the probiotic *dahi* group than in the control group. Hence, the probiotic *dahi* decreased diet-induced hypercholesterolemia and reduced the atherogenic index by increasing HDL and attenuating the rise in TAG on the hypocholesterolemic diet. Sinha and Yadav (2007) studied the antiatherogenic effect of probiotic *dahi* supplemented with *Lb. acidophilus* and *Lb. casei* in rats fed with a cholesterol rich diet. They found that the total plasma cholesterol, low density lipoprotein, and plasma triglycerides were suppressed and HDL cholesterol was not affected. Moreover, the atherogenic index reduced significantly in probiotic dahi and culture fed groups when compared with the reference diet fed group. Therefore, ethnic dairy foods supplemented with beneficial organisms can be an excellent alternative control for the problem of hypercholesterolemia and the atherogenic effect.

8.17 Antidiabetic Effect

Diabetes is a looming epidemic worldwide, affecting almost all major sections of society, creating burdens on global health and economy. Diabetes and hypertension are comorbidity diseases that occur together in the same species. There is a complex relationship between insulin resistance diabetes and essential hypertension. An induction in insulin resistance often leads to diabetic dyslipidemia, which is highly increased by high levels of plasma total cholesterol, LDL cholesterol, and very low density lipoprotein (VLDL) cholesterol (Yadav et al. 2007). A wide range of antihypertensive drugs is available in the market but not all offer beneficial effects in hypertensive diabetes. Therefore, the development of new therapy methods is needed in order to produce an efficient method for preventing or reducing the occurrence of diabetes and hypertension with the least side effects. The consumption of ethnic fermented dairy foods is a new therapeutic strategy in preventing or delaying the onset of diabetes and subsequently reducing the incidence of hypertension. The antidiabetic effect of *dahi* containing *Lc. lactis* was observed on high fructose-induced diabetic rats. The fasting blood glucose, glycosylated hemoglobin, insulin, free fatty acids, and triglyceride levels of the *dahi* fed group animals were significantly lower than those of control group (Yadav et al. 2006). Moreover production of free fatty acids and CLA in the probiotic *dahi* containing *Lb. acidophilus* and *Lb. casei* during fermentation and storage was reported by Yadav et al. (2007). The CLA content increased in probiotic *dahi* during fermentation and remained stable during storage, whereas no change was observed in the control. Probiotic lactobacilli appeared to increase the production of FFAs by lipolysis of milk fat and produced CLA by using internal linoleic acid, which may confer nutritional and therapeutic value to the product. The effect of fermented milk products containing probiotic strains (*Lb. acidophilus* and *Lb. casei*) demonstrated that a number of diabetes-associated parameters, that is, glucose intolerance, hyperglycemia, hyperinsulemia, dyslipidemia, and oxidative stress could be improved by the ingestion of probiotics.

8.18 Anticarcinogenic Effect

Cancer usually defined as "uncontrolled cell growth" is one of the leading causes of death worldwide. Mutations in key regulatory genes alter the behavior of cells and can potentially cause cancer. As many human cancers are caused from preventable factors such as infection, inflammation, smoking and diet; preventive strategies might be the most effective to reduce cancers. A proper diet may be one of the critical strategies for reducing the risk of cancers. Lactic acid bacteria (LAB) have been shown to be an effective chemopreventive food ingredient against many cancer types including colorectal, bladder, liver, breast, and gastric cancer. The polysaccharide component of the bacterial cell wall or the bacterial metabolites of LAB are known to mediate a nonspecific host immune modulation and control the growth of and inhibit cancer cells. These effects act via diverse mechanisms including alteration of gastrointestinal microflora, enhancement of the host's immune response, antioxidative, and antiproliferative activities. The lactic fermentation of milk in *dahi* making also leads to the conversion of some fatty acids into CLA that has cancer prevention virtues. Rajpal and Kansal (2008) demonstrated the reduction of gastrointestinal cancer in rats fed with buffalo milk probiotic *dahi* containing selected strains of *Lb. acidophilus* and *Bif. bifidum* and using *dahi* culture (*Lc. lactis* spp. *cremoris* and *Lc. lactis* spp. *lactis biovar. diacetylactis*). Probiotic *dahi* decreased lipid peroxidation and beta-glucuronidase activity in the gut and increased glutathione-S-transferase (GST), a carcinogen detoxifying enzyme activity in the liver, which resulted in attenuation of carcinogenesis in the GI tract. Moreover, in the Ayurvedic system, *ghee* is considered to induce several beneficial effects on human health and is used extensively for therapeutic purposes such as in the preparation of a number of formulations for treating skin allergy and respiratory diseases. *Ghee* is considered capable of increasing mental powers and improving physical appearance and also considered curative of ulcers and eye diseases (Kansal and Ekta 2008). Studies revealed that milk fat contains several components such as (CLA, sphingomyelins, butyric acid, and β carotene) which have therapeutic potential against carcinogenesis (Parodi 1997). CLA, besides being a powerful anticarcinogen, has antiatherogenic, immunomodulating, and lean body mass enhancing properties (Pariza 1997). In view of the role of diet in chronic diseases, such as cancer, the potential of dietary probiotics in preventing cancers is promising and thus is of great interest. One recent study found that dietary supplementation with a strain of *Lb. acidophilus* significantly suppressed the total number of colon cancer cells in rats in a dose-dependent manner (Kim et al. 2007).

8.19 Conclusions

The cow and its milk have been held sacred in the world since the dawn of human civilization. Milk has been considered one of the most natural and highly nutritive parts of a balanced daily diet. Currently, the integration of advanced scientific knowledge with traditional information is gaining incredible momentum toward developing the concept of potential therapeutic foods and it has long been believed that the consumption of ethnic Indian fermented milk products provides various health benefits. The purposeful application of fermentation for food preservation, palatability, and other reasons is an ancient art. The consumption of ethnic fermented milk products may be beneficial in a multitude of disorders both inside and outside the GI tract combating the problem of lactose intolerance, carcinogenesis, diabetes, and hypertension by releasing certain bioactive peptides; defining their immense importance for the individual in the future. These findings are interesting and should encourage future studies to (1) substantiate or extend these findings by using animal models and clinical trials; (2) ascertain whether these effects are age-specific or can be observed across all age groups. Though the manufacture of these fermented dairy foods in the organized sector is picking up, there is a dire need to evaluate and understand the health aspects of these products and also to further enhance their value through the use of proven strains of probiotics and other functional starter lactic cultures. Science-based evidence would further accentuate their value as dairy health foods.

References

Abdel-Salam, A.M. 2010. Functional foods: Hopefulness to good health. *American Journal of Food Technology* 5: 86–99.

Achaya, K.T.A. 1998. *Historical Dictionary of Indian Food.* Oxford University Press, Delhi.

Adolfsson, O., S.N. Meydani, and R.M. Russel. 2004. Yogurt and gut function. *American Journal of Clinical Nutrition* 80(2): 245–256.

Akalin, A.S., O. Tokusolu, S. Gonc, and S. Aycan. 2007. Occurrence of conjugated linoleic acid in probiotic yogurts supplemented with fructooligosaccharide. *International Dairy Journal* 17: 1089–1095.

Alaiz, M., M. Beppu, K. Ohishi, and K. Kikugawa. 1994. Modification of delipidated apoprotein B of low density lipoprotein in by lipid oxidation products in relation to macrophage scavenger receptor binding. *Biological and Pharmaceutical Bulletin* 17: 51–57.

Ames, B.N. 1999. Micronutrient deficiencies: A major cause of DNA damage. *Annals of the New York Academy of Sciences* 889(1): 87–106.

Anantakrishnan C.P. and M.R. Srinivasan. 1964. *Milk Products of India: Dahi.* Indian Council of Agricultural Research, New Delhi, pp. 15–18.

Anantakrishnan C.P. and M.R. Srinivasan. 1964. *Milk Products of India: Buttermilk.* Indian Council of Agricultural Research, New Delhi, India, pp. 54–57.

Aneja, R.P., B.N. Mathur, R.C. Chandan, and A.K. Banerjee. 2002. Cultured/fermented products. Technology of Indian milk products. *Handbook on Process Technology Modernization for Professionals, Entrepreneurs and Scientists.* Dairy India Yearbook, New Delhi, India, pp. 133–157.

Aneja, R.P., M.N. Vyas, D. Sharma, and S.K. Samal. 1989. A method for manufacturing lassi. Indian Patent No. 17374.

Aso, Y. and H. Akazan. 1992. Prophylactic effect of a *Lactobacillus casei* preparation on the recurrence of superficial bladder cancer. *Urologia Internationalis* 49: 125–129.

Atanasova, J. and I. Ivanova. 2010. Antibacterial peptides from goat and sheep milk proteins. *Biotechnology & Biotechnological Equipment* 24(2): 1799–1803.

Ayebo, A.D. and K.M. Shahani. 1980. Role of cultured dairy products in diet. *Cultured Dairy Products* 15: 21–29.

Bagnicka, E., N. Strzałkowska, A. Jóźwik, J. Krzyżewski, J.O. Horbańczuk, and L. Zwierzchowski. 2010. Defensins in farm animals, their expression and polymorphism. *Acta Biochimica Polonica* 57(4): 487–497.

Balasubramanyam, N.N., A.M. Natarajan, R.V. Rao. 1984. Studies on the nutritional quality of yogurt. *Cherion* 13: 62–66.

Belury, M.A. 2002. Inhibition of carcinogenesis by conjugated linoleic acid: Potential mechanisms of action. *Journal of Nutrition* 132: 2995–2998.

Bharti, S.K., N.K. Sharma, K. Murari, and A. Kumar. 2012. Functional aspects of dairy foods in human health: An overview. *Critical Review in Pharmaceutical Sciences* 1: 35–42.

Bhattacharya, A., J. Banu, M. Rahman, J. Causey, and G. Fernandes. 2006. Biological effects of conjugated linoleic acids in health and disease. *Journal of Nutritional Biochemistry* 17: 789–810.

BIS. 1980. *Specifications for dahi*. Bureau of Indian Standards: 9617. Manak Bhawan, New Delhi.

Bourlioux, P. and P. Pochart. 1988. Nutritional and health properties of yogurt. *World Review of Nutritional and Dietetics* 56: 217–258.

Bronner, F. and D. Pansu. 1999. Nutritional aspects of calcium absorption. *Journal of Nutrition* 129: 9–12.

Burgess, C., M. O' Connell-Motherway, W. Sybesma, J. Hugenholtz, and D. van Sinderan. 2004. Riboflavin production in *Lactococcus lactis*: Potential for *in situ* production of vitamin-enriched foods. *Applied and Environmental Microbiology* 70: 5769–5777.

Buttriss, J. 1997. Nutritional properties of fermented milk products. *International Journal of Dairy Technology* 50(1): 21–27.

Chandan, R.C., C.H. White, A. Kilara, and Y.H. Hui. 2006. *Manufacturing Yogurt and Fermented Milks*. Blackwell Publishing Ltd., Iowa, USA, pp. 89–115.

Cho, H.J., W.K. Kim, E.J. Kim, K.C. Jung, S. Park, H.S. Lee, A.L. Tyner, and J.H. Park. 2003. Conjugated linoleic acid inhibits cell proliferation and erbB3 signaling in HT-29 human colon cell line. *American Journal of Physiology- Gastrointestinal and Liver Physiology* 284: G996–G1005.

Cho, H.J., W.K. Kim, J.I. Jung, E.J. Kim, S.S. Lim, D.Y. Kwon, and J.H. Park. 2005. Trans-10, cis-12, not cis-9, trans-11, conjugated linoleic acid decreases ErbB3 signaling in HT-29 human colon cell line. *World Journal of Gastroenterology* 11: 5142–5250.

Coakley, M., M.C. Johnson, E. McGarth, S. Rahman, R.P. Ross, G.F. Fitzgerald, R. Devery, and C. Stanton. 2006. Intestinal bifidobacteria that produce trans-9, trans-11 conjugated linoleic acid: A fatty acid with antiproliferative activity against human colon SW480 and HT-29 cancer cells. *Nutrition and Cancer* 56: 95–102.

Coakley, M., R.P. Ross, M. Nordgren, G.F. Fitzgerald, R. Devery, and C. Stanton. 2003. Conjugated linoleic acid biosynthesis by human derived *Bifidobacterium* species. *Journal of Applied Microbiology* 94: 138–145.

Collins, K. 1994. Folic acid supplements provide useful benefits. *Better Nutrition for Today Living* 56: 18–19.

Crittenden, R.G., N.R. Martinej, and M.J. Playne. 2003. Synthesis and utilization of folate by yogurt starter cultures and probiotic bacteria. *International Journal of Food Microbiology* 80: 217–222.

Dashper, S.G., N.M. O'Brien-Simpson, K.J. Cross, R.A. Paolini, B. Hoffmann, D.V. Catmull, M. Malkoski, and E.C. Reynolds. 2005. Divalent metal cations increase the activity of the antimicrobial peptide kappacin. *Antimicrobial Agents and Chemotherapy* 49: 2322–2328.

De, S. 1980. *Outlines of Dairy Technology: Makkhan*. Oxford University Press, New Delhi, pp. 428–432.

De, S. 2002. *Out Lines of Dairy Technology*. Oxford University Press, Delhi.

De Rodas, B.Z., S.E. Gilliland, and C.V. Maxwell. 1996. Hypocholesterolemic action of *Lactobacillus acidophilus* ATCC 43121 and calcium in swine with hypercholesterolemia induced by diet. *Journal of Dairy Science* 79: 2121–2128.

Dewan, S. and J.P. Tamang. 2006. Microbial and analytical characterization of *Chhu*, a traditional fermented milk product of the Sikkim Himalayas. *Journal of Scientific and Industrial Research* 65: 747–752.

Dewan, S. and J.P. Tamang. 2007. Dominant lactic acid bacteria and their technological properties isolated from the Himalayan ethnic fermented milk products. *Leeuwenhoek International Journal of General and Molecular Microbiology* 92: 343–352.

Donkor, O., A. Henriksson, T. Vasiljevic, and N.P. Shah. 2007. Proteolytic activity of dairy lactic acid bacteria and probiotics as determinant of growth and *in vitro* angiotensin-converting enzyme inhibitory activity in fermented milk. *Lait* 86: 21–38.

FAO, 1990. Importance, technology and economics of traditional milk products. *Food and Agriculture Organization of the United Nations, Rome.* M-26, ISBN 92-5-102899-0.

Finglas, P.M., A.J. Wright, C.A. Wolfe, D.J. Hart, D.M. Wright, and J.R. Dainty. 2003. Is there more to folates than neural-tube defects? *Proceedings of Nutrition Society* 62: 591–598.

Fitzgerald, R.J. and B.A. Murray. 2006. Bioactive peptides and lactic fermentations. *International Journal of Dairy Technology* 59: 118–125.

Fitzgerald, R.J. and H. Meisel. 2003. Milk protein hydrolysates and bioactive peptides. In: Fox, P.F. McSweeney, P.L.H. (Eds.), *Advanced Dairy Chemistry*, Vol. 1: *Proteins*, 3rd edition. Kluwer Academic/ Plenum Publishers, New York, NY, USA, pp. 675–698.

FSSR. Food Safety and Standards (Food products Standards and Food Additive) Regulations. http://fssai.gov.in/gazatted Notification aspx. 2011, Accessed on Jan 10th, 2014.

Garg, S.K., P. Bhale, and R.S. Rawat. 1983. Shrikhand—An indigenous fermented milk product. *Indian Dairyman* 35: 657–662.

German, J.B. 1999. Butyric acid: A role in cancer prevention. *Nutrition Bulletin* 24: 203–209.

German, J.B. and C.J. Dillard. 2006. Composition, structure and absorption of milk lipids: A source of energy, fat-soluble nutrients and bioactive molecules. *Critical Reviews in Food Science and Nutrition* 46: 57–92.

Ghosh, J. and G.S. Rajoria. 1990. Technology for production of *misti dahi*—A traditional fermented milk product. *Indian Journal of Dairy Science* 43: 239–246.

Gifford, J.L., H.N. Hunter, and H.J. Vogel. 2005. Lactoferricin: A lactoferrin-derived peptide with antimicrobial, antiviral, antitumor and immunological properties. *Cellular and Molecular Life Science* 62: 2588–2598.

Gobbetti, M., F. Minervini, and C.G. Rizzello. 2007. Bioactive peptides in dairy products. In: *Handbook of Food Products Manufacturing*, ed. Y. H. Hui, John Wiley and Sons, Inc., Hoboken, New Jersey, pp. 489–517.

Gobbetti, M., F. Minervini, C.G. Rizzello. 2004. Angiotensin I converting- enzyme-inhibitory and antimicrobial bioactive peptides. *International Journal of Dairy Technology* 57: 172–188.

Haque, E. and R. Chand. 2008. Antihypertensive and antimicrobial bioactive peptides from milk proteins. *European Food Research and Technology* 227: 7–15.

Hata, Y., M. Yamamoto, H. Ohni, K. Nakajima, Y. Nakamura, and T. Takano. 1996. A placebo-controlled study of the effect of sour milk on blood pressure in hypertensive subjects. *American Journal of Clinical Nutrition* 64: 767–771.

Hayes, M., R.P. Ross, G.F. Fitzgerald, C. Hill, and C. Stanton. 2005. Casein-derived antimicrobial peptides generated by *Lactobacillus acidophilus* DPC6026. *Applied and Environmental Microbiology* 72: 2260–2264.

Hirota, T., K. Ohki, R. Kawagishi, Y. Kajimoto, S. Mizuno, Y. Nakamura, and M. Kitakaze. 2007. Casein hydrolysate containing the antihypertensive tripeptides Val-Pro-Pro and Ile-Pro-Pro improves vascular endothelial function independent of blood pressure-lowering effects: Contribution of the inhibitory action of angiotensin-converting enzyme. *Hypertension Research* 30: 489–496.

Hugenholtz, J. and E.J. Smid. 2002. Nutraceutical production with food grade microorganisms. *Current Opinion in Biotechnology* 13: 497–507.

Hugenholtz, J., W. Sybesma, M.N. Groot, W. Wisselink, V. Ladero, K. Burgess, D. van Sinderen, J.C. Piard, G. Eggink, E.J. Smid, G. Savoy, F. Sesma, T. Jansen, P. Hols, and M. Kleerebezem. 2002. Metabolic engineering of lactic acid bacteria for production of neutraceuticals. *Antonie van Leewenhoek* 82: 217–235.

Ip, C., Y. Dong, and M.M. Ip. 2002. Conjugated linoleic acid isomers and mammary cancer prevention. *Nutrition and Cancer* 43: 52–58.

Islam, M.N., F. Akhter, A.K.M. Mausam, M.A.S. Khan, and M. Asaduzzaman. 2010. Preparation of dahi for diabetic patient. *Bangladesh Journal of Animal Science* 39(1&2):144–150.

Joshi, K.S. 2014. Docosahexaenoic acid content is significantly higher in ghrita prepared by traditional Ayurvedic method. *Journal of Ayurveda and Integrative Medicine* 5(2): 85–88.

Kamau, S.M., S.C.H. Cheison, W.Chen, X.M. Liu, and R.R.Lu. 2010. Alpha-Lactalbumin: Its production technologies and bioactive peptides. *Comprehensive Reviews in Food Science and Food Safety* 9: 197–212.

Kansal, V.K. and B. Ekta. 2008. Nutraceutical properties of dairy ghee. In: *Proceedings on International Conference on Traditional Dairy Foods*. November 14–17, (IFCON-93) held at CFTRI, Mysore, pp. 151–159.

Khurana, H.K. and S.K. Kanawjia. 2007. Recent trends in development of fermented milks. *Current Nutrition and Food Science* 3: 91–108.

Kim, E.J., P.E. Holthuizen, H.S. Park, Y.L. Ha, K.C. Jung, and J.H. Park. 2002. Trans-10, cis-12-conjugated linoleic acid inhibits Caco-2 colon cancer cell growth. *American Journal of Physiology—Gastrointestinal and Liver Physiology* 283: 357–367.

Kim, J.E., J.Y. Kim, K.W. Lee, and H.J. Lee. 2007. Cancer chemopreventive effects of lactic acid bacteria. *Journal of Microbiology and Biotechnology* 17: 1227–1235.

Korhonen, H. 2009. Milk derived bioactive peptides: From science to applications. *Journal of Functional Foods* 1(2): 177–187.

Korhonen, H. and A. Pihlanto. 2003. Food derived bioactive peptides opportunities for designing future foods. *Current Pharmaceutical Design* 9: 1297–1308.

Koutelidakis, I., B. Papaziogas, E.J. Giamarellos-Bourboulis, J. Makris, T. Pavlidis, H. Giamarellou, and T. Papaziogas. 2003. Systemic endotoxaemia following obstructive jaundice: The role of lactulose. *Journal of Surgical Research* 113(2): 243–247.

Kritchevsky, D., S.A. Tepper, S. Wright, S.K. Czarnecki, T.A. Wilson, and R.J. Nicolosi. 2004. Conjugated linoleic acid isomer effects in atherosclerosis: Growth and regression of lesions. *Lipids* 39: 611–616.

Lefranc, C. 2001. Cool, calm and collected. *Dairy Industries International* 66(6): 36–37.

Lin, M.Y. and C.M. Young. 2000. Folate levels in cultures of lactic acid bacteria. *International Dairy Journal* 10: 409–413.

Lopez-Exposito, I., and I. Recio. 2008. Protective effect of milk peptides: Antibacterial and antitumor properties. In: *Bioactive Components of Milk. Advances in Bladder Research* 606: 271–294.

Lourens-Hattingh, A. and B.C. Viljoen. 2001. Yogurt as probiotic carrier food. *International Dairy Journal* 11(1): 1–17.

Luzzana, M., D. Agnellini, P. Cremonesi, G. Caramenti, and S. de Vita 2003. Milk lactose and lactulose determination by the differential pH technique. *Le Lait* 83(5): 409–416.

Malik, R.K., S. Garg, T.P. Singh. 2014. *Probiotics in Combating Lifestyle Disorders*. Indian Dairy Association, New Delhi, India, pp. 138–141.

Mann, G.V. 1974. Studies of a surfactant and cholesteremia in the Maasai. *American Journal of Clinical Nutrition* 27: 464–469.

Martini, M.C., D. Kukielka, D.A. Savaiano. 1991. Lactose digestion from yogurt: Influence of a meal and additional lactose. *American Journal of Clinical Nutrition* 53: 1253–1258.

Matar, C., J.G. LeBlanc, L. Martin, G. Perdigón. 2003. Biologically active peptides released in fermented milk: Role and functions. In: *Handbook of Fermented Functional Foods. Functional Foods and Nutraceuticals Series* (Ed. Farnworth, E.R.). Florida: CRC Press, Florida, pp. 177–201.

Meisel, H. and E. Schlimme. 1990. Milk proteins: Precursors of bioactive peptides. *Trends in Food Science and Technology* 1(2): 41–43.

Meisel, H. and R.J. Fitzgerald. 2003. Biofunctional peptides from milk proteins: Mineral binding and cytomodulatory effects. *Current Pharmaceutical Design* 9: 1289–1295.

Meisel, H. and W. Bockelman. 1999. Bioactive peptides encrypted in milk proteins: Proteolytic activation and thropho-functional properties. *Antonie van Leeuwenhoek* 76: 207–215.

Minkiewicz, P., C.J. Slangen, J. Dziuba, S. Visser, and H. Mioduszewska. 2000. Identification of peptides obtained via hydrolysis of bovine casein by chymosin using HPLC and mass spectrometer. *Milchwissenschaft* 55(1): 14–17.

Mogra, R. and M. Choudhry. 2008. Effect of starter culture on the development of curd. *Journal of Dairying, Foods & Home Science* 27(2): 130–133.

Möller, N.P., K.E. Scholz-ahrens, N. Roos, and J. Schrezenmeir. 2008. Bioactive peptides and proteins from foods: Indication for health effects. *European Journal of Nutrition* 47: 171–182.

Morishita, T., N. Tamura, T. Makino, and S. Kudo. 1999. Production of menaquinones by lactic acid bacteria. *Journal of Dairy Science* 82: 1897–1903.

Nakamura, Y., M. Yamamoto, K. Sakai, A. Okubo, S. Yamazaki, and T. Takano. 1995a. Purification and characterization of angiotensin I converting enzyme inhibitors from sour milk. *Journal of Dairy Science* 78: 777–783.

Nakamura, Y., N. Yamamoto, K. Sakai, and T. Takano. 1995b. Antihypertensive effect of sour milk and peptides isolated from it that are inhibitors to angiotensin I-converting enzyme. *Journal of Dairy Science* 78: 1253–1257.

Nargunde, A.S. 2013. Role of dairy industry in rural development. *International Journal of Advanced Research in Engineering and Technology* 4(2): 8–16.

Oo, T.Z., N. Cole, L. Garthwaite, D. Mark, P. Willcox, and H. Zhu. 2010. Evaluation of synergistic activity of bovine lactoferricin with antibiotics in corneal infection. *Journal of Antimicrobial Chemotherapy* 65: 1243–1251.

Otani, H., K. Yukihiro, and P. Minkyu. 2000. The immuno enhancing property of a dietary casein phosphopeptide preparation in mice. *Food and Agricultural Immunology* 12(2): 165–173.

Padghan, P. V. and B. Mann. Biofunctional properties of traditional Indian lassi prepared from buffalo milk. 2012. PhD thesis, National Dairy Research Institute, deemed university, Karnal. [Unpublished data].

Pal, D. and P.N. Raju. 2007. Indian traditional dairy products: An overview. InSovenir, *International Conference on "Traditional dairy foods" held at National Dairy Research Institute*, Karnal, November, pp. 14–17.

Pariza, M. 1997. Conjugated linoleic acid, a newly recognized nutrient. *Chemistry and Industry* (London) (United Kingdom) 12: 464–466.

Parodi, P.W. 1997. Milk fat components: Possible chemopreventive agents for cancer and other diseases. *Australian Journal of Dairy Technology* 51: 24–32.

Parodi, P.W. 1999. Symposium: A bold new look at milk fat. Conjugated linoleic acid and other anticarcinogenic agents of bovine milk fat. *Journal of Dairy Science* 82: 1339–1349.

Parodi, P.W. 2004. Milk in human nutrition. *Australian Journal of Dairy Technology* 59: 3–59.

Patel, R.S. and B.K. Chakraborty. 1998. Shrikhand—A review. *Indian Journal of Dairy Sciences* 41: 109–115.

Pometto, A., K. Shetty, G. Paliyath, and R.E. Levin (Eds.) 2005. *Food Biotechnology*. CRC Press, Boca Raton, Florida, USA.

Prasad, S., R.K. Dhiman, A. Duseja, Y.K. Chawla, A. Sharma, and R. Agarwal. 2007. Lactulose improves cognitive functions and health-related quality of life in patients with cirrhosis who have minimal hepatic encephalopathy. *Hepatology* 45 (3): 549–559.

Prashant, S.K. Tomar, R. Singh, S.C. Gupta, D.K. Arora, B.K. Joshi, and D.K. Kumar. 2009. Phenotypic and genotypic characterization of lactobacilli from Churpi cheese. *Dairy Science and Technology* 89: 531–540.

Quesada-Chanto, A., A.S. Afschar, and F. Wagner. 1994. Microbial production of propionic acid and vitamin B12 using molasses or sugar. *Applied Microbiology and Biotechnology* 41: 378–383.

Rajpal, S. and V.K. Kansal. 2008. Buffalo milk probiotic dahi containing *Lactobacillus acidophilus*, *Bifidobacterium bifidum* and *Lactococcus lactis* reduces gastrointestinal cancer induced by dimethyl hydrazine dihydrochloride in rats. *Milchwissenschaft* 63(2): 122–125.

Rajpal, S. and V.K. Kansal. 2009. Probiotic dahi containing *Lactobacillus acidophilus*, *Bifidobacterium bifidum* stimulates immune system in mice. *Milchwissenschaft* 64(2): 147–150.

Ramamurthy, M.K. and K.M. Narayanan. 1971. Fatty acid composition of buffalo and cow milk fats by gas-liquid chromatography (GLC). *Milchwissenschaft* 26: 693–697.

Rangappa, K. S. and K.T. Achaya. 1974. *Indian Dairy Products*. Asia Publishing House, Bombay, India, pp. 386.

Rao, K.H. and P.N. Raju. 2003. Prospects and challenges for Indian dairy industry to export dairy products. *Indian Journal of Dairy and Biosciences* 14(2): 72–78.

Reddy, B.S. and A. Rivenson. 1993. Inhibitory effect of *Bifidobacterium longum* on colon, mammary, and liver carcinogenesis induced by 2-amino-3-methylimidazo [4, 5-f] quinoline, a food mutagen. *Cancer Research* 53(17): 3914–3918.

Reddy, P.B. 2010. Growth and trend discerning of Indian dairy industry. *Asia Pacific Journal of Social Science* 2(2): 105–125.

Rogelj, I. 2000. Milk, dairy products, nutrition and health. *Food Technology and Biotechnology* 38: 143–147.

Sarkar, S. 2008. Effect of probiotics on biotechnological characteristics of yogurt: A review. *British Food Journal* 110: 717–740.

Sarkar, S. and A.K. Mishra. 1998. Effect of feeding propiono-acido-aifido (PAB) milk on the nutritional status and excretory patterns in rats and children. *Milchwissenschaft* 53: 666–668.

Schumann, C. 2002. Medical, nutritional and technological properties of lactulose. An update. *European Journal of Nutrition* 41(1): i17–i25.

Schuster, G.S., T.R. Dirksen, A.E. Ciarlone, G.W. Burnett, M.T. Reynolds, and M.T. Lankford. 1980. Anticaries and antiplaque potential of free fatty acids *in vitro* and in vivo. *Pharmacology and Therapeutics in Dentistry* 5: 25–33.

Seki, N., H. Hamano,Y. Iiyama, Y. Asano, S. Kokubo, K. Yamauchi, Y. Tamura, K. Uenishi, and H. Kudou. 2007. Effect of lactulose on calcium and magnesium absorption: A study using stable isotopes in adult men. *Journal of Nutritional Science and Vitaminology* 53(1): 5–12.

Shantha, N.C., L.N. Ram, J. O' Leary, C.L. Hicks, and E.A. Decker. 1995. Conjugated linoleic acid concentrations in dairy products as affected by processingand storage. *Journal of Food Science* 60: 695–698.

Sharma, R. and D. Lal. 1997. Effect of dahi preparation on some water soluble vitamins. *Indian Journal of Dairy Science* 50: 318–320.

Sharma, S.K. and H. Reuter. 1993. Quarg making by ultrafiltration using polymeric and mineral membrane module: A comparative performance study. *Lait* 73: 303–310.

Silva, S.V. and F.X. Malcata. 2005. Caseins as source of bioactive peptides. *International Dairy Journal* 15: 1–15.

Singh, R. 2007. Characterization and technology of traditional Indian cultured dairy products. *Bulletin of the International Dairy Federation* 415: 11–20.

Sinha, P.R.V. and H. Yadav 2007. Antiatherogenic effect of probiotic *dahi* in rats fed cholesterol enriched diet. *Journal of Food Science and Technology* 44(2): 127–129.

Smacchi, E. and M. Gobbetti. 1998. Peptides from several Italian cheeses inhibitory to proteolytic enzymes of lactic acid bacteria, *Pseudomonas fluorescence* ATCC 948 and to the angiotensin I converting enzyme. *Enzyme and Microbial Technology* 22: 687–694.

Soel, S.M., O.S. Choi, M.H. Bang, J.H. Park, W.K. Kim. 2007. Influence of conjugated linoleic acid isomers on the metastasis of colon cancer *in vitro* and in vivo. *Journal of Nutritional Biochemistry* 18: 650–657.

Srinivas, S. and V. Prakash. 2010. Bioactive peptides from bovine milk a-casein: Isolation, characterization and multifunctional properties. *International Journal of Peptide Research and Therapeutics* 16: 7–15.

Srinivasan, D. 1979. *Concept of Cow in the Rigveda.* Motilal Banarasidas, Delhi, p. 4.

Srinivasan, M.R. and C.P. Anantakrishnan. 1979. *Milk Products of India.* ICAR, New Delhi,

Stanton, C., J. Murphy, E. McGarth, and R. Devery. 2003. Animal feeding strategies for conjugated linoleic acid enrichment of milk. In: Sebedio, J.L., Christie, W.W., Adolf, R.O. (Eds.) *Advances in Conjugated Linoleic Acid Research*, AOCS Press, Champaign, IL, pp. 123–145.

Sun, C.Q., C.J. O' Connor, and A.M. Roberton. 2002. The antimicrobial properties of milk fat after partial hydrolysis by calf pregastric lipase. *Chemico Biological Interactions* 140: 185–198.

Sybesma, W., C. Burgess, M. Starrenberg, D. van Sinderen, and J. Hugenholtz. 2004. Multivitamin production in *Lactococcus lactis* using metabolic engineering. *Metabolic Engineering* 6: 109–115.

Szwajkowska, M., A. Wolanciuk, J. Barłowska, J. Król, and Z. Litwinczuk. 2011. Bovine milk proteins as the source of bioactive peptides influencing the consumers' immune system—A review. *Animal Science Paper and Reports* 29: 269–280.

Taha, S., M. Mehrez, M. Sitohy, A.G. Abou Dawood, M. ABD-El Hamid, and W. Kilany. 2010. Effectiveness of esterified whey proteins fractions against Egyptian Lethal Avian Influenza A (H5N1). *Virology* 7(1): 330–334.

Tamang, J.P. 2010. *Himalayan Fermented Foods: Microbiology, Nutrition, and Ethnic Values*. CRC Press, Taylor & Francis Group, New York.

Tamang, J.P., S. Dewan, S. Thapa, N.A. Olasupo, U. Schillinger, A. Wijaya, and W.H. Holzapfel. 2000. Identification and enzymatic profiles of predominant lactic acid bacteria isolated from soft-variety *chhurpi*, a traditional cheese typical of the Sikkim Himalayas. *Food Biotechnology* 14: 99–112.

Tamime, A.Y. and R.K. Robinson. 1985. *Yoghurt: Science and Technology, Background to Manufacturing Practice*, 11–107. Pergamon Press Ltd, Oxford.

Thapa, T.B. 2002. Diversification in processing and marketing of yak milk based products, TAAAS/IYIC/Yak foundation/FAOROAP/ICIMOD/ILR/Workshop, pp. 484–489.

Thormar, H. and H. Hilmarsson. 2007. The role of microbicidal lipids in host defense against pathogens and their potential as therapeutic agents. *Chemistry and Physics of Lipids* 150: 1–11.

Van der Kraan, M.I.A., K. Nazmi, A. Teeken, J. Groenink, W. van 't Hof, E.C. Veerman, J.G. Bolscher, and A.V. NieuwAmerongen. 2005. Lactoferrampin, an antimicrobial peptide of bovine lactoferrin, exerts its candidacidal activity by a cluster of positively charged residues at the C-terminus in combination with a helix-facilitating N-terminal part. *The Journal of Biological Chemistry* 386: 137–142.

Whigham, L.D., M.E. Cook, and R.L. Atkinson. 2000. Conjugated linoleic acid: Implications for human health. *Pharmacological Research* 42: 503–510.

Wong, N.P., D.K. Walton, and G.R. Beechen. 1993. A preliminary comparison of the plasma amino acids of rats fed milk or yogurt. *Federation Proceedings* 42: 555.

Wright, G., A. Chattree, and R. Jalan. 2011. Management of hepatic encephalopathy. *International Journal of Hepatology*. Article ID 841407, 10 pages, doi:10.4061/2011/841407

Yadav, H., S. Jain, and P.R. Sinha. 2006. Antidiabetic effect of probiotic dahi containing Lactobacillus acidophilus and Lactobacillus caseiin high fructose fed rats. *Nutrition* 23: 62–68.

Yadav, H., S. Jain, and P.R. Sinha. 2007. Evaluation of changes during storage of probiotic *dahi* at 78°C. *International Journal of Dairy Technology* 60(3): 205–210.

Yadav, H., S. Jain, and P.R. Sinha. 2007. Production of free fatty acids and conjugated linoleic acid in probiotic dahi containing *Lactobacillus acidophilus* and *Lactobacillus casei* during fermentation and storage. *International Dairy Journal* 17(8): 1006–1010.

Yegna Narayan Aiyar, A.K. 1953. Dairying in ancient India. *Indian Dairyman* 5: 77–83.

Chapter 9

Health Benefits of Fermented Vegetable Products

S. V. N. Vijayendra and Prakash M. Halami

Contents

9.1 Introduction

Fermentation is a process, mediated by microorganisms that are present naturally or added intentionally, in which organic substrates, such as complex carbohydrates, are converted into either alcohol or acids (Paulová et al. 2013). The production of lactic acid (LA) by lactic acid bacteria (LAB) and alcohol by yeasts are examples of fermentation. Foods such as vegetables, fruits, and milk undergo some beneficial biochemical changes along with some significant modifications when treated with microorganisms or enzymes (Campbell-Platt 1994). Fermentation of foods extends shelf-life, and produces flavor compounds, which help to increase organoleptic properties of the foods and improves their nutritional value besides providing therapeutic benefits to consumers (Parvez et al. 2006). LAB are found to influence the texture, flavor, nutritive properties, health attributes, and shelf-life of food products (Devi et al. 2012) and also act as a source of functional ingredients (Florou-Paneri et al. 2013). Fermentation of foods can add value in terms of providing antimicrobial and antioxidant properties, producing essential amino acids and bioactive compounds, as well as enhancing bioavailability of the mineral. As a result, these foods can be used as therapeutic agents for humans (Tamang 2007). It is a general observation that eating fermented foods keeps people healthy. The regular consumption of fermented foods helps in reducing harmful and pathogenic flora in the intestine and improves the immune system.

Fermented foods are a major source of beneficial probiotic flora, besides; they contain several enzymes that help in the digestion of food carbohydrates and proteins thus helping better absorption in the intestine (Reddy and Pierson 1994). Around the world, the fermentation of foods has been practised for centuries in the traditional way, and their health benefits are well-known. Fermentation is the oldest and cheapest process for the preservation of foods. Among dairy products, the application of fermented milks in treating gastrointestinal disorders was recorded by the Romans in 76 AD (Stanton et al. 2005). However, the beneficial effects and the enhanced longevity gained through the consumption of fermented foods have been scientifically documented only after 1900 by Metchnikoff (Mackowiak 2013). The health benefits of traditional fermented foods especially dairy products have been known for a long time (Naidu et al. 1999, Hutkins 2006, Klaenhammer 2007). However, traditional fermented foods of vegetable origin, that are a rich source of LAB and bioactive molecules have not yet been explored for their health potential (Peres et al. 2012, Kumar et al. 2013).

Several plant-based foods have biological properties that can be exploited as a source of functional agents while preparing health foods. In the human diet, vegetables play a major role in providing a good amount of nutrients such as proteins, dietary fiber, phytochemicals, minerals, vitamins, and phytosterols. The role of vegetables and fruits in reducing hypertension (Dauchet et al. 2007) and heart diseases (He et al. 2007) have been well documented. The low sugar content, neutral pH, and the composition of vegetables do not favor spontaneous growth of LAB. However, vegetables have been fermented for centuries mainly to extend their shelf life and for use during the off season. Various vegetables-based fermented foods prepared in Indian subcontinent (Rati Rao et al. 2006) and in Asia (Swain et al. 2014) have been extensively reviewed. Fermentation of vegetables is known to enhance the nutritional value of vegetables in addition to providing health benefits. Fermentation of fruits and vegetables using LAB is a simple, economical, and cheap process to enhance the nutritional, sensory quality, and safety of the finished product (Steinkraus 1996, Demir et al. 2006).

In the recent past, the consumption of processed vegetables and fruits has increased (McFeeters 2004) due to rapid developments in the field of biotechnology in combination with traditional lactic fermentation. The exploitation of LA fermentation for the processing of fruits and vegetables (Di Cagno et al. 2013) and the use of vegetable products as a source of probiotic bacteria (Martins et al. 2013) have been recently reviewed. Fang (2013) has reviewed various aspects of fermented vegetables such as production methods, fermentation engineering, functional properties, and safety. Among the people of North East India, there are some general beliefs on the health benefits of consuming traditionally fermented vegetables. *Chyang* or fermented finger millet or *kodo ko jaanr* are given to postnatal women in the Himalayas to regain their strength (Thapa and Tamang 2004).

Sinki, a fermented product of radish tap-root, is very effective in curing diarrhea and stomach-related ailments (Tamang 2010) and *iromba*, which is prepared from the tree bean (*Parkia roxburghii*) is considered to be an appetizer (Singh et al. 2007). Certain fermented vegetable products (*gundruk, sinki,* and *iniziangsang*) are said to be good appetizers, and the ethnic people of the North-East India use these foods as remedies for indigestion (Tamang and Tamang 2009a). The extensive and detailed ecology of LAB associated with Vietnamese fermented vegetables was explored recently (Nguyen et al. 2013). This chapter mainly focuses on various health benefits offered by fermented vegetables, which have been reported in recent times.

9.2 Fermented Vegetables as Functional Foods for Health Benefits

Functional food is defined as food that contains known biologically active compounds which when ingested in defined quantity and quality provides a clinically proven and documented health benefit, and thus, an important source in the prevention, management, and treatment of chronic diseases of the modern age (Anon 2014). Consumer awareness toward functional foods is increasing with the progress of time, and people are expecting more and more health benefits that can decrease the risk of diseases with lesser side effects apart from enhanced nutritional value. Health benefits provided by foods may be categorized into three areas: direct health benefits, reduced risk of diseases, and improved life condition (van Kleef et al. 2005). The development of functional foods is considered to be an interesting area in the present scenario due to the increase in processing of foods (Annunziata and Vecchio 2011). The role of functional foods, the result of an innovative trend in the food industry, in nutrition and health have recently been exhaustively reviewed (Bigliardi and Gulati 2013). Fermentation of vegetables such as bamboo shoots enhances their therapeutic and nutritional value, thus making them an ideal functional food (Nirmala et al. 2014). Young bamboo shoots have several health benefits and these are attributed to the bioactive compounds present such as phenols, phytosterols, and dietary fibers and minerals, which can provide protection against many chronic and degenerative diseases (Nirmala et al. 2014). Similarly, phenolic compounds present in bamboo shoots may also have multiple biological effects such as antioxidation, antiaging, antifatigue, antimicrobial, and the prevention of cardiovascular diseases. Fermentation enhances these attributes further making bamboo shoots products more of a functional food (Nirmala et al. 2014).

Table 9.1 summarizes the several health benefits reported from fermented vegetables, especially *kimchi* and *sauerkraut*. In addition, *kimchi* exhibits several health benefits such as anticancer, antiobesity, anticonstipation, colorectal health promotion, probiotic properties, cholesterol reduction, fibrinolytic effect, antioxidative and antiaging properties, brain health promotion, immune enhancement, and skin health promotion (Park et al. 2014). Fermented bamboo shoots (FBS) are well-known for their antioxidant, antiaging, and anticancer activities. It was observed that, upon fermentation, the phytosterol level in succulent bamboo shoots in *Bambusa balcooa* increased from 0.12% to 0.62% dry weight (Sarangthem and Singh 2003).

9.2.1 Anticholesterolemic Activity

This refers to preventing the build-up of cholesterol in the blood. Elevated levels of cholesterol are considered to be a major risk factor for coronary heart diseases, and are also known to induce colon cancer. Certain LAB including strains of *Lactobacillus acidophilus* are capable of reducing cholesterol by assimilation mechanisms. Besides cholesterol degradation, cholesterol oxidase activity and bile salt hydrolase activity are also known to contribute anticholesterolemic activity by LAB. Since most fermented vegetables are known to harbor a large number of LAB, it is possible that they possess anticholesterolemic activity. The lipid lowering effect of *kimchi* has been reported recently

Table 9.1 Health Benefits of Fermented Vegetables

Name of Product	*Active Ingredients*	*Pronounced Health Benefits*	*References*
Kimchi	Isocyanate and sulfide indole-3-carbinol	Prevention of cancer, detoxification of heavy metals in liver, kidney, and small intestine	Park and Kim (2010)
	Vitamin A, vitamin C, and fibers	Suppression of cancer cells	Cheigh (1999)
	Organic acids, lactobacilli	Suppression of harmful bacteria, stimulation of beneficial bacteria, prevention of constipation, cleaning the intestine, and prevention of colon cancer	-do-
	Capsaicin, allicin	Prevention of cancer, suppression of *Helicobacter pylori*	An et al. (2014)
	Chlorophyll	Helps in prevention of absorbing carcinogen	Ferruzzi and Blakeslee (2007)
	Vitamin U	Inhibition of free radical production	Lee et al. (2014)
Saurkraut	LAB	Probiotics	Beganović et al. (2011)
	Vitamin C	Scurvy	Peñas et al. (2013)
	Isothiocynate	Prevention of cancer	Higdon et al. (2007)
	Glucosinolates	Activation of natural antioxidant enzymes	Martinez-Villaluenga et al. (2012)
Inziangsang	LAB	Probiotics, appetizers	Tamang et al. (2009)
Gundruk	Organic acids	Appetizer, improves milk efficiency	Tamang et al. (2009)
Sinki	LAB	Biopreservative, probiotics, antidiarrheal, stomach pain, etc.	Tamang et al. (2009)
Khalpi	LAB	Biopreservative, probiotics	Tamang et al. (2009)
Fermented *Gherkin*	LAB Vitamin K Potassium Vinegar	Probiotics Blood clot normally Intracellular electrolyte for reducing blood pressure Appetite stimulant	Breidt et al. (2013)

Table 9.1 (*Continued*) Health Benefits of Fermented Vegetables

Name of Product	*Active Ingredients*	*Pronounced Health Benefits*	*References*
Fermented bamboo shoots	Phenolics, flavonoids, tannin, crude fiber	Antioxidants, anti-free radicals, anticancer, and antiaging activity. Also minerals, fibers and probiotic bacteria as a health-enhancing food	Tamang and Tamang (2009b)
Beetroot *kanji*	Minerals	Prevention of infection and malignant diseases	Winkler et al. (2005)
	Betacyanin	Anticancer agent for colon cancer	

(Choi et al. 2013). More profound activity was noticed in the subjects with higher total cholesterol (>190 mg/dL) and LDL-C content (>130 mg/dL) in young healthy adults. Significantly decreased fasting blood glucose content in high *kimchi* intake group (>210 g/day) was observed.

9.2.2 Anticancer Effect

Certain fruits and vegetables which are rich in polyphenols, glucosinolates, and fibers can control colorectal cancer, which is a diet-related cancer more common in people who consume more red meat and foods high in saturated fats and consume less of plant-based foods (Gingras and Béliveau 2011). Eid et al. (2014) have reviewed the role of fruits and vegetables in reducing bowel cancer progression and how the polyphenols present in these foods can shift the gut ecology to give a beneficial effect to consumers. Chang et al. (2010) reported that *Lb. acidophilus* KFRI342 strains displayed the greatest ability to reduce the growth of cancer cells, SNU-C4, and were found to be useful probiotics with dairy starter culture properties. Besides *kimchi*, sauerkraut in the diet can also contribute to healing cancer due to the high levels of glucosinolate, the compound known to contribute to anticancer activity (Martinez-Villaluenga et al. 2012). It is known that the breakdown products of glucosinolates can modulate the initiation phase of carcinogenesis and are also known to inhibit programmed cell death.

9.2.3 Vitamin Production

Vitamins are one of the essential micronutrients for the growth of all living cells. Human beings cannot synthesize vitamins *in situ* and thus depend on external sources (LeBlanc et al. 2013). Some of the LAB and bifidobacteria are known to produce or convert metabolites into vitamins (Pompei et al. 2007, Chen et al. 2010). Several of the bifidobacteria species isolated from the gut are capable of synthesizing folate *in vivo* and *in situ* in humans (Strozzi and Mogna 2008). Riboflavin is another vitamin produced by lactic cultures. A riboflavin producing *Lactobacillus fermentum* was isolated from sourdough, and the yield could be enhanced by the mutants obtained by growing this isolate in increased levels of roseoflavin (Russo et al. 2014). The two fold increase in riboflavin content in bread fermented using these mutant cultures was noticed. The production of vitamin B12 (cobalamin) by *Lactobacillus reuteri* is reported (Taranto et al. 2003). However, there are very few reports available to date on the use of such type of cultures for the production of fermented vegetables, which can provide vitamins in the natural way. Production of folate by *Lactobacillus sakei* and riboflavin by *Leuconostoc mesenteroides* during *kimchi* fermentation was noticed (Jung et al. 2013), thus making *kimchi* a potential source of dietary vitamins. The vitamin content in bamboo shoot is less when compared to that of FBS products, which is due to the production of vitamins by LAB during fermentation (Chen et al. 2010). Several strains of *Saccharomyces cerevisiae, Candida tropicalis, Aureobasidium* sp., and *Pichia manschuria* isolated from Indian fermented foods like *idli* and *jalebi* batter were found to produce vitamin B12 (Syal and Vohra 2013). Hence, there is vast scope for the use of such probiotic cultures in vegetable fermentation to enhance the health of consumers. Fermentation of vegetables like carrot and beetroot by lactic cultures has a positive effect with an increase in levels of vitamins such as vitamin C, folate, and cobalamin (Martín et al. 2005, Jägerstad et al. 2006, Rakin et al. 2007).

9.3 Lactic Fermentation of Vegetables

A starter culture is defined as the microbial preparation of a large number of cells of at least one or more microorganisms to be added to raw material to produce fermented food by accelerating and steering its fermentation process (Holzapfel 2002). LAB found in raw material act as starter cultures during vegetable fermentation. Fermentation of vegetables is mostly a lactic fermentation that refers to the involvement of LAB to produce LA and to carry out the fermentation (Table 9.2). Vegetables act as an excellent source and a rich substrate for fermentation, wherein sugars such as glucose, fructose, and sucrose get converted into LA. Most vegetables are fermented by the addition of NaCl as brine (2%–5%) where it creates an osmotic condition and thus prevents the growth of spoilage bacteria. Salted fermented vegetables include, sauerkraut, *kimchi,* and *gherkin* (Breidt et al. 2013) and there are several nonsalted, acidic fermented vegetables, including *gundruk, khalpi, sinki, sunki, ingiangang* and also the fermented vegetables of Turkey, and so on (Tamang and Sarkar 1993, Endo et al. 2008, Rhee et al. 2011). Traditionally, fermented vegetables have been produced by taking advantage of the natural, resident microflora present in the raw material. This practice was found to yield a product with uncertain quality that may require a longer fermentation time. Subsequently, upon evaluating the complexity of the microflora, potential starter cultures identified and defined inoculum was developed for fermentation especially for sauerkraut and *kimchi.* Identifying the dominant LAB during different stages of fermentation resulted in the development of a defined starter culture with desirable properties such as proteolytic activity, survival in high salt concentration, and through the stress of freeze-drying, and also the ability to produce a high amount of organic acids, aromatic compounds, or antimicrobial compounds such as bacteriocin and metabolite such as exopolysaccharide (Patel et al. 2014). Several of these attributes are particularly important for obtaining high-quality finished products of fermented vegetables (Gardner et al. 2001). LAB associated with fermented vegetables are known to carry out two important types of fermentation, homo and heterofermentation. During homofermentation, LA is the principal end product obtained from glucose metabolism. However, in heterofermentation, besides LA, other organic acids, such as acetic acid and propionic acid are produced besides the evolution of CO_2.

9.3.1 Probiotics and Antimicrobial Peptides in Fermented Vegetables

Similar to dairy products, fermented vegetables also act as a desirable source for the growth of LAB exerting beneficial health. Probiotic bacteria colonize the intestinal mucus layer and affect

Table 9.2 Major LAB in Fermented Vegetables and Their Role in the Fermentation

LAB	*Possible Role*	*Fermented Vegetable/s*	*References*
Homofermenter/s *Ent. faecium* *Ent. faecalis*	Citrate metabolism, bacteriocin production	Green olive fermentation	Montaño et al. (2000)
Ped. acidilactici	Production of typical flavor due to lipase and peptidase activity	*Inziangsang*	Tamang et al. (2009)
	Hydrolysis of raffinose oligosaccharide	*Ingiangsang, Khalpi,* and fermented bamboo shoots	Tamang et al. (2009)
Lb. plantarum	Production of antifungal compound (3,6 bis (2-methylpropyl)-2 piperazinedien)	*Kimchi*	Yang and Chang (2010)
	Probiotic properties due to lactose hydrolysis and high hydrophobicity	Fermented Turkish vegetables	Karasu et al. (2010)
Lb. brevis	Typical flavor development due to peptidase, esterase, and lipase activity	*Sinki*	Tamang et al. (2009)
Lb. casei	LA production	Green olive of Sicily	Randazzo et al. (2004)
Obligate heterofermenter *Leuconostoc kimchi* sp. Nov.,	Maturation and flavor development	*Kimchi*	Kim et al. (2000)
Leuc. mesenteroides	Malolactate reaction	*Sauerkraut*	Johanningsmeier et al. (2004)
Leuc. fallax	LA and acetic acid, CO_2, mannitol production	*Sauerkraut*	Barrangou et al. (2002)
Leuc. citreum	Early and mid-stages of *kimchi* fermentation at 15°C	*Kimchi*	Choi et al. (2003)
Lb. delbrueckii, Lb. fermentum, and *Lb. plantarum*	LA	*Sunki*	Endo et al. (2008)

the immune system, inhibit the colonization of enteric pathogens, and play a major role in the cell signaling process (Kanmani et al. 2013). Tamang et al. (2009) reported that the LAB isolated from several Himalayan fermented vegetables exhibit probiotic properties such as high hydrophobicity associated with their colonizing ability in the GI tract of the host. Among the fermented vegetables, *kimchi* has been referred as a potential system for the delivery of probiotics (Parvez et al. 2006, Park et al. 2014). A novel culture of *Lb. acidophilus* KFRI342 obtained from *kimchi* was found to exhibit interesting probiotic characteristics such as protection against tumor initiation, imparting immunostimulation, and also had the ability to protect DNA damage as evaluated by comet assay (Chang et al. 2010). Recently, Sonar and Halami (2014) reported the potential of lactobacilli obtained from fermented bamboo shoot for their probiotic properties as well as technological attributes.

LAB cultures are being used as starter cultures for fermentation of meat, vegetable, milk, and cereals to enhance flavor and aroma, to protect the products from spoilage microorganisms and to extend the shelf-life (Kleerebezem and Hugenholtz 2003). Several LAB cultures with functional properties were isolated from FBS that were naturally fermented in North East India (Goveas et al. 2012, Tamang et al. 2012). A vancomycin-sensitive strain of *Pediococcus pentosaceus* producing heat stable bacteriocin with antilisterial activity was isolated from beans (Venkatheswari et al. 2010). We have also reported a *Ped. pentosaceus* producing cell lytic, heat-stable (121°C for 15 min), and pH (3–5) stable bacteriocin having antilisterial activity from a locally available cucumber (Halami et al. 2011). This bacteriocin had a broad spectrum of activity against Gram-positive and Gram-negative pathogens as well as spoilage LAB with cell lytic activity. Prior to this, we isolated an antilisterial bacteriocin strain of *Pediococcus acidilactici* K7 (NCIM5424) from fermented cucumbers (Halami et al. 2005). It produced pediocin PA-1 like bacteriocin that had stability at a broad pH range (2–9) and had strong antibacterial activity against *Listeria*, selected strains of *Lactobacillus* spp., *Pediococcus* spp., and *Enterococcus* spp. Several pediocin PA-1 like bacteriocin producers were isolated from vegetable sources that are known to be intergeneric and interspecific PA-1 producers that have strong antilisterial activity (Devi et al. 2012). An exopolysaccharide producing *Weissella cibaria* 92 isolated from fermented cabbage was found to have considerable antimicrobial activity against Gram-positive and Gram-negative pathogens such as *Staphylococcus aureus* and *Escherichia coli*, respectively (Patel et al. 2014). Several lactic cultures were isolated from traditional Romanian fermented fruits and vegetables such as cucumbers, cauliflower, green tomatoes, cabbage, carrots, celery, paprika, apples, plums, and pears. Some of these were found to have antimicrobial activity against *Listeria monocytogenes*, *E. coli*, *Salmonella*, and *Bacillus* (Grosu-Tudor and Zamfir 2013). Similarly, several LAB producing bacteriocins with antimicrobial activity have been isolated from *kimchi* (Rhee et al. 2011) and other fermented vegetables (Joshi et al. 2006).

Antimicrobial peptides, also known as bacteriocins, have potential application in food preservation and for therapeutic purposes in health care. Microbial-derived bioactive peptides with an antimicrobial property such as those produced by LAB in fermented foods are good candidates as food additives (Gálvez et al. 2008). Table 9.3 lists the bacteriocins produced by various LAB cultures. The benefits of antimicrobial peptides over chemical preservatives include minimized adverse effects, the requirement of low intensity heat treatment (minimal processing), and the retention of organoleptic quality and nutritional properties of foods (Gálvez et al. 2007). To improve the vegetable fermentation process, the addition of bacteriocins or bacteriocin producing starter cultures during fermentation, which can increase the quality of the fermented product, besides controlling the growth of spoilage and pathogenic microorganisms during fermentation, can be tried. Thus, consistent quality in the end product can be achieved. In *kimchi* the growth of *Lis. monocytogenes* was inhibited by a bacteriocinogenic strain of *Ped. acidilactici*

Table 9.3 Bacteriocinogenic LAB from Fermented Vegetables

LAB	*Source*	*Bacteriocin Type*	*Activity Against*	*References*
Lactococcus lactis subsp. *lactis* strains, NCK400 and 1JH80	Commercial sauerkraut fermentation	Nisin	*B. cereus, Lis. monocytogenes, Staphylococcus aureus*	Harris et al. (1992)
Lc. lactis	Vegetables	Nisin-like bacteriocin	Variety of LAB, but also to *Staph. aureus* and *Lis. monocytogenes*	Franz et al. (1997)
Lc. lactis KC24	*Kimchi*	Bacteriocin KC24	*Lis. monocytogenes*	Han et al. (2013)
Ped. pentosaceus K23-2	*Kimchi*	Pediocin K23-2	*Listeria* spp., LAB	Shin et al. (2008)
Ped. parvulus	Minimally processed vegetables	Pediocin PA-1	*Lis. monocytogenes, C. botulinum*	Bennik et al. (1997)
Leuc. citreum GJ7	*Kimchi*	Kimchicin GJ7	Gram+ve and Gram-ve bacteria including *E. coli*	Chang and Chang (2010)
Ped. pentosaceus NCIM 5420	Fermented cucumber	Pediocin PA-1 like	*Lis. monocytogenes*	Devi and Halami (2011) Devi et al. (2014)
Lb. plantarum Acr2	Fermented carrot	-do-	*Lis. monocytogenes, ALB*	-do-
Ent. faecium NCIM 5423	-do-	-do-	*Do*	-do-
Ent. mundt	Minimally processed vegetables	Mundticin	*Lis. monocytogenes, C. botulinum*, and a variety of LAB	Bennik et al. (1998)
Lb. plantarum 163	Chinese fermented vegetables	Plantaricin 163	*Staphylococcus, Listeria, Bacillus*, and *E. coli*	Hu et al. (2013)

(Choi and Beuchat 1994). A report by Kwak et al (2014) describing the dipeptide from LAB isolated from Korean traditional fermented vegetables with antifungal activity, suggests the possible production of an array of antimicrobial substances by these bacteria.

9.3.2 Role of Probiotic Bacteria

The WHO/FAO (2001) group of experts on probiotics has defined probiotics as live microorganisms which, when administered in adequate amounts, confer a health benefit on the host. Species of lactobacilli and bifidobacteria have been claimed to provide health benefits when consumed. Most acidic fermented vegetables are known to be treasures for obtaining probiotic cultures. The probiotic strain plays a crucial role, as these bacteria can survive and colonize the gastrointestinal tract (GIT) to confer functional properties and health benefits (Suskovic et al. 2010). The ability to tolerate acid and bile conditions, the adherence to intestinal surfaces, the exhibition of antimicrobial activity against pathogens, and the possession of technological properties are considered as the main criteria in the selection of probiotic bacteria (Naraida et al. 2012). Several strains of non-hemolytic LAB such as *Lactobacillus pentosus*, *Lactobacillus plantarum*, and *Lactobacillus paracasei* subsp. *paracasei* isolated from traditionally fermented olives are found to possess desirable *in vitro* probiotic properties like acid resistance (more than 3 h at pH 3.0), resistance to bile salt, and bile salt hydrolyzing activity, which can be explored for the exploitation of health benefits from these probiotic isolates when used as starter cultures for commercial applications (Argyri et al. 2013). However, 50%–70% reduction in the adhesion of lactobacilli grown in fermented carrot juice over that grown in a laboratory medium was reported (Tamminen et al. 2013). A link between probiotics and lower levels of stress hormones, and the protective effect of probiotics against depression are reported (Bravo et al. 2011).

9.3.3 Biogenic Amines

Biogenic amines are organic basic compounds which are present in various types of foods like *sauerkraut*, fishery products, cheese, wines, dry sausages, and fermented vegetables (Suzzi and Gardini 2003). Histamine has a heterocyclic structure, whereas tyramine has an aromatic structure. These are generated by the decarboxylation of corresponding amino acids by the microorganisms present in these foods (Tamang et al. 2008), which is not a desirable property of any starter culture to be used for food fermentation (Tamang and Tamang 2009b). However, some species of LAB can produce biogenic amines. Their presence indicates the deterioration of the foods or their defective preparation and is considered to be a health risk to sensitive individuals. The major symptoms of their consumption are cold sweat, hot flushes, headache, red rash, nausea, respiratory distress, hypertension, and hypotension. Tyramine is the major biogenic amine present in *tarhana*, a cereal-based food of Turkey fermented mainly by LAB and yeasts. On the average 92.8 and 55.0 mg/kg tyramine is reported from homemade and commercially prepared *tarhana* (Özdestan and Üren 2013). Halász et al. (1994) indicated a maximum limit of 100 mg/kg of histamine as a safe level in foods. High levels (>100 mg/kg) of histamine and tyramine can cause adverse effects to human health (Rauscher-Gabernig et al. 2009). Fermentation of cabbage with certain lactic starters such as *Lb. casei* subsp. *casei, Lb. plantarum,* and *Lb. curvatus* could reduce the biogenic amine content of sauerkraut (Rabie et al. 2011). They have noticed 161–165 mg/kg DW of biogenic amines in cabbage fermented by *Lb. casei* subsp. *casei* and *Lb. curvatus* and slightly higher content (220 mg/kg) in that fermented with *Lb. plantarum* when compared with natural fermented cabbage which had 804 mg/kg of biogenic amines after 1 month of storage. Control *sauerkraut* had six major biogenic amines (putrescine, tyramine, histamine, cadaverine, spermidine, and spermine), whereas, only putrescine, spermidine, and spermine were detected in sauerkraut fermented by these lactic cultures.

9.3.4 Fermented Vegetables as a Source of Bioactive Peptides

Bioactive peptides are short chain peptides generally consisting of 3–20 amino acids and these are formed by degradation of the original protein (Szwajkowska et al. 2011), due to the action of digestive enzymes or by microbial fermentation or during food processing. Bioactive peptides play an important role in metabolic regulation and modulation. Some of the vegetables harbor LAB as natural flora, and some of these can produce bioactive peptides (Hebert et al. 2008, 2010). Bioactive proteins and peptides have several health benefits such as antihypertensive, antilipemic, antioxidative, antimicrobial, immunomodulating, osteoprotective and opiate effect, and so on. Various health effects of bioactive peptides and proteins derived from different types of foods have been reviewed (Möller et al. 2008). A review on vegetable foods as a cheap source of bioactive peptides with health benefits has been recently published (Garcìa et al. 2013). Different thermophilic strains of *Lactobacillus delbrueckii* subsp. *bulgaricus, Lb. acidophilus,* and *Lb. helveticus* were found to hydrolyze soy bean protein to form bioactive peptides (Aguirre et al. 2008, Pescuma et al. 2013).

Angiotensin I converting enzyme (ACE) inhibitory peptides are bioactive peptides with potential antihypertensive properties *in vivo.* Mushrooms like *Tricholoma giganteum* and *Pleurotus cornucopiae* are a major source of a naturally occurring bioactive peptide that has ACE inhibitory activity (Lee et al. 2004). An ACE inhibitor peptide (Tyr-Pro-Lys) having IC_{50} of 10.5 mg/mL was isolated from broccoli and purified (Lee et al. 2006). This enzyme is also present in potato (Pihlanto et al. 2008). Bioactive peptides with other properties are also reported to exist in vegetables. Dioscorin (32 kDa) a peptide with antioxidant activity was isolated from a yam tuber (Hou et al. 2001). The hypocholesterolemic activity of potato hydrolysates has been demonstrated by the *in vivo* method and a peptide with higher hypocholesterolemic activity was obtained after 16 h of hydrolysis (Liyanage et al. 2010). Fermented soybean product *tofoyu* was found to have hypocholesterolemic effects (Kuba et al. 2004).

9.3.5 Reduction of Antinutritional Compounds

Some vegetables inherently contain naturally occurring toxic substances. Among these, the presence of cyanogenic glycoside causes major diseases of the nervous system, goiter, and miscarriage. Though bamboo shoots are rich in both amino acids and antioxidants, the cyanogenic glycoside present in bamboo shoots is a health concern. However, the fermentation of bamboo shoots by lactic cultures like *Lb. lactis* reduces this cyanogenic glycoside (Singh et al. 2007).

Phytic acid, also known as inositol hexakisphosphate (IP6), is a strong chelator of cations and known to bind several minerals resulting in decreased bioavailability of those nutrients and is hence referred to as an antinutritional factor. Phytate levels can be reduced by the enzyme phytase produced by microorganisms present in food (Raghavendra and Halami 2009). Degradation of phytic acid by the lactic cultures obtained from fermented vegetables is considered as a functional property. In this context, Tamang et al. (2009) evaluated several LAB obtained from fermented Himalayan vegetable products. It was found that most of *Lb. brevis* cultures followed by *Ped. pentosaceus* and *Lb. plantarum* were found to exhibit phytate degradation ability.

9.4 Conclusions

Fermented vegetables offer several health benefits and thus are truly referred to as functional foods or health-enhancing foods. There is consumer demand for organic food with the minimum use of chemical preservatives, hence, fermented vegetables can fulfill this requirement. As such fermentation of vegetables with LAB increases the safety aspects of the vegetables by way of producing acids and antimicrobial compounds like bacteriocins. Increase in the antioxidant activity due to fermentation was also seen. Fermentation also decreases the antinutritional factors and toxic metabolites present in some vegetables. At present, there are defined starter cultures only for a limited number of fermented vegetables. Therefore, there is a need to evaluate the microflora associated with fermented vegetables and identify the suitable cultures for large-scale production. Identifying the nonculturable bacterial cultures and studying their functionality could be carried out for the commercialization of fermented vegetables to fulfill market demand. The large-scale production of fermented vegetables can pave the way for the increased consumption of these products thereby leading to the formation of a healthy society. In addition, increasing vegetarianism and consumer demand for alternatives to dairy-based probiotic foods due to their high fat and cholesterol content or lactose content may lead to increased demand for fermented vegetables, which are also equally good in terms of providing health benefits. Hence, there will be a good demand for fermented vegetables in the near future.

References

Aguirre, L., Garro, M.S., and de Giori, G.S. 2008. Enzymatic hydrolysis of soybean protein using lactic acid bacteria. *Food Chemistry* 111: 976–982.

An, J., Jung, S.M., Chan, K., and Tam, C.F. 2014. Development of a 28-day *kimchi* cyclic menu for health. *Journal of Culinary Science and Technology* 12: 43–66.

Annunziata, A. and Vecchio, R. 2011. Functional foods development in the European market: A consumer perspective. *Journal of Functional Foods* 3(3): 223–228.

Anon. 2014. Functional food center. 2014. Web. 28 May 2014. (http://functionalfoodcenterdallas.wordpress.com/tag/nutrition/)

Argyri, A.A., Zoumpopoulou, G., Karatas, K.A.G., Tsakaliou, E., Nychas, G.J.E., Panagou, E. Z., and Tassou, C.C. 2013. Selection of potential probiotic LAB from fermented olives by *in vitro* tests. *Food Microbiology* 33: 282–291.

Barrangou, R., Yoon, S.S., Breidt, F., Jr., Fleming, H.P., and Klaenhammer, T.R. 2002. Identification and characterization of *Leuconostoc fallax* strains isolated from an industrial sauerkraut fermentation. *Applied and Environmental Microbiology* 68: 2877–2884.

Beganović, J., Pavunc, A.L., Gjuračić, K., Špoljarec, M., Šušković, J., and Kos, B. 2011. Improved sauerkraut production with probiotic strain *Lactobacillus plantarum* L4 and *Leuconostoc mesenteroides* LMG 7954. *Journal of Food Science* 76: M124–M129.

Bennik, M.H.J., Smid, E.J., and Gorris, L.G.M. 1997. Vegetable associated *Pediococcus parvulus* produces pediocin PA-1. *Applied and Environmental Microbiology* 63: 2074–2076.

Bennik, M.H.J., Vanloo, B., Brasseur, R., Gorris, L.G.M., and Smid, E.J. 1998. A novel bacteriocin with a YGNGV motif from vegetable-associated *Enterococcus mundtii*: Full characterization and interaction with target organisms. *Biochemical Biophysical Acta* 1373: 47–58.

Bigliardi, B. and Gulati, F. 2013. Innovation trends in the food industry: The case of functional foods. *Trends in Food Science and Technology* 31: 118–129.

Bravo, J.A., Forsythe, P., Chew, M.V., Escaravage, E., Savignac, H.M., Dinan, T.G., Bienenstock, J., and Cryan, J.F. 2011. Ingestion of *Lactobacillus* strain regulates emotional behavior and central GABA receptor expression in a mouse via the vagus nerve. *Proceedings of National Academy of Sciences, U.S.A.* 108: 16050–16055.

Breidt, F., McFeeters, R.F., Perez-Diaz, I., and Lee, C.H. 2013. Fermented vegetables. In: Doyle M. P. and Buchanan R. L., eds. *Food Microbiology: Fundamentals and Frontiers*, 4th ed, Washington, D.C.: ASM Press, 841–855, doi:10.1128/9781555818463.ch33.

Campbell-Platt, G. 1994. Fermented foods—A world perspective. *Food Research International* 27: 253–257.

Chang, J.Y. and Chang, H.C. 2010. Improvements in the quality and shelf life of *kimchi* by fermentation with the induced bacteriocin-producing strain, *Leuconostoc citreum* GJ7 as a starter. *Journal of Food Science* 75: M103–M100.

Chang, J.H., Shim, Y.Y., Cha, S.K., and Chee, K.M., 2010. Probiotic characteristics of lactic acid bacteria isolated from *kimchi*. *Journal of Applied Microbiology* 109: 220–230.

Cheigh, H. 1999. Production, characteristics and health functions of *kimchi*. *Acta Horticulture* (ISHS) 483: 405–420.

Chen, Y.S., Wu, H.C., Liu, C.H., Chen, H.C., and Yanagida, F. 2010. Isolation and characterization of lactic acid bacteria from *jiang-sun* (fermented bamboo shoots), a traditional fermented food in Taiwan. *Journal of Science Food and Agriculture* 90: 1977–1982.

Choi, S.Y. and Beuchat, L.R., 1994. Growth inhibition of *Listeria monocytogenes* by a bacteriocin of *Pediococcus acidilactici* M during fermentation of *kimchi*. *Food Microbiology* 11: 301–307.

Choi, I.K., Jung, S.H., Kim, B.J., Park, S.Y., Kim, J., and Han, H.U. 2003. Novel *Leuconostoc citreum* starter culture system for the fermentation of kimchi, a fermented cabbage product. *Antonie van Leeuwenhoek* 84: 247–53.

Choi, H., Noh, J.S., Han, J.S., Kim, H.J., Han, E.S., and Song, Y.O. 2013. Kimchi, a fermented vegetable, improves serum lipid profiles in healthy young adults: Randomized clinical trial. *Journal of Medicinal Food* 16: 223–229.

Dauchet, L., Kesse-Guyot, E., Czernichow, S., Bertrais, S., Estaquio, C., Peneau, S., Vergnaud, A.C., Chat-Yung, S., Castetbon, K., Deschamps, V., Brindel, P., and Hercberg, S. 2007. Dietary patterns and blood pressure change over 5-y follow-up in the SU.VI.MAX cohort. *American Journal of Clinical Nutrition* 85: 1650–1656.

Demir, N., Bachçeci, K.S., and Acar, J. 2006. The effects of different initial *Lactobacillus plantarum* concentrations on some properties of fermented carrot juice. *Journal of Food Processing and Preservation* 30: 352–363.

Devi, S.M. and Halami, P.M. 2011. Detection and characterization of pediocin PA-1/AcH like bacteriocin producing LAB. *Current Microbiology* 63: 181–185.

Devi, S.M., Asha, M.R., and Halami, P.M. 2014. *In situ* production of pediocin PA-1 like bacteriocin by different genera of LAB in soymilk fermentation and evaluation of sensory properties of the fermented soy curd. *Journal of Food Science and Technology* 51: 3325–3332.

Di Cagno, R., Coda, R., De Angelis, M., and Gobbetti, M. 2013. Exploitation of vegetables and fruits through lactic acid fermentation. *Food Microbiology* 33: 1–10.

Endo, A., Mizuno, H., and Okada, S. 2008. Monitoring the bacterial community during fermentation of *sunki*, an unsalted, fermented vegetable traditional to the Kiso area of Japan. *Letters in Applied Microbiology* 47: 221–226.

Eid, N., Walton, G., Costabile, A., Kuhnle, G.G.C., and Spencer, J.P.E. 2014. Polyphenols, glucosinolates, dietary fibre and colon cancer: Understanding the potential of specific types of fruit and vegetables to reduce bowel cancer progression. *Nutrition and Aging* 2: 45–67.

Fang, F. 2013. Fermented vegetables. In: Chen, J. and Zhu, Y. eds. *Solid State Fermentation for Foods and Beverages*, CRC Press, Boca Raton, USA, 199–216.

Ferruzzi, M.G. and Blakeslee, J. 2007. Digestion, absorption, and cancer preventative activity of dietary chlorophyll derivatives. *Nutrition Research* 27: 1–12.

Florou-Paneri, P., Christaki, E., and Bonos, E. 2013. LAB as source of functional ingredients. In: Kongo, M. LAB- R & D for Food, Health and Livestock Purposes, InTech, Croatia, 589–614.

Franz, C.M., Du Toit, M., Von Holy, A., Schillinger, U., and Holzapfel, W.H. 1997. Production of nisin-like bacteriocins by *Lactococcus lactis* strains isolated from vegetables *Journal of Basic Microbiology* 37: 187–196.

Gálvez, A., Abriouel, H., López, R.L., and Omar, N.B. 2007. Bacteriocin-based strategies for food biopreservation. *International Journal of Food Microbiology* 120: 51–70.

Gálvez, A., López, R.L., Abriouel, H., Valdivia, E., and Omar, N.B. 2008. Application of bacteriocins in the control of foodborne pathogenic and spoilage bacteria. *Critical Reviews in Biotechnology* 28: 125–152.

García, M.C., Puchalska, P., Esteve, C., and Marina, M.L. 2013. Vegetable foods: A cheap source of proteins and peptides with antihypertensive, antioxidant, and other less occurrence bioactivities. *Talanta* 106: 328–349.

Gardner, J.N., Savard, T., Obermeier, P., Caldwell, G., and Champagne, P.C. 2001. Selection and characterization of mixed starter cultures for lactic acid fermentation of carrot, cabbage, beet and onion vegetable mixtures. *International Journal of Food Microbiology* 64: 261–275.

Gingras, D. and Béliveau, R. 2011. Colorectal cancer prevention through dietary and lifestyle modifications. *Cancer Microenvironment* 4: 133–139.

Goveas, L.C., Selvajeyanthi, S., Vijayendra, S.V.N., Tamang, J.P., and Halami, P.M. 2012. Functional properties of LAB isolated from naturally fermented bamboo shoots of North East India. Abstract No. FMM5 of the paper in ICFOST held at CFTRI, Mysore, December 6–7, 2012.

Grosu-Tudor, S.S. and Zamfir, M. 2013. Functional properties of LAB isolated from Romanian fermented vegetables. *Food Biotechnology* 27: 235–248.

Halami, P.M., Ramesh, A., and Chandrashekar, A. 2005. Fermenting cucumber, a potential source for the isolation of pediocin-like bacteriocin producers. *World Journal of Microbiology and Biotechnology* 21: 1351–1358.

Halami, P.M., Badarinath, V., Devi, S.M., and Vijayendra, S.V.N. 2011. Partial characterization of heat-stable, antilisterial and cell lytic bacteriocin of *Pediococcus pentosaceus* CFR SIII isolated from a vegetable source. *Annals of Microbiology* 61: 323–330.

Halász, A., Bárath, A., Simon-Sarkadi, L., and Holzapfel, W. 1994. Biogenic amines and their production by microorganisms in food. *Trends in Food Science and Technology* 5: 42–49.

Han, E.J., Lee, N.K., Choi, S.Y., and Paik, H.D. 2013. Bacteriocin KC24 produced by *Lactococcus lactis* KC24 from kimchi and its antilisterial effect in UHT milk. *Journal of Dairy Science* 96: 101–104.

Harris, L.J., Fleming, H.P., and Klaenhammer, T. R. 1992. Characterization of two nisin-producing *Lactococcus lactis* subsp. *lactis* strains isolated from a commercial sauerkraut fermentation. *Applied and Environmental Microbiology* 58: 1477–1483.

He, F.J., Nowson, C.A., Lucas, M., and MacGregor, G.A. 2007. Increased consumption of fruit and vegetables is related to a reduced risk of coronary heart disease: Meta analysis of cohort studies. *Journal of Human Hypertension* 21: 717–728.

Hebert, E.M., Mamone, G., Picariello, G., Raya, R.R., Savoy, G., Ferranti, P., and Addeo, F. 2008. Characterization of the pattern of αs1- and β-casein breakdown and release of a bioactive peptide by a cell envelope proteinase from *Lactobacillus delbrueckii* subsp. lactis CRL 581. *Applied and Environmental Microbiology* 74: 3682–3689.

Hebert, E.M., Saavedra, L., and Ferranti, P. 2010. Bioactive peptides derived from casein and whey proteins. In: Mozzi, F., Raya, R., and Vignolo, G. eds. *Biotechnology of LAB: Novel Applications*, Ames, Wiley-Blackwell, 233–249.

Higdon, J.V., Delage, B., Williams, D.E., and Dashwood, R.H. 2007. Cruciferous vegetables and human cancer risk: Epidemiologic evidence and mechanistic basis. *Pharmacological Research* 55: 224–236.

Holzapfel, W.H. 2002. Appropriate starter culture technologies for small-scale fermentation in developing countries. *International Journal of Food Microbiology* 75: 197–212.

Hou, W.C., Lee, M.H., Chen, H.J., Liang, W.L., Han, C.H., Liu, Y.W., and Lin, Y.H. 2001. Antioxidant activities of dioscorin, the storage protein of yam (*Dioscorea batatas* Decne) tuber. *Journal of Agriculture and Food Chemistry* 49: 4956–4960.

Hu, M., Zhao, H., Zhang, C., Yu, J., and Lu, Z. 2013. Purification and characterization of plantaricin 163, a novel bacteriocin produced by *Lactobacillus plantarum* 163 isolated from traditional Chinese fermented vegetables. *Journal of Agricultural and Food Chemistry* 61: 11676–11682.

Hutkins, R.W. 2006. *Microbiology and Technology of Fermented Foods.* Oxford: Blackwell Publishing Ltd.

Jägerstad, M., Jastrebova, J., and Svensson, U. 2006. Folates in fermented vegetables—A pilot study. *LWT Food Science and Technology* 37: 603–611.

Johanningsmeier, S.D., Fleming, H.P., and Breidt, R. 2004. Malolactic activity of lactic acid bacteria during sauerkraut fermentation. *Journal of Food Science* 69: M222–M227.

Joshi, V.K., Sharma, S., and Rana, N.S. 2006. Production, purification, stability and efficacy of bacteriocin from isolates of natural lactic acid fermentation of vegetables. *Food Technology and Biotechnology* 44: 435–439.

Jung, J.Y., Lee, S.H., Jin, H.M., Hahn, Y., Madsen, E.L., and Jeon, C.O. 2013. Metatranscriptomic analysis of lactic acid bacterial gene expression during *kimchi* fermentation. *International Journal of Food Microbiology* 163: 171–179.

Kanmani, P., Kumar, R.S. Yuvaraj, N., Paari, K.A., Pattukumar, V., and Arul, V. 2013. Probiotics and its functionality valuable products—A review. *Critical Reviews in Food Science and Nutrition* 53: 641–658.

Karasu, N., Simsek, Ö., and Con, A.H. 2010. Technological and probiotic characteristics of *Lactobacillus plantarum* strains isolated from traditionally produced fermented vegetables. *Annals of Microbiology* 60: 227–234.

Kim, J., Chun, J., and Han, H.U. 2000. *Leuconostoc kimchii* sp. nov., a new species from kimchi. *International Journal of Systematic and Evolutionary Microbiology* 50: 1915–1919.

Klaenhammer, T.R. 2007. Probiotics and prebiotics. In: Doyle, M.P. and Beuchat, L.R. eds. *Food Microbiology: Fundamentals and Frontiers*, ASM Press, Washington, D.C., 891–907.

Kleerebezem, M. and Hugenholtz, J. 2003. Metabolic pathway engineering of LAB. *Current Opinion in Biotechnology* 14: 232–237.

Kuba, M., Shinjo, S., and Yasuda, M. 2004. Antihypertensive and hypocholesterolemic effects of tofuyo in spontaneously hypertensive rats. *Journal of Health Sciences* 60: 670–673.

Kumar, R.S., Kanmani, P., Yuvaraj, N., Paari, K.A., Pattukumar, V., and Arul, V. 2013. Traditional Indian fermented foods: A rich source of LAB. *International Journal of Food Sciences and Nutrition* 64: 415–428.

Kwak, M.K., Liu, R., Kim, M.K., Moon, D., Kim, A.H.J., Song, S.H., and Kang, S.O. 2014. Cyclic dipeptides from lactic acid bacteria inhibit the proliferation of pathogenic fungi. *Journal of Microbiology* 52: 64–70.

LeBlanc, J.V., Milani, C., de Giori, G.S., van Sinderen, F.S.D., and Ventura, M. 2013. Bacteria as vitamin suppliers to their host: A gut microbiota perspective. *Current Opinion in Biotechnology* 24: 160–168.

Lee, D.H., Kim, J.H., Park, J.S., Choi, Y.J., and Lee, J.S. 2004. Isolation and characterization of a novel angiotensin I-converting enzyme inhibitory peptide derived from the edible mushroom *Tricholoma giganteum*. *Peptides* 25: 621–627.

Lee, H.R., Cho, S.D., Lee, W.K., Kim, G.H., and Shim, S.M. 2014. Digestive recovery of sulfur-methyl-l-methionine and its bio-accessibility in *Kimchi* cabbages using a simulated *in vitro* digestion model system. *Journal of Science Food and Agriculture* 94: 109–112.

Lee, J.E., Bae, I.Y., Lee, H.G., and Yang, C.B. 2006. Tyr-Pro-Lys, an angiotensin I-converting enzyme inhibitory peptide derived from broccoli (*Brassica oleracea Italica*). *Food Chemistry* 99: 143–148.

Liyanage, R., Minamino, S., Nakamura, Y., Shimada, K., Sekikawa, M., Sasaki, K., Ohba, K., Jayawardana, B.C. Shibayama, S., and Fukushima, M., 2010. Preparation method modulates hypocholesterolaemic responses of potato peptides. *Journal of Functional Foods* 2: 118–125.

Mackowiak, P.A. 2013. Recycling Metchnikoff: Probiotics, the intestinal microbiome and the quest for long life. *Frontier in Public Health*, 1, Article 52, 1–3. doi: 10.3389/fpubh.2013.00052. Accessed on 10th Feb. 2014.

Martín, R., Olivares, M., Marín, M.L., Xaus, J., Fernández, L., and Rodríguez, J.M., 2005. Characterization of a reuterin-producing *Lactobacillus coryniformis* strain isolated from a goat's milk cheese. *International Journal of Food Microbiology* 104: 267–277.

Martinez-Villaluenga, C., Peñas, E., Sidro, B., Ullate, M., Frias, J., and Vidal-Valverde, C., 2012. White cabbage fermentation improves ascorbigen content, antioxidant and nitric oxide production inhibitory activity in LPS-induced macrophages. *LWT-Food Science and Technology* 46: 77–83.

Martins, E.M.F., Ramos, A.M., Vanzela, E.S.L., Stringheta, P.C., Pinto, C.L.O., and Martins, J.M. 2013. Products of vegetable origin: A new alternative for the consumption of probiotic bacteria. *Food Research International* 51: 764–770.

McFeeters, R.F. 2004. Fermentation microorganisms and flavor changes in fermented food. *Journal of Food Science* 69: 35–37.

Möller, N.P., Scholz-Ahrens, K.E., Roos, N., and Schrezenmeir, J. 2008. Bioactive peptides and proteins from foods: indication for health effects. *European Journal of Nutrition* 47: 171–182.

Montaño, A., Sánchez, A.H., and Castro, A. 2000. Changes in the amino acid composition of green olive brine due to fermentation by pure culture of bacteria. *Journal of Food Science* 65: 1022–1027.

Naidu, A.S., Bidlack, W.R., and Clemens, R.A. 1999. Probiotic spectra of lactic acid bacteria (LAB). *Critical Reviews in Food Science and Nutrition* 39: 13–126.

Naraida, L., Susanti, N.S.P., Hana, R.R.B,, Priscilia, D., and Nurjanah, S. 2012. Evaluation of probiotic properties of LAB isolated from breast milk and their potency as starter culture for yogurt fermentation. *International Journal of Food Nutrition and Public Health* 5: 33–60.

Nirmala, C., Bisht, M.S., and Laishram, M. 2014. Bioactive compounds in bamboo shoots: Health benefits and prospects for developing functional foods. *International Journal of Food Science and Technology* 49: 1425–1431.

Nguyen, D.T.L., Van Hoorde, K., Cnockaert, M., De Brandt, E., Aerts, M., Thanh L.B., and Vandamme, P. 2013. A description of the LAB microbiota associated with the production of traditional fermented vegetables in Vietnam. *International Journal of Food Microbiology* 163: 19–27.

Winkler, C., Wirleitner, B., Schroecksnadel, K., Schennach, H., and Fuchs, D. 2005. *In vitro* effects of beetroot juice on stimulated and unstimulated peripheral blood mononuclear cells. *American Journal of Biochemistry and Biotechnology* 1: 180–185.

WHO/FAO. 2001. Health and nutritional properties of probiotics in food including powder milk with live lactic acid bacteria. Report of a joint FAO/WHO expert consultation on evaluation of health and nutritional properties of probiotics in food including powder milk with live lactic acid bacteria. Argentina: FAO/WHO.

Yang, E.J. and Chang, H.C. 2010. Purification of a new antifungal compound produced by *Lactobacillus plantarum* AF1 isolated from kimchi. *International Journal of Food Microbiology* 139: 56–63.

Chapter 10

Health Benefits of *Kimchi*

Eung Soo Han, Hyun Ju Kim, and Hak-Jong Choi

Contents

10.1 Introduction

Kimchi is a typical Korean fermented vegetable food and was introduced as one of the fermented food of the world (Cheigh and Park 1994, Tamang and Kailasapathy 2010).

10.1.1 History

Dangun, founder of the Chosun country on the Korean peninsula 4346 years ago (2333 BC), was born as the son of a bear-woman and the God Hwanung (Kwon 2010). The bear was transformed into a human female body by eating mugwort (*Chrysanthemum coronarium*) and garlic in a dark cave without light for 21 days. It was believed that the mugwort and garlic should have been fermented as *kimchi* in the dark cave during this time. *Kimchi* was developed during ancient times in the Korean peninsula (Kim et al. 1997a). When available, Koreans cultivated and consumed fresh vegetables, however, in preparation for winter, they developed a pickling method to preserve the harvest (Korean Restaurant Guide 2009). *Kimchi* was at first only a salted vegetable; in the twelfth century spices and seasonings were added; in the eighteenth century red pepper became one of the major spices for *kimchi*; and in the nineteenth century *kimchi* cabbages were introduced to produce the dish as it is known today (Korean Restaurant Guide 2009).

Kimchi is produced from a variety of *kimchi* cabbages (*Brassica rapa* L. sub-species *pekinensis*) that must be free from significant defects, and trimmed to remove inedible parts. *Kimchi* cabbage is salted, washed with fresh water, and drained to remove excess water, then may or may not be cut into suitable sized pieces/parts for processing with a seasoning mixture consisting mainly of red pepper (*Capsicum annuum* L.) powder, garlic, ginger, and edible allium varieties. These ingredients may be chopped, sliced, or broken into pieces for fermentation, before or after being packaged into appropriate containers to ensure proper ripening and preservation.

Kimchi, a spicy fermented pickled vegetable, is a generic term used to denote a variety of fermented *kimchi* cabbage, radish, and garlic foods in Korea; the word is thought to come from "chimchae," which means salting of vegetables. The flavor of *kimchi* is dependent upon the vegetable ingredients, fermentation conditions, and the lactic acid bacteria (LAB) involved in the fermentation process (Lee et al. 2005). *Kimchi* is stored for several months and the process of fermentation results in lactic acid formation (Lee and Lee 2006).

10.1.2 Market and Trade

A typical adult Korean consumes 50–200 g of *kimchi* per day (Current of Kimchi Industry, 2011). Currently, more than 1.5 million tons of *kimchi* are consumed each year in South Korea with a market value exceeding 230 million USD in 2010 (Current of Kimchi Industry, 2011). *Kimchi* consumption is a rapidly growing phenomenon that has spread to other countries of the world such as China, Russia, Japan, and the United States. With the introduction of *kimchi* by Korean immigrants abroad, it is now considered a global food (Korean Restaurant Guide 2009) and is served in many Korean restaurants around the world. Thirty thousand tons of *kimchi* are exported to 47 countries, mainly Japan, Hong Kong, Taiwan, Russia, China, and the United States (Current of Kimchi Industry, 2011). *Kimchi* is such an important food to the nation's culture and cuisine, that a dehydrated *kimchi* preparation, the so-called "space *kimchi*" was sent into space with the first Korean astronaut (Song et al. 2009).

10.1.3 Preparation and Culinary Process

More than 100 different types of vegetables can be used to prepare *kimchi* (Kim and Chun 2005). *Kimchi* cabbage, radish, and cucumber, with a seasoning mixture made of red pepper powder, garlic, ginger, and green onion are among the ingredients used (Nam et al. 2009). *Kimchi* cabbage was developed in Korea for making *kimchi* cultivars in the nineteenth century. Without starter cultures, *kimchi* is made through lactic acid fermentations of *kimchi* cabbage at low temperatures to ensure proper ripening and preservation. Since *kimchi* is representative of a typical open ecosystem, each bath of the fermented product has a different composition of bacteria depending on the fermentation conditions and the ingredients which can be highly variable.

There are 336 kinds of *kimchi* in Korea, see Figure 10.1 (Jo 2000a). The main types are whole-cabbage *kimchi* (*pogikimchi*), diced-radish *kimchi (kakdugi)*, and water *kimchi (nabakkimchi)*.

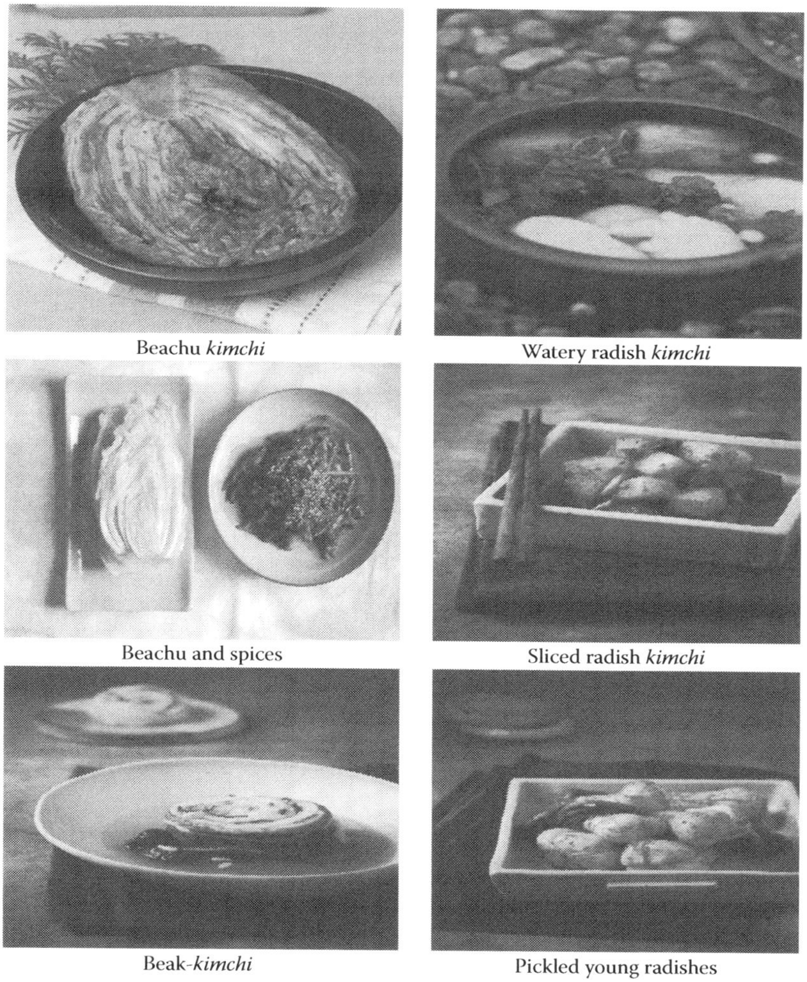

Figure 10.1 Different types of *kimchi*.

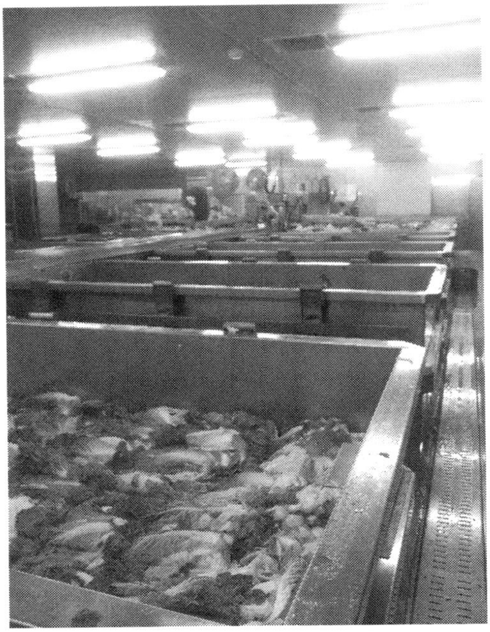

Figure 10.2 Manufacturing process of *kimchi* in the factory. Photo shows salted cabbage.

Kimchi is prepared as follows: First, cut well-washed cabbage and radish into small pieces and salt this for some hours. Second, after washing the salted materials, mix them with red pepper powder, garlic, dropwort, leaf mustards, and some gluey starch paste. Third, boil fermented fish in some water and cool. Fourth, add the fermented fish to the above blended stuff and store the mixture in a pot to ferment at *kimchi* refrigerator (Figure 10.2).

10.1.4 Fermentation and Microbiology

Phytolactic acid bacteria are the most important microorganisms in *kimchi* fermentation. Using conventional methods of isolation and phenotypic identification, the following species are found to be responsible for *kimchi* fermentation: *Leuconostoc mesenteroides*, *Leuconostoc citreum*, *Leuconostoc gasicomitatum*, *Lactobacillus plantarum*, *Lactobacillus sakei*, *Weissella koreensis*, and *Weissella cibaria* (Jo 2000b). Commercial *kimchi* with a consistent quality was produced by a starter culture consisting of *Leu. mesenteroides* and *Lb. sakei* in Korea. *Leu. citreum* HJ-P4, a strain with high dextran sucrase activity that was isolated from naturally fermented *kimchi* and adapted to grow at low temperature, has been proposed as a starter culture to produce commercial *kimchi* (Yim et al. 2008).

10.1.5 Safety and Hygiene

Lactic fermentation of *kimchi* protects microbial spoilage, and pathogenic bacteria are inhibited by acids and bacteriocins (Lee and Lee 2009). Lee et al. (1995) studied the fate of *Listeria monocytogenes* during *kimchi* fermentation. The viable cell count of *Listeria* increased during the first 2 days of fermentation but decreased with time while viable cells remained after 10 days at 35°C. The relationship between the concentration of LAB or pH and growth of three Gram-positive food-borne pathogens, *Bacillus cereus*, *L. monocytogenes*, and *Staphylococcus aureus*, were evaluated. Heating (85°C for 15 min) or neutralization (pH 7.0) was conducted on days 0 and 5 of fermentation and it was found that pathogenic bacteria were inhibited by *kimchi* (Kim et al. 2008c). Lee and Lee (2009) investigated the antimicrobial activity of *kimchi* against *L. monocytogenes*, *Staphy. aureus*, *Escherichia coli* O157:H7, and *Salmonella typhimurium*. The effect of different incubation temperatures (0°C, 4°C, 10°C, and 20°C) on the antimicrobial activity of the fermented *kimchi* was studied (Lee and Lee 2009). Higher acidity values were obtained when the fermentation temperature was higher. The greatest inactivation of *S. typhimurium* occurred in *kimchi* fermented at 20°C, while *L. monocytogenes* was inactivated in *kimchi* fermented at 0°C for 2 weeks. Raw garlic showed strong antimicrobial activity against the pathogens (Lee and Lee 2009).

A number of bacteriocin-producing LAB that make this natural biological method of preservation possible have been isolated from *kimchi*. *Leuconostoc* sp. produces a bacteriocin called leuconocin J, which is active against some LABs and food-borne pathogens (Choi et al. 1999). *Lactococcus lactis* BH5 produces a bacteriocin with a broad spectrum of activity against pathogenic and nonpathogenic microorganisms (Hur et al. 2000). A bacteriocin-producing *Lc. lactis* subsp. *lactis* from *kimchi* inhibited strains of *Clostridium perfringens*, *Clostridium difficile*, *L. monocytogenes*, vancomycin resistant *Enterococcus* and one out of four *Staphy. aureus* strains resistant to the antibiotic methicillin as well as some closely related LAB (Park et al. 2003). Pediocin A, a bacteriocin produced by *Pediococcus pentosaceus* (Shin et al. 2008), could be another possibility. Microbial interactions have been found to be important, and LAB sensitive to a bacteriocin produced by *Leuc. citreum* GJ7 enhance the bacteriocin production (Chang et al. 2008).

10.1.6 Nutrition and Biochemistry

The composition of *kimchi* depends on the variety of vegetables used, the process, and the fermentation and preservation methods. Complex biochemical changes occur before during and after fermentation. These include changes in carbohydrates, vitamins, accumulation of organic acids and sugar alcohols, and tenderization of texture. *Kimchi* is an important source of vitamins (especially ascorbic acid), minerals, dietary fiber, and other nutrients (Cheigh and Park 1994). Several organic acids such as lactic, citric, acetic, and succinic acids are produced during *kimchi* fermentation. Kim and Kim (1989) developed a sensor that detected pH values during *kimchi* fermentation at temperature 25°C, 10°C, and 4°C. After 8 days of storage, the pH values of the fermented product were 3.8, 3.7, and 3.3 at 25°C, 10°C, and 4°C, respectively (Kim and Kim 1989). Owing to its high consumption (100 g/day), *kimchi* is included in a food composition database of Korean foods (Lee et al. 2008c). Dietary fiber is especially important for the prevention of chronic diseases as its effects include reducing blood cholesterol, stabilizing blood sugar, and regulating bowel movements (Lee et al. 2008c).

The role of amino acids as the major structural and functional components of the body is well-known. Amino acid composition determines the protein quality of foods, and recent investigations have shown the benefits of a balance between essential and nonessential amino acids as well as the effect of amino acid supplements on muscle strength (Kim et al. 2009). One hundred and fifty high-protein foods were selected. According to the 2001 National Health and Nutrition Survey, the major foods contributing to protein intake were rice, beef, pork, chicken, egg, milk, soybean curd, and *kimchi*. Some of these foods are low in protein content, but their contribution is important because they are consumed in large amounts (100 g/day). The average protein intake for Koreans was 127% of the recommended level (Korean Nutrition Society 2000) and even higher for children.

10.1.7 Health Benefits

Kimchi was selected as one of the world's healthiest foods in 2006 by *Health* magazine due to its many beneficial properties (Nam et al. 2009). The functional components are derived from the raw materials, fermentation metabolites, and microbiota of *kimchi*. These include β-carotene, chlorophyll, vitamin C, and dietary fiber derived from raw materials such as *kimchi* cabbage, radish, red pepper, garlic, ginger, green onion, and leaf mustards. Organic acids, amino acids, peptides, vitamins, ornithine, and mannitol are produced during *kimchi* fermentation. Different types of probiotics are produced in *kimchi* such as *Lc. mesenteroides*, *Leu. citreum*, *Leu. gasicomitatum*, *Lb. sakei*, *W. koreensis*, and *W. cibaria*. Viable cells and cell wall components show health functional properties in the human body.

Lactic acid treatment from *kimchi* was found to play a role in the prevention of fat accumulation and in the improvement of obesity-induced cardiovascular disease, particularly atherosclerosis, by attenuating the TNF-α-induced changes of adipokines (Park et al. 2008). Glycoprotein antimutagenic substances have been isolated from the *Lb. plantarum* supernatant culture produced from *kimchi* (Rhee and Park 2001); antioxidants also have been isolated from *kimchi* (Sim and Han 2008). It has been reported that the consumption of *kimchi* causes weight loss; prevents constipation and colon cancer; reduces serum cholesterol (Park et al. 2006); and exerts beneficial antistress principles (Lee and Lee 2009) because *kimchi* contains *S*-adenosyl-L-methionine (SAM), a bioactive material used in the treatment of depression. *Kimchi* prevents osteoarthritis and liver disease (Lee et al. 2008b), demonstrates antiobesity effects (Kong et al. 2008), and inhibits atherosclerosis (Kim et al. 2007). A potential probiotic strain of *Lb. plantarum* isolated from *kimchi* inhibits the growth and adherence of *Helicobacter pylori* in an MKN-45 cell line with small peptides as possible inhibitors (Lee and Lee 2006).

10.2 Source of Phytochemicals

Phytochemicals, chemical compounds that occur naturally in plants (phyto means "plant" in Greek), are responsible for the color, smell, and functionality of *kimchi*. *Kimchi* contains many kinds of phytochemicals, such as phenolic compounds, terpenoids, organosulfides, indols, glucosinolates, and organic acids via its plant ingredients. Natural antioxidants contained in kimchi include phenol, phenolic acid, hydroxycinnamic acid derivatives, flavonoids, and ascorbic acid, which eradicate reactive oxygen species (ROS) or free radicals. *Kimchi* is also known as a relatively strong antioxidant activator, an action that is influenced by the relative amounts of each ingredient and the duration of fermentation (Park and Cho 1995). About 10,000 different phytochemicals have the potential to affect diseases such as cancer, stroke, or metabolic syndrome. Phytochemicals derived from plants are shown in Table 10.1.

In the preparation of *kimchi* the ingredients consist of major raw materials, spices, and additional materials. *Kimchi* cabbage and radish are the most important ingredients in the major raw materials group. *Baechu kimchi* is the typical *kimchi* and is often referred to simply as *kimchi*. Excepting *baechu kimchi*, *kimchi* is classified as *kakdugi*, *dongchimi*, mustard leaf, *yeolmoo*, green onion, and cucumber *kimchi*. The spices are garlic, red pepper, green onion, ginger, mustard, and onion. Additional materials including other vegetables (leaf mustard, watercress, carrot), fruits (pear, apple), nuts (ginkonut, chestnut, pine nut), and cereals (rice, barley, wheat flour) are optional. All the ingredients of *kimchi* such as red pepper powder, garlic, ginger, green onion, *kimchi* cabbage, and radish are the source of phytochemicals and contribute to its numerous health benefits (Park et al. 2014).

Table 10.1 Classification of Phytochemicals

Classification		*Phytochemicals*	
Phenolic compound	Flavonoids	Anthocyanidins	Cyanidin, delphinidin, malvidin, pelargonidin, peonidin, petunidin
		Flavanols	Monomer (catechins): catechin, epicatechin, epigallocatechin, epicatechingallate Dimer and polymer: theaflavin, proanthocyanidin
		Flavanones	Hesperetin, naringenin, eriodictyol
		Flavonols	Quercetin, kaempferol, myricetin, isorhamnetin, rutin
		Flavones	Apigenin, luteolin, limonin, nomilin
		Isoflavones	Daidzein, genistein, glycitein
	Phenolic acids	Hydroxybenzoic acids	Ellagicacid, gallicacid, salicylic acid, tannic acid, vanillin, capsaicin, curcumin, gingerol
		Hydroxycinnamic acids	Caffeicacid, chlorogenic acid, cinnamic acid, ferulic acid, coumarin
	Lignans		Silymarin, matairesinol, pinoresinol
	Stilbenoids		Resveratrol, pterostilbene, piceatannol
Terpenes (Isoprenoids)	Carotenoids	Carotenes	α- and β-Carotene, lycopene
		Xanthophylls	Canthaxanthin, lutein, cryptoxanthin, zeaxanthin, astaxanthin, fucoxanthin
	Saponins		
	Lipids	Phytosterols	Campesterol, β-sitosterol, γ-sitosterol, stigmasterol
		Tocopherols	Vitamin E
		Fatty acids	Omega-3,6,9
Organosulfides	ITCs		Sulforaphane
	Thiosulfonates		Allyl methyl trisulfide, diallyl sulfide
Indoles, glucosinolates			Allicin, alliin, allylisothiocyanate, piperine
Organic acids			Oxalic acid, phytic acid, tartaric acid, propionic acid

Source: From Cora J.D. and German, J.B. 2000. *Journal of the Science of Food and Agriculture* 80: 1744–1756.

Glucosinolates found in cruciferous vegetables such as *kimchi* cabbage are hydrolyzed by the enzyme myrosinase. Isothiocyanates (ITCs) are the glucosinolate degradation products which have anticarcinogenic properties (Cheigh and Park 1994). Jang et al. (2010) evaluated the antibacterial activity of 3-butenyl, 4-pentenyl, 2-phenylethyl, and benzyl isothiocyanate in brassica vegetables. In addition, Hong and Kim (2006) investigated the changes in ITCs levels in *kimchi* cabbage during *kimchi* storage. β-Sitosterol is the major phytochemical in higher plants, including fruits and vegetables. The compound has been shown to have the potential for prevention and therapy of human cancer. Choi et al. (2004) investigated the effects of β-sitosterol on the cell proliferation of HCT116 human colon cancer cells to understand its antiproliferative mechanism. Park et al. (2003) also studied *kimchi* and an active component, β-sitosterol, on the signaling pathway of oncogenic H-Ras(v12)-induced DNA synthesis.

Chlorophylls and carotenoids in mustard leaf *kimchi* have been reported to have antioxidant effects, and methanol extract of onion *kimchi* may have anticancer and immune activity. Capsaicin in red pepper powder can increase lipid metabolism. Lim et al. (1997) reported that capsaicinoids in red pepper powder has a liver glycogen sparing effect, increases the breakdown of fat in adipose tissues, and increases the release of free fatty acid by increasing insulin and catecholamine concentrations in serum. However, *kimchi* has other compounds that lower lipids in liver even more effectively than red pepper or capsaicin alone.

Garlic has a certain level of allicin and sulfur containing compounds, which possess antimicrobial and anticancer effects. Garlic, an important secondaryingredient in *kimchi* contains allyl sulfide, which exerts a regulatory influence on lipid metabolism. It has been reported that the administration of garlic decreases blood cholesterol and triglyceride levels in both humans and rats (Ried et al. 2013). The effects of 3-(4′-hydroxyl-3′, 5′-dimethoxyphenyl) propionic acid (HDMPPA), an active principle in Korean cabbage *kimchi* have been investigated. Results suggest that synthetic HDMPPA, as an antioxidant, may have a therapeutic application in human atherosclerosis (Kim et al. 2007).

10.3 Nutrient Synthesis and Bioavailability

The composition of *kimchi* depends on the variety of vegetables used, the fermentation process, the preservation methods as well as the complex biochemical changes in carbohydrates and vitamins, the accumulation of organic acids, and the texture degradation and softening. *Kimchi* is an important source of vitamins (especially ascorbic acid), minerals, dietary fiber, and other nutrients. The nutritional components of *kimchi* varieties are shown in Tables 10.2 through 10.4.

Table 10.2 General Components of *Kimchi* (per 100 g of Edible Portion)

Components	*Baechu Kimchi*	*Kaktugi*	*Gat Kimchi*	*Pa Kimchi*	*Baek Kimchi*	*Yeolmoo Kimchi*	*Dongchimi*	*Nabak kimchi*
Calorie (kcal)	18	33	41	52	8	38	11	9
Moisture (%)	90.8	88.4	83.2	80.7	95.7	84.5	94.2	95.1
Crude protein (g)	2	1.6	3.9	3.4	0.7	3.1	0.7	0.8
Crude lipid (g)	0.5	0.3	0.9	0.8	0.1	0.6	0.1	0.1
Crude ash (g)	2.8	2.3	3.5	3.3	1.5	3.2	2	1.5
Carbohydrate (g)	3.9	7.4	8.5	11.8	2	8.6	3	2.5
Dietary fiber (g)	3	2.8	4	5.1	1.4	3.3	0.8	1.5

Source: From Lee, H.G. 2006. *Food Composition Table*. National Academy of Agricultural Science Rural Resources Development Institute, Korea.

Table 10.3 Mineral Content of *Kimchi* (per 100 g of Edible Portion)

Minerals	*Baechu Kimchi*	*Kaktugi*	*Gat Kimchi*	*Pa Kimchi*	*Baek Kimchi*	*Yeolmoo Kimchi*	*Dongchimi*	*Nabak Kimchi*
Calcium (RE)	47	37	118	70	21	116	18	36
Phosphorus (μg)	58	40	64	55	25	51	17	7
Iron (μg)	0.8	0.4	1.3	0.9	0.3	1.9	0.2	0.1
Sodium (mg)	1146	596	911	876	422	622	609	1256
Potassium (mg)	300	400	361	336	116	606	120	66
Magnesium (mg)	30	13	–	–	–	32	7	6
Manganese (mg)	0.2	0.5	–	–	–	0.3	0.1	0.1
Zinc (mg)	0.5	0.4	–	–	–	0.7	0.2	0.2
Copper (μg)	0.08	0.07	–	–	–	0.07	0.04	0.02

Source: From Lee, H.G. 2006. *Food Composition Table*. National Academy of Agricultural Science Rural Resources Development Institute, Korea.

RE: retinol equivalent.

Not detected: cobalt, molybdenum, selenium, fluorine, iodine.

Table 10.4 Vitamin Content of *Kimchi* (per 100 g of Edible Portion)

Vitamins	*Baechu Kimchi*	*Kaktugi*	*Gat Kimchi*	*Pa Kimchi*	*Baek Kimchi*	*Yeolmoo Kimchi*	*Dongchimi*	*Nabak Kimchi*
Vitamin A (RE)	48	38	390	352	9	595	15	77
Vitamin A (β-carotene) (μg)	290	226	2342	2109	53	3573	88	460
Vitamin B_1 (mg)	0.06	0.14	0.15	0.14	0.03	0.15	0.02	0.03
Vitamin B_2 (mg)	0.06	0.05	0.14	0.14	0.02	0.29	0.02	0.06
Niacin (mg)	0.8	0.5	1.3	0.9	0.3	0.6	0.2	0.5
Vitamin C (mg)	14	19	48	19	10	28	9	10
Vitamin B_6 (mg)	0.19	0.13	–	–	–	–	–	–
Folic acid (μg)	43.3	58.9	74.8	–	–	–	–	–
Vitamin E (mg)	0.7	0.2	1.3	–	–	–	–	–

Source: From Lee, H.G. 2006. *Food Composition Table*. National Academy of Agricultural Science Rural Resources Development Institute, Korea.

Not detected: vitamin A (retinol), pantothenic acid, vitamin B_{12}, vitamin K.

Vitamins may undergo various biochemical changes because of the chemical enzyme reactions in microorganisms during fermentation and preservation. The changes in vitamin content during *baechu kimchi* fermentation (3.5% salt concentration at pH 7) are shown in Figure 10.3 (Cheigh and Park 1994). Vitamin B groups (B_1, B_2, B_{12}) were produced in *kimchi* during fermentation and increased twofold at 20 days, the optimum ripening stage of *kimchi* (Cheigh and Park 1994).

Depending on the type of fermentation and related microorganisms, ascorbic acid contents have a general tendency to decrease in the beginning, increase during active fermentation, and then decrease later. In model systems, the total vitamin C content also decreases initially, increases

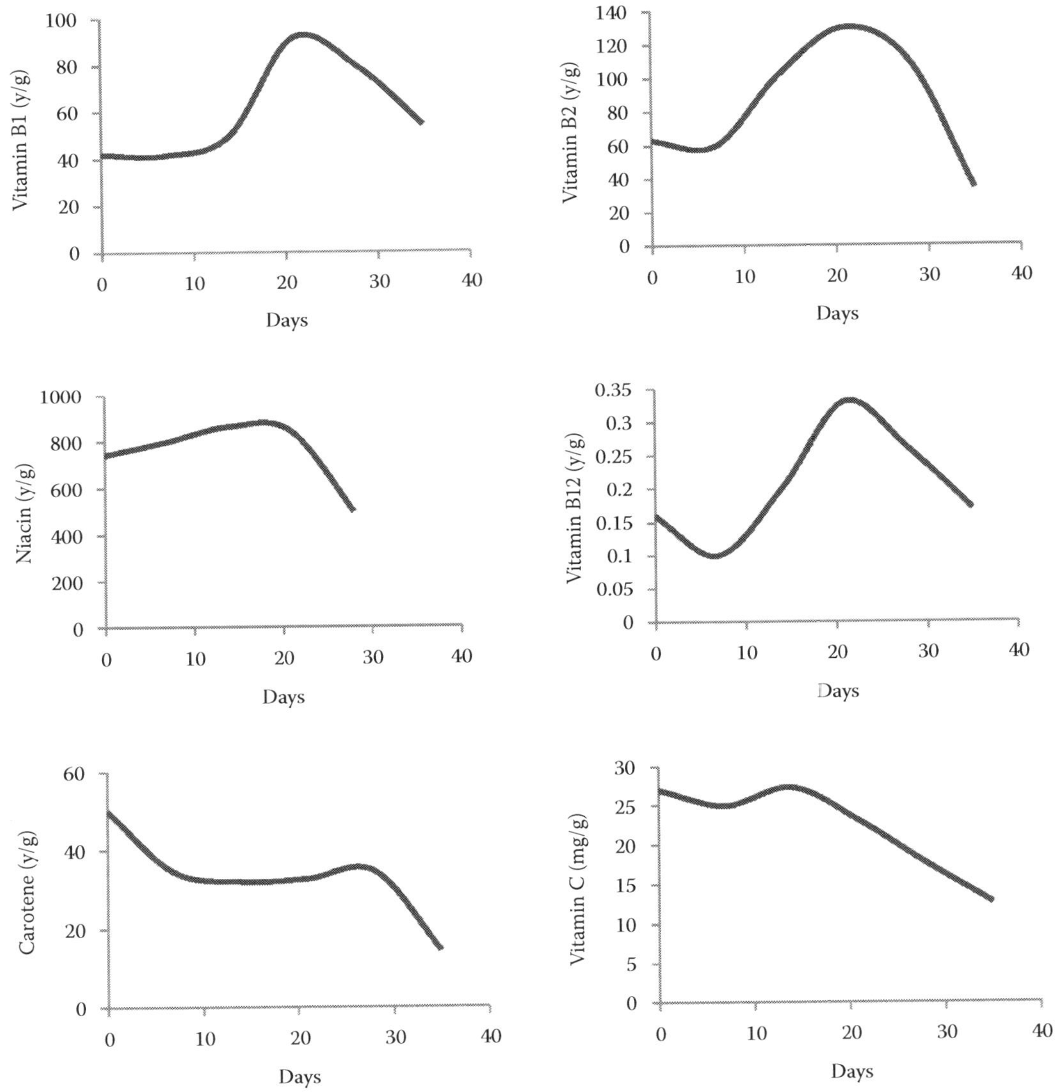

Figure 10.3 Changes in the vitamin content in *kimchi* during fermentation. (From Cheigh, H.S. and Park, K.Y. 1994. *Critical Reviews in Food Science and Nutrition* 34: 175–203.)

to the initial level or more at a certain time, and then gradually decreases later during the fermentation of *baechu kimchi*. In these studies, the absolute amount of biochemically synthesized ascorbic acid was about 52.1% of the initial value, and the addition of galacturonic acid enhanced ascorbic acid synthesis (Cheigh et al. 1996). Therefore, galacturonic acid may play a role as the precursor of ascorbic acid synthesis. The total vitamin C content under aerobic fermentation with the addition of galacturonic acid in this model is lower than under anaerobic fermentation without the addition of galacturonic acid (Lee and Lee 1981). The destruction of ascorbic acid when in contact with air may lead to a low potential of biological synthesis in aerobic conditions. In the *kimchi* model, a pH range of 4.0–4.5 is considered favorable for the biosynthesis and stability of ascorbic acid. The stability of ascorbic acid in *kimchi* is affected by pH, dissolved oxygen, garlic, and preservatives, therefore, changes in ascorbic acid content in *kimchi* during preparation and preservation would be influenced by the *kimchi* variety, recipe ingredients, microorganisms, and environmental conditions (Lee and Lee 1981).

The content of vitamin B groups increases gradually with time. From the initial fermentation stage, accumulation reaches the maximum level on day 21, and then drastically decreases afterwards (Lee et al. 1989). The increase in the vitamin B groups during the initial fermentation stage of *kimchi* may occur by biochemical synthesis due to microorganisms that have not been fully identified. Therefore, the vitamin B synthesis rate would be affected by the species of microorganisms and the fermentation conditions (Rhie and Chun 1982). A specific *kimchi*, which was inoculated with one strain of *Propionibacterium freundenreic hiissshermani* and fermented at 4°C, produced as much as four times the vitamin B_{12} as did normal *kimchi* fermentation (Kwak et al. 2008).

Kimchi is also an important source of carotene. Carotene content is affected more by the raw ingredients. This decreases slowly during the fermentation and is reduced to about 50% of the initial value after optimum fermentation (Ro et al. 1979). Organic acids such as lactic, acetic, and succinic acid are produced during *kimchi* fermentation. The total acidity increases from 0.1% in the initial stage to 1.0% at the final stage (Mheen and Kwon 1984). The kind of organic acid varies according to salt concentrations, fermentation temperature, and microorganisms (Table 10.5) (Kim and Kim 1989).

The World Institute of Kimchi studied the characteristics of the fermented vegetable foods in the world. They selected *kimchi, paocai, tsukemono, sauerkraut*, pickle, and *gundruk* as typical products (Table 10.6). They analyzed macronutrients (Table 10.7), minerals, and vitamins (Table 10.8). *Kimchi* has a balanced nutritional composition compared with other fermented vegetable foods, especially in minerals and vitamins (Han 2012). In addition, the safety of various salted vegetable foods in the world was evaluated by heavy metals (Jang et al. 2014).

10.4 Health Benefits

10.4.1 Immunomodulatory Effects

LAB participate in a major part of the commensal microbial flora of the human gastrointestinal tract, and reinforce the host defense systems by inducing mucosal immune responses. A number of reports have shown that LAB, such as *Lactobacillus* and *Bifidobacterium*, and their fermented products are effective at enhancing innate and adaptive immunity, preventing gastric mucosal lesion development, alleviating allergies, and mounting defenses against intestinal pathogen infection. Since *kimchi* is naturally fermented by a variety of LAB and *kimchi* LAB have been shown to modulate the host's immune responses, *kimchi* as a source of beneficial LAB has been in the

Table 10.5 Nonvolatile Organic Acid Content of Kaktuki

	Salt Concentration					
	1%		*2%*		*3%*	
	Fermentation Period					
Organic Acids	*4 Days*	*8 Days*	*4 Days*	*8 Days*	*4 Days*	*8 Days*
Lactic acid	21.38	57.98	24.42	40.94	19.52	31.58
Oxalic acid	0.02	0.24	0.28	0.28	0.32	0.22
Malonic acid	0.02	0.06	ND	0.02	ND	0.04
Fumaric acid	0.01	0.20	0.02	0.18	ND	0.14
Succinic acid	3.86	11.58	3.12	6.24	2.82	4.88
Maleic acid	0.02	0.02	0.02	0.04	0.02	0.04
Malic acid	0.06	3.88	0.04	3.16	0.04	3.26
Citric acid	2.16	10.8	5.78	9.06	4.34	4.81
Total	27.71	84.76	33.68	59.92	27.06	44.98

Source: From Kim, S.Y. and Kim, K.O. 1989. *Korean Journal of Food Science and Technology* 21: 370–374.

Note: ND = not detectable.

spotlight. Furthermore, phytochemicals present in *kimchi* also have shown beneficial effects on the host's immunity. In this chapter, we describe the immunomodulatory effects of *kimchi* and the several LAB strains isolated from *kimchi*.

10.4.1.1 Modulation of Immunity

The innate immune response serves not only as the first line of defense but also plays a crucial role in the development of subsequent adaptive immune responses. Several studies have described that intake of *kimchi* controls innate and adaptive immunity in animal models. Kim and Lee (1997) reported that the diet of freeze-dried *kimchi* fermented at 3 and 6 weeks at 4°C resulted in enhanced proliferation of rat splenocytes compared to controls fed unfermented *kimchi,* indicating that the intake of fermented *kimchi* upregulates the proliferation of spleen cells (Kim et al. 1997a,b). A similar study showed that treatment of the methanol extract of onion *kimchi* induces the enhanced proliferation of splenocytes and increases production of nitric oxide (NO) by macrophages (Park et al. 2004). Another study investigated the effect of *kimchi* on the culture of immune cells. In the presence of *kimchi* extracts, rat splenocytes, thymocytes, and bone marrow cells grew better than negative controls treated with phosphate-buffered saline, suggesting that *kimchi* may affect differentiation and growth of immune cells as well as immune responses (Kim et al. 1997a,b). As innate immune cells, macrophages enhance phagocytosis, pinocytosis, and the production of lysozyme, and cytoplasmic granules upon activation by external stimuli such as pathogenic infections. Treatment of murine macrophages with *kimchi* extracts from 3-week-fermented *kimchi* increases the capability of phagocytosis against *Candida albicans* (Choi et al. 1997).

Table 10.6 Packaging and Components of Fermented Vegetables in the World

	Package	*Component*
Kimchi	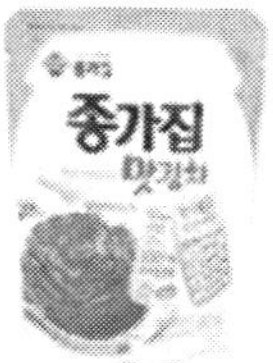	Salted cabbage, radish, salted shrimp, salted anchovies, kelp, powdered red pepper, garlic, ginger, spring onion, onion, chives
Paocai	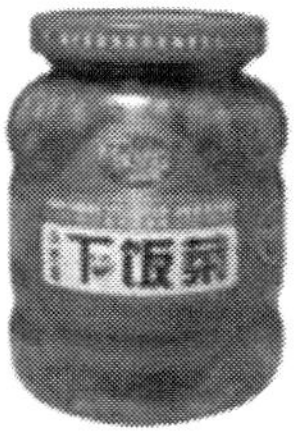	*Zhacai*, radish, cowpea, rapeseed oil, refined salt, salted pepper, cooking wine, lactic acid, MSG, 5′-IMP, 5′-GMP, turmeric
Tsukemono	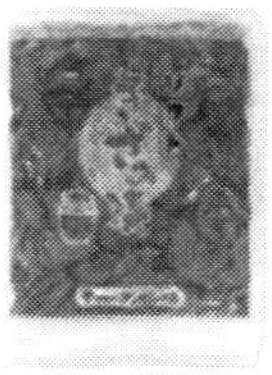	Salted radish, salt purified water, glucose–fructose, soy sauce, MSG, citric acid, succinic acid, DL-malic acid, sodium saccharin, potassium sorbate, powdered rice bran
Sauerkraut	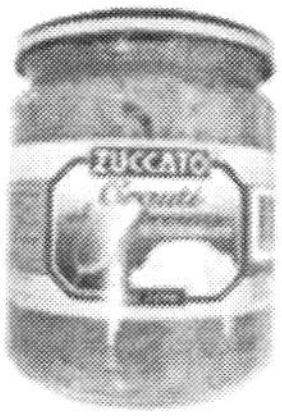	Cabbage, white wine, refined salt
Pickle	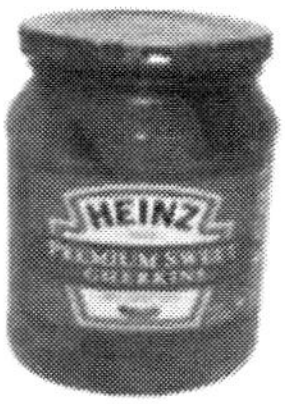	Cucumber, refined salt, fructose syrup, white vinegar
Gundruk	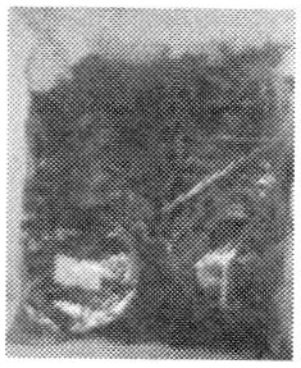	Leafy vegetables, mustards, cauliflower

Source: From Han, E.S. 2012. Overview of Kimchi. *The 4th International Kimchi Conference*, Washington DC.

Table 10.7 Macronutrient Content of Fermented Vegetable Foods in the World (g%)

	Protein	*Lipid*	*Carbohydrate*	*Dietary Fiber*	*Crude Ash*
Kimchi	18.2	2.0	56.6	29.3	23.2
Paocai	8.4	42.2	27.9	29.3	21.5
Tsukemono	7.8	1.0	53.4	20.7	37.9
Sauerkraut	12.8	2.3	66.3	34.0	18.6
Pickle	1.3	0.7	92.4	38.4	5.6
Gundruk	20.0	2.1	60.9	4.7	17.0

Source: From Han, E.S. 2012. Overview of *kimchi*. *The 4th International Kimchi Conference*, Washington DC.

Note: Calculated from average macronutrient measured in dried sample and drying yield.

Several studies have reported that LAB involved in *kimchi* fermentation also display immunomodulatory effects (Table 10.9). Chae et al. (1998) investigated the effect of oral administration of a LAB homogenate on various immune responses. Mice fed a LAB homogenate show: (1) enhanced proliferation of splenocytes and intestinal cells; (2) increased NO production by peritoneal macrophages; (3) increased production of intestinal IgA levels; (4) increased levels of tumor necrosis factor (TNF)-α and IL-2 in serum; and (5) increased number of specific antibody-producing B cells. The results of this study imply that the oral administration of LAB homogenate is capable of inducing intestinal immune responses as well as systematic immunity as detected by elevated levels of cytokines in the blood (Chae et al. 1998). Cellular fractions (whole cells, cell wall, and cytosol fraction) of *Lb. brevis* FSB-1 isolated from *kimchi* were tested for their ability to stimulate various immune responses. While *Lb. brevis* FSB-1 did not show direct activity on

Table 10.8 Mineral and Vitamin Content of Fermented Vegetable Foods in the World (mg%)

	Calcium	*Sodium*	*Phosphorus*	*Zinc*	*Iron*	*β-Carotene*	*Ascorbic Acid*	*Tocopherol*
Kimchi	488.9	6565.7	389.9	3.0	6.1	12.1	68.7	4.0
Paocai	204.0	7529.5	116.3	1.2	6.8	10.8	0.0	15.9
Tsukemono	165.0	13738.8	302.9	1.0	5.8	0.0	0.0	0.0
Sauerkraut	693.0	4208.1	295.3	2.3	12.8	0.0	88.4	0.0
Pickle	94.0	1914.6	27.6	0.0	1.0	1.3	0.0	0.0
Gundruk	2896.3	251.8	473.5	4.2	107.0	4.3	0.0	0.2

Source: From Han, E.S. 2012. Overview of *kimchi*. *The 4th International Kimchi Conference*, Washington, DC.

Note: Calculated from average general component measured in dried sample and drying yield.

Table 10.9 Various Immunomodulatory Effects of Different LAB Isolated from *Kimchi*

	Immunomodulatory Effects			
LAB	*Innate Immunity*	*Adaptive Immunity*	*Symptoms Improvement*	*References*
Lactobacillus brevis FSB-1	Induce proliferation and activation of macrophages	Enhance proliferation of bone marrow cells		Kim et al. (2004)
Lb. plantarum CJLP133	Upregulate expression of costimulatory molecules on macrophages	Adjust Th1/Th2 balance	Reduce hypersensitive reaction caused by Th2 cells	Won et al. (2010)
Lb. plantarum CJLP243		Enhance IFN-γ secretion and lymphocyte proliferation		Lee et al. (2011)
Lb. sakei proBio65		Induce Foxp3^{+} Treg differentiation Inhibit IgE and Th2 cytokine production	Alleviate atopic dermatitis	Park et al. (2008), Lim et al. (2011)
Lb. plantarum K8		Inhibit IgE and Th2 cytokine production	Alleviate atopic dermatitis	Lee et al. (2008)
Lb. plantarum	Enhance NO production by peritoneal macrophages	Enhance intestinal secretory IgA production		Chae et al. (1998)

the proliferation of bone marrow cells, all cellular fractions induced the activation of macrophages (Kim et al. 2004b). In particular, the cytosol fraction of *Lb. brevis* FSB-1 showed a strong capability of complement activation (Kim et al. 2004b). Seo and Lee (2007) also investigated the immune stimulating effects of cytosol and cell wall fractions of the *Lactobacillus acidophilus* strain isolated from *kimchi*. In contrast to a cytosol fraction, which showed comparable intestinal immune modulating activity to LPS used as a positive control, the cell wall fraction displayed weak activity. Both cell wall and cytosol fractions had a low capability on the proliferation of splenocytes. However, the levels of macrophage proliferation by both fractions were higher than those in the positive control group (Seo and Lee 2007). Several *Lactobacillus* strains from *kimchi* had the effect of skewing T cells from T helper 2 (Th2) toward Th1 responses, thus promoting humoral immunity. Won et al. (2011) demonstrated that *Lb. plantarum* was able to polarize the subsequent T cell activity toward Th1, resulting in the inhibition of Th2 responses. The study demonstrated that lactobacilli from *kimchi* may modulate the Th1/Th2 balance via macrophage activation in the hypersensitive reaction caused by Th2 cells (Won et al. 2011).

Probiotic bacteria demonstrate benefits in the treatment of human inflammatory bowel diseases as they induce the differentiation and activation of regulatory T (Treg) cells and are able to enhance the secretion of anti-inflammatory cytokine such as interleukin (IL)-10 by Treg in the gut. A recent study showed that the *Lb. sakei* proBio65 strain isolated from *kimchi* induces IL-10 production in response to mesenteric lymphocytes. Interestingly, the phenomenon mediated by this probiotic bacterium also increases the population of $Foxp3^+$ cells, which are designated as Treg (Lim et al. 2011). This study highlights that like other LAB that induce the differentiation of Treg by the activation of toll-like receptor (TLR)2 and TLR6 signaling pathways (Kwon et al. 2010, Konieczna et al. 2012), LAB from *kimchi* may be used as a therapeutic to control inflammatory disorders such as atopic dermatitis and inflammatory bowel disease (Lim et al. 2011).

10.4.1.2 Alleviation of Immune Disorders

Many types of LAB products have antiallergic effects in a murine model. For example, heat-killed LAB suppress specific immunoglobulin (Ig) E synthesis and alleviate allergic symptoms in animals (Tsai et al. 2012). The probiotic extracts of *kimchi* also suppress antiatopic dermatitis, which is characterized by the chronic relapsing inflammation associated with hyperproduction of IgE. The ral administration of *Lb. plantarum* K8 extracts showed effectiveness in 1-chloro-2,4-dinitrobenzene (DNCB)-treated NC/Nga mice, an animal model of atopic dermatitis, via modulation of the IgE level and the production of IL-4 and IL-5 which are recognized as Th2 cytokines (Lee et al. 2008a). In addition, *Lb. sakei* proBio65 induces the differentiation of Treg as described above. This *kimchi* microorganism was shown to be effective in reducing allergen-induced skin inflammation (Park et al. 2008). Oral administration of *Lb. sakei* proBio65 in mice treated with DNCB showed a more rapid recovery from allergic dermatitis compared with control mice through the regulation of both elevated IgE and IL-4 (Park et al. 2008, Kim et al. 2013). Table 10.9 shows the immunomodulatory effects of different LAB strains on innate or adaptive immune responses as a function of health benefits.

10.4.2 Pathogen Preventing Effects

Probiotics beneficially affect the host by improving the balance of the intestinal flora. Probiotic intake leads to the creation of gut microbiology conditions that suppress harmful microorganisms and favor beneficial microorganisms, ultimately enhancing gut health (Mountzouris et al. 2007). Park et al. (2008) have reported that *Lb. sakei* proBio65 has a broad antimicrobial spectrum against various pathogenic microorganisms, including *E. coli*, *S. typhimurium*, and *Shigella flexneri*, and strongly inhibits the growth of *Staphy. aureus*, which is known to be a factor in severe atopic dermatitis (Park et al. 2008). Several probiotic *Lb. plantarum* strains isolated from *kimchi* also have been shown to inhibit the growth of intestinal pathogens, such as *E. coli*, *Staphy. aureus*, *Yersinia enterocolitica*, *S. typhimurium*, and *L. monocytogenes* (Lee et al. 2011a). The protective role of these *kimchi* LAB in a pathogenic infection model has not been investigated, however, it is expected that probiotic *kimchi* LAB contribute to the protection of the host against pathogenic infections since *kimchi* LAB strains have a direct microcidal function and are able to enhance the production of IL-12 and interferon (IFN)-γ (Park et al. 2008, Lee et al. 2011a), which are essential Th1 cytokines for immune responses to clear pathogen-infected cells. Further studies are required to confirm the protective effects of *kimchi* LAB using appropriate animal models. Figure 10.4 presents the immunomodulatory effects of LAB isolated *kimchi*.

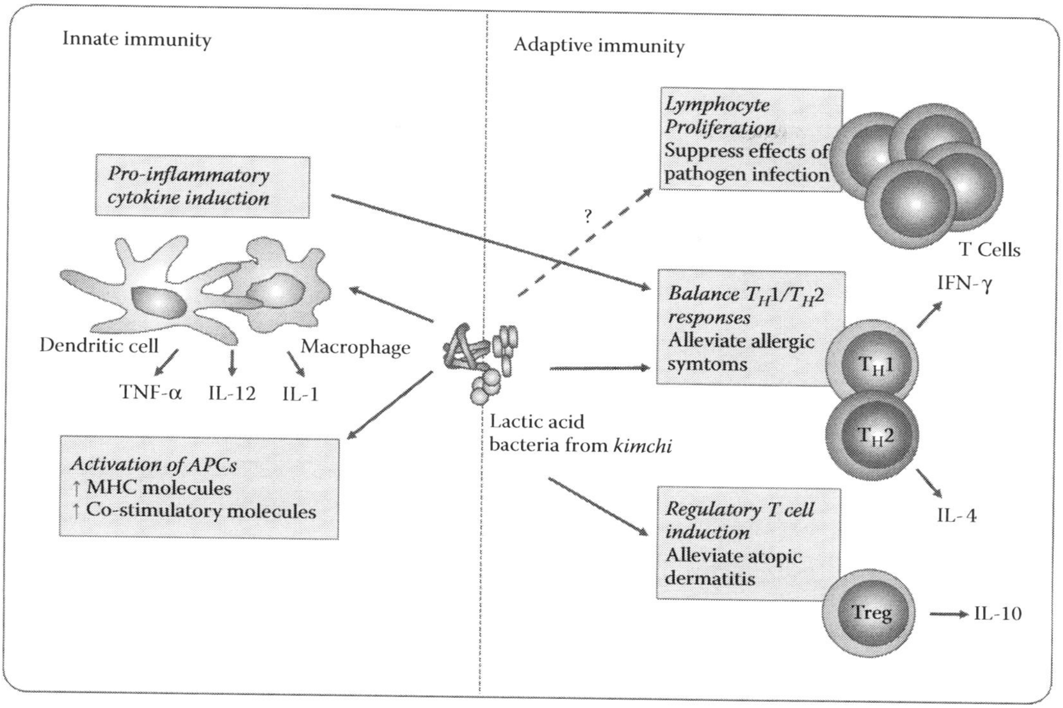

Figure 10.4 Immunomodulatory effects of LAB isolated from *kimchi* on different health benefits. LAB exerts health benefit effects by inducing either innate response or adaptive immune response. APCs, antigen-presenting cells; MHC, major histocompatibility complex; TNF, tumor necrosis factor; IL, interleukin; IFN, interferon; T_H, T helper; Treg, regulatory T cell. (Adapted from Yoon, S.S., Park, Y.S., and Choi, H.J. 2013. *Current Topic of Lactic Acid Bacteria Probiotics* 1: 9–19.)

10.4.3 Antioxidative Effects

The antioxidant properties of *kimchi* are derived from the ingredients used to make *kimchi* and other biological compounds produced during fermentation. The antioxidant effect of *kimchi* has been confirmed *in vitro*, *in vivo*, and in clinical studies (Cheigh and Hwang 2000). Carotenoids, flavonoids, polyphenols, vitamin C, vitamin E, and chlorophyll present in *kimchi* ingredients are known to be primary antioxidants (Cheigh and Park 1994). HDMPPA in optimally fermented *baechu kimchi* was identified as an active principle and shown to have a free radical scavenging effect and retard low density lipoprotein (LDL) oxidation (Lee et al. 2004, Kim et al. 2007) (Figure 10.5 and Table 10.10).

Kimchi retards linoleic auto-oxidation (Hwang and Song 2000) and LDL oxidation (Kwon 1998), and scavenges free radicals (Ryu et al. 1997, 2004a,b). Red mustard leaf *kimchi* shows a higher inhibition rate of peroxide formation in linoleic acid autoxidation system (Cheigh 2003). Also, mustard leaf *kimchi* shows a good antioxidant activity in cooked ground pork without antioxidant during refrigerated storage (Lee et al. 2010, 2011b). The antioxidant activity of the overripened *kimchi* (greater than 2 years) is significantly higher than the short-term fermented *kimchi* (less than 7days) (Park et al. 2011). Many researchers have suggested that the antioxidative

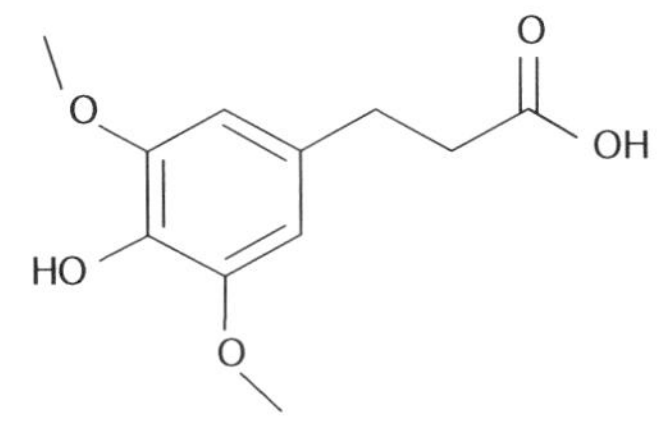

Figure 10.5 HDMPPA. (From Lee, Y.M. et al. 2004. *Korean Journal of Food Science and Technology* 36: 129–133.)

Table 10.10 DPPH Free Radical Scavenging and LDL-Oxidation Activity of *Kimchi*

Sample	*50% Reductase (SC_{50}) μ/mL*	*LDL Oxidation*
MeOH ext.	77.12 ± 4.12	50.6 ± 2.16
Vit. C	2.68 ± 1.28	12.9 ± 0.3
HDMPPA	0.784.19	1.4 ± 0.1

Source: From Lee, Y.M. et al. 2004. *Korean Journal of Food Science and Technology* 36: 129–133.

property of *kimchi* is one of the mechanisms for antimutagenicity/anticancer, antiatherogenecity (Kwon 1998b, Kim et al. 2004b) and antiaging (Ryu et al. 1997, 2004a).

10.4.4 Antiaging Effects

The free radical theory is one of the most acceptable hypotheses that explain the aging process. The ROS or lipid radicals react with biochemicals in the cell resulting in damage and cell death. Thus, cells try to reserve antioxidants and antioxidative enzyme systems to get rid of free radicals. *Kimchi* and its ingredients enhance the activities of antioxidative enzymes, such as superoxide dismutase, catalase, glutathione reductase/peroxidase as well as increase vitamin E and carotene levels in the plasma and liver (Kwon et al. 1998, Kim et al. 2000). The concentration of total free radicals and hydroxyl radicals in the plasma of the elderly who consume more than 112 g of *kimchi* per day is lower than that of the elderly who consume less *kimchi*, however, GSH and GSH/GSSG are higher. These results demonstrate that *kimchi* may play a role either by inhibiting the production of free radicals or discarding the free radicals more efficiently (Kim et al. 2002b). This observation is confirmed in the senescence-accelerating animal (SAM) model study. Free radical production in the brain of SAM decreases and the activities of the antioxidative enzymes increase with *kimchi* consumption for 1 year (Kim et al. 2002a).

Kimchi contains many of the antioxidative compounds that show antiaging effects on the skin. Ryu et al. (2004a) investigated the morphological changes of the skin in hairless mice fed diets containing Korean cabbage, mustard leaf, and *baechu kimchi* for 16 weeks. *Kimchi* consumption retarded skin aging due to the presence of antioxidant and antiaging compounds. In particular, some components of mustard leaf *kimchi* may have had a large effect on skin rejuvenescence (Ryu et al. 2004b).

10.4.5 Weight-Controlling Effects

Kimchi is a low-calorie food with 30 kcal/100 g (Cheigh and Park 1994). Since *kimchi* has low carbohydrate and fat content and a high content of vitamin, minerals, dietary fiber, and phytochemicals, it helps weight control. The body weight reduction of rats by *kimchi* positively correlates with the amount of *kimchi* intake (Sheo and Seo 2004). Rats fed 10% *kimchi* for 4 weeks showed significant reduction in body weight but this phenomenon was not observed in rats fed lesser amounts of *kimchi*, suggesting that *kimchi* taken in large doses over a long period has a dietary effect (Sheo and Seo 2004). The size and number of adipocytes of rats fed a high fat diet were reduced by *kimchi*, especially with fermented *kimchi*. This research group emphasized that the duration of fermentation was more important than the amount of *kimchi* intake on reducing the epididymal fat pan size and adipose cell number (Kim et al. 1997a,b). The lipolytic activity of red pepper in adipocytes was observed. The activity increased with the degree of pungency of the red pepper suggesting that capsaicin is the compound responsible for this activity (Do et al. 2004). Capsaicin in red pepper is known to promote metabolism and burn fat, and thus helps in weight control (Kang et al. 2011). Capsaicin reduces metabolic dysregulation in obese/diabetic mice by enhancing expression of adiponectin and its receptor (Kang et al. 2011). Capsaicin is a pungent principle of hot red pepper that has long been used to enhance food palatability, and is used medicinally as a counterirritant. Early studies with animals have shown that rats fed high-fat diets with added capsaicin gain less weight than controls have lower plasma triglyceride levels (Kawada et al. 1986a) and oxidize more lipids (Kawada et al. 1986b). In addition, red pepper ingestion seems to increase carbohydrate oxidation more than it does fat (Lim et al. 1997).

In a clinical trial obese girls who had a body mass index (BMI) of over 25 consumed 3 g of freeze-dried *kimchi* for 6 weeks in pill form. Total body fat content decreased (−5.11%) but changes in body weight and abdominal fat were not significant (Baek et al. 2001). This result is in agreement with the observation from the animal study. Therefore, large doses and long-term intake of *kimchi* are recommended for weight reduction. It is a known fact that the consumption of properlyfermented *kimchi*, not freshly prepared *kimchi*, helps prevent obesity and adult diseases by reducing body fat, blood pressure, blood sugar, and serum lipid levels (Kim et al. 2011). In addition, it has been proven that LAB separated from *kimchi* has an "ornithine" producing capacity from natural sea salt, an aminoacid with antiobesity efficacy (Moon et al. 2012, Park et al. 2012).

10.4.6 Lipid-Lowering Effects

The biologically active compounds in *kimchi* ingredients known to have lipid-lowering effects are β-sitosterol in *kimchi* cabbage; S-methylcysteinesulfoxide, and S-allylcysteine sulfoxide in garlic; and capsaicin in red pepper (Cheigh and Park 1994). The LAB in *kimchi* also are known to have a lipid-lowering effect, especially cholesterol lowering activity. The mechanisms of these compounds for lowering lipids have been studied extensively. β-Sitosterol isaphyto-cholesterol competes with cholesterol for absorption in the intestine. The alliin in onions enhances the lipolytic activity through hormonal regulation by increasing adrenalin and glucagon secretion. The allicin in garlic inhibits cholesterol synthesis by inhibiting acetyl-CoA synthetase or HMG-CoA reductase activity. Capsaicin stimulates α-hydroxylase activity by converting cholesterol into bile acids (Srinivasan and Sambaiah 1980), and it increases energy expenditure via thyroid hormone regulation (Yoshioka et al. 1998). Certain LAB strains such as *Lb. acidophilus* can bind cholesterol in their cell wall as well as decompose cholesterol for assimilation, and de-conjugate bile acids (Gilliland and Speck 1977, Gilliland et al. 1985). Based on the accumulated evidence, the effects of individual *kimchi*

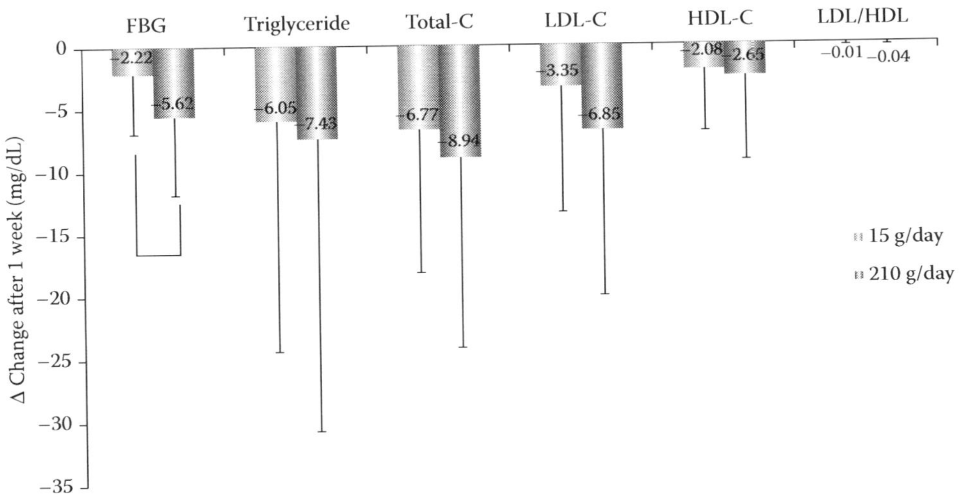

Figure 10.6 Changes in plasma biochemical parameters of the subjects after 7 days of *kimchi* consumption. (From Choi, I.H. et al. 2013. *Journal of Medicinal Food* 16: 223–229.)

ingredients and *kimchi* should have hypolipidemic effects. A nutritional survey of *kimchi* intake and lipid analysis showed that daily *kimchi* consumption levels and HDL cholesterol concentration positively correlated while LDL cholesterol negatively correlated in 102 healthy Korean men between 40 and 64 years of age (Kwon et al. 1999). Research on the lipid-lowering effects of dry *kimchi* has been extensively carried out with various kinds of *kimchi* consumed by animals and human subjects (Kwon et al. 1999, Choi et al. 2001). These results conclude that *kimchi* has lipid-lowering effects in the plasma, liver, and other organs. *Kimchi* decreases triglyceride, cholesterol, and LDL cholesterol in the plasma and HDL cholesterol increases in SAM (Kim 2001), rats (Kim et al. 1997a,b, Kwon et al. 1997, Sheo and Seo 2004), and rabbits (Kwon 1998, Hwang and Song 2000, Jeon et al. 2002). HMG-CoA reductase, cholesterol ester transfer protein (CETP), and acyl cholesterol acyltransferase (ACAT) activity in the liver of rats and rabbits decrease with a *kimchi* diet. The lag phase duration of LDL oxidation at week 2 was twice that of the baseline in Caucasians never exposed to *kimchi*. However, plasma lipid profiles, vitamins C, E, and homocysteine in the plasma did not change. High *kimchi* intake (210 g/day) improved fasting blood glucose and total serum cholesterol compared to low *kimchi* intake (15 g/day) in young healthy adults (Choi et al. 2013) (Figure 10.6).

10.4.7 Antiartherogenic Effects

Oxidized LDL and hypercholesterolemia are one of the major symptoms in the development of atherosclerosis. The functional properties of *kimchi* and its ingredients such as antioxidant activity, free radical scavenging activity, and hypolipidemic activity are responsible for retarding atherosclerosis. Rabbits fed a high cholesterol diet for 12 weeks developed atherosclerosis; however, *kimchi* ingredients prevented atherosclerosis. The lipid deposition in the aorta arch of rabbits fed *kimchi* cabbage (Kwon 1998), red pepper powder (Kwon et al. 2003b), and garlic (Kwon et al. 2003a) decreased. These results showed that these ingredients may have antiatherogenic effects. The active principle, HDMPPA in *baechu kimchi* responsible for lipid-lowering activity also showed antiatherogenic effects. HDMPPA showed both preventive and therapeutic effects on hypercholesterolemia in rabbits and these beneficial effects were comparable to that of Simvastatin, which is a widely used drug for treating hypercholesterolemia in the clinic (Kim et al. 2004a). The plasma cholesterol and LDL cholesterol decreased while HDL cholesterol increased due to the decrease of HMG-CoA reductase. CETP and ACAT of plasma (Kim et al. 2004b) and the thickness of the aorta arch in rabbits fed a cholesterol diet were significantly reduced (Kim et al. 2004b). The mechanisms of HDMPPA in the prevention of atherosclerosis are not fully understood. However, HDMPPA appears to inhibit cell formation in the smooth muscle cell of the aorta by increasing NO synthesis and inhibiting COX-2 expression (Figure 10.7) (Kim et al. 2004b, Noh et al. 2013). HDMPPA increased GSH level and suppressed NO production in a murine macrophage cell line (Song et al. 2004). HDMPPA could maintain NO bioavailability by increasing nitric oxide synthase (NOS) expression and preventing NO degradation by ROS. Furthermore, HDMPPA treatment in apoE KO mice inhibited eNOS (endothelial NOS) uncoupling through an increase in vascular tetrahydrobiopterin content and a decrease in serum asymmetric dimethylarginine levels. Moreover, HDMPPA ameliorated inflammatory-related protein expression in the aorta of apoE KO mice (Noh et al. 2013). Therefore, HDMPPA, the active compound of *kimchi* may exert its vascular protective effect through the preservation of NO bioavailability and the suppression of the inflammatory response (Noh et al. 2013).

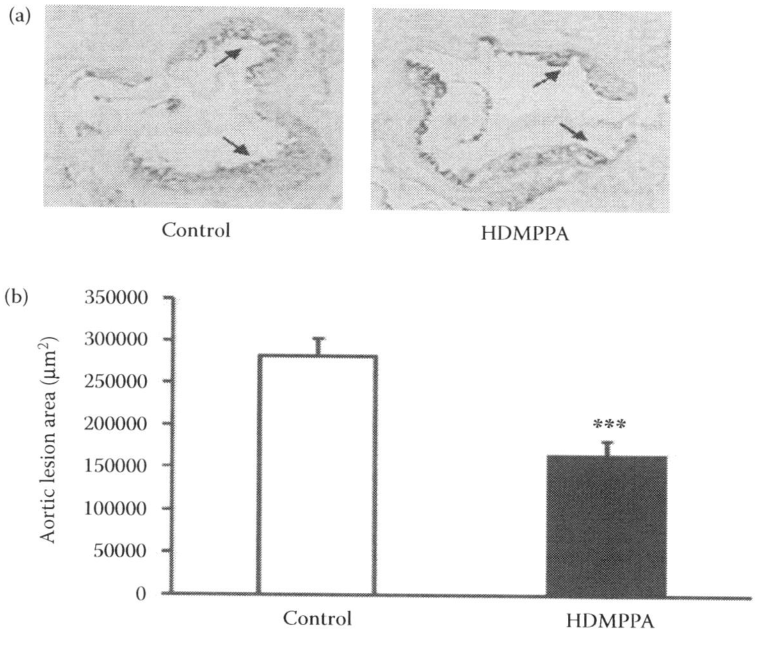

Figure 10.7 (a) Representative photomicrographs of the aortic sinus from apoE KO mice. Animals in the control and HDMPPA groups were killed after an 8-week experimental period, and the aortic roots were stained with oil red O and hematoxylin. The arrow indicates the site of the atherosclerotic lesion. (b) Atherosclerotic lesions were quantified as lesion areas of each group. The HDMPPA group showed 40% less atherosclerosis compared with the control group. Data are mean ± SEM values ($n = 10$). ***$P < 0.001$ versus control group. (Adapted from Noh, J.S., Choi, Y.H., and Song, Y.O. 2013. *British Journal of Nutrition* 109: 17–24.)

Nonlipidemic Caucasians (4 individuals) consuming 150 g of *kimchi* (1/2 cup) daily with their regular meal for 2 weeks showed that the lag phase duration of LDL oxidation was extended twice as much compared with that of the baseline suggesting that *kimchi* may have the ability to reduce the incidence of arteriosclerosis. A *kimchi* pill supplementation (3 g/day) study with 12 middle aged healthy Korean adults showed the atherogenic index for the *kimchi* group decreased compared to the placebo group (Choi et al. 2001).

10.4.8 Anticancer Effects

Kimchi contains high contents of nutrients such as vitamins (ascorbic acid, b-carotene, and vitamin B complex), minerals (calcium, potassium, iron, and phosphorus), essential amino acids, and dietary fiber (Cheigh and Park 1994). *Kimchi* also contains high levels of LAB, allicin, capsaicin, organic acid, phenol compounds, flavonoid, and sulfur compounds. Dietary fiber and LAB isolated from *kimchi* show anticancer activity (Lee and Jeong 1999). The components isolated from culture supernatant of *Lb.casei* show anticancer activity (Kim et al. 2008b) and CBT-AK5 purified from *Lb.casei* (LAFTI L26) shows excellent antitumor activity against Sarcoma-180 infected ICR mice (Yeo et al. 2008). The consumption of *Lb. plantarum* cell lysate isolated from *kimchi* can induce a strong stimulation of mucosal or systemic immune system and these effects result in an efficient antitumor activity (Shin et al. 1998).

Kimchi and its active components including β-sitosterol have potential in both the prevention and treatment of cancer, and present convincing evidence that their anticancer effects may be a result of an inhibition of *Ras* oncogene signaling (Park et al. 2003). High levels of NaCl used when preparing *kimchi* in a warm region can be a problem, since high concentrations of NaCl (>9.5%) in *kimchi* may be comutagenic to the mutagen N-methyl-N'-nitro-N-nitrosoguanidine (MNNG). Bamboo salt has the most potent *in vitro* anticancer effect, induces apoptosis, anti-inflammatory activities, and exerts *in vivo* antimetastatic effect (Zhao et al. 2013).

The methanol extract of *kimchi*, red pepper powder, garlic, and lactic bacteria show antimutagenic or anticancer activities. The *kimchi* extract also inhibits the growth of various human cancer cells (Park, 1995).

10.5 Therapeutic Values

Korea has a two-track food administration system: one is a general food control system under the food code; the other is a health functional food register system under the jurisdiction of the Korean Food and Drug Administration. Some functional components such as terpenes, phenolics, fatty acids, lipids, sugars and carbohydrates, amino acid and proteins, and probiotics are registered on the health functional food register system. Health functional components can be registered under the admission of the Korean Food and Drug Administration after the examination of clinical data. General *kimchi* may forever remain as a storage food in Korea, and health functional *kimchi* may emerge in Korea in the near future. There is extensive evidence of the health functional properties of *kimchi* from studies that have investigated antioxidants, vitamin synthesis, modulation of immunity, alleviation of immune disorders, treatment of gastrointestinal disorders, prevention against inflammatory bowel disease, protection from microbial infection, lowering blood cholesterol and antiatherosclerosis, increased antiaging, protection from obesity, cancer prevention, and protection from hypertension.

We have proposed research to understand the health functional properties of *kimchi* for protection against diabetes, osteoporosis, rheumatoid arthritis, coronary heart disease, hepatic disease, stress, and fatigue, prevention against constipation, increased memory, eye protection, increased muscle activity, prevention against sexual dysfunction, hangover relief, and the prevention of dental disease.

10.6 Conclusions

The health benefits of *kimchi* have been recognized either directly through the interaction of ingested live microorganisms (bacteria or yeast) or indirectly through the ingestion of microbial metabolites produced during the fermentation process (biogenic effect). As we understand more about the role of microorganisms in human nutrition, immune function, and disease prevention, the market size of *kimchi* will increase in the world. *Kimchi* therapy has been applied to a wide range of health disorders such as obesity and gastrointestinal disorders. New strains will be identified and various types of *kimchi* will be developed to fulfill the needs of the world consumer. In addition, industry-based probiotic research is focusing on increasing the shelf-life of *kimchi* and increasing the survival rate of probiotics through the intestinal tract, and improving handling and packing procedures to ensure that the desired health benefits are delivered to the consumer. Introduction of new types of *kimchi* containing beneficial bacteria such as probiotics *kimchi*, kim-cheese, disease-specific medicinal *kimchi*, and infant *kimchi* will serve to accelerate the development of a range of new healthy fermented foods. *Kimchi* has been a part of the worldwide human diet, and may become important in the diets of future space travelers.

References

Baek, Y.H., Kwak, J.R., Kim, S.J., Han, S.S., and Song, Y.O. 2001. Effects of *kimchi* supplementation and/or exercise training on body composition and plasma lipids in obese middle school girls. *Journal of Korean Society of Food Science and Nutrition* 30: 906–912.

Chae, O., Shin, K., Chung. H., and Choe, T. 1998. Immunostimulation effects of mice fed with cell lysate of *Lactobacillus plantarum* isolated from kimchi. *Korean Journal of Biotechnology and Bioengineering* 13: 424–430.

Chang, J.Y., Lee, H.J., and Chang, H.C. 2008. Identification of the agent from *Lactobacillus plantarum* KFRI464 that enhances bacteriocin production by *Leuconostoccitreum* GJ7. *Journal of Applied Microbiology* 103: 2504–2515.

Cheigh, H.S. 2003. Antioxidative activities of anthocyanins in red mustard leaf kimchi. *Journal of the Korean Society of Food Science and Nutrition* 32: 937–941.

Cheigh, H.S. and Hwang, J.H. 2000. Antioxidative characteristics of kimchi. *Food Industry and Nutrition* 5: 52–56.

Cheigh, H.S. and Park, K.Y. 1994. Biochemical, microbiological, and nutritional aspects of kimchi (Korean fermented vegetable products). *Critical Reviews in Food Science and Nutrition* 34: 175–203.

Cheigh, H.S., Yu, R., and Choi, H.J. 1996. Biosynthesis of L—Ascorbic acid by microorganisms in kimchi fermentation process. *Journal of Food Science and Nutrition* 1: 37–40.

Choi, S.H., Kim, H.J., Kwon, M.J., Baek, Y.H., and Song, Y.O. 2001. The effects of kimchi pill supplementation on plasma lipid concentration in healthy people. *Journal of the Korean Society of Food Science and Nutrition* 30: 913–920.

Choi, M.W., Kim, K.H., and Park, K.Y. 1997. Effects of kimchi extracts on the growth of Sarcoma-180 cells and phagocytic activity of mice. *Journal of the Korean Society of Food Science and Nutrition* 26: 254–260.

Choi, Y.H., Kim, Y.A., Park, C., Choi, B.T., Lee, W.H., Hwang, K.M.H., Jung, K.O., and Park, K.Y. 2004. β-Sitosterol induced growth inhibition is associated with up-regulation of Cdk inhibitor p21WAF1/CIP1 in human colon cancer cells. *Journal of the Korean Society of Food Science and Nutrition* 33: 1–6.

Choi, H.J., Lee, H.S. Her, S., Oh, D.H., and Yoon, S.S. 1999. Partial characterization and cloning of leuconocin J, a bacteriocin produced by *Leuconostoc*sp. J2 isolated from the Korean fermented vegetable Kimchi. *Journal of Applied Microbiology* 86: 175–181.

Choi, I.H., Noh, J.S., Han, J.S., Kim, H.J., Han E.S., and Song, Y.O. 2013. Kimchi, a fermented vegetable, improves serum lipid profiles in healthy young adults: Randomized clinical trial. *Journal of Medicinal Food* 16: 223–229.

Cora, J.D. and German, J.B. 2000. Phytochemicals: Nutraceuticals and human health. *Journal of the Science of Food and Agriculture* 80: 1744–1756.

Current of Kimchi Industry. 2011. World Institute of Kimchi. Korea.

Do, M.S., Hong, S.E., Ha, J.H., Choi, S.M., Ahn, I.S., Yoon, J.Y., and Park, K.Y. 2004. Increased lipolytic activity by high-pungency red pepper extract in rat adipocytes in vitro. *Journal of Food Science and Nutrition* 9: 34–38.

Gilliland, S.E., Nelson, C.R., and Maxwell, C. 1985. Assimilation of cholesterol by *Lactobacillus acidophilus. Applied and Environmental Microbiology* 49: 377–381.

Gilliland, S.E. and Speck, M.L. 1977. Deconjugation of bile acids by intestinal lactobacilli. *Applied and Environmental Microbiology* 33: 15–18.

Han, E.S. 2012. Overview of kimchi. *The 4th International Kimchi Conference*, Washington DC.

Hong, E.Y. and Kim, G.H. 2006. Changes in isothiocyanate levels in Korean Chinese cabbage leaves during kimchi storage. *Food Science and Biotechnology* 15: 688–693.

Hur, J.W., Hyun, H.H., Qyun, Y.R., Kim, T.S., Yeo, I.H., and Park, H.D. 2000. Identification and partial characterization of lacticin BH5, a bacteriocin produced by *Lactococcus lactis* BH5 isolated from Kimchi. *Journal of Food Protection* 63: 1707–1712.

Hwang, J.H., Song, Y.O., and Cheigh, H.S. 2000. Fermentation characteristics and antioxidative effect of red mustard leaf kimchi. *Journal of the Korean Society of Food Science and Nutrition* 29: 1009–1015.

Hwang, J.W. and Song, Y.O. 2000. The effects of solvent fractions of kimchi on plasma lipid concentration of rabbit fed high cholesterol diet. *Journal of the Korean Society of Food Science and Nutrition* 29: 204–210.

Jang, M., Hong, E., and Kim, G.H. 2010. Evaluation of antibacterial activity of 3-butenyl, 4-pentenyl, 2-phenylethyl, and benzyl isothiocyanate in Brassica vegetables. *Journal of Food Science* 75: 412–416.

Jang, J.Y., Kim, T.W., Park, H.W., Park, S.H., Lee, J.H., Choi, H.J., Han, E.S., Kang, M.R., and Kim, H.J. 2014. Safety evaluation of heavy metal in salted vegetable foods from diverse origin in Korea. *Journal of Food Hygiene and Safety* 29: 1–6.

Jeon, H.N., Kwon, M.J., and Song, Y.O. 2002. Effects of kimchi solvent fractions on accumulation of lipids in heart, kidney, and lung of rabbit fed high cholesterol diet. *Journal of the Korean Society of Food Science and Nutrition* 31: 814–818.

Jo, J.S. 2000a. *Study of Kimchi.* Korea: Yurim Publishing company, pp. 83–86.

Jo, J.S. 2000b. *Study of Kimchi.* Korea: Yurim Publishing company, pp. 225–256.

Kang, J.H., Tsuyoshi, G., Le Ngoc, H., Kim, H.M., Tu, T.H., Noh. et al. 2011. Dietary capsaicin attenuates metabolic dysregulation in genetically obese diabetic mice. *Journal of Medicinal Food* 14: 310–315.

Kawada, T., Hagihara, K., and Iwai, K. 1986a. Effects of capsaicin on lipid metabolism in rats fed high fat diet. *Journal of Nutrition* 116: 1272–278.

Kawada, T., Watanabe, T., Takaishi, T., Tanaka, T., and Iwai, K. 1986b. Capsaicin-induced β-adrendergic action on energy metabolism in rats: Influence of capsaicin on oxygen consumption, respiratory quotient, and substrate utilization. *Experimental Biology and Medicine* 183: 250–256.

Kim, H.J. 2004. The preventive and therapeutic effects of 3-(4′-hydroxyl-3′5′-dimethoxyphenyl) propionic acid, an active principle in kimchi, on atherosclerosis in rabbits. PhD Dissertation, Pusan National University, Korea.

Kim, J.H. 2001. The effect of kimchi intake on antiaging characteristics in SAM and human. PhD Dissertation, Pusan National University, Korea.

Kim, E.K., An, S.Y., Lee, M.S., Kim, T.H., Lee, H.K., Hwang, W.S. et al. 2011. Fermented kimchi reduces body weight and improves metabolic parameters in overweight and obese patients. *Nutrition Research* 31: 436–443.

Kim, M. and Chun, J. 2005. Bacterial community structure in kimchi, a Korean fermented vegetable food, as revealed by 16S rRNA gene analysis. *International Journal of Food Microbiology* 103: 91–96.

Kim, S.Y. and Kim, K.O. 1989. Effect of sodium chloride concentrations and storage periods on characteristics of kakdugi. *Korean Journal of Food Science and Technology* 21: 370–374.

Kim, H.J., Kim, D.M., Baek, H., Lee, S.H., and Chung, M.J. 2008b. Anti-cancer effects of peptides purified from culture supernatant of *Lactobacillus casei*. *Journal of Korean Dairy Technology and Science Association* 26: 5–10.

Kim, H.J., Lee, J.S., Chung, H.Y., Song, S.H., Suh, H., Noh, J.S., and Song, Y.O. 2007. 3-(4′-Hydroxyl-3′, 5′-dimethoxyphenyl) propionic acid, an active principle of Kimchi, inhibits development of atherosclerosis in rabbits. *Journal of Agricultural and Food Chemistry* 55: 10486–10492.

Kim, J.Y. and Lee, Y.S. 1997. The effects of kimchi intake on lipid contents of body and mitogen response of spleen lymphocytes in rats. *Journal of the Korean Society of Food Science and Nutrition* 26: 1200–1207.

Kim, B.H., Lee, H.S., Jang, Y.A., Lee, J.Y., Cho, Y.J., and Kim, C.I. 2009. Development of amino acid composition database for Korean foods. *Journal of Food Composition and Analysis* 22: 44–52.

Kim, M.J., Lee, K.T., and Lee, O.Y. 1997a. *Kimchi, Thousand Years*. Korea: Designhouse, pp.110–137.

Kim, H.J., Kwon, M.J., Seo, J.M., Kim, J.K., Song, S.H., Suh, H.S., and Song, Y.O. 2004a. The effects of 3-(4′-hydroxyl-3′5′-dimethoxyphenyl) propionic acid in Chinese cabbage kimchi on lowering hypercholesterolemia. *Journal of the Korean Society of Food Science and Nutrition* 33: 52–58.

Kim, H.J., Kwon, M.J., and Song, Y.O. 2000. Effects of solvent fraction of Korean cabbage kimchi on antioxidative enzyme activities and fatty acid composition of phospholipids of rabbit fed 1% cholesterol diet. *Journal of the Korean Society of Food Science and Nutrition* 29: 900–907.

Kim, M.J., Kwon, M.J., Song, Y.O., Lee, E.K., Youn, H.J., and Song, Y.S. 1997b. The effects of kimchi hematological and immunological parameters *in vivo* and *in vitro*. *Journal of the Korean Society of Food Science and Nutrition* 26: 1308–1214.

Kim, J.H., Ryu, J.D., Lee, H.G., Park, J.H., Moon, G.S., Cheigh, H.S., and Song, Y.O. 2002a. The effect of kimchi on production of free radicals and anti-oxidative enzyme activities in the brain of SAM. *Journal of the Korean Society of Food Science and Nutrition* 31: 117–123.

Kim, J.H, Ryu, J.D., and Y.O. Song. 2002b. The effect of kimchi intake on free radical production and the inhibition of oxidation in young adults and the elderly people. *Korean Journal of Community Nutrition* 7: 257–265.

Kim, J.Y., Park, B.K., Park, H.J., Park, Y.H., Kim, B.O., and Pyo, S. 2013. Atopic dermatitis-mitigating effects of new *Lactobacillus* strain, *Lactobacillus sakei* probio 65 isolated from Kimchi. *Journal of Applied Microbiology* 115: 517–526.

Kim, S.Y., Shin, K.S., and Lee, H. 2004b. Immunopotentiating activities of cellular components of *Lactobacillus brevis* FSB-1. *Journal of the Korean Society of Food Science and Nutrition* 33: 1552–1559.

Kim, Y.S., Zheng, Z.B., and Shin, D.H. 2008c. Growth inhibitory effects of Kimchi (Korean traditional fermented vegetable product) against *Bacillus cereus, Listeria monocytogenes*, and *Staphylococcus aureus*. *Journal of Food Protection* 71: 325–332.

Kong, Y.H., Cheigh, H.S., Song, Y.O., Jo, Y.O., and Choi, S.Y. 2008. Anti-obesity effects of Kimchi tablet composition. *Journal of the Korean Society of Food Science and Nutrition* 36: 1529–1536.

Konieczna, P., Groeger, D., Ziegler, M., Frei, R., Ferstl, R., Shanahan, F., Quigley, E.M., Kiely, B., Akdis, C.A., and O'Mahony. L. 2012. *Bifidobacterium infantis* 35624 administration induces Foxp3 T regulatory cells in human peripheral blood: Potential role for myeloid and plasmacytoid dendritic cells. *Gut* 61: 354–366.

Korean Nutrition Society. 2000. *Recommended Dietary Allowances for Koreans*, 7th ed. Seoul, Korea: The Korean Nutrition Society.

Korean Restaurant Guide. 2009. Kimchi stories. Http://www.koreanrestaurantguide.com/kimchi/kimchi_0.htm (accessed March 29, 2009).

Kwak, C.S., Hwang, J.Y., Watanabe, F., and Park, S.C. 2008.Vitamin B12 contents in some Korean fermented foods and edible seaweeds. *Korean Journal of Nutrition* 41: 439–447.

Kwon, M.J. 1998. Antiatherogenic effect of baechu kimchi. PhD Dissertation, Pusan National University, Korea.

Kwon, J.R. 2010. Samkukusa: 53–54, Korea. Origin; Ilyeon, Samkukusa. (a.d. 1281), Koryo.

Kwon, H.K., Lee, C.G., So, J.S., Chae, C.S., Hwang, J.S., Sahoo, A., Nam, J.H., Rhee, J.H., Hwang, K.C., and Im, S.H. 2010. Generation of regulatory dendritic cells and CD4+Foxp3+ T cells by probiotics administration suppresses immune disorders. *Proceedings of the National Academy of Science* 107: 2159–2164.

Kwon, M.J., Chun, J.H., Song, Y.S., and Song, Y.O. 1999. Daily kimchi consumption and its hypolipidemic effect in middle-aged men. *Journal of the Korean Society of Food Science and Nutrition* 28: 1144–1150.

Kwon, M.J., Song, Y.S., Choi, M.S., Park, S.J., Jeong, K.S., and Song, Y.O. 2003a. Cholesteryl ester transfer protein activity and atherogenic parameters in rabbit supplemented with cholesterol and garlic powder. *Life Sciences* 72: 2953–2964.

Kwon, M.J., Song, Y.S., Choi, M.S., and Song, Y.O. 2003b. Red pepper attenuates cholesteryl ester transfer protein activity and atherosclerosis in cholesterol-fed rabbits. *Clinica Chimica Acta* 332: 37–44.

Kwon, M.J., Song, Y.O., and Song, Y.S. 1997. Effects of kimchi on tissue and fecal lipid composition and apolipoprotein and thyroxine levels in rats. *Journal of the Korean Society of Food Science and Nutrition* 26: 507–513.

Kwon, M.J., Song, Y.S., and Song, Y.O. 1998. Antioxidative effect of kimchi ingredients on rabbits fed cholesterol diet. *Journal of the Korean Society of Food Science and Nutrition* 27: 1189–1196.

Lee, H.G. 2006. Food composition table. National Academy of Agricultural Science Rural Resources Development Institute, Korea.

Lee, M.A., Choi, J.H., Choi, Y.S., Han, D.J., Kim, H.Y., Shim, S.Y., Chung, H.K., and Kim, C.J. 2010. The antioxidative properties of mustard leaf (*Brassica juncea*) kimchi extracts on refrigerated raw ground pork meat against lipid oxidation. *Meat Science* 84: 498–504.

Lee, M.A., Choi, J.H., Choi, Y.S., Kim, H.Y., Kim, H.W., Hwang, K.E., Chung, H.K., and Kim, C.J. 2011b. Effects of kimchi ethanolic extracts on oxidative stability of refrigerated cooked pork. *Meat Science* 89: 405–11.

Lee, J.J. and Jeong, Y.K. 1999. Cholesterol-lowering effect and anticancer activity of kimchi and kimchi ingredients. *Korean Journal of Life Science* 9: 743–752.

Lee, S.H., Kim, M.K., and Frank, J.F. 1995. Growth of *Listeria monocytogenes* Scott A during kimchi fermentation and in the presence of kimchi ingredients. *Journal of Food Protection* 58: 1215–1218.

Lee, M., Kim, M.K., Vancanneyt, M., Swings, J., Kim, S.H., Kang, M.S., and Lee, S.T. 2005. *Tetragenococcus Koreensis* sp. nov., a novel rhamnolipid-producing bacterium. *International Journal of Systematic and Evolutionary Microbiology* 55: 1409–1413.

Lee, Y.M., Kwon, M.J., Kim, J.K., Suh, H.S., Chio, J.S., and Song, Y.O. 2004. Isolation and identification of active principle in Chinese cabbage kimchi responsible for antioxidant activity. *Korean Journal of Food Science and Technology* 36: 129–133.

Lee, H.M. and Lee, Y. 2006. Isolation of *Lactobacillus plantarum* from kimchi and its inhibitory activity on the adherence and growth of *Helicobacter pylori*. *Journal of Microbiology and Biotechnology* 16: 1513–1517.

Lee, H.R. and Lee, J.M. 2009. Anti-stress effects of kimchi. *Food Science and Biotechnology* 18: 25–30.

Lee, T.Y. and Lee, J.W. 1981. The changes of vitamin C content and effect of galacturonic acid addition during kimchi fermentation. *Journal of Korean Society of Agricultural Chemistry and Biotechnology* 24: 139–144.

Lee, Y., Lee, H.J., Lee, H.S., Jang, Y.A., and Kim, C.I. 2008. Analytic dietary fiber database for the national health and nutrition survey in Korea. *Journal of Food Composition and Analysis* 21: S35–S42.

Lee, I.H., Lee, S.H., Lee, I.S., Park, Y.K., Chung, D.K., and Choue, R. 2008. Effects of probiotic extracts of kimchi on immune function in NC/Nga mice. *Korean Journal of Food Science and Technology* 40: 82–87.

Lee, M.K., Lee, J.K., Son, J.A., Kang, M.H., Koo, K.H., and Suh, J.W. 2008. S-Adenosyl-L-methionine (SAM) production by lactic acid bacteria strains isolated from different fermented Kimchi products. *Food Science and Biotechnology* 17: 857–860.

Lee, S.K., Shin, M.S., Jhong, D.Y., Hong, Y.H., and Lim, H.S. 1989. Changes of kimchi contained different garlic contents during fermentation. *Korean Journal of Food Science and Technology* 21: 68–74.

Lee, J., Yun, H.S., Cho, K.W., Oh, S., Kim, S.H., Chun, T., Kim, B., and Whang, K.Y. 2011. Evaluation of probiotic characteristics of newly isolated *Lactobacillus* spp.: Immune modulation and longevity. *International Journal of Food Microbiology* 148: 80–86.

Lim, J., Seo, B.J., Kim, J.E., Chae, C.S., Im, S.H., Hahn, Y.S., and Park, Y.H. 2011. Characteristics of immunomodulation by a *Lactobacillus sakei* proBio65 isolated from Kimchi. *Korean Journal of Microbiology and Biotechnology* 39: 313–316.

Lim, K., Yoshioka, M., Kikuzato, S., Kiyonaga, A., Tanaka, H., Shido, M., and Suzuki, M. 1997. Dietary red pepper ingestion increases carbohydrate oxidation at rest and during exercise in runners. *Medicine and Science in Sports and Exercise* 29: 355–361.

Mheen, T.I. and Kwon, T.W. 1984. Effect of temperature and salt concentration on kimchi fermentation. *Korean Journal of Food Science and Technology* 16: 443–448.

Moon, Y.J., Soh, J.R., Yu, J.J., Sohn, H.S., Cha, Y.S., and Oh, S.H. 2012. Intracellular lipid accumulation inhibitory effect of *Weissella koreensis* OK1-6 isolated from Kimchi on differentiating adipocyte. *Journal of Applied Microbiology* 113: 652–658.

Mountzouris, K.C., Tsirtsikos, P., Kalamara, E., Nitsch, S., Schatzmayr, G., and Fegeros, K. 2007. Evaluation of the efficacy of a probiotic containing *Lactobacillus, Bifidobacterium, Enterococcus,* and *Pediococcus* strains in promoting broiler performance and modulating cecal microflora composition and metabolic activities. *Poultry Science* 86: 309–317.

Nam, Y.D., Chang, H.W., Kim, K.H., Roh, S.W., and Bae, J.W. 2009. Metatranscriptome analysis of lactic acid bacteria during kimchi fermentation with genome-probing microarrays. *International Journal of Food Microbiology* 130: 140–146.

Noh, J.S., Choi, Y.H., and Song, Y.O. 2013. Beneficial effects of the active principle component of Korean cabbage kimchi via increasing nitric oxide production and suppressing inflammation in the aorta of apoE knockout mice. *British Journal of Nutrition* 109: 17–24.

Park, K.Y. 1995. The nutritional evaluation, and antimutagenic and anticancer effects of kimchi. *Journal of the Korean Society of Food Science and Nutrition* 24: 169–182.

Park, S.G. and Cho, Y.S. 1995. Changes in the contents of sugar, organic acid, free amino acid, and nucleic acid-related compounds during fermentation of leaf mustard kimchi. *Journal of the Korean Society of Food Science and Nutrition* 24: 48–53.

Park, K.Y., Cho, E.J., Rhee, S.H., Jung, K.O., Yi, S.J., and Jhun, B.H. 2003. Kimchi and an active component, beta-sitosterol, reduce oncogenic H-Ras(v12)-induced DNA synthesis. *Journal of Medicinal Food* 6: 151–156.

Park, K.Y., Jeong, J.K., Lee, Y.E., and Daily, J.W. 2014. Health benefits of kimchi (Korean ferrnented vegetables) as a probiotic food. *Journal of Medicinal Food* 17: 6–12.

Park, K.U., Kim, J.Y., Cho, Y.S., Yee, S.T., Jeong, C.H., Kang, K.S., and Seo, K.I. 2004. Anticancer and immuno-activity of onion kimchi methanol extract. *Journal of the Korean Society of Food Science and Nutrition* 33: 1439–1444.

Park, K.Y., Kil, J.H., Jung, K.O., Kong, C.S., and Lee, J. 2006. Functional properties of Kimchi (Korean fermented vegetables). *Acta Horiculturae* 706: 167–172.

Park, C.W., Youn, M., Jung, Y.M., Kim, H., Jeong, Y., Lee, H.K. et al. 2008. New functional probiotic *Lactobacillus sakei* Probio 65 alleviates atopic symptoms in the mouse. *Journal of Medicinal Food* 11: 405–412.

Park, J.A., Tirupathi Pichiah, P.B., Yu, J.J., Oh, S.H., Daily, J.W.3rd, and Cha, Y.S. 2012. Anti-obesity effect of kimchi fermented with *Weissella koreensis* OK1–6 as starter in high-fat diet-induced obese C57BL/6 J mice. *Journal of Applied Microbiology* 113: 1507–1516.

Park, J.M., Shin, J.H., Gu, J.G., Yoon, S.J., Song, J.C., Jeon, W.M., Suh, H.J., Chang, U.J., Yang, C.Y., and Kim, J.M. 2011. Effect of antioxidant activity in kimchi during a short-term and over-ripening fermentation period. *Journal of Bioscience and Bioengineering* 112: 356–359.

Rhee, C.H. and Park, H.D. 2001. Three glycoproteins with antimutagenic activity identified in *Lactobacillus plantarum* KLAB21. *Applied and Environmental Microbiology* 67: 3445–3449.

Rhie, S.G. and Chun, S.K. 1982. The influence of temperature on fermentation of kimchi. *Korean Journal of Nutrition and Food* 11: 63–66.

Ried, K., Toben, C., and Fakler, P. 2013. Effect of garlic on serum lipids: An updated meta-analysis. *Nutrition Reviews* 71: 282–299.

Ro, S.L., Woodburn, M., and Sandine, W.E. 1979. Vitamin B12 and ascorbic acid in kimchi inoculated with *Propionibacterium freudenreichii* ss. *shermanii*. *Journal of Food Science* 44: 873–877.

Ryu, B.M., Ryu, S.H., Jeon, Y.S., Lee, Y.S., and Moon, G.S. 2004a. Inhibitory effect of solvent fraction of various kinds of kimchi on ultraviolet B induced oxidation and erythema formation of hairless mice skin. *Journal of the Korean Society of Food Science and Nutrition* 33: 785–790.

Ryu, B.M., Ryu, S.H., Lee, Y.S., Jeon, Y.S., and Moon, G.S. 2004b. Effect of different kimchi diets on oxidation and photooxidation in liver and skin of hairless mice. *Journal of the Korean Society of Food Science and Nutrition* 33: 291–298.

Ryu, S.H., Jeon, Y.S., Kwon, M.J., Lee, Y.S., and Moon, G.S. 1997. Effect of kimchi extracts to reactive oxygen species in skin cell cytotoxicity. *Journal of the Korean Society of Food Science and Nutrition* 26: 814–821.

Seo, J.H. and Lee, H. 2007. Characteristics and immunomodulating activity of lactic acid bacteria for the potential probiotics. *Korean Journal of Food Science and Technology* 39: 681–687.

Sheo, H.J. and Seo, Y.S. 2004. The effects of dietary Chinese cabbage kimchi juice on the lipid metabolism and body weight gain in rats fed high-calories-diet. *Journal of Society of Food Science and Nutrition* 33: 91–100.

Shin, K., Chae, O., Park, I., Hong, S., and Choe, T. 1998. Antitumor effects of mice fed with cell lysate of *Lactobacillus plantarum* isolated from kimchi. *Korean Journal of Biotechnology and Bioengineering* 13: 357–363.

Shin, M.S., Han, S.K., Ryu, J.S., Kim, K.S., and Lee, W.K. 2008. Isolation and partial characterization of a bacteriocin produced by *Pediococcus pentosaceus* K23-2 isolated from Kimchi. *Journal of Applied Microbiology* 105: 331–339.

Sim, K.H. and Han, Y.S. 2008. Effect of red pepper seed on Kimchi antioxidant activity during fermentation. *Food Science and Biotechnology* 17: 295–301.

Song, B.S., Park, J.G., Park, J.N., Han, I.J., Kim, J.H., Choi, J.I., Byun, M.W., and Lee, J.W. 2009. Korean space food development: Ready-to-eat Kimchi, a traditional Korean fermented vegetable, sterilized with high-dose gamma irradiation. *Advances in Space Research* 44: 162–169.

Song, Y.S., Choi, C.Y., Suh, H., and Song, Y.O. 2004. 3-(4′-hydroxyl-3′5′-dimethoxyphenyl) propionic acid suppresses NO production and elevates GSH levels in murine macrophage. *Journal of Food Science and Nutrition* 9: 270–275.

Srinivasan, K. and Sambaiah, K. 1980. Hypocholesterolemic effect of red pepper and capsaicin. *Indian Journal of Experimental Biology* 18: 898–899.

Tamang, J.P., and Kailasapathy, K. 2010. *Fermented Foods and Beverages of the World*. New York: CRC Press, Taylor & Francis Group.

Tsai, Y.T., Cheng, P.C., and Pan, T.M. 2012. The immunomodulatory effects of lactic acid bacteria for improving immune functions and benefits. *Applied Microbiology and Biotechnology* 96: 853–862.

Won, T.J., Kim, B., Song, D.S., Lim, Y.T., Oh, E.S., Lee, D.I., Park, E.S., Min, H., Park, S.Y., and Hwang, K.W. 2011. Modulation of Th1/Th2 balance by *Lactobacillus* strains isolated from kimchi via stimulation of macrophage cell line J774A.1 *in vitro*. *Journal of Food Science* 76: H55–H61.

Yeo, M.H., Kim, D.M., Kim, Y.H., Kim, J.H., Baek, H., and Chung, M.J. 2008. Antitumor activity of CBT-AK5 purified from *Lactobacillus casei* against Sarcoma-180 infected ICR mice. *Korean Journal of Dairy Science Technology* 26: 23–30.

Yim, C.Y., Eom, H.J., Jin, Q., Kim, S.Y., and Han, N.S. 2008. Characterization of low temperature-adapted *Leuconostoc citreum* HJ-P4 and its dextransucrase for the use of kimchi starter. *Food Science and Biotechnology* 17: 1391–1395.

Yoon, S.S., Park, Y.S., and Choi, H.J. 2013. Genetics and research revolutions in the lactic acid bacteria: Focused on probiotics and immunomodulation. *Current Topic of Lactic Acid Bacteria Probiotics* 1: 9–19.

Yoshioka, M., St-Pierre, S., Suzuki, M., and Tremblay A. 1998. Effects of red pepper added to high-fat and high-carbohydrate meals on energy metabolism and substrate utilization in Japanese women. *British Journal of Nutrition* 80: 503–510.

Zhao, X., Kim, S.Y., and Park, K.Y. 2013. Bamboo salt has *in vitro* anticancer activity in HCT-116 cells and exerts anti-metastatic effects in vivo. *Journal of Medicinal Food* 16: 9–19.

Chapter 11

Health Benefits of *Tempe*

Mary Astuti

Contents

11.1 Introduction

Food has played a major role in human life since ancient times. Millions of people suffered from health problems because of overeating, or because of unbalanced, or nutrient-deficient diets. The problems of nutritional imbalances are mainly due to bad food choices or habits and possibly occur in both developed and developing countries. The manifestations of food imbalance may appear similar to the symptoms of deficiency, while overeating may cause some degenerative or noncommunicable diseases. Soybeans are the most important leguminous source of protein and oil in human food. The role of soybeans in the form of traditional food items such as *tofu, miso, natto, kinema, tempe*, and soysauce in many parts of Asia is well recognized (Nagai and Tamang 2010). Soybeans, which were originally developed in the Orient, are now gaining popularity in Western countries and in other parts of the world, including Indonesia.

In Indonesia, soybeans are consumed mainly in the form of traditional foods consisting of fermented or non-fermented products. Commercially fermented soybeans are *tempe*, soysauce, and *tauco*, whereas *tofu* is made of nonfermented soybeans. *Tempe* is fermented soybeans prepared by *Rhizopus* (*Rhi.*) spp., *Rhizopus oligosporus, Rhizopus oryzae, or Rhizopus stolonifer* (Steinkraus 1983). *Tempe* has different characteristics from soybeans. The texture of *tempe* is compact, it does not easily disintegrate even when cut with a knife, the color is white, and it has an aroma of mold and boiled soybeans. Actually, there are many kinds of *tempe* (fermented leguminous) depending on the raw materials from which *tempe* is prepared. *Tempe* from soybeans is called *tempe*, from velvet beans *tempe benguk*, from sword beans *tempe koro* and from waste *tofu tempe gembus*.The most popular raw material for *tempe* preparation is soybeans. For that reason the word *tempe* is preferred to soybean *tempe*. To prepare *tempe*, soybeans are washed, cleaned, and soaked overnight, the soaking water is then discarded and the beans are boiled for 30 min. The next process is dehulling to separate the seed coat. Then, the beans are again soaked in water for about 20–24 h until the pH is 4.5–5.0. Next, the beans are washed and boiled for 60 min. The cooked beans are drained and spread out until the temperature is around 30°C. The beans are then inoculated with *tempe* inoculum powder or *tempe* starter or mixed culture which usually contains *Rhi. oligosporus* and *Rhi. oryzae*. The inoculum powder added is about 1 g mix culture powder/kg soybean. The beans are wrapped in materials such as banana or teak leaves, or in perforated plastic bags. The next step is incubation at room temperature (27–30°C) for about 36–48 h. Generally, *tempe* fermented for 48 h is consumed as a source of protein in Indonesian diets. *Tempe* is also served as the cheapest source of protein. The physical characteristics of *tempe* are shown in Table 11.1.

Table 11.1 Physical Characteristic of Fresh *Tempe*

Fermentation Time (h)	*Color*	*Flavor*	*Texture*	*Surface Appearance*
0	Yellowish	Strong beany	Not compact	Not covered with mold mycelia
24	Grayish	Less beany flavor	Less compact	Partly covered with mycelia
48	White	Strong *tempe*	Compact	Entirely covered with mycelia
72	Yellowish-white	Less ammonia smell	Less compact	Moderately Covered with mycelia. Yellowish spots and moist
96	Brownish-white	Strong ammonia smell	Less compact and brittle	Covered with mycelia less entirely, brownish spots and moist

Source: From Astuti, M. 1992. *Iron Bioavailability in Traditional Indonesian Soybean Tempe.* Doctoral thesis, Tokyo University of Agriculture, Tokyo.

Tempe is not consumed as raw food but in the form of cooked *tempe*. Frying is the most popular cooking method to serve *tempe* as a dish or snack. After frying, the color changes from white to goldenbrown. This color distinguishes fried *tempe*. Other *tempe* dishes which are commonly consumed are *tempe* chips, *tempe* sambal (*tempe* cooked with chili and garlic and then pulverized together), barbeque *tempe* or sate *tempe*, *tempe* curry, and so on. *Tempe* is not only known in Indonesia but also in another countries such as Japan, Holland, Belgium, Turkey, Australia, Singapore, Malaysia, the United States, Italy, and others. In other countries, *tempe* maybe served as *tempe* burgers, *tempe* hotdogs, *tempe tempura*, *tempe* soups, and so on.

11.2 Nutrition Aspect of *Tempe*

11.2.1 Protein

Protein is an important macronutrient contained in food. Protein contains amino acids that are needed by the body. The quality of the protein in food is largely determined by its amino acid composition. High-quality protein depends on the completeness of essential amino acids, whether in their type or in their amounts. (Dideriksen et al. 2013) Usually, animal-based food is known as a better source of protein than vegetable-based food. However, *tempe* is included as a vegetable-based food containing a good source of protein for the Indonesian diet. *Tempe* is a good source of protein that has a lower price than another food source of protein, including meat, fish, and others. In *tempe* production, some soybean nutrition including protein is changed during the fermentation process (Astuti 1994). Nevertheless, the change in protein is not significant, which is about 46.86 g (dB) in unfermented soybean and 47.10 g (dB) in *tempe* fermented for 48 h, although the soluble nitrogen may increase. The increase in soluble nitrogen indicates that during the fermentation process, the protein in the soybeans is digested by the protease enzyme produced by the microbes. Murata et al. (1967) found that during the fermentation process, the soluble nitrogen increased from 0.5% to 2.0%.

Negishi and Sugahara (1996) reported that *tempe* prepared from *Rhi. oligosporus* has a higher protein content than *tempe* prepared from traditional inoculum namely *usar* and commercial *tempe* produced in Japan. The glutamic acid (Glu) content was found to be the highest, followed by aspartic acid (Asp), leucine (Leu), and lysine (lys), in order of decreasing content (Astuti 1994). Regarding the amino acid score, the first limiting amino acid was identified to be sulfur-containing amino acids (SAA). Jense and Donath in 1924 (Steinkraus 1983) found that *tempe* protein was highly nutritious when fed to animals. In 1955, Auret and VanVeen (1955) published their findings on the importance of *tempe* protein for the feeding of children in developing countries. Steinkraus et al. (1960) and Murata et al. (1967) reported that the protein content in unfermented soybean and *tempe* was approximately the same. However, the soluble nitrogen increased with fermentation time. The quality of protein was studied by Hackler et al. (1964), who discovered that the protein efficiency ratio (PER) of unfermented soybeans and fermented soybeans was not significantly different, therefore fermentation did not significantly improve the quality of the protein. In contrast with Hackler's experiment, Gyorgy et al. (1964) demonstrated that rats which are fed with 10% of protein of *tempe* and with skim milk for 10 weeks showed equal PER values. Bai et al. (1975) reported that the protein quality in terms of net protein utilization (NPU) of unfermented soybeans was 56.7 as compared to 58.7 for soy *tempe*. Sudarmadji (1977) observed that there were no statistically significant differences in PER value for fried unfermented soybean and fried *tempe*. Using *tempe* as a source of protein in baby formula, Astuti (1982) found that the growth rate of rats fed with this formula was not different from rats fed with a commercial baby-food formula. Investigation into the role of *tempe* in preventing nutrition problems in Indonesia, that is, in protein calorie malnutrition for preschool children by Hermana (1983), stated that food supplementation with a formulation of 70% rice and 30% *tempe* flour had a beneficial effect on the nutritional status as well as on protection from gastrointestinal infections.

11.2.2 Carbohydrates

Tempe processing has a beneficial effect on carbohydrates, such as oligosaccharides, especially in the decrease of raffinose and stachiose content (Gyorgy et al. 1964). Moreover, Vander Riet et al. (1987) reported that starch, stachyose, raffinose, and sucrose levels decreased. The level of glucose increases sharply during *tempe* fermentation, and this might be the product of the digestion from complex to simple carbohydrates. In unfermented soybeans the level of glucose was 0.315 g/100 g and in *tempe* 1.24 g/100 g (Astuti 1994).

11.2.3 Lipids

Lipids are an important nutrient contained in soybeans. The lipids contained in *tempe* are lower than in unfermented soybeans. It has been shown that during soybean fermentation the lipase enzyme hydrolyze triacyl glycerol into free fatty acids. These fatty acids are used as a source of energy for mold growth in the lower lipid content of *tempe* (Astuti 1994). Wagenknecht et al. (1961) and Sudarmadji (1977) also stated that the fermentation of *tempe* is able to increase free fatty acid content. The levels of palmitic acid were 1585.5 mg/100 g in soybeans and decreased to 580.2 mg/100 g in *tempe*. Furthermore, palmitic acid rapidly decreased about 41% during 24 h of *tempe* fermentation (Astuti 1994). Compared to other fatty acids in *tempe*, stearic acid was found only in small concentrations. The levels of stearic acid were 146.23 mg/100 g in unfermented soybeans and 72.04 mg/100 g in *tempe*. During the first 24 h of fermentation, stearic acid decreased about 41.14%. Oleic acid decreased about 59.25 mg/100 g in *tempe* fermented for 48 h. Among the polyunsaturated fatty acids, the lowest was linolenic acid and the highest was linoleic acid. The declining rate of fatty acids during the 24 and 48 h fermentation is possibly related to the growth of mold, because in 48 h fermentation the mold grows rapidly. The decreasing of lipid and fatty acids in *tempe* indicate that lipid and fatty acids were used as the main source of energy for the growth and metabolism of mold. That statement confirms the previous study by Hering et al. (1990).

11.2.4 Vitamins

The level of vitamin B-complexes increases except vitamin B_1. The work of Jense in 1924 (Shurtleff and Aoyagi 1979) showed that the thiamine content in *tempe* was less than in unfermented soybeans. A study by Steinkraus et al. (1960), Murata et al. (1967), and Liem et al. (1977) showed a dramatic rise of vitamin B_{12} content from 0.15 mcg in 100 g of unfermented soybeans to 3.9 mcg in *tempe*. Suparmo (1988) found that *tempe* prepared with a mixed culture of *Rhi. oligosporus* and *Bacillus megaterium* produced a higher vitamin B_{12} level than with using *Rhi. oligosporus* alone. Okada (1989) who analyzed commercial *tempe* in Bogor, West Java, reported that the vitamin B_{12} content was in the range of 0.07–4.6 mcg/100 g of fresh *tempe*. The range of vitamin B_{12} from *tempe* prepared with *Rhi. oligosporus* NRRL2710 in Japan was 0.03–0.06 mcg/100 g. It seems that vitamin B_{12} is mainly produced by bacteria rather than mold. During the overnight soaking of cooked soybeans, the growth of *Klebsiella pneumonia* increased and produced vitamin B_{12} (Okada 1989). Ginting and Arcot (2004) reported that folic acid in unfermented soybeans was 71.6 μg/100 g and increased to 416.4 μg/100 g in *tempe*. Khasanah (2013) found that during *tempe* fermentation the folic acid increased from 0.64 to 1.02 mg/kg. Khasanah (2013) reported that folic-deficient rats fed with 125 g/kg *tempe* in a feeding trial for 5 weeks increased serum folic acid in the *tempe* diet to about 14.42 μg/L compared to the folic-deficient diet whose content was 8.43 μg/L. The hemoglobin content was respectively 14.42 and 7.76 g/dL in the *tempe* diet and the folic-deficient diet of rats.

Asmoro (unpublished data 2014) found that black soybean *tempe* fermented with *Rhi. oligosporus* for 48 h has a higher folic acid content than *tempe* fermented with *Rhi. stolonifer* or *Rhi. oryzae*. The results were 2.0, 1.1, and 0.9 mg/kg, respectively, for *tempe* fermented with *Rhi. oligosporus, Rhi. stolonifer,* and *Rhi. oryzae*. By using the averted intestine method the absorption of folic acid in *tempe* fermented for 48 h was 38.6%. Tocopherol composition changed during *tempe* fermentation. Except for alpha tocopherol, the levels of beta, gamma, and delta tocopherol increased. Even though beta tocopherol has only 40% of the biological activity of alpha tocopherol, an increase of 225% betatocopherol (Astuti 1994) added value to the natural antioxidant activity in *tempe*.

11.2.5 Minerals

The levels of minerals in *tempe* were not influenced the fermentation process. The iron content in unfermented soybeans was 9.34 mg/100 g and in *tempe* 9.39 mg/10 g. Vander Riet et al. (1987) reported that during fermentation the iron, copper, and zinc contents in *tempe* remained constant. According to Murata et al. (1967), some of the protein was broken down into simple protein, peptides, and amino acids during fermentation. As a result, iron was released from the iron–protein complex, thus increasing soluble iron. According to Astuti (1994) the soluble iron was distributed in the protein fraction with a molecular weight in the range of 5000–70,000 Da. Iron in protein fractions with a molecular weight of 70,000 Da significantly decreased along with the length of fermentation time, whereas iron in fractions with a molecular weight of 5000 Da sharply increased. *Tempe* is therefore a good source of available iron.

Calcium and magnesium levels in unfermented soybeans were 226.69 and 124.11 mg/100 g compared to 198.00 and 130.46 mg/100 g in *tempe* (Astuti 1994). Calcium content decreased during fermentation, but the process is not clearly understood. Calcium is possibly released from the bridge of phytate protein during the digestion of complex compounds and lost together with bound water, which may be released during fermentation. According to Sudarmadji and Markakis (1977), *Rhi. oligosporus* produced phytase enzymes which release phytate–Ca–protein from the complex compound. Watanabe et al. (2008) reported that calcium absorption ratio in rats fed with a *tempe* diet was significantly higher than the other diets (*tempe* fermented by anaerobic fermentation and soybean diets). This result might be caused by the low phytate content in *tempe*.

11.2.6 Antioxidant Enzyme SOD

Oxygen is vital for life, yet is potentially toxic when reduced to superoxide anions. Superoxide anions are known to be capable of stimulating lipid peroxidation (Thomas et al. 1985). One of the terminal products of lipid peroxidation is malondialdehyde (MDA), which can reach into cells and tissues which cause not only damage of lipid molecules but also of nonlipid biomolecules, such as proteins or DNA that cause cell mutation. Since lipid peroxides are suggested as one of the substances responsible for degenerative diseases, more attention should be paid to foods which have a beneficial effect on lipid peroxide prevention. Soybean *tempe* has been observed by Gyorgy et al. (1964) to contain antioxidant isoflavones.

Astuti et al. (1996a) reported that in the early stages of *tempe* fermentation (0–12 h) SOD activity was not detected, but after 12 h of fermentation SOD activity gradually increased upto 48 h of fermentation, and then gradually decreased. The highest specific activity of SOD was found in *tempe* inoculated with *Rhi. oryzae* followed by commercial mixed inoculum and then *Rhi. oligosporus*. The increase of SOD during fermentation indicated that SOD production was concomitant with the growth of mold. The reason remains unclear. One possibility is that during fermentation, aerobic SOD is produced by the cells to protect them against an excess of superoxide anions produced from reduced oxygen. Every normal cell will have a defense system to protect the cell against the action of free radicals such as superoxide anions. Rukmini et al. (1997) reported that SOD was developed in *tempe* made of pigeon peas.

11.2.7 Antinutrients

Soybeans contain a wide range of antinutritional factors such as phytate, saponin, hemagglutinins, flatus factors, and antitrypsin. Some of the anti-nutritional factors in soybeans are difficult to remove in the usual process of cooking due their heat stable properties. *Tempe* processing has a beneficial effect on carbohydrates, that is, oligosaccharides, especially the decrease of raffinose and stachiose content. The decrease of raffinose and stachiose during *tempe* processing eliminates exactly the flatulence problems experienced after consuming soybeans. Callowy et al. (1971) reported that *tempe* essentially decreases flatulence when it is consumed by human subjects. Fermentation of *tempe* decreases phytic acid content, as was found by Sudarmadji and Markakis (1977). Phytic acid is an antinutrient which inhibits the absorption of divalent minerals, thus decreasing the availability of those minerals. The contents of phytate in soybean and *tempe* were 18.4 and 13.4 g/kg, respectively (Watanabe 2011).

11.3 Health Benefits of *Tempe*

11.3.1 Tempe *and Diarrhea*

In Southeast Asia, the top three causes of death in children under 5 years old are prenatal disorders, respiratory infections, and diarrhea (Budiningsari et al. 2010). Diarrhea is defined as an abnormal condition of stool discharge which is frequent (Harries 1977). The causes of diarrhea were infection, malabsorption, allergy, poison, immunodeficiency, and others (Sudigbia 1990). The synergetic mechanism between infection and diarrhea looks to increase the degree and duration of diarrhea. Sudigbia (1982) found that 50% of the pediatric diarrhea death rate at Karyadi Hospital, Central Java, Indonesia was accompanied by encephalitis and bronchopneumonia. The consequences of diarrhea were loss of water and electrolytes, which usually cause dehydration and nutrients imbalance. The relationship between *tempe* consumption and the immune system were first stated by Van Veen and Schaefer (1950). Based on his investigation, the prisoners of World War II in Java who ate *tempe* everyday were saved from dysentery when there was an outbreak in the prison. Dysentery is a kind of gastrointestinal disease caused by infection by dysentery amoeba. On the basis of his/their observation, people who often ate *tempe* have better immunity against amoebic infections than those that eat *tempe* rarely.

Karmini (1987) used rabbits as hosts to receive infection and also used enteropathogenic *Escherichia coli* bacteria as an infectious agent, which has been proved to infect rabbits. The results showed that based on histopathological characteristics, there was no damage to the mucosal layer of epithelial cells in the stomach, small intestine, and colon of the rabbits treated with *tempe*, whereas there was damage to untreated rabbits. It may be concluded that *tempe* can influence enteropathogenic bacterial infections.

Sibarani (1991) reported that experimental rabbits fed with *tempe* were able to produce SIgA immunoglobulin, a cellular immunity component which is not found in untreated rabbits. Soemantri and Sudigbia (1985) described that when preschool children with chronic diarrhea treated with the *tempe* best formula (composed of 58% *tempe*, 23% wheat flour, 2% cornoil, 15% salt, and 0.5% emulsifier) had a significantly shorter recovery duration from diarrhea than those who consumed a milk-based formula. Most chronic cases indicated an increase in weight after the second week of treatment with the *tempe* formula.

Diarrhea episodes have their impact on the nutritional status through the increase of loose stools, vomiting, anorexia, the withholding of food due to ignorance, mucosal intestinal damage, and the catabolic effect of infections (Soenarto et al. 1997). The proper feeding of children with diarrhea has to fulfill the following requirements. The food must be easily digested and absorbed. It must contain high-quality protein, for example, hydrolyzed protein, and have a low lactose content. The study to evaluate the effect of the *tempe* formula was done by Soenarto et al. and the study was carried out at the Karyadi Hospital in Semarang, Indonesia and the Sardjito Hospital in Yogyakarta, Indonesia. Children aged 6–24 months suffering from acute diarrhea were enrolled if they fulfilled the following criteria: (1) purging soft or watery stools more than thrice a day, (2) diarrhea before admission that has lasted less than 7 days, (3) living less than 17 km from the hospital, (4) willing to stay in the hospital until the diarrhea was resolved, and (5) their parents or caregivers agreed to sign an informed consent. Patients who had severe diarrhea and had experienced other episodes of diarrhea in the previous 2 weeks were excluded. The research protocol was approved by the Ethics Committee of the Universitas Gadjah Mada.

The researcher prepared three kinds of formulas, a soy-based food formula, an industrial *tempe* formula, and a traditional *tempe* formula. Each formula was packed in a 25 g sachet. The patients were randomly assigned to three treatment groups. The feeding formula was started when there was no sign of dehydration. Each patient was given two sachets of formula in addition to the normal daily menu provided by the hospital. The *tempe* formula was equal to 37.5 g of fresh *tempe*. The formulas were served as porridge by dissolving them in 100–120 mL water. The outcomes of the study show that the traditional *tempe* formula had the best effect on the duration of the diarrhoea. The differences in the duration of the diarrhea were not significant. This study indicates that *tempe*, a popular protein source in Indonesian cuisine, is able to reduce the duration of diarrhea and improve the nutritional status of children.

The effect of soybean fermentation as antidiarrhea was studied by Kiers et al. (2003) in weaned pigs as animal models. In pig production, Weaning is a critical phase in pig production and is associated with digestive disorders causing reduction in growth and diarrhea which is often associated with *E. coli* bacteria (enterotoxigenic *E. coli* [ETEC]) and causes mortality in weaned piglets (Hampson 1994). Preventing diarrhea is very important in the pig industry to reduce economic losses. ETEC are not only the most common type of colibacillosis in young animals especially in pigs and calves, but also occur in human beings. ETEC is the predominant causative microorganism of severe diarrhea in children in developing countries (Nagy and Fekete 1999, Kiers et al. 2003).

Kiers et al. (2003) replaced the piglet diet (toasted full-fat soybeans) with cooked soybeans or *Rhi. microporus* or *Bacillus subtilis*-fermented soybeans. The effect on the incidence, severity, and duration of diarrhea in ETEC-challenged weaned piglets was determined. The results showed that the severity of diarrhea was significantly less on the diet with *Rhizopus*-fermented soybeans compared with the control diet of toasted soybeans. Piglets fed fermented soybeans showed the increased in feed intake, daily weight gain, and feed efficiency.

In conclusion, fermented soybean has beneficial effect in the control of ETEC inducing diarrhea.

Nutrition therapy is the most important aspect of diarrhea management for improving the nutritional status of the diarrhea patient. Two important points in diarrhea management are (1) rehydration and (2) early refeeding. Thus, nutritional support provided during and after diarrhea will help the healing process. To consider the positive impact of *tempe* consumption for children suffering from diarrhea, a case study was conducted in Wirosaban Hospital, Yogyakarta, Indonesia. Children between the ages of 1.5 and 10 years with acute diarrhea who fulfilled the inclusion criteria were divided into two groups, there was the control group and the treatment group. The treatment group was provided with *tempe* porridge that met the standard of diet, taste, and organoleptic properties, and was acceptable to the diarrhea patients. The *tempe* porridge was prepared with 200 g rice porridge, 70 g *tempe,* and 30 g vegetables including carrot and pumpkin. To improve the taste, a little coconut milk, vegetable oil, and sweet soy sauce was added to the porridge. The amount of rice porridge mixed with *tempe* for children aged 1–3, 4–6, and 7–9 years was 200, 250, and 300 g, respectively. The average of diarrhea frequency was measured based on the number of diarrhea cases in each subject for a minimum 2 days observation and then divided by the number of hospitalization days. The average duration of diarrhea was measured based on the length of diarrhea occurrence in each interval of diarrhea in 1 day for a minimum of 2 days observation and then divided by the number of hospitalization days.

In previous research, Mahmud (1987) reported that *tempe* has compounds which are able to inhibit the pathogenic bacteria causing diarrhea. *Tempe* is a kind of probiotic food that possibly influences the growth of pathogenic bacteria. Therefore, immunity toward pathogenic bacteria will increase and shorten the time of hospitalization. Frequency of diarrhea for the group provided *tempe* porridge compared with the group provided with the usual diet from the hospital showed significantly different results. The research conducted by Budiningsari et al. (2010) in accordance with the previous research conducted in Sardjito Hospital, Yogyakarta, Indonesia. Giving *tempe* porridge as nutritional support during and after diarrhea will improve the absorption capacity of intestinal mucosa, thus reducing the frequency of diarrhea and pain, and preventing the decrease in nutritional status.

The problems of diarrhea and refeeding also occurred in India. Although Indian society did not recognize and had never consumed *tempe* before, knowing about the potential of *tempe* as a food that may help in the recovery from diarrhea led to the development of oral rehydration therapy (ORT) based on *tempe*. According to Vaidehi (1995), *tempe* made in Bogor, Indonesia using *Rhi. oligosporus* and *Rhi. oryzae* powdered and packed as *tempe* flour. ORT *tempe* was prepared by mixing 65 g *tempe* flour, with 140 g wheat flour, 30 g milk powder, 125 g sugar, a little baking powder, and some drops of cardamom essence. All ingredients were mixed together and sieved, after which100 mL water was added and the mixture prepared as dough, rolled into flat round leaves and cut into pieces. The leaves are then spread on a greased tray, baked at 120°C for 45 min and removed from the oven when the color changed to golden brown. Pour the powder into fine mix (100 mesh) and store in plastic containers. This product is called *tempe* porridge powder. To prepare *tempe* Superoralitmix, 3.5 g sodium chloride, 1.3 g potassium chloride, and 2.25 g sodium citrate were ground together and sieved 3–4 times and added to 45 g of *tempe* porridge powder and 2.95 g glucose. Then all was mixed well and packed in triple laminated foil packs. The entire pack was dissolved in 1 L of boiled and cooled water before serving. *Tempe* Superoralitmix was evaluated for patients aged 1–5 years old at Bowring and Lady Curzon Hospital, Bangalore, India and compared to WHO-ORT. The patients were administered ORT according to the state of dehydration under the guidance of the hospital pediatrician. Evaluation was done on the intake of ORT, number of diarrheal days, frequency of loose stools, and the status of dehydration recovery.

Patients treated with *tempe*-ORT consumed a smaller amount of ORT for their recovery compared to the WHO-ORT. This maybe influenced by the organoleptic properties of *tempe*-ORT. The number of loose stools per patients per day was less in *tempe*-ORT than in WHO-ORT. The weight gain of patients (n-42) was much higher in *tempe*-ORT than in WHO-ORT. The differences may be caused by the higher nutritive value of *tempe*-ORT than WHO-ORT. *Tempe*-ORT contains 4.9 g protein, 38.75 g carbohydrate, and 143 cal while WHO-ORT contains 20 g carbohydrate and 80 cal.

Patients treated with *tempe*-ORT were 100% recovered compared with patients treated with WHO-ORT. *Tempe* Superoralite has a beneficial effect on weight gain and recovery from diarrhea. From this study, it is recommended that *tempe* be prepared with balanced cereals and pulses and used to solve the problems of malnutrition and micronutrient deficiency diseases. Measures to popularize *tempe* technology should be undertaken by arranging training programs in both rural and urban areas besides encouraging industrial manufacture for easy availability for the use and benefit of consumers (Vaidehi 1995). To observe the extent to which *tempe* is capable of inducing the human immune system, Nurrahman et al. (2013) conducted a research study of 21 male subjects, aged 19–24 years who lived in a dormitory. None of the subjects smoked, took alcohol or drugs, and did not take antioxidant supplements during the intervention periods. The subjects were healthy (as stated by a medical doctor) and had a normal body mass index (BMI). The respondents were divided into three groups, each group consisting of seven people. The first group was determined as a control group, they did not consume *tempe* or *tempe* extract, the second group consumed black soybean *tempe* extract in the form of capsules, and the third group consumed cooked black soybean *tempe* seasoned with garlic and salt. The intervention was conducted for 28 days. During intervention all the respondents only consumed food provided by the researcher. Except for the placebo group, each respondent in group 3 consumed *tempe* as much as100 g/day while group 2 consumed three capsules per day equivalent to 100 g of fresh *tempe*. One week before the intervention the respondents were not allowed to consume any soyfood product for 1 week. Blood samples were drawn at 0, 14, and 28 days for all subjects. The blood was analyzed for the proliferation of T and B cell. The results are shown in Table 11.2.

As shown in Table 11.2, after 14 days intervention, the average stimulation index for T cell proliferation were 1.950, 1.49, and 1.834 for control, *tempe* extract, and *tempe* groups, respectively. The data show there was no significant difference across the groups. However, in 28 days of intervention the stimulation index of T cell of *tempe* group increased sharply from 2.207 to 3.600. A previous study by Nurrahman et al. (2011) reported that the increased ability of T cells to proliferate after consuming *tempe* was due likely to some components in *tempe* such as antioxidant isoflavones, unsaturated fatty acids, and free amino acids. *Tempe* contains the highest level of Glu. According to Grimble and Grimble (1998), beside glutamine, sulfur amino acids such as methionine, cysteine, and cystine are required by T cells to function in the immune system. *Tempe* also contains genistein, and among soybean products, the genistein content in *tempe* is the highest. A measure of 100 g of *tempe* contains 1.4515 mg genistein (Siregar and Pawiroharsono 1997). It is possible that the genistein in *tempe* interacts with receptors on the surface of T cells

Table 11.2 Effect of *Tempe* Consumption on T and B Cell Proliferation

Groups of Respondents	*Time of Intervention (Days)*			*Time of Intervention (Days)*		
	0	*14*	*28*	*0*	*14*	*28*
Control	2.0051 ± 0.477	1.950 ± 0.369	2.775 ± 0.300	1.042 ± 0.091	1.007 ± 0.010	1.100 ± 0.122
Tempe extract	1.797 ± 0.469	1.490 ± 0.239	2.004 ± 0.533	1.062 ± 0.002	1.003 ± 0.009	1.099 ± 0.201
Tempe	2.207 ± 0.593	1.834 ± 0.255	3.600 ± 0.301	1.065 ± 0.048	1.002 ± 0.008	1.097 ± 0.152

Source: From Nurrahman, M., A. Suparmo, and Soesatyo, M.H.N.E. 2013. *International Journal of Current Microbiology and Applied Sciences* 2(9):316–327.

thus activating proliferation. The components in *tempe* are very complex, which may be able to stimulate the formation of lymphokine especially interleukin1 (IL-1) and interleukin2 (IL-2). IL-1 is produced by macrophage which affects to increase proliferation. To prove the above suggestion, further research is needed. The increase of the T cells stimulation index after consuming *tempe* and its extract indicated *tempe* has a positive effect on the cellular immune system. Differently from the index stimulation of T cells, after 28 days intervention in B cell proliferation, the increase index was not significantly different. This indicated that consuming *tempe* and its extracts are not able to increase B cell proliferation.

11.3.2 Tempe *and Lipid-Related Disease*

In recent years, deaths due to noncommunicable diseases such as coronary heart disease have been increasing rapidly. Lipid-related diseases are not only found in industrialized countries but also in developing countries. Diet is one of the most important factors in these noncommunicable diseases. Food with high-fat (HF) content and low in antioxidant content tends to results in deposition of excess lipid in the body thus developing oxidative stress. Imbalances of pro-oxidant and antioxidant may produce free radicals and reactive oxygen species (ROS) which caused early aging. To prevent oxidative cell damage and early aging, the diet must provide adequate quantities of antioxidants. *Tempe* is a fermented food which has a high content of antioxidants such as genestein, daidzein, and tocopherol that can be used for preventing lipid-related diseases.

Mangkuwidjoyo et al. (1985) reported that *tempe* had a positive effect on cholesterol levels and histopathogical changes in the livers and arteries of rats after a feeding trial of 4 months. It was suggested that *tempe* constituents inhibit the enzyme which is responsible for the formation and biosynthesis of cholesterol and prevents oxidation of LDL cholesterol thus minimizing the production of plaque in the arteries. The hypocholesterolemic effect of *tempe* indicates a potential use for diets in the affluent to prevent cardiovascular diseases.

The high level of triacylglycerol in serum and the liver are not only caused by the high intake of lipid in the diet but also caused by iron-deficiency anemia. The high levels of triacylglycerol in serum and the liver in the case of iron-deficiency anemia is due to the inability of enzyme stearoyl CoA desaturase to function (Rao et al. 1983). Stearoyl CoA desaturase enzyme has a role in the desaturation of long-chain fatty acids. Astuti (1992) reported that triacylglycerol of the casein group, unfermented soybean group, and *tempe* groups were not significantly different. The levels were 213.45, 118.07, and 124.64 mg/dL, respectively, for the casein, unfermented soybean, and *tempe* diets.

The cholesterol levels of anemic rats fed with the casein, unfermented soybean, and *tempe* diets were 89.42, 64.15, and 63.92 mg/dL, respectively. The high cholesterol levels of the casein group support the previous study by Nagata et al. (1980), who found that cholesterol levels in rats fed with a casein diet were higher than a *tempe* diet. This finding indicated that *tempe*, a product of mold fermentation, influenced cholesterol metabolism.

The mechanism of the hypocholesterolemic effect of soy protein has been studied by Sugano et al. (1982) who claimed possible participation of hormonal control in the cholesterol metabolism of soy protein diets. According to Nagata et al. (1982) soybean protein reduced cholesterol absorption and enhanced fecal excretion of steroids. Moreover, Astuti et al. (1996b) reported their study on the effect of the *tempe* diet of hyperlipidemic rats on the lipid profile, the lipid peroxides in rats' serum, and the mechanism of cholesterol reduction. Thirty-five male Sprague–Dawley rats, 60 days old were made hyperlipidemic by feeding a HF diet for 1 month. The cholesterol concentration was evaluated in the serum of rats before and after feeding the HF diet. The rats were then divided into five groups and fed with casein (C), *tempe* T-25, T-50, T-75, and T-100% as a source of protein. The lipid profile evaluated in serum was measured enzymatically and the lipid peroxide was assayed using the fluorometric method developed by Yagi (1982). The levels of lipid peroxide were expressed as malondialdehyde (MDA) nmol/mL serum and SOD activity was assayed in serum using the nitrobluetetrazolium method (Oyanagui 1984). The results are shown in Tables 11.3 and 11.4.

As shown in Table 11.3, the serum total cholesterol of rats fed with 100% *tempe* diet was the lowest. The substitution of casein with 50% *tempe* showed significant difference with the casein diet for total cholesterol and LDL cholesterol. Astuti (1998) found that feeding *tempe* to the rats increased biliary cholesterol. According to Garcia et al. (1993) fatty acids in *tempe*, that is, palmitic, stearic, oleic, linoleic, arachidic, and behenic acids inhibited the rats liver microsomal enzyme 3-hydroxy-3-methylglutaryl-coenzymeA reductase (HMG-CoA reductase). The greatest inhibition was done by linolenic acid followed by oleic acid and then arachidic acid.

Table 11.3 Serum Lipid Profile in Rats

	Lipid Concentration (mg/dL)			
Diets	*Tot-chl*	*HDL-chl*	*LDL-chl*	*Triacylglycerol*
Casein	106.4 ± 7.8^{a}	71.4 ± 7.8^{a}	35.0 ± 13.4^{a}	267.9 ± 33.2^{a}
Casein + *Tempe* 25	97.4 ± 8.6^{ab}	64.1 ± 3.4^{a}	33.3 ± 7.6^{ab}	202.6 ± 20.5^{ab}
Casein + *Tempe* 50	91.7 ± 4.6^{b}	67.2 ± 2.6^{a}	24.5 ± 3.5^{ab}	144.2 ± 12.7^{b}
Casein + *Tempe* 75	93.7 ± 4.7^{b}	64.4 ± 3.8^{a}	29.3 ± 4.8^{ab}	127.4 ± 10.7^{b}
Casein + *Tempe* 100	88.8 ± 2.6^{b}	67.3 ± 2.8^{a}	21.5 ± 4.2^{b}	118.81 ± 8.6^{c}

Source: From Astuti, M., Y. Marsono, and N. Sukana. 1996b. *Technical Bulletin American Soybean Association MITA (P) No. 044/11/96.*

Note: Values are means of seven rats ± SD. Values not labeled with the same superscript in the letter in the same column indicate significant differences (P 0.05, ANOVA, and DMRT).

Table 11.4 Serum Lipid Peroxidation (MDA) and SOD Inhibition in Rats

Diets	*MDA (nmol/mL Serum)*	*SOD Inhibition (%)*
Casein	11.61 ± 0.97^{a}	20.83 ± 1^{a}
Casein + *Tempe* 25	10.42 ± 1^{a}	33.97 ± 2^{b}
Casein + *Tempe* 50	8.10 ± 1^{b}	33.37 ± 2^{b}
Casein + *Tempe* 75	4.91 ± 0^{c}	41.31 ± 2^{bc}
Casein + *Tempe* 100	3.69 ± 0^{c}	48.57 ± 1^{c}

Source: From Astuti, M., Y. Marsono, and N. Sukana. 1996b. *Technical Bulletin American Soybean Association MITA (P) No. 044/11/96.*

Note: Values are means of seven rats ± SD. Values not labeled with the same superscript in the letter in the same column indicate significant differences (P 0.05, ANOVA, and DMRT).

The substitution of *tempe* in the diets did not affect the concentration of HDL cholesterol. This finding is consistent with the observation of Aljawad et al. (1990). Serum triacylglycerol of rats fed with the *tempe* diet was the lowest among the five groups of rats. Feeding 100% of *tempe* in hyperlipidemic rats decreased triacylglycerol 56.68%. This result was suggested due to the amino acid and fatty acid composition in *tempe*.

Table 11.4 shows that lipid peroxides in the serum of rats fed with the 100% *tempe* diet was the lowest among the five groups of rats. The results indicated that *tempe* has the highest prevention on lipid peroxidation. This finding supports the previous study by Astuti (1994). *Tempe* contains natural antioxidants tocopherol, isoflavonoids, and SOD. These antioxidants can prevent lipid oxidation induced by free radicals as well as free iron. In the majority of organisms, SOD performs a vital function in the defense mechanism system against the toxic effects of oxygen. The highest activity of SOD in rats fed with the 100% *tempe* probably correlated to trace minerals copper and zinc. It was known that copper and zinc were the active side of this enzyme (Astuti et al. 1996a).

The hypocholesterolemic properties of *tempe* in human subjects were studied by Arsiniati (1997) who developed a *tempe* formula, namely, *Tempe* A-5. The nutrition content of *Tempe* A-5 consist of protein 26.65 g, lipid 18.17 g, carbohydrate 46.71 g/100 g of formula and the energy was 455.01 cal. The subjects were 75 hyperlipidemic adult men, aged 40–65 years old with total cholesterol ≥220 mg/dL and/ or triacylglycerol levels >175 mg/dL. They were divided into three groups and were given different diets for 2 weeks. Group 1 were given a standard diet and *tempe* formula, group 2 were given a standard diet and *tempe* and group 3 were given a standard diet. All of the three diets were isocaloric. Respondents in group1 were given *Tempe* A-5 thrice daily each 67.50 g. *Tempe* A-5 was diluted in warm water before being consumed. During the treatment diet none of the respondents were allowed to consume soybean and soybean products. All food consumed was measured and listed in a food record. The lipid profiles and serum uric acid levels were evaluated. The results are shown in Tables 11.5 through 11.7. SD means standard diet.

Total cholesterol and LDL cholesterol of the subject taking *Tempe* A-5 decreased about 18.56% and 16.81%. The decreasing of total and LDL cholesterol support the previous study by Sugiyarto (1990). The HDL cholesterol increased 24.19%. This has a greatest meaning because HDL cholesterol was known as good cholesterol.

Serumuric acid in subjects who consumed *Tempe* A-5 was not significantly different from the other diet.

Table 11.5 Total Cholesterol, LDL-chol, and HDL-chol of the Subjects

	Total Cholesterol (mg/dL)		*LDL Cholesterol (mg/dL)*	
Treatments	*Pre*	*Post*	*Pre*	*Post*
SD + *Tempe*A-5	234.96 ± 41.39	191.28 ± 43.6	151.12 ± 46.74	125.72 ± 39.44
SD + *Tempe*	224.84 ± 38.48	206.00 ± 40.28	134.08 ± 40.20	122.96 ± 56.95
SD	213.24 ± 43.00	203.88 ± 45.43	142.72 ± 32.91	136.40 ± 40.24
	HDL Cholesterol (mg/dL)		*Triacylglycerol (mg/dL)*	
SD + *Tempe*A-5	37.95 ± 11.07	47.14 ± 13.16	255.56 ± 103.07	221.04 ± 87.30
SD + *Tempe*	41.70 ± 7.73	45.23 ± 14.29	230.68 ± 88.69	209.48 ± 89.45
SD	38.74 ± 8.11	40.10 ± 8.99	227.00 ± 81.96	187.08 ± 7.59

Source: From Arsiniati, M.A. 1997. *Reinventing the Hidden Miracle of Tempe Proceedings International Tempe Symposium.* Jakarta: Yayasan *Tempe* Indonesia, pp. 187–198.

Table 11.6 Changes in Lipid Profile (%)

Treatments	*Total Cholesterol*	*LDL Cholesterol*	*HDL Cholesterol*	*Triacylglycerol*
SD + *Tempe*A-5	18.56	16.81	24.19	13.76
SD + *Tempe*	8.38	8.29	8.47	9.19
SD	4.36	4.32	5.51	7.59

Source: From Arsiniati, M.A. 1997. *Reinventing the Hidden Miracle of Tempe Proceedings International Tempe Symposium.* Jakarta: Yayasan *Tempe* Indonesia, pp. 187–198.

Table 11.7 Serum Uric Acid Level of the Subjects

Treatments	*Pretreatment (mg/dL)*	*Posttreatment (mg/dL)*	*Changes (mg/dL)*	*Changes (%)*
SD + *Tempe*A-5	7.08 ± 1.52	6.84 ± 1.49	0.23	3.39
SD + *Tempe*	6.73 ± 1.48	6.39 ± 1.07	0.34	5.05
SD	6.54 ± 1.34	6.47 ± 1.21	0.07	1.07

Source: From Arsiniati, M.A. 1997. *Reinventing the Hidden Miracle of Tempe Proceedings International Tempe Symposium.* Jakarta: Yayasan *Tempe* Indonesia, pp. 187–198.

The hypocholesterolemic properties of *tempe* in human subjects were also studied by Astuti (1998, unpublished) who developed a formula-based *tempe* namely over-forty *tempe* (OFT *Tempe*). Twenty-four hypercholesterolemic subjects (6 female and 18 male) consumed OFT *Tempe* for 3 months. Everyday all subjects took 20 g of OFT *tempe*, mixed with 200 mL of warm water. At the initial phase of the experiments and every month after consuming OFT *tempe* formula the blood samples were collected and analyzed for total cholesterol and LDL cholesterol, uric acid, and lipid peroxidation in serum. Serum cholesterol was evaluated by the spectrophotometric method and the lipid profile using fluorometric method developed by Yagi (1982) expressed by MDA nmol/mL serum.

The results show that during the feeding trial (consuming OFT *tempe* 20 g/day) the total cholesterol in male subjects decreased from 240.5 to 215 mg/dL or decreased about 10.38% and in female subjects decreased from 233 to 205 mg/dL or decreased about 12.01%. For LDL cholesterol for male subjects the decrease was from 160 to 148 mg/dL or a decrease of about 7.5% and for female subjects the decrease was from 155 to 145 mg/dL, a decrease of about 6.45%. The decreasing total cholesterol and LDL cholesterol supported the previous study by Arsiniati (1997). In the male subjects, the serum uric acid decreased from 5.66 to 4.75 mg/dL during the 1 month of consuming OFT-*Tempe* and in female subjects decreased from 4.35 to 3.50 mg/dL. All of the subjects had normal values of uric acid. This study indicates that the normal uric acid can be maintained by consuming *tempe* formula. The normal levels of uric acid in the males was 3.4–7.0 mg/dL and in the females was 2.4–5.7 mg/dL.

Lipid peroxide which expresses as MDA in male and female subjects tend to decrease in the normal range. According to Yagi (1993), the level of MDA in normal healthy subjects was not exceeding 4 nmol/mL. Our study shows that the MDA level in male subjects before consumption of OFT *Tempe* was 4.95 nmol/mL and for female subjects was 5.10 nmol/mL.The higher concentration of MDA in all subjects was because all of the subjects were hypercholesterolemic. Plachta et al. (1992) found an increase in the level of lipid peroxide in patients suffering from atherosclerosis. After 1 month of consuming OFT *tempe*, the level of MDA for males was 3.8 nmol/mL and for females was 3.92 nmol/mL. MDA is one of the products of decomposition of fatty acid in lipid peroxidation. It is able to reach cells and tissue, thus resulting in cell damage. It was shown that consuming OFT *tempe*, the MDA level decreased to normal level. This study indicated that *tempe* has a positive effect on the preventing of oxidation may be by the antioxidants in *tempe* and the components in *tempe* that work on the repair system. Using human subjects our study supported the previous study using animal models (Astuti 1992) that showed that *tempe* contains bioactive substances which are able to inhibit lipid peroxidation.

11.3.3 Tempe *and Anemia*

Iron-deficiency anemia is one of the most prevalent nutritional problems in the world. It is estimated that at least 1 billion individuals are anemic because of insufficient iron. Iron-deficiency anemia is found in all countries, but it is most prevalent and of greatest severity in developing countries. It is particularly prevalent among infants, young children, pregnant women, and lactating mothers. The most important cause of iron deficiency in developing countries is poor absorption of iron or bio-unavailability of iron from the diets. Dietary iron that has low availability comes predominantly from cereals and vegetables (Layrisse et al. 1968). One of the alternatives to solve this problems in developing countries is to explore foods which are potentially rich sources of iron and to improve the availability of iron in food. *Tempe* a fermented soybean food is a source of protein and iron but in the diet *tempe* is consumed together with staple foods, especially rice. Only a little *tempe* is consumed as a snack food. The effect of mixing *tempe* and the Indonesian staple food of rice on iron availability has not yet been investigated. A previous study by Hermana (1983) demonstrated that the mixing of rice with soybeans in the ratio 7:3 can improve the protein malnutrition of children under 5 years.

To prevent anemia, food not only rich in iron but also which has a high availability should be consumed. Iron availability is the proportion of iron which is absorbed and utilized by the body (Erbersdobler 1989). To predict the availability of iron, the *in vitro* and *in vivo* method can be used. Astuti (1992) reported that the iron availability of rice is lower than that of *tempe*. The iron availability of *tempe* was 59.17% compared to 51.64% in rice. The mixing of rice with *tempe* increases the iron availability of mixed foods. The highest level was found in the ratio of rice:*tempe* = 5:5. The addition of 1 part of *tempe* increased 10% the iron availability of rice.

Using anemic rats, Astuti (1992) reported her study on iron bioavailability of *tempe*. The rats were made moderately anemic by feeding them iron-deficient diets (11 ppm Fe) for 14 days. The blood from the tail vein of the rats was taken for hemoglobin determination. The anemic rats were randomly assigned to three groups of seven rats each. During the 11 days repletion period, the Casa control group were fed with a casein diet which contained 54 ppm Fe, group US were fed with an unfermented soybean diet which contained 33 ppm Fe and group T were fed with a *tempe* diet which contain 34 ppm Fe. Iron intake during repletion and hemoglobin levels were evaluated and the hemoglobin regeneration was calculated. The results showed that at the end of the repletion period, the hemoglobin levels of the casein, the unfermented soybean, and the *tempe* diets were 14.69, 11.76, and 12.04 g/dL, respectively. The high hemoglobin level in the casein group was due to the higher iron content in their diet. The hemoglobin level of rats fed with the *tempe* diet showed a normal level. This indicates that *tempe* contains a good nutrient for hemoglobin synthesis.

Hemoglobin regeneration efficiency was used to estimate iron availability in moderately anemic rats. Body weight and blood hemoglobin levels were used to calculate the initial and final hemoglobin iron contents. It shows that the hemoglobin regeneration was 45.64%, 44.76%, and 44.79%, respectively, for the casein, unfermented soybean, and *tempe* groups. Hemoglobin regeneration of the three groups of rats was not significantly different. The results indicate that iron in both unfermented soybean and *tempe* can be categorized as a good iron source. However, boiled soybeans are very rarely consumed in the diet due to the problem of flatulence.

11.3.4 Tempe *and Menopausal Symptoms*

Menopause marks the end of a woman's menstrual cycles and her fertility. It happens when the ovaries no longer make estrogen and progesterone, two hormones needed for a woman's fertility. Menopause occurs when the ovaries no longer release an egg every month and menstruation stops. Menopause happens naturally with age. When it occurs after the age of 50, is considered a normal part of aging. However, some women experience menopause early because of surgery or treatment of disease or because of illness; or belatedly at more than 60 years old.

Symptoms of menopause can include abnormal ones such as vaginal bleeding. Other symptoms are hot flushes, insomnia, thinning hair, drying skin, vaginal dryness, and itching and also complications that women may develop after menopause including osteoporosis and heart disease. To prevent the symptoms of menopause, it is very important to consume a diet which is rich in compounds like estrogen.

Tempe a product of soybean fermentation contains isoflavone antioxidants which are structurally similar to estrogen. Isoflavone content in *tempe* was 12.7294 mg/100 g dB. The highest Aglicon isoflavone in *tempe* was daidzein (Siregar and Pawiroharsono 1997), followed by glycetein, genestein and factor II. The isoflavone content in *tempe* was 7.7184, 3.3464, 1.4515, and 0.2131 mg/100 g dB for daidzein, glycetein, genestein, and factor II, respectively. Genestein has been proved to process antitumor activity (Jha 1997).

Tempe and soybean products are consumed in high levels by the Asian population. The estrogenic compounds may play an important role in the prevention of menopausal symptoms. Unfortunately, there is no epidemiological data specifically on menopausal disorders in populations with a very high intake of *tempe* (Astuti et al. 2000).

Sapbamrer et al. (2013) reported that the Thais consumed soybean with a content of isoflavone higher than *meju* (130 μg/g) and *doenjang* (193 μg/g) from Korea, but lower than *douchi* (530 μg/g) from China, *tempe* (660 μg/g) from Indonesia, and *miso* (1260 μg/g) from Japan, respectively. The health effect of dietary fermented soybean among Thai women was studied by Sapbamrer et al. (2013) in northern Thailand. The women subjects who live in Baan Tham village of Phayao province had their last menstrual period at least 12 months prior to their participation in the study. A total of 60 women were divided into two groups, that is, experimental group ($n = 31$) and reference group ($n = 29$). The women preferring to eat *tempe* were chosen for experimental group. The fermented soybean (*tempe*) provided approximately 60 mg of isoflavone a day which was the range recommended for their daily isoflavone intake. The reference group was permitted to continue their usual diet, but was not permitted to consume fermented soybean. They were permitted to consume soy or soy products no more than in three meals per week. During the intervention period, both the reference and the experimental group were asked weekly about the frequency of soy and soy product consumption.

Five milliliters of fasting blood was obtained on the first day of the experiment as baseline data and after 6 months of intervention they were evaluated for their reproductive hormones (estradiol and progesterone), lipids, and glucose. According to Sapbamrer et al. (2013) fermented soybeans contain 132 ± 95.4 μg/g genestein and 63.0 ± 44.6 μg/g daidzein. Extradiol remained stable in the experimental group but progesterone increased significantly. The amount of dietary soy isoflavone might be an important factor affecting reproductive hormone mechanism. It is also suggested that isoflavone in fermented soybean may mimic estrogen by binding to its receptor sites, and consequently elevate or maintain reproductive circulation. In lipids profile, the cholesterol for the experimental group reduced significantly, but triglycerides did not change. Blood glucose in the experimental group did not change, but the glucose in the reference group increased significantly. It seems that the amount of isoflavone and protein consumed was an important factor influencing glucose level.

In conclusion, traditional fermented dietary soybean have favorable effects on progesterone and cholesterol, but have no effects on estradiol, glucose, and triglycerides. Another study was designed by Haron (2013) in postmenopausal Malay women. Postmenopausal Malay women had low calcium intake that achieved only 40%–50% of the Malaysian RNI. The low intake of calcium among these subjects may be due to their predominantly non-milk-based diet where 30–40% of them did not take any milk. In this study, fractional calcium absorption from *tempe* was compared to that observed from milk, using a dual stable isotope approach in a randomized crossover design. Subjects consumed the same calcium load (130–150 mg Ca) from either milk or *tempe* with a 1-month washout period between each test meal. 42 Ca (0.036 mg/kg) was administered intravenously to subjects prior to oral administration of 44 Ca (0.272 mg/kg) in milk.

The results show that calcium absorption from *tempe* (36.9 ± 10.4%) was not significantly different from milk (34.3 ± 8.4%), but calcium balance in *tempe* (108 ± 63 mg/day) was significantly higher compared with milk (71 ± 64 mg/day). This study indicates that the calcium bioavailability of *tempe* is similar to that of milk. *Tempe* may have potential to contribute significantly to the calcium needs of these postmenopausal Malay women who were at risk of low bone mass and had insufficient vitamin D levels.

11.3.5 Possible Role of Tempe *in Cancer Prevention*

Recently, attention was also focused on the potential role of soybean and soybean products including *tempe* on reducing the cancer risk factor. Several compounds with anticarcinogenic activity are found in relatively high concentration in soybean and soybean products. Asian countries have the lowest rates of cancers that are common in Western society such as breast, prostate, and colon cancer (Kiriakidis et al. 1997). The protective effect of the diet containing soy may partly explain the epidemiological study on colorectal cancer in Japan which found that the frequent consumption of soybean and soybean products such as *tofu* or *miso* markedly decreased the risk of both rectal and colon cancer (Watanabe et al. 1984). Cassidy et al. (1994) showed that premenopausal women fed textured soy products will increase menstrual cycle length approximately two and a half days. This finding is supported by an epidemiological study conducted in Singapore by Lee et al. (1991) which showed that 50% decreased risk of breast cancer associated with regular soy consumption in premenopausal women. Isoflavone in soybean products is suggested to play a role in estrogen receptor. Genestein and daidzein, an isoflavon aglycon, have potential to inhibit tyrosine protein kinase which is involved in cancer development.

Messina et al. (1994) reported that genestein added in cancer cells *in vitro* are able to inhibit the growth of cancer cells. Moreover, genestein also showed the ability to inhibit the angiogenesis *in vitro.* Angiogenesis is necessary for tumor growth. The effect of soybean *tempe* on tumor development was studied by Kiriakidis et al. (1997), who demonstrated that the glucolipids in *tempe* inhibit the proliferation of tumor cells in mice. The inhibition of the *tempe* isoflavone was studied by Lu et al. (2009). The isoflavone extracted from soybean and *tempe* was evaluated for its capacity in inhibition of SP2/0 (mouse myeloma cell) and HeLa (uterus cancer cell) cell lines. The criterion of inhibition is as follows: (1) week, inhibition <30%, (2) medium, inhibition >30 – <50 and (3) strong, inhibition >50%. The result is shown in Table 11.8.

Results in Table 11.8 showed that the isoflavone extracted from *tempe* produces better inhibition for cancer cells only at higher concentration. According to Liu et al. (2009), the effect of *tempe* isoflavone is stronger than soybean isoflavone as anticancer. The effect of *tempe* as anticolon cancer was evaluated in Sprague–Dawley rats by Hsu et al. (2009) from Taiwan. They found that intake of *tempe* was able to inhibit colon cancer by elevating SOD activity in liver tissue. Astuti et al. (1996a) reported that the highest SOD level occurred in *tempe* fermented for 60 h. Utama et al. (2013) reported that HF-diet rats fed with *tempe* increase cecal acetate, butyrate, propionate,

Table 11.8 The Inhibition of *Tempe* Isoflavone on SP2/0 and HeLa Cell Lines

Sample Concentration (μg/mL)	*Inhibition Ratio, % in SP2/0 Cell Lines*		*Inhibition Ratio, % in HeLa Cell Lines*	
	Tempe	*Soybean*	*Tempe*	*Soybean*
20	96.90	83.16	69.5	60.5
10	47.45	26.47	47.7	43.0
5	20.79	16.75	37.5	33.9
2.5	7.80	–	36.3	30.0
1.25	–	–	34.3	23.4

Source: From Liu, Y. et al. 2009. *Japan Agricultural Research Quarterly* 43(4): 301–307.

and succinate concentration. Organic acids such as butyrate and propionate were known as anti-tumor agents. The increasing of organic acids in cecal has a positive effect on cancer prevention. Moreover, they reported that *tempe* has a potential role to depress several risk factors such as lithocholic acid which are related to colon disease. The increasing of intestinal mucins and IgA supported the possible role of *tempe* in reducing the risk of colon cancer. Indonesians are known as the largest *tempe* consumers in the world; however, studies of the prevalence of cancer have not yet been conducted.

11.3.6 Tempe *and Inflammation (Neuroinflammation)*

Inflammation occurring in tissues of the body is caused by infections, trauma, metabolites toxicity, or autoimmunity. The inflammation can occur in all cells of the body including neuro cells. Aging is a normal process in human life. Some elderly people suffer from neurodegenerative diseases. The homeostatic imbalance between anti-inflammatory and pro-inflammatory cytokines in aging becomes one factor that increases the risk for neurodegenerative disease. Neurodegenerative disease is a series of neuron dysfunctions due to the continuous death of neurons. Developing neurodegenerative diseases such as dementia or Alzheimer's disease (AD) frequently occur in elderly people and cause a reduction in the ability to form memories or a loss of memory. At the mild stage of AD, the deficits only affect short-term memory but over time it leads to severe dementia (Park et al. 2012). The lack of a neurotransmitter such as acetylcholine (Ach) which is involved in the transmission of the information causes memory impairment. The excessive amount of Ach esterase results in a low level of Ach. Oxygen is vital for life but it becomes potentially toxic when reduced to superoxide anions. ROS is a product of oxidative stress which normally occurs in the human body. Maintaining the balance of pro-oxidants and antioxidants can reduce oxidative stress. Healthy habits such as regular exercise, healthy diet, mental stimulation, stress management, quality sleep, and an active social life reduce the risk of oxidative stress. By leading a brain-healthy lifestyle, elderly people may be able to prevent AD diseases.

Many dietary factors have been postulated to play a role in the prevention of cognitive decline and dementia in the elderly. Consuming foods such as ginger, green tea, fatty fish, blueberries, and soy products may protect neuron cells from damage. Soybean and fermented soybean such as *tempe* have been linked to many health benefits mainly in lowering incidence of diarrhoea, lipid-related disease (Astuti et al. 1996b, Soenarto et al. 1997). *Tempe* contain isoflavone genestein and daidzein in high amounts, it also contains folic acid, vitamin B_{12}, magnesium, and other nutrients which can potentially improve brain health. *Tempe* has been studied mostly for antioxidant properties but the neuroprotective potential and mechanism involved remain poorly understood.

Indonesians not only consume *tempe* but also tofu in similar amount. The percentage of household consumption of soybean products in Indonesia, according to Hardinsyah (2010) are as follows: *Tempe* 69.89%, *tofu* 63.72%, soy sauce 42.5%, *oncom* 2.76%, *tauco* 0.85%, and soy milk 0.90%.*Tempe* and *tofu* consumption were 8.5 kg/cap/year and 7.5 kg/cap/year, respectively. *Tempe* and *tofu* as soybean products contain phytoestrogen. Phytoestrogen can protect the brain through complex mechanisms. A previous study in Honolulu stated that Japanese who consumed *tofu* in higher levels and more than twice a week had a lower risk of dementia, brain atrophy, and cognitive function compared to people who consumed tofu in lower amounts (White et al. 2000). This may be caused by phytoestrogen in *tofu* which could protect apoptosis of rats' neurons. This finding is different from the previous report which suggested that frequent and high tofu consumption is associated with a worse cognitive function in the East Asian elderly (Hogervorst et al. 2008). A previous study conducted by Hogervorst et al. (2008) consisted of 719 male and female participants in the age of 52–98 years old from two different villages in Central Java and West Java. Hopkins verbal learning test (HVLT) was used to evaluate the memory and and learning ability, with every sentence repeated 3 times to get immediate recall (IR). Memory loss was the main indicator of the accident of dementia. Food intake and frequency especially of *tofu* and *tempe* was calculated every week. The results showed that high *tofu* consumption was associated with worse memory, while high *tempe* consumption was related to better memory especially in participants over 68 years old. It may be due to the differences in isoflavone content. Some *tofus* in the market contain formaldehyde. The presence of formaldehyde in *tofu* is used to preserve the freshness of *tofu* (Setiawati, 2008). The presence of formaldehyde in fresh *tofu* may cause neurotoxic effects. In this study, the researcher has not analyzed the formaldehyde content in *tofu*.

Neuroprotective effects between total isoflavones from soybean and *tempe* against scopolamine-induced cognitive dysfunction was studied by Ahmad et al. (2014). At neuroinflammation condition, pro-inflammatory cytokines and ROS produce an activated microglia and astrocytes which may result in apoptosis and necrosis (Glass et al. 2010). According to Ahmad et al. (2014), the rats consuming isoflavones from soybean and *tempe* at 40 mg/kg significantly reversed the scopolamine effect and improved memory. Intake of *tempe* isoflavones in the concentration of 10, 20, and 40 mg/kg significantly increased Ach and reduced Ach esterase. Meanwhile, only a high dose (40 mg/kg) of isoflavone soybean showed significant improvement. Ach is an important neurotransmitter in the preganglionic sympathetic and parasympathetic neurons. Ach is also the neurotransmitter at the adrenal medulla and serves as the neurotransmitter at all the parasympathetic innervated organs and also sweat glands. Ach esterase is an enzyme involved in Ach synthesized. The presence of acyltransferase is the marker that the neuron is cholinergic. Cholinergic neurons of the brain play a vital role in the cognitive deficits related to aging and neurodegenerative diseases. The study of Ahmad et al. (2014) showed that the *tempe* isoflavone at 40 mg/kg was able to reduce inflammation better than the soybean isoflavone.

11.3.7 Tempe *and Diabetes Mellitus*

The incidence of type 2 diabetes mellitus in Asian populations is suggested to be lower than in Western countries. One possible reason is that most of the Asian population consumes soybean products including fermented soybean. Soybean protein and peptides from fermented soybean prevent and postpone the progression of type 2 diabetes. SOD has important factors which prevent the damage of the pancreas. The antioxidative effect of soybeans, soybean protein fraction, and *tempe* were studied by Wulan (2000) using diabetic rats induced by alloxan. The results showed that the highest activity of SOD was found in diabetic rats fed with a *tempe* diet and the lowest was found in diabetic rats fed with a soybean diet. Histological observation of the pancreatic islet showed that the most heavy cell damage was found in rats fed with soybean. The rats fed with soybean protein faction and *tempe* diets showed little cell damage. This indicated that *tempe* has a beneficial effect on improving the pancreatic beta cell of diabetic rats.

Suarsana (2009) studied about hypoglycemic and antioxidative activities of the methanol extract of *tempe* on diabetic rats. He reported that boiling and frying processes are able to decrease the isoflavone in *tempe* 18.20% and 39.15%. The methanol extract of *tempe* at dose 300 ppm/kg bw/day showed a high antioxidant activity similar to 200 ppm of butylated hydroxy toluene (BHT) and had a similar hypoglycemic effect to acarbose at dose 4.5 mg/kg bw. The administration of methanol extract of *tempe* in normal rats improved glycogen level in the liver (9.29%), muscle (18.27%), SOD activity (21.2%), glutathione peroxidase (GPx) activity (6.6%), catalase (10.3%) and reduced MDA level (5.07%) in the pancreas. The administration of methanol extract of *tempe* in diabetic rats was able to inhibit the increase of blood glucose level (67.36%), MDA level (34.5%); maintain intracellular antioxidant enzyme activity (SOD, GPx, and catalase) in the pancreas and it also inhibited the rate of pancreatic beta cells damage.

11.4 Conclusion

During soybeans fermentation by mold of *Rhizopus* spp., there are a lot of nutritional changes which make *tempe* more nutritious. *Tempe* has a good quantity and quality of protein, and contains vitamin B_{12} in adequate amount. Several studies showed that *tempe* can be used to improve health. *Tempe* improves the immune system and is able to inhibit the pathogenic bacteria causing diarrhea. *Tempe* which contains the antioxidants genestein, daidzein, tocopherol, and also SOD has a good capability to prevent oxidative stress causing noncommunicable disease such as hyperlipidemia, diabetes mellitus type 2, cancer (breast and colon), cognitive decline, and dementia. *Tempe* consumption is able to prevent the damage of the pancreatic beta cell. The structure of the isoflavone in *tempe* is similar to the estrogen hormone. Therefore, *tempe* consumption has a positive effect for women to prevent menopausal symptoms. Metabolites of *tempe* in the intestinal tract such as butyrate and propionate are known as antitumor agents. Consuming *tempe* can maintain the normal level of human blood uric acid. Bioavailability of iron in *tempe* is very good, so *tempe* consumption is able to inhibit iron-deficiency anemia. *Tempe* not only contains calcium in adequate amounts but also has a good bioavailability. Based on nutritional aspects and health benefits, *tempe* which is originally from Indonesia and categorized as a traditional food, can be developed as a functional food to prevent non-communicable disease and infectious disease caused by pathogenic bacteria. Exploration is still needed to promote *tempe* which has a potential role in reducing non-communicable disease all over the world.

References

Ahmad, A., Ramasamy, K., Jaafar, S.M., Majeed, A.B.A., and Mani, V. 2014. Total isoflavones from soybean and *tempeh* reversed scopolamine-induced amnesia, improved cholinergic activities and reduced neuro-inflammation in brain. *Food and Chemical Toxicology* 65:120–128.

Aljawad, N.S., Fryer, E.B., and Fryer, H.C. 1990. Effects of casein, soy, and whey proteins and aminoacid supplementation on cholesterol metabolism in rats. *The Journal of Nutritional Biochemistry* 2(3):150–155.

Arsiniati, M.A. 1997. The effect of *tempe* diet on uric acid and plasma lipid level. In Sudarmadji, S., Suparmo, and S. Raharjo (Eds.), *Reinventing the Hidden Miracle of Tempe.* Proceedings International *Tempe* Symposium. Jakarta: Yayasan *Tempe* Indonesia, pp. 187–198.

Asmoro, N.W. 2014. Pengaruh Jenis Inokulumdan Lama Fermentasi *Tempe* Kedelai Hitam terhadap Kandungan Asam Folat dan Absorbsinyapada Usus Tikus (*Sprague Dawley*) secara In Vitro. Unpublished Data.

Astuti, M. 1982. *Tempe* as protein source in baby food formula. Report, 10–12. Universitas Gadjah Mada, Yogyakarta.

Astuti, M. 1992. *Iron bioavailability in traditional Indonesian soybean tempe.* Doctoral thesis, Tokyo University of Agriculture, Tokyo.

Astuti, M. 1994. *Iron bioavailability of traditional Indonesian soybean tempe*, Vol. XXXV. Memoirs of the Tokyo University of Agriculture.

Astuti, M. 1998. Soy and heart disease—Effects independent of cholesterol reduction: The role of tempe on lipid profile and lipid peroxidation (Abstract). In the role of soy in preventing and treating chronic disease. *Proceedings of a Symposium.* Brussels, Belgium, September 15–19, 1996. *American Journal of Clinical Nutrition* 68(6S):1522S–1523.

Astuti, M. 1998. Over Forty *Tempe* (OFT). Unpublished Data.

Astuti, M., Marseno, D.W., Marsono, Y., and Gitawati, I. 1996a. Development of antioxidant enzyme superoxide dismutase in soybean *tempe*. Report. Unpublished Data.

Astuti, M., Marsono, Y., and Sukana, N. 1996b. The role of *tempe* on lipid performance and lipid peroxides in hyperlipidemic rats. Technical Bulletin American Soybean Association MITA (P) No. 044/11/96.

Astuti, M., Meliala, A., Dalais, F.S., and Wahlqvist, M.L. 2000. *Tempe*, anutritious and healthy food from Indonesia. *Asia Pacific Journal of Clinical Nutrition* 9(4):322–325.

Auret, M. and VanVeen, A.G. 1955. Possible sources of proteins for child feeding in underdeveloped countries. *The American Journal of Clinical Nutrition* 3:234–243.

Bai, R.G., Prabha, T.N., Rao, T.N.R., Sreedhara, V.P., and Sreedhara, N. 1975. Studies on *tempeh*. Part I. Processing and nutritional evaluation of *tempeh* from a mixture of soybean and groundnut. *Journal of Food Science and Technology* 12(3):135–138.

Budiningsari, D., Susanti, E., and Renaningtyas, D. 2010. The effect of *tempe* porridge modification treatment on food intake, length of hospitalization, frequency and duration of diarrhea in hospitalized children with diarrhoea in Wirosaban Hospital Yogyakarta. Presented in *Green Mega Food Workshop*, Copenhagen, October 15.

Callowy, D.H., Hickey, C.A., and Murphy, E.L. 1971. Reduction of intestinal gas-forming properties of legumes by traditional and experimental food processing method. *Journal of Food Science* 36:251–255.

Cassidy, A., Bingham, S., and Setchell, K.D.R. 1994. Biological effectsof a dietof soy protein rich in isoflavones on the menstrual cycle of premenopausal women. *The American Journal of Critical Nutrition* 60:333–340.

Dideriksen, K., Reitelseder, S., and Holm, L. 2013. Influence of amino acids, dietary protein, and physical activity on muscle mass development in humans. *Nutrients* 5:852–876.

Erbersdobler, H. 1989. Factors influencing uptake and utilization of macronutrients. A *Paper in the Proceeding of Nutrient Availability: Chemical and Biochemical Aspects*. Henry Ling Ltd, Great Britain.

Garcia Hermosilla, J.A., Jha, H.C., Egge, H., Mahmud, M., Hermana, S., and Rao, G. 1993. Isolation and characterization of hydroxymethylglutaryl coenzyme A reductase inhibitors from fermented soybean extracts. *Journal of Clinical Biochemistry and Nutrition* 15:163–174.

Ginting, E. and Arcot, J. 2004. High-performance liquid chromatographic determination of naturally occurring folates during *tempe* preparation. *Journal of Agricultural and Food Chemistry* 52:7752–7758.

Glass, C.K., Saijo, K., Winner, B., Marchetto, M.C., and Gage, F.H. 2010. Mechanisms underlying inflammation in neurodegeneration. *Cell* 140:918–934.

Grimble, R.F. and Grimble, G.K. 1998. Immunonutrition: Role of sulfur aminoacids, related amino acids, and polyamines. *Nutrition* 14:605–670.

Gyorgy, P., Murata, K., and Ikehata, H. 1964. Antioxidants isolated from fermented soybeans. *Nature* 203:870–872.

Hackler, L.R., Steinkraus, K.H., Van Buren, J.P., and Hand, D.B. 1964. Studies on the utilization of *tempeh* protein by weanling rats. *The Journal of Nutrition* 82(4):452–456.

Hampson, D.J. 1994. Postweaning *Escherichia coli* diarrhea in pigs. In Gyles C.L. (Ed.), *Escherichia coli in Domestic Animals and Humans*. Guildford: CAB International, pp. 171–191.

Hardinsyah. 2010. Soy foods consumption in Indonesia. *Presented in 3rd Soy Symposium*, Surabaya, August 2–3.

Haron, H. 2013. *Tempeh*: A source of isoflavones and calcium for postmenopausal Malay women at risk of bone loss. *Presented in 8th SE Asia Soy Foods Seminar and Trade Show*, Bali, May 21–23.

Harries, J.T. 1977. *Essential of Pediatrics Gastroenterology*. United Kingdom: Churchill Livingstone.

Hering, I., Bisping, B., and Rehm, H.J. 1990. Fatty acid composition during *tempe* fermentation. *Presented in Second Asian Symposium on Non-Salted Soybean Fermentation*, Jakarta, Indonesia, February 13–15.

Hermana, 1983. *Pengaruh konsumsi bahan makanan campuran dengankedelai atautempe terhadapanak balita penderita KKP*. PhD thesis, Bogor Agricultural University, Bogor.

Hogervorst, E., Sadjimim, T., Yesufu, A., Kreager, P., and Rahardjo, T.B. 2008. High tofu intake is associated with worse memory in elderly Indonesian men and women. *Dementia and Geriatric Cognitive Disorders* 26(1):50–57.

Hsu, C.K.,Yu, Y.P., and Chung, Y.C. 2009. Effect of *tempeh* on the intestinal microbiota and colon cancer in rats. *New Biotechnology* 25:S205.

Jha, H.C., Kiriakidis, S., Hoppe, M., and Egge, H. 1997. Antioxidative Constituents of *Tempe*. In Sudarmadji, S., Suparmo, and S. Raharjo (Eds.), *Reinventing the Hidden Miracle of Tempe Proceedings International Tempe Symposium*. Jakarta: Yayasan *Tempe* Indonesia, pp. 73–84.

Karmini, M. 1987. *The effect of tempe on the control of enteropathogenic diarrhea*. Doctoral thesis, Bogor University, Bogor.

Khasanah,Y. 2013. *Pengaruh Asupan Tempe Terhadap Status Folatpada Tikus (Sprague Dawley)*. Thesis, Universitas Gadjah Mada, Yogyakarta.

Kiers, J.L., Meiler, J.C., Nout, M.J.R., Rombouts, F.M., Nabuurs, M.J.A., and Vander Meulen, J. 2003. Effect of fermented soybeans on diarrhea and feed efficiency in weaned piglets. *Journal of Applied Microbiology* 95:545–552.

Kiriakidis, S., Stathi, S., Jha, H.C., Hartmann, R., and Egge, H. 1997. Fatty acid esters of sitosterol 3β-glucoside from soybeans and *tempe* (fermented soybeans) as antiproliferative substances. *Journal of Clinical Biochemistry and Nutrition* 22:139–147.

Layrisse, M., Martinez-Torres, C., and Roche, M. 1968. Effect of interaction of various foods on iron absorption. *American Journal of Clinical Nutrition* 10: 1175–1182.

Lee, H.P., Gourley, L., Duffy, S.W., Esteve, J., Lee, J., and Day, N.E. 1991. Dietary effects on breast cancer risk in Singapore. *Lancet* 337:1197–1200.

Liem, T.H. Irene, Steinkraus, K.H., and Cronk, T.C. 1977. Production of vitamin B12 in *tempeh*, a fermented soybean food. *Applied and Environmental Microbiology* 34(6):773–776.

Liu,Y., Wang, L., Cheng, Y., Saito, M., Yamaki, K., Qiao, Z., and Li, L. 2009. Isoflavone content and anti-acetylcholinesterase activity in commercial Douchi (a traditional Chinese salt-fermented soybean food). *Japan Agricultural Research Quarterly* 43(4):301–307.

Lu, Y., Wang, W., Shan, Y., Zhiqiang, E., and Wang, L. 2009. Study on the inhibition of fermented soybean to cancer cells. *Journal of Northeast Agricultural University* 16(1):25–28.

Mahmud, M.K. 1987. Peranan Makanan Bayi Formula *Tempe* dalam Penanggulangan Masalah Diarepada Anak Balita. Thesis, Institut Pertanian Bogor, Bogor.

Mangkuwidjoyo, S., Pranowo, D., Nitisuwiryo, S., and Noor, Z. 1985. Pengamatan daya hipokolesterolemikpada *tempe. Presented in Simposium Pemanfaatan Tempe dalam Peningkatan Upaya Kesehatan dan Gizi*, Jakarta.

Messina, M.J., Perksy, V., Setchell, K.D.R., and Barnes, S. 1994. Soy intake and cancer risk: A review of the in vitro and in vivo data. *Nutrition and Cancer* 21(2):113–131.

Murata, K., Ikehata, K., and Miyamoto, T. 1967. Studies on the nutritional value of *tempeh*. *Journal of Food Science* 32(5):580–586.

Nagai, T. and Tamang, J.P. 2010. Fermented soybeans and non-soybeans legume foods. In Tamang, J.P. and Kailasapathy, K. (Eds.), *Fermented Foods and Beverages of the World*. New York: CRC Press, Taylor & Francis Group, pp. 191–224.

Nagata, Y., Imaezumi, K., and Sagano, M. 1980. Effect of soya bean protein and casein on serum cholesterol levels in rats. *British Journal of Nutrition* 44(2):113–121.

Nagata,Y., Ishikami, N., and Sugano, M. 1982. Studies on the mechanism of antihipocholesterolemic action of soy protein and soy protein-type amino acid mixtures in relation to the casein counterparts in rats. *The Journal of Nutrition* 112:1614–1625.

Nagy, B. and Fekete, P.Z. 1999. Enterotoxigenic *Escherichia coli* (ETEC) in farm animals. *Veterinary Research* 30:259–284.

Negishi,Y. and Sugahara, T. 1996. Protein content and amino acid composition of *tempe* prepared from beans of various origins with different seed molds. *Journal of International Society for Southeast Asian Agricultural Sciences* 2:30–42.

Nurrahman, Astuti, M., Suparmo, and Soesatyo, M.H.N.E. 2011. The effect of black soybean *tempe* and its ethanol extract on lymphocyte proliferation and IgA secretionin *Salmonella typhimurium* induced rat. *African Journal of Food Science* 5(14):775–779.

Nurrahman, Astuti, M., Suparmo, and Soesatyo, M.H.N.E. 2013. The role of black soybean *tempe* in increasing antioxidant enzyme activity and human lymphocyte proliferation in vivo. *International Journal of Current Microbiology and Applied Sciences* 2(9):316–327.

Okada, N. 1989. Role of microorganism in *tempeh* manufacture. Isolation of vitamin B12 producing bacteria. *Japan Agricultural Research Quarterly* 22(4):310–316.

Oyanagui, Y. 1984. Reevaluation of assay methods and establishment of Kit for superoxide dismutase activity. *Analytical Biochemistry* 142:290–296.

Park, S.J., Kim, D.H., Jung, J.M., Kim, J.M., Cai, M., Liu, X., Hong, J.G., Lee, C.H., Lee, K.R., and Ryu, J.H. 2012.The ameliorating effects of stigmasterol on scopolamine-induced memory impairments in mice. *European Journal of Pharmacology* 676:64–70.

Plachta, H., Bartnikoswa, E., and Obara, A. 1992. Lipid peroxides in blood from patients with atherosclerosis of coronary and peripheral arteries. *Clinical Chemical Acta* 211:101–112.

Rao, G.A., Crane, R.T., and Larkin, E.C. 1983. Reduction of hepatic stearoylcoAdesaturase activity in rats fed iron deficient diets. *Lipids* 18:573–575.

Rukmini, H.S., Subardjo, B., and Astuti, M. 1997. Development of superoxide dismutase during pigeon pea *tempe* fermentation. In Sudarmadji, S., Suparmo, and S. Raharjo (Eds.), *Reinventing the Hidden Miracle of Tempe Proceedings International Tempe Symposium* .Jakarta: Yayasan *Tempe* Indonesia, p. 264.

Sapbamrer, R., Visavarungroj, N., and Suttajit, M. 2013. Effects of dietary traditional fermented soybean on reproductive hormones, lipids, and glucose among postmenopausal women in northern Thailand. *Asia Pacific Journal of Clinical Nutrition* 22(2):222–228.

Setiawati, I. 2008. Formaldehyde-laced tofu still selling despite raids. Accessed from http://www.thejakartapost.com.

Shurtleff, W. and Aoyagi, A. 1979. *The Book of Tempeh.* NewYork, Hagerstown, SanFrancisco, London: Harper & Row Publisher.

Sibarani, S. 1991. *The effect of tempe on preventing diarrhea of rabbits against Escherichia coli.* Doctoral thesis, Universitas Diponegoro, Semarang.

Siregar, E. and Pawiroharsono, S. 1997. Inocula formulation and its role for biotransformation of isoflavonoid compounds. In Sudarmadji, S., Suparmo, and S. Raharjo (Eds.), *Reinventing the Hidden Miracle of Tempe Proceedings International Tempe Symposium.* Jakarta: Yayasan *Tempe* Indonesia, pp. 85–98.

Soemantri, A. and Sudigbia, I. 1985. Management of chronic diarrhea witha *tempe* based formula. Presented in National Symposium of Tempe, Jakarta, April, 15–16.

Soenarto, Y., Sudigbia, Hermana, I., Karmini, M., and Karyadi, D. 1997. Antidiarrheal characteristics of *tempe* produced traditionally and industrially in children aged 6–24 months with acute diarrhea. In S. Sudarmadji, S., Suparmo, and S. Raharjo (Eds.), *Reinventing the Hidden Miracle of Tempe Proceedings International Tempe Symposium,* eds. Jakarta: Yayasan *Tempe* Indonesia, pp. 174–186.

Steinkraus, K.H., Hwa, J.B., Van Buren, J.P., Prowidenti, M.I., and Hand, D.B. 1960. Studies on *tempeh* and Indonesian fermented soybeans food. *Journal of Food Science* 25:777–788.

Steinkraus, K.H. (Ed.) 1983. Indonesian *tempe* and related fermentations. In *Handbook of Indigenous Fermented Food* ed. Kh. H. Steinkraus, 1–94. New York, Basel: Marcel Dekker, Inc, pp. 1–94.

Suarsana, I.N. 2009. Aktivitas Hipoglikemikdan Antioksidatif Ekstrak Metanol *Tempe*pada Tikus Diabetes. Accessed from http://repository.ipb.ac.id.

Sudarmadji, S. 1977. *Certain chemical and nutritional aspects of soybean tempeh.* PhD thesis, Michigan State University.

Sudarmadji, S. and Markakis, P. 1977. The phytate and phytase of soybean *tempeh. Journal of the Science of Food and Agriculture* 28:381–383.

Sudigbia, I. 1982. Pengobatan rehidrasi intravenapadapenderita gastroenteritis. *Presented in Pertemuan ilmiah Penelitian Penyakit Diared iIndonesia,* Jakarta.

Sudigbia, I. 1990. Pengaruh Suplementasi *Tempe* Terhadap Kecepatan Tumbuh padaPenderita Diare anak umur 6–24 bulan. Thesis, Universitas Diponegoro, Semarang.

Sugano, M., Tanaka, K., and Ide, T. 1982. Secretion of cholesterol, triglyceride and apolipoproteinA-1by isolated perfused liver from rats fed soybean protein and casein or their amino acid mixture. *The Journal of Nutrition* 112:1166–1169.

Sugiyarto. 1990. Pengaruh *Tempe* Kedele terhadap Profil Lipid Penderita-Penderita Hiperkolesterolemiayang BerobatdiBagianIlmuPenyakitDalamFK UI/RSCM Jakarta. Pascacarjana, Universitas Indonesia.

Suparmo 1988. Mixed-culture fermentation for vitamin B12 synthesis in tempeh. Doctoral thesis, Michigan State University.

Thomas, C.E., Morehouse, L.E., and Aust, S.D. 1985. Ferritin and superoxide-dependent lipid peroxidation. *The Journal of Biological Chemistry* 260:3275–3280.

Utama, Z., Okazaki, Y., Tomotake, H., and Kato, N. 2013. *Tempe* consumption modulates fecal secondary bile acids, mucins, immunoglobulin a, enzyme activities, and cecal microflora and organic acids in rats. *Plant Foods for Human Nutrition* 68:177–183.

Vaidehi, M.P. 1995. Tempe technology for Indian situation, Report, University of Agricultural Sciences, Bangalore, India.

Vander Riet, W.B., Wight, A.W., Cilliers, J.J.L., and Datel, J.M. 1987. Foodchemical analysis of *tempeh* prepared from South Africa. *Food Chemistry* 25:197–208.

Van Veen, A.G. and Schaefer, G. 1950. The influence of *tempeh* fungus on the soyabean. *Documenta Neerlandica et Indonesica de Morbis Tropicis* 2:270–281.

Wagenknecht, A.C., Mattick, L.R, Lewin, L.M., Hand, D.B., and Steinkraus, K.H. 1961. Changes in soybean lipid during *tempeh* fermentation. *Journal of Food Science* 26:373–376.

Watanabe,Y., Tada, S., Kawamoto, I., Uozumi, G., Kajiwara, J., Yanaguchi, Y., Murakami, K., Misaki, F., Akasaka, Y., and Kawai, K. 1984. Epidemiologic study of colorectal cancer in Japan. Case control study of background factors in rectal and colon cancers. *Nippon Sokakilogo Gakkai Zasshi* 81:185–193.

Watanabe, N. 2011. Tempe and mineral availability. In Tzi-BunNg (Ed.), *Soybean—Biochemistry, Chemistry and Physiology*. Croatia: Tech, pp. 189–200. ISBN: 978-953-307-219–7. Available from: http://www.intechopen.com/books.

Watanabe, N., Aoki, H., and Fujimoto, K. 2008. Fermentation of soybean by *Rhizopus* promotes the calcium absorption ratio in rats. *Journal of the Science of Food and Agriculture* 88:2749–2752.

White, L.R., Petrovitch, H., Ross, G.W., Masaki, K., Hardman, J., Nelson, J., Davis, D., and Markesbery, W. 2000. Brain aging and midlife tofu consumption. *Journal of the American College of Nutrition* 19(2): 242–255.

Wulan, S.N. 2000. Pengujian Efek Antioksidatif dan Hipoglisemik Kedele, Fraksi Protein Kedele dan *Tempe* padaTikus yang Diinduksi Diabetes dengan Injeksi Alloxan. Thesis, Universitas Gadjah Mada, Yogyakarta.

Yagi, K. 1982. *Lipid Peroxides in Biology and Medicine*. NewYork, London: Academic Press.

Yagi, K. 1993. Lipid peroxide, free radicals and diseases. In *Active Oxygens, Lipid Peroxides and Antioxidants*. Tokyo: Japan Scientific Societies Press.

Chapter 12

Health Benefits of Korean Fermented Soybean Products

Dong-Hwa Shin, Su-Jin Jung, and Soo-Wan Chae

Contents

12.1 Introduction

Although fermented soybean products are not well-known on a global level, they are very popular in Asian countries, such as Korea, China, Japan, and the countries of Southeast Asian (Kwon et al. 2010). Most products are used as condiments for preparing the cuisines of these countries and for daily table foods like soups. The products are good sources for side dishes accompanying boiled rice, which is a main dish in these countries. The fermented soybean products are now becoming more popular in many countries throughout the world. The manufacturing procedure of fermented soybean products shows little difference across countries. Soybeans are usually soaked in water for a certain period of time and are boiled in a kettle. Then, they are mashed to allow easy fermentation by pure strains for inoculated or induced natural fermentation. After the fermentation, *meju* or *koji* is steeped in brine for some months to leach the ingredients in fermented soybeans digested by enzymes, which are produced by many different varieties of microbes including mold, yeast, and bacteria. The specific strains concerned in this process will be presented in each sector.

12.2 Cheonggukjang

Cheonggukjang is one of the essential side dishes of the Korean table and a representative traditional Korean food made from fermented soybeans (Lee et al. 2011). Although it is similar to Japanese *natto*, these two products are not classified in the same category due to differences in production procedures, contributed strains, and intake methods. *Cheonggukjang* can be made in the shortest period of time (2–3 days) and has a peculiar flavor. Also it is most effective way to keep the health in view of nutritional and economic view of point to Korean people. Though *cheonggukjang* is fermented in a short period of time, there are significant changes during fermentation. In particular, some sticky mucilaginous substances are created during its fermentation process and a savory flavor is generated through pulverizing proteins. It is one of the fermented soybean products with a unique flavor that has never been experienced in the West. In addition, *cheonggukjang* plays an important role in supplying proteins to Asians who eat rice.

12.2.1 History

Although the history of manufacturing *cheonggukjang* in Korea goes back to the history of using soybeans, *Samguk Sagi* (683 AD) that is, the oldest record of fermented soybean products has a record of *meju*. *Cheonggukjang* was first introduced in *Sallimgyeongje* (Hong 1715) with the name of *Jeongukjangm* in which the production process is almost the same as the present process. It is presented as *Dusi* in ancient documents and there is a record that Japanese *natto* was propagated by *Gamjinhoejang* who was a monk in the time of the Tang dynasty in 756 AD.

12.2.2 Preparation and Culinary Process

As *cheonggukjang* is produced in a short period of time, it is usually made from just harvested soybeans (late fall to winter and early spring) in every household (Shin 2011). In recent years, *cheonggukjang* can be made regardless of the seasons. In particular, because *cheonggukjang* can be produced in factories at all times instead of processing it at home, it can be consumed through the year by purchasing it in a market. In a method of producing *cheonggukjang*, soybeans are steamed for 5–6 h after steeping them in water (10–16°C, for 10–16 h). In a factory, soybeans are thermally processed using pressured steam (1.5–2 kg) for 30 min and fermented in a container after dehydration. Rice straw is used as a starter in the fermentation process. The fermentation is usually processed at 42–43°C for 2 days. Some sticky mucilaginous substances and a distinct savory flavor are created during this fermentation process. The fermentation is performed through primary (42–43°C) and secondary fermentation (52–53°C) processes. After completing the fermentation processes, some spices including salt and garlic are added to the *cheonggukjang* in order to finish it as a product. *Cheonggukjang* is usually distributed at ambient or cold storage. It is not much consumed as raw *cheonggukjang* but is cooked as a pot stew with some spices (garlic, green onion, red pepper, etc.) and usually taken as a side dish with boiled rice (Figures 12.1 and 12.2). The production process of *cheonggukjang* is presented in Figure 12.3.

12.2.2.1 Socioeconomy

Cheonggukjang is one of popular fermented soybean products and protein suppliers to Koreans etc. It is usually taken as a side dish with boiled rice. The fermentation of *cheonggukjang* is less than

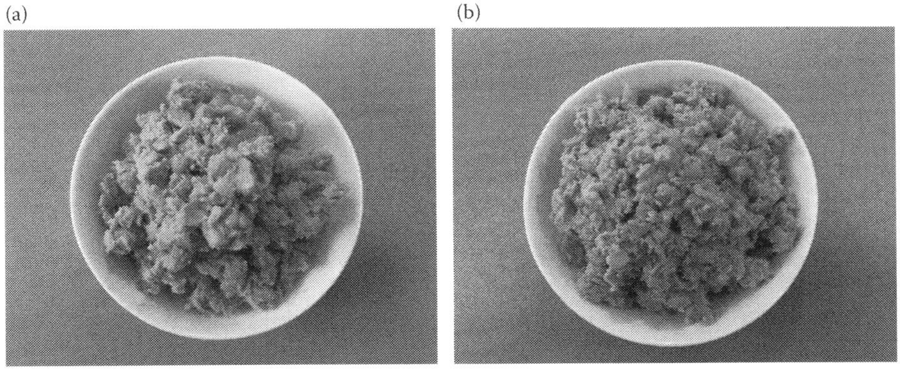

Figure 12.1 ***Cheonggukjang*** **(a) traditional and (b) commercial.**

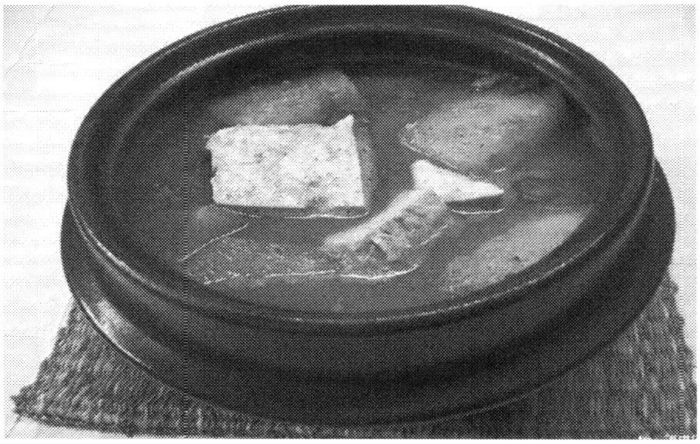

Figure 12.2 ***Cheonggukjang*** **pot stew.**

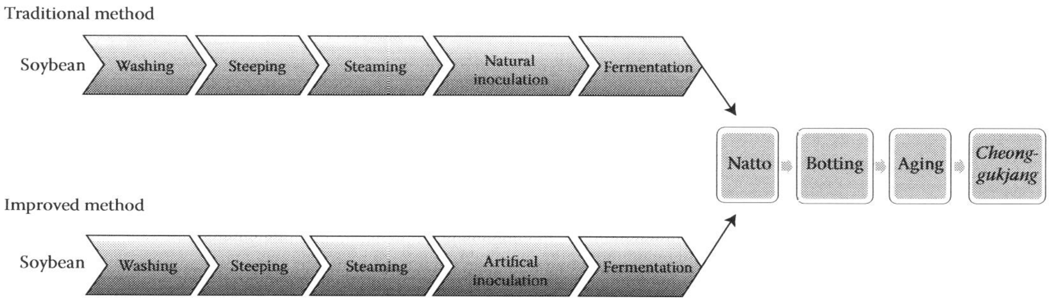

Figure 12.3 **Production process of *cheonggukjang*.**

that of other fermented soybean products and it is largely consumed by the aged as it is recognized as healthy food for this age group. As the younger generation avoid *cheonggukjang* on account of its distinct flavor, there is a trend to producing it with a softening of its taste and flavor for all kinds of people. It is expected that the consumption of *cheonggukjang* will increase as a traditional fermented soybean product, which suits boiled rice perfectly, as it improves in quality. Regarding its industrial scale in Korea, the annual production of *cheonggukjang* is about 8723 tons and the value of shipments are about 32,672 million won ($1 = 1100 won). Also, the value of exports is about $156,039 (Ministry of Food and Drug Safety 2012).

12.2.3 Microbiology and Food Safety

It is clear that *Bacillus subtilis* contributes to *cheonggukjang*, which has been made over thousands of years based on natural fermentation (Chung et al. 2006). The identification of the main microbes which are responsible for *cheonggukjang* fermentation is less than 100 years. Sawamura of Japan isolated the *Bacillus* from *natto* in 1961 (William and Aoyagi 2012). This is similar to *Bacillus mesentericus* and was named *Bacillus natto* Sawamura. It is temporarily acknowledged but commonly accepted that *B. subtilis* is the major bacillus in fermenting *cheonggukjang*. Although, the *cheonggukjang* bacillus grows well in steamed soybeans, it is decomposed through its proliferation in grains, meats, fishes and shellfish, and so on. Also, its mucilaginous substances are more fluently produced in a vegetable medium. This bacterium uses glucose, sucrose, and fructose well as a carbon source and contributes to create mucilaginous substances (Baek et al. 2010). Also, it usually uses glutamic acid, arginine, aspartic acid, and proline as nitrogen sources.

Although most of nonspore-forming vegetative cells are destroyed as soybeans are steamed, spore formers survive at a specific temperature of around 40°C. Then, these spore formers are germinated and proliferated. Thus, all of the nonspore formers in *cheonggukjang* are destroyed and the genus of *Bacillus* that is the largest inclusion in soybeans is selectively proliferated (Kwon et al. 2006). This bacillus mainly contributes to the fermentation process in *cheonggukjang*. In natural fermentation, although spore formers, which survive thermal treatments, are proliferated, selective proliferation can be carried out using a starter.

Several types of biogenic amines are created through pulverizing proteins by microorganisms (Cho et al. 2006) and the type and amount (mg/kg) of creation are determined as tyramine (133.8) > tryptamine (133.8) > puricine (26.4). In addition, spermidine (52.0) and others are also created (Lee et al. 2011). It is necessary to reduce foreign bodies by managing fermentation according to the universal needs of reducing amounts of biogenic amines in fermented protein foods.

12.2.4 Nutritional Composition and Functional Properties

General ingredients in *cheonggukjang* consist of 48%–60% of moisture, about 17% of protein, about 5% of fat, and about 5% of fiber (Park 2009). Different water-soluble nutrients are produced according to decomposition in soybean ingredients by some enzymes generated by microorganisms, which contribute to the fermentation process of *cheonggukjang* (Lim et al. 2009). Soybean proteins produce peptone, polypeptide, and several types of amino acids by protease. The total amount of amino acids is about 12% and presented by the order of glutamic > aspartic > leucine > arginine > valine. Also, carbohydrates are decomposed to saccharides by amylase. It has been known that the major substance of mucilaginous substances in *cheonggukjang* is levan, which is a polymerization of fructose and glutamic acid (Baek et al. 2010).

During the fermentation of *cheonggukjang*, vitamin B_2 is increased by 5–10 times and vitamin K is also created. In particular, it has been identified that vitamin K_2 is 5–10 times greater than in other vegetables compared with vitamin K_1 (Jung et al. 1990, Wu and Yong 2011). Also, vitamin B_1 and vitamin B_2 in soybeans create small amounts of other nutrients including vitamins in addition to water-soluble essential amino acids during the fermentation process of *cheonggukjang* (Kim et al. 1999, Kim and Hahm 2002). In addition, the mucilaginous substance, which has been known to have different functionalities, is one of distinctive characteristics in *cheonggukjang* (Table 12.1).

Table 12.1 Proximate Composition of *Cheonggukjang*

	Protein (g)	*Lipid (g)*	*Carbohydrate (g)*	*Fiber (g)*	*Ca (mg)*	*Fe (mg)*	*K (mg)*	*VitB1 (mg)*	*VitB2 (mg)*
Steamed soybean	16.0	9.0	7.6	2.1	70	2.0	570	0.22	0.09
Cheonggukjang	16.5	10.0	9.8	2.3	90	3.3	660	0.70	0.56

Source: From Kim, K.Y. and Y.T. Hahm. 2002. *The Institute of Molecular Biology and Genetics* 16: 1–18.

Cheonggukjang includes well-known healthy functional substances, such as dietary fiber, phospholipids, isoflavones, phenolic acid, polyglutamic acid (gamma-PGA), saponin, trypsin inhibitor, and some bioactive substances including phytic acid in addition to soybean nutrients (Sung et al. 2005). It has been known that these ingredients represent various functionalities such as antiobesity, glycemic control, fibrinolytic activity, blood pressure control, lipid improvement, anticancer, bowel function improvement, and immune function control (Kim et al. 2009).

12.2.4.1 Digestion Improvement and Rich Nutrients

The fiber and carbohydrate that compose soybean skins or cell membranes are decomposed to saccharides by β-amylase and soybean proteins are decomposed to amino acids by *B. subtilis.* In particular, *cheonggukjang* includes rich dietary fibers, which do not exist in meats (Lee et al. 2005). In addition, the sticky mucilaginous substance in *cheonggukjang* includes a combined substance of levan type fructan, which is polymerized by fructose and glutamic acid, and polyglutamic acid. Although there is almost no vitamin K_2 in soybeans, vitamin K can be generated through a fermentation process and vitamin B_{12}, which does not exist in soybeans, is generated by bacilli during such a fermentation process and this leads to increased mineral contents and digestive absorption rates. Although, the protein absorption rate of soybeans in the small intestine is just about 65%, it can be increased up to 95% as in the case of *cheonggukjang* (Kim et al. 1994). Isoflavones included in soybeans are presented as genistin, daidzin, and glycitin which are increased in *cheonggukjang* to about 21 times greater than in raw soybeans (Lee et al. 2007). Also, the absorption rate of the isoflavones is decreased as these are combined with saccharides. As these are fermented, however, bioactive functions are increased because of increasing such digestive absorption rates through turning them into genistaein and daidzein, which are types of aglycones, by enzymes, which remove saccharides (Table 12.2).

Table 12.2 Changes in Bioactive Substances after Fermenting Steamed Soybeans to *Cheonggukjang*

Phytochemical			*Steamed Soybean*	*Cheonggukjang*
Isoflavone	Glucoside	Daidzin	15–57	79–93
		Genistin	36–86	87–91
		Glycitin	2–6	10–12
	Aglycone	Daidzein	0.3–5	4–7
		Genistaein	0.2–5	3–4
		Glycitein	0.1–0.6	11–13
Gamma-PGA			–	↑
Ammonia			–	↑
Protein absorption (%)			65	95

Source: From Kwon, D.Y. et al. 2010. *Nutrition Research* 30: 1–13.

12.2.4.2 Blood Pressure Lowering Effect

Angiotensin II that is the strongest blood pressure increasing substance in a living body is generated by the angiotensin converting enzyme (ACE). The antihypertensive agents that have been most widely used in recent clinics are such ACE inhibitors. It has been known that the amino acids, valine and tyrosine, generated by the fermentation process exhibit the function of inhibiting ACE enzyme activations (Okamoto et al. 1995). In a spontaneously hypertensive rat (SHR) model that shows an increase in blood pressure according to an advance in age, the model that consumes *cheonggukjang* shows no increases in blood pressure. A control group (casein) that consumes steamed soybeans represents more increases in blood pressure compared to its initial level (Yang et al. 2003) (Table 12.3). This reveals that ingesting *cheonggukjang* over a long period of time inhibits an increase in blood pressure and exhibits a more blood pressure lowering effect than steamed soybeans. As mentioned above, the reason that ingesting *cheonggukjang* shows a better blood pressure lowering effect than steamed soybeans is due to the peptide, which is a hydrolyzate that inhibits ACE activations during the fermentation process of *cheonggukjang*.

The methanol extract of autoclaved soybeans, *cheonggukjang*, and acarbose are dissolved in dimethylsulfoxide (DMSO) at a concentration of 5 mg/mL, respectively.

12.2.4.3 Antiatherogenic Effect

Regarding blood cholesterol, it is important to maintain a normal plasma cholesterol level because the blood cholesterol becomes a lipid supplier. The substance produced by the *Bacillus licheniformis* CK 11–4 strain, which represents an excellent thrombolytic activity, extracted from *cheonggukjang* shows a plasminogen activation effect, which is a thrombolytic enzyme, as alkaline and thrombophilic eire protease (Kim et al. 1996). It is reported that the thrombolytic enzyme in *cheonggukjang* represents 3–4 times higher activation levels than the strains extracted from *natto*, which is a fermented soybean food in Japan (Kim 1998). *Cheonggukjang* fermentation bacillus creates protease, which is a protein decomposition enzyme, and the enzyme plays a role in dissolving thrombus in the human body. The protein decomposition enzyme included in *cheonggukjang* significantly inhibits the composition of cholesterols through reducing the activation of HMG-Co reductase. Also, it is expected that the enzyme prevents heart disease through a function of melting thrombus, which stick in the blood vessels. In addition, a group that consumes *cheonggukjang* for a long period of time shows an increase in the level of plasminogen, which melts thrombus, of about 40%, compared to a group not consuming *cheonggukjang* (Yang et al. 2003). This is due to the fact that the fibrinolytic system, which supports smooth blood circulation, plays an important role in melting thrombus and inhibiting excessive thrombus. In addition, regarding the protein decompositions, dietary fibers, and indigestible saccharides generated during the fermentation of

Table 12.3 Inhibitory Activities of the Methanol Extract of Autoclaved Soybeans and *Cheonggukjang* against α-Glucosidase (%)

	Autoclaved Soybean	*Cheonggukjang*	*Acarbose*
Activity	43.6	62.7	22.8

Source: From Yang, J., S. Lee, and Y. Song. 2003. *Journal Korean Society Food Science Nutrition* 32: 899–905.

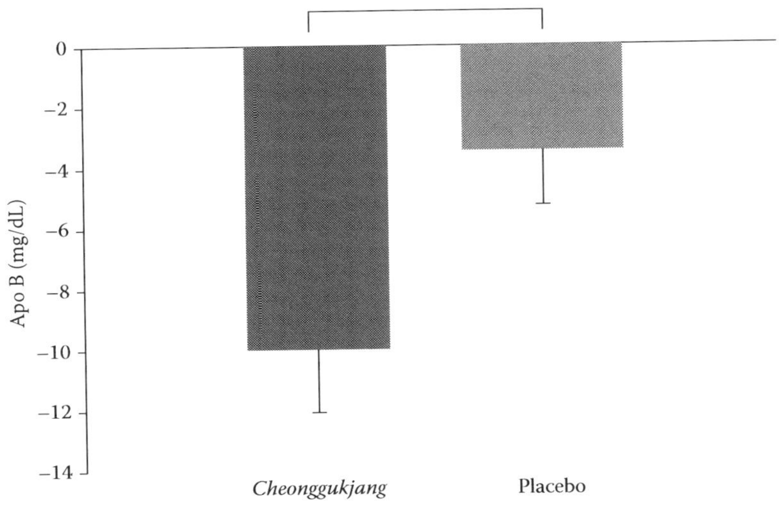

Figure 12.4 Changes in Apo B during the intervention period $p < 0.05$.

cheonggukjang that inhibit absorptions of intestinal neutral lipids and cholesterols, it is possible to prevent arteriosclerosis by increasing an excretion of lipids to the feces (Lae 2005). In a mature rat that is induced to hyperlipidemia through a high fat diet, there is an antiatherogenic effect by feeding *cheonggukjang* powder for 5 weeks where serum TG, TC, LDL-C, VLDL-C concentrations, and atherogenic indexes are decreased (Koh 2006). In recent years, ingesting *cheonggukjang* for a long period of time in overweight and obese adults represents significant decreases in Apolipoprotein B, which is an atherogenic index, compared to other control groups (Back et al. 2011) (Figure 12.4). Also, there is a report that the concentration rate of Apolipoprotein B and Apolipoprotein A1 for adults who show impaired fasting glucose and take *cheonggukjang* for 8 weeks is significantly decreased (Shin et al. 2011). In a clinical manner, the Apolipoprotein B has been considered as an important estimation factor in diagnosing risk factors of arteriosclerosis and cardiovascular diseases. Also, the Apolipoprotein B is related to potential causes in all arteriosclerosis and cardiovascular diseases and shows a better diagnostic capability than LDL-C. The lower level of the Apolipoprotein B, the lower the possibility of causing arteriosclerosis is ensured (Back et al. 2011).

12.2.4.4 Antioxidant Effect

Antioxidative substances in *cheonggukjang* are isoflavones, phenolic, chlirogenic, isochlorogenic, amino acids, tocopherol, peptides, saponins, and so on (Lee et al. 2001). As soybeans are fermented to *cheonggukjang*, the antioxidative level in isoflavones is increased by about twice that of raw soybeans (Lee et al. 2007) and the genistein in isoflavones represents an antioxidative effect through inhibiting the generation of superoxide anions and removing hydrogen peroxide, which is a growth factor of tumors (Ryu et al. 2007). Such an antioxidative characteristic of *cheonggukjang* exhibits a resistivity for oxidative stresses in a living body and that leads to the delay in or prevention of various diseases or aging due to such oxidation in a living body. In addition, ingesting *cheonggukjang* represents an antioxidative effect through inhibiting peroxidation effectively in

LDL-C and erythrocytes in a living body. Also, as the antioxidative capability in *cheonggukjang* extracts is proportionate to the contents of polyphenols and isoflavones (Devi et al. 2009), and it is more effective to take a type of *cheonggukjang* than to consume soybeans.

12.2.4.5 Blood Glucose Control

Because *cheonggukjang* has rich cellulous it helps to smooth absorptions of saccharides and is effective in the control of blood glucose levels due to its low blood glucose indexes. It is reported that the concentrations of blood glucose and plasma insulin in a rat with type-2 diabetes were significantly decreased by consuming *cheonggukjang,* compared to the control group that takes steamed soybeans and casein (Kim et al. 1996) (Figure 12.5). The reason is that the trypsin, which is an inhibitor, in *cheonggukjang,* affects the pancreas and causes an acceleration in the secretion of insulin.

The concentrations of serum TC, LDL-C, and FBG in adults who represent actual FBG are significantly decreased by ingesting *cheonggukjang* for 8 weeks compared with other control groups (Shin et al. 2011). It reveals that the intake of *cheonggukjang* inhibits the activation of a-glucosidase in the small intestine and helps to prevent and improve diabetes by improving the insulin resistivity based on delaying the movement rate of soluble dietary fibers in the digestive tract (Kim et al. 2003). In addition, there is a report that dietary fibers create short chain fatty acids and that this decreases blood glucose levels by secreting GLP-1 (glucose peptide-1) (Tolhurst et al. 2012).

12.2.4.6 Body Weight Control

For preventing and treating obesity, proper exercise and dietary habits without overeating are necessary. The ingesting of fiber rich foods, such as brown rice, whole grain, beans, and *cheonggukjang,* helps to prevent and treat obesity. By ingesting such fiber rich foods, overeating will be

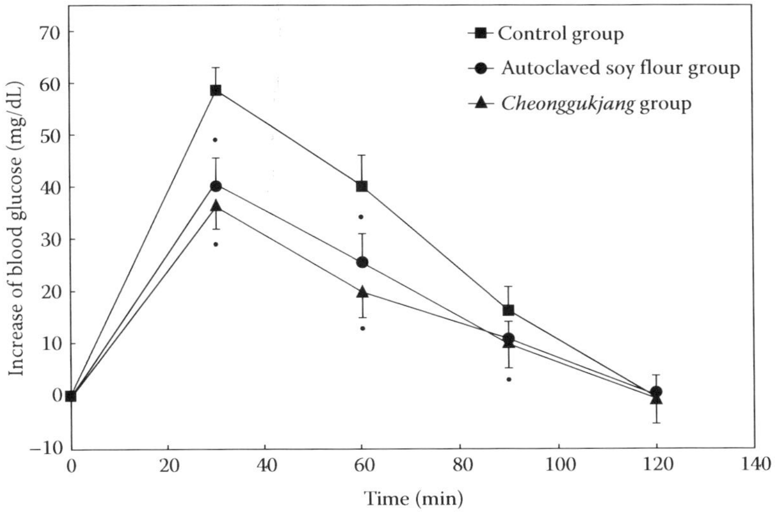

Figure 12.5 Antidiabetic effects in soybeans and *cheonggukjang*. (From Kim W. et al. 1996. *Applied and Environmental Microbiology* 62: 2482–2488.)

avoided, due to the water absorption characteristics of fiber itself and this will also help to prevent colon cancer (Burkitt 1971). In addition, *cheonggukjang* decreases cholesterol levels. In a rat that is induced to hyperlipidemia, ingesting *cheonggukjang* for 5 weeks represents decreases in body weight and body fat percentage (Kim 1998, Lee et al. 2001, Koh 2006). It reveals that the dietary fiber and indigestible saccharide in *cheonggukjang* represent an obese inhibitory effect by inhibiting absorptions of lipids in intestines and increasing excretions. Some adults who show BMI more than 23 kg/m^2 exhibit significant decreases in visceral fat areas as raw *cheonggukjang* of about 70 g (dried weight of 26 g) is taken for 12 weeks (Back 2009).

12.2.4.7 Anticancer Effect

Recently, Western-style colon cancers have been increasing in Asian countries. It is estimated that excessive intakes of meat and the lacks of ingesting fibers cause such cancers. Also, instant foods, refined sugar and flour, food additives, and preservatives play an important factor of causing sudden increases in cancers. That is, foods play an important role in causing and preventing cancers. It is considered that the low incidence rate of breast cancer and prostate cancer in Korea is related to the habit of ingesting a large volume of soybeans and fermented soybean foods. In addition, there are several reports on the excellent anticancer effects of genistein, which is the major ingredient of fermented soybean foods, on breast cancer and prostate cancer (Wei et al. 1993, Tiisala et al. 1994).

Cancers are classified into two different stages; a stage of genetic damage and a stage of accelerating cell division rates. In animal tests, it shows that ingesting the genistein in *cheonggukjang* inhibits the processing of malignant tumor cells and prevents an acceleration of cancer-causing cell divisions (Kwak et al. 2002). Moreover, it has been known that ingesting *cheonggukjang* shows an effect on preventing colon cancer, rectal cancer, stomach cancer, lung cancer, prostate cancer, and breast cancer. The saponic substances in *cheonggukjang* decrease cancer-causing substances and cancer-accelerating factors during cancer-causing processes and represent different influences of raw soybean types and fermentation strains on antimutation. In the case of the *cheonggukjang* extracts produced by adding rice straw, they shows excellent antimutation activation effect for aflatoxin B_1 (Lee and Kim 2012).

12.2.4.8 Bowel Function Improvement

Modern man suffers from constipation. Constipation is a signal from the human body that alerts one to an unhealthy bowel. The causes of constipation are the lack of exercise, the abuse of laxatives, and the decrease in feces due to the lack of fiber rich food. Fibers contain moisture 40 times more than its own weight. *Cheonggukjang* contains rich fibers, such as insoluble fiber (cellulose), hemicelluloses, and soluble fiber (pectin), and that increases the viscosity of intestinal contents and decreases a gastric emptying rate (Lee and Hwang 1997, Kim et al. 2006). In addition, it stimulates the large intestine wall and that leads to a reduction in the transit time of feces through the large intestine and to an increase in beneficial intestinal microorganisms (Kim 2009). Also, it improves bowel function (Table 12.4) (Lae 2005). Moreover, the bacillus in *cheonggukjang* shows an excellent bowel cleansing effect and some soybean oligo-saccharides in *cheonggukjang*, such as stachyose, raffinose, and so on, facilitate the composition of vitamins in the bowel together with dietary fibers. The oligo-saccharides do not use harmful bacilli but use bifidobateria (Inoguchi et al. 2012).

Table 12.4 Changes in Transit Times through the Large Intestine before and after Taking *Cheonggukjang*

Large Intestine	*Before (n = 10)*	*After (n = 10)*	*p-value*
Rt. colon	15.0 ± 14.3[a]	10.2 ± 11.9	0.313
Lt. colon	8.4 ± 9.4	6.9 ± 8.2	0.549
RS. colon	19.2 ± 13.4	9.1 ± 7.8	0.008[b]
Total colon	42.2 ± 20.1	26.2 ± 20.3	0.000[c]

Source: From Lae, P. 2005. The effect of fermented soybean powder on improvement of constipating patients receiving maintenance hemo dialysis. MS thesis, Kyung Buk National University Daegu, Korea.

[a] Mean ± SD.
[b] $p < 0.01$.
[c] $p < 0.001$.

About 100 billion bacilli are included in 100 g *cheonggukjang*. In particular, a beneficial bacillus, bifidobacteria that facilitates digestion and absorption through accelerating the peristaltic movement in the intestinal canal inhibits proliferations of intestinal harmful bacilli and external intrusion bacilli. Also, it inhibits and reduces ammonia, amine, and indole generated by putrefactive bacteria and acts as a growth facilitating factor (Park et al. 1998).

12.2.4.9 Immune Control Improvement

It has been known that nucleic acid foods have an effect on enhancing the immune function. *Cheonggukjang* contains the polymer nucleic acid, γ-polyglutamic acid (γ-PGA), generated by the fermentation bacilli in *cheonggukjang* (Lee et al. 2010). Also, it has been reported that γ-PGA improves immunities through activating a secretion of IFN-γ in the Th_1 lymphocyte (Hahm et al. 2004, Jang et al. 2008). In addition, in people who have skin allergies ingesting *cheonggukjang* for a long period of time (raw *cheonggukjang* of 27 g/d) represents positive effects on improving immune control and skin nervousness. In particular, the size of wheals induced by antigens is largely decreased. Also, interferon-γ, which is an immune index, and interlukin-4, which is a type of cytokines, are significantly increased in a group ingesting *cheonggukjang*. It reveals that taking *cheonggukjang* for a long period of time increases immunities (Chang et al. 2005, Jang et al. 2008, Kwon et al. 2011b) (Table 12.5).

12.3 Doenjang

12.3.1 Mold and Bacillus-Mixed Fermented Soybean Foods

In natural fermented foods using soybeans, the fermentation is not performed by a single microorganism but by a complex fermentation process with molds and bacilli, even yeasts (Kim et al. 2010b). Regarding the various fermented foods of the world, most of their fermentations are carried out by such complex fermentation processes, except for the complete management of fermentation bacilli. The characteristics of complex fermentation represent deep and peculiar flavors due

Table 12.5 Changes in Interferon-γ and Interlukin-4 during the Intervention Period

	Cheonggukjang (n = 29)			*Placebo (n = 28)*			
Items (unit)	*(0 wk)*	*(12 wk)*	*p-value*[a]	*(0 wk)*	*(12 wk)*	*p-value*[a]	*p-value*[b]
Interferon-γ (IU/mL)	14.56 ± 3.1	17.57 ± 1.9	<0.001***	15.63 ± 5.5	18.1 ± 2.2	0.020*	0.620
Interlukin-4 (pg/mL)	0.17 ± 3.1	0.26 ± 0.2	0.016*	0.55 ± 1.6	0.45 ± 0.8	0.506	0.323

Source: From Kwon, D.Y. et al. 2011b. *BMC Complementary Alternative of Medicine* 11 2011 Dec 5;11:125. doi: 10.1186/1472-6882-11-125.

Note: Values are presented as mean ± SD.

[a] A linear mixed model for repeatedly measured data.
[b] Paired t-test (*$p < 0.05$, ***$p < 0.001$).

to the generating of various substances compared to that of single fermentation. However, it makes it difficult to maintain uniform quality due to the difficulties in managing uniform fermentation.

Doenjang is one of traditional fermented soybean foods in Korea. It is one of the Korean spices and is represented as a type of yellowish brown paste. *Doenjang* has a peculiar flavor due to the fermentation of soybeans. In the traditional method of making *doenjang, meju* is first made from steamed soybeans and separated into *ganjang* and *meju* paste after steeping in salt water (Kim et al. 2011a). Then, the solid paste is matured to obtain *doenjang*. In an industrial manner, *koji* is made from flour in which molds are inoculated to steamed soybeans and the *koji* is mixed with steamed soybeans and salt water. Then, the mixture is fermented as a spice, *doenjang* (improved method) (Figures 12.6 and 12.7).

Although, *doenjang* has been traditionally made using *meju*, other improved methods have also been introduced in industries. As the functionality and nutritional value of *doenjang* has been known based on the fact that the amino acids and other related substances are generated from soybean proteins by microorganisms, it has become one of the seasoning foods that shows increased consumption throughout the world.

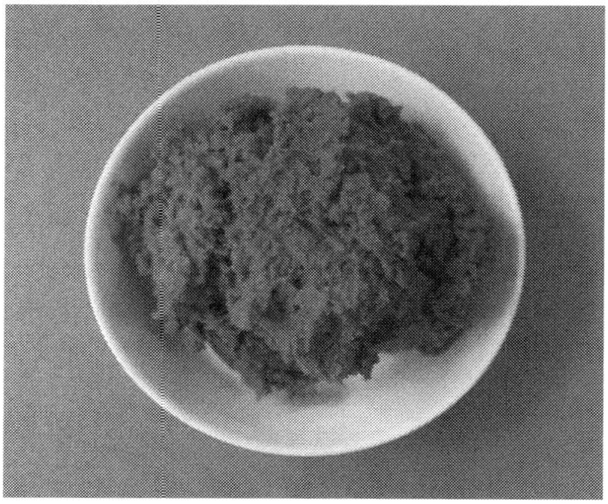

Figure 12.6 ***Doenjang*** **(traditional).**

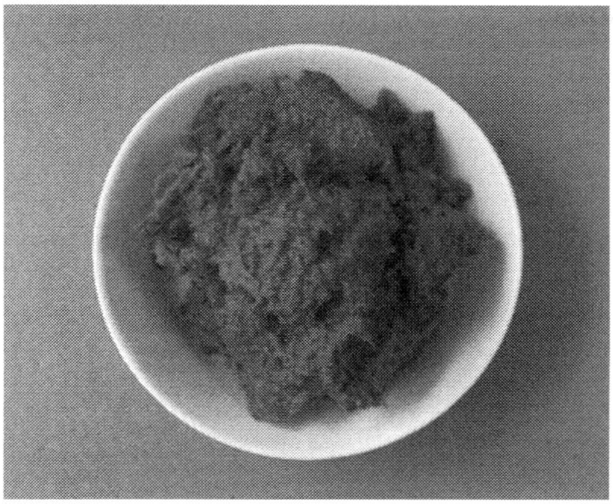

Figure 12.7 ***Doenjang*** **(commercial).**

12.3.2 History

Fermented soybean products in Korean dietary life were introduced before the birth of Christ. Although the dietary history of *doenjang* estimated in Korean dietary life goes back to before the period of the Three Kingdoms, the recorded document shows that the "Si," which is the raw material of soybean fermented products, was presented in the 3rd year of King *Sinmun* (683 AD) (Cho 1980). Also, it is considered that such a record is also mentioned in *Chea Mihn Yho Suli* where *meju* and soybean fermented products are generalized in this period. The raw material of *doenjang* is *meju* and these are closely related. *Doenjang* is also introduced with the making of *meju*.

12.3.3 Preparation and Culinary

Doenjang is classified into rice *doenjang* and barley *doenjang* based on starches used in its making and is also divided into *makdoenjang, tojang, makjang*, and *jeupjang* according to its processing methods. In addition, there are two different methods in producing *doenjang*; the traditional way in which *doenjang* is made from *meju* and an improved method that mixes flour *koji* with steamed soybeans and ferments the mixture. In Korea, both the traditional and improved methods are used to produce *doenjang*. The production process of *meju*, which is the major raw material, is presented in Figure 12.8.

The *meju* produced by this process is dried in the sun and fermented in salt water. The process of making *doenjang* using this *meju* is presented in Figure 12.9 (Shin 2011).

After steeping *meju* in salt water for 3–4 months, the sap of the *meju* is to be separated for use as *ganjang* and the other solid parts of the *meju* are used to make *doenjang* with some additives

Soybean → Steeping (12 hours) → Steaming (6 hours) → Cooling (about 40°C) → Pulverizing → Shaping (Block type)

→ Rice straw → Drying (about 1 week) → Hanging and fermentation (1 month) → Post fermentation (1 month) → *Meju*

Figure 12.8 ***Meju*** **production process.**

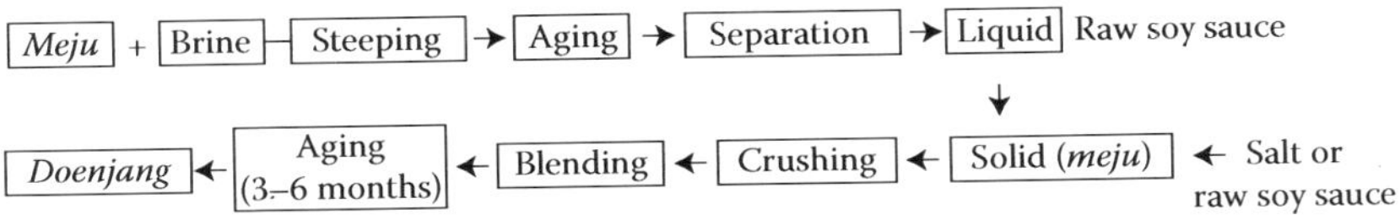

Figure 12.9 Traditional *doenjang* production process.

(*meju* powder, steamed rice, barley, etc.). Then, the *doenjang* mixture is to be matured for 3–6 months in order to obtain complete *doenjang*. The taste of *doenjang* is varied according to the qualities of *meju* and the separation methods applied to the process of obtaining the sap from the *meju* steeped in salt water.

Doenjang has been served as soup almost every day in Korea with some spices (garlic, red pepper, etc.) and bean curd, and tofu. The *doenjang* soup is a side dish for rice. It is similar to Japanese *doenjang* soup, *misosiru*, using japanese *doenjang*. In addition, *doenjang* is used to make *ssamjang* with other additives and as a supplement in order to remove the odor of fish. Also, *doenjang* has been used as other different foodstuffs including dressings for salad.

12.3.4 Socioeconomy

An average of 8.8 g *doenjang* is consumed by a person in Korea and fermented soybean products form a large market in Korea. A larger *doenjang* market is presented by Japan and the market has been increasing throughout the world as the healthy food image of *Doenjang* grows. The *doenjang* market in Korea shows the annual gross production of about 101,395 tons and the values of shipments reach to about 142,302 million won ($1 = 1100 won; Ministry of Food and Drug Safety 2012). Also, the value of exports is about 4.9 million dollars. As fermented soybean products do not require large-scale production facilities they can be operated as a family business. Thus, farm families that produce the raw materials, soybeans, are competing with large-scale enterprises through their own particular products. Because there are differences in tastes between traditional and factory made products, such small-scale traditional family products are also consumed in markets.

12.3.5 Microbiology and Food Safety

Korea's traditional *doenjang* induces natural fermentation instead of managing fermentation bacilli, and various microorganisms contribute to the process of fermentation according to given environments. In the traditional method, microorganisms well implanted to pulverized *meju* are first proliferated and other microorganisms are induced according to conditions. The genus of microorganisms that contribute to the fermentation of *meju* is classified into different categories; *Mucor* and *Aspergillus* for molds, *Bacillus* for a bacillus, *Lactobacillus* and *Streptococcus* for lactic acids, and *Saccharomyces, Zygosaccharomyces, Pichia, Hansenula,* and *Devaryomyces* for yeasts (Park 2009). The major strains in this genus are summarized in Table 12.6.

In *doenjang*, biogenic amines that contribute to its safety are created (Cho et al. 2006) and its amounts (mg/kg) are determined by the order of tyramine (669.5) > histidine (569.4) > putreseine (462.6) > 2-phenyl ethyl amine (244.7) in which the *doenjang* processed by traditional methods represents higher levels than the improved *doenjang* that manages its strains. The biogenic amines are generated as a raw matter, which contains proteins, used as a fermentation matrix and representing a possibility of reducing its generation through managing strains or

Table 12.6 Microorganisms Isolated from Traditional *Meju*

Fungi	• *Aspergillus flavus, Asp. fumigatus, Asp. niger, Asp. oryzae, Asp. retricus, Asp. spinosa, Asp. terreus, Asp. wentii Botrytis cineara* • *Mucor adundans, Mucor circinelloides, Mucor griseocyanus, Mucor hiemalis, Mucor jasseni, Mucor racemosus Penicillium citrinum, Pen. griseopurpureum, Pen. griesotula, Pen. Kaupscinskii, Pen. lanosum, Pen. Thomii, pen. Turalense* • *Rhizopus chinencis, Phi. nigricans, Rhi. oryzae, Rhi. sotronifer*
Yeast	• *Candida edax, Candida incommenis, Candida utilis Hansenula anomala, Hansenula capsulata, Hansenula holstii Rhodotorula flava, Rhodotorula glutinis* • *Saccharomyces* sp., *Saccharomyces exiguus, Saccharomyces cerevisiae, Saccharomyces kluyveri* • *Zygosaccharomyces japonicus, Zygosaccharomyces rouxii*
Bacteria	• *Bacillus citreus, Bac. circulans, Bac. licheniformis, Bac. megaterium, Bac. mesentricus, Bac. subtilis, Bac. pumilis Lactobacillus* sp. • *Pedicocus* sp., *pedicoccus acidilactici*

Source: From Choi, S.H. et al. 1995. *Journal of Agricultural Science*. Chungnam National University, Korea 22: 188–197.

improving fermentation conditions. In addition, the generation of aflatoxin by *Aspergillus flavus* is determined as a meager level or destroyed in the fermentation and maturation process (Kim et al. 2011b, Lee 2012).

12.3.6 Nutritional Composition and Functional Properties

Soybeans contain about 20% of milk fats and about 40% of proteins. Also, they include specific ingredients. For instance, they include isoflavones as a phytoestrogen and 12 different isomers including daidzein, genistein, and glycitein are largely indicated (Banaszkilwicz 2011). In particular, it has also been known that these elements contribute to various bioactive functions.

12.3.6.1 Anticancer Operation

It has been known that anticancer effects in traditional *doenjang* are due to nutritional factors, such as trypsin inhibitor, isoflavone, vitamin E, and unsaturated fatty acids like linoleic acid and bioactive substances (Kwon et al. 2011a). In recent years, it is indicated that *doenjang* extracts increase the glutathione S-transferase activity, which contributes to the detoxification of the liver, and have an effect on increasing the natural killer cell activity that removes cancer cells (Choi et al. 1998). Also, the biological activity in *doenjang* is stable to heat and able to sustain effects of preventing and resisting cancers as it is taken as *doenjang* soup or *doenjang* pot stew. In addition, as the fermentation period of *doenjang* is getting longer, the chances of transforming isoflavones to genistein and dadzein, which are aglycones, are increased. Thus, *doenjang* which is fermented over a long period of time represents more anticancer effects where the weights of tumors and the inhibition rates of tumor activities are decreased (Son 1995, Jung et al. 2006) (Table 12.7). In particular, fermented *doenjang* has an antibacterial effect for *Bacillus cereus*, colon bacilli, *Listeria monocytogenes*, *Streptococcus faecalis*, *Escherichia coli* O157:H7, and so on (Cha et al.

Table 12.7 Antitumor Activity in *Doenjang*

Sample	*Tumor Weight (g)*	*Inhibition Rate (%)*
Sarcoma 180 cancer cell(A) + PBS	5.8 + 0.3[a]	–
(A) + Fermented *doenjang* (3 months)	5.4 ± 0.2[a]	7
(A) + Fermented *doenjang* (6 months)	4.7 ± 0.3[b]	19
(A) + Fermented *doenjang* (24 months)	3.6 ± 0.2[c]	38

Source: From Jung, K.O., S.Y. Park, and K.Y. Park. 2006. *Nutrition* 22: 539–545.

[a–c] Significant differences based on the Duncan's multiple range test ($p < 0.05$).

1999). However, it is indicated that unfermented *doenjang* has no such antibacterial effect. It has also been recognized that the antibacterial effect is due to antibacterial substances, which are generated during the fermentation process of *doenjang*, such as peptide, 4-hydroxy benoic acid, and benzoic acid. It is indicated that *doenjang* methanol extracts have effects on inhibiting cancer cell growth in the human body and antimutation for degrading DNA syntheses (Jung et al. 2006). The *doenjang* a fermented products show some anticancer effect and inhibition of DNA synthesis compared to raw soybean. The reason is that *deonjang* has more bioactive components produced during fermentation process which are not in raw soybeans, and can be generated and increased during its fermentation period of more than 3 months (Jung et al. 2006).

12.3.6.1.1 Antioxidation and Aging Inhibition

Human beings produce energy required for vital activities by oxidizing organic matter through oxygenic respiration in which process some oxygen free radicals are generated even though it is in relatively small quantities (Velichkovskii 2001). The oxygen free radicals cause several disorders for destroying DNA, proteins, or fat molecules in cell membranes and are generated by some environmental pollutants and cancer-causing substances. Thus, it is important to take antioxidant substances or antioxidant agents in order to remove such oxygen-free radicals in the body. The browning substances and phenol compounds generated during the fermentation and maturing processes represent a strong antioxidant function for unsaturated fatty acids like linoleic acid. Such a function increases the contents of free amino acids, such as glutamic acid, lysine, tryptophan, histidine, and tyrosine, according to increases in fermentation periods (Lee et al. 2014). Also, increases in amino acids will increase antioxidant effects.

12.3.6.1.2 Lowering Blood Pressure

Hypertension is a state that represents a higher blood pressure level than normal values. Although it is varied according to body weights and ages, the normal blood pressure is determined by more than 140 and 90 mmHg for systolic and diastolic blood pressures, respectively. Because hypertension shows no symptoms, it is known as the silent killer. It may cause hypertensive heart failure, arteriosclerosis, and renal failure. A factor causing hypertension in the human body is an angiotensin converting enzyme (ACE). The most largely used antihypertension agent in clinics is an inhibitor of this enzyme. The substance that shows an inhibitory function of ACE activation in *doenjang* is a dipeptide, arginine-proline (Kim et al. 1999). That is, *doenjang* increases peptide contents because of decomposing soybean proteins during its fermentation process and ingesting *doenjang* decreases blood pressure through inhibiting the activation of ACE (Yang 2000). The inhibitory function of ACE is varied according to fermentation periods. Unfermented *doenjang* shows a low ACE inhibitory activation level but increases in fermented periods exhibit high blood pressure control effects (Shin et al. 2011) (Figures 12.10 and 12.11). These characteristics represent decreases in blood pressure in which the peptide that is a fermented product of proteins, which are increased during the fermentation process of *doenjang*, inhibits the activation of ACE (Yang 2000).

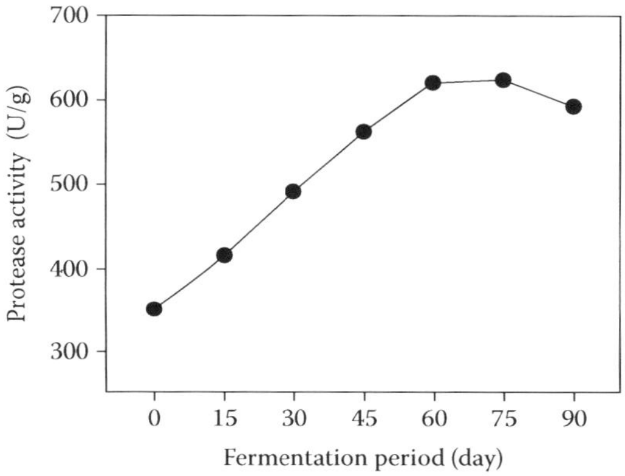

Figure 12.10 Fermentation period and protease activation. (From Shin, D.H. et al. 2012. *Public Health Education* 10–133.)

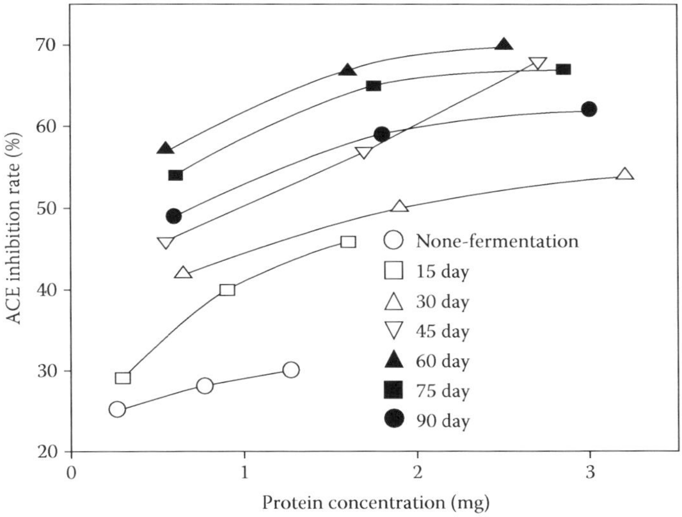

Figure 12.11 ACE inhibition rate according to fermentation periods of *doenjang*. (From Yang, B. 2000. *Korean Journal Microbiology and Biotechnology* 28: 228–232.)

12.3.6.1.3 Antiatherogenic Effect

Increases in serum cholesterol levels and LDL-C play a major risk role in causing arteriosclerosis and myocardial infarction. Cholesterol synthesis rates in its initial stage are controlled by the activation of HMG-CoA reductase. It is reported that such a controlling function is due to the substance generated during the process in which the ingredient of *doenjang* that decreases serum cholesterol levels is changed to isoflavones and nonglycosides (aglycone, genistein, daidzein, and glycitein) through the fermentation process of *doenjang* (Shin et al. 2011). This substance decreases the activation of HMG-Co A reductase (Forsythe 1995). In particular, *doenjang* shows that the substance generated by the transformation from a glucoside type, which is one of isoflavones, to an aglycone type during its fermentation process decreases serum cholesterol levels and LDL-C oxidations and that leads to lowering dangerous levels of cardiovascular diseases. In recent clinical studies, ingesting *doenjang* for some overweight adults for 12 weeks exhibits improvement in lipid metabolism but there are no significant differences in results (Cha et al. 2012). It is considered that ingesting *doenjang* shows a positive effect on lipid metabolism by lowering the synthesis of VLDL-C and LCL-C rather than the synthesis of HDL-C. In addition, in various animal tests there is an effect on improving hyperlipidemia based on decreases in serum neutral fats and total cholesterol levels (Lee and Lee 2002). The reason that there are no significant improving effects in clinical studies differed from animal tests is because of serving ordinary diet instead of controlled dietary conditions and maintains a regular diet. Also, significant improvements in serum lipids are not expected because the subjects participated in studies represent normal serum lipid and lipid protein concentration levels. The isoflavones in *doenjang* increase the activation of an LDL-C receptor, which becomes a cause factor in vascular diseases, and increase an HDL-C level, which is beneficial to prevent vascular diseases and that plays an important role in preventing cardiovascular diseases (Choi et al. 2010, Kwak et al. 2012).

12.3.6.1.4 Antithrombolytic Effect

Although blood coagulation and hemolysis operations in the human body are maintained at an equal level, several factors cause an increase in hemolysis and that leads to present thrombus. The thrombus increases blood pressure by cutting supplies of nutrients and oxygen to biological tissues, due to the cutting of blood circulation by accumulating it in the fine blood vessels particularly including the cerebral vessels, and this will cause cardiovascular diseases such as stroke. The blood coagulation inhibitory activation of *doenjang* is due to the contents of fibrinolytic enzymes and thrombin inhibitors in *doenjang* (Jang et al. 2004). The fibrinolytic capability of the *B. subtilis* strain that secrete a strong antifibrinolytic enzyme separated from *doenjang* is 3–4 times higher than *cheonggukjang* and Japanese *natto* and the enzyme separated from the *Bacillus amyloliquefaciens* represents stabilities in pH and heat. That is, the peptide that inhibits the activation of thrombin, which is a blood coagulation enzyme, in *doenjang* inhibits such thrombin that contributes to make thrombus and plays a role in fibrin coagulation inhibitors. The *doenjang* that is fermented for 6 months to 2 years shows a high effect on inhibiting blood coagulation because of increasing peptide levels (Jang et al. 2004).

12.3.6.1.5 Antiobesity

Based on reports that the genistein included in soybeans and fermented soybean products facilitates the α-oxidation of fatty acid, it has been highlighted as a beneficial substance in reducing

Table 12.8 Antiobesity Effects in Rats for Ingesting Different Soybean Fermented Products Including *Doenjang* (Ingesting for 30 Days)

(g)	*Normal Rat*	*High-Fat Diet*	*High-Fat Diet + Doenjang*	*High-Fat Diet + Cheonggukjang*	*High-Fat Diet + Gochujang*	*High-Fat Diet + Ssamjang*
Initial weight	143.7 ± 3.9	143.7 ± 3.9	143.8 ± 4.1	143.7 ± 3.9	143.9 ± 4.5	143.7 ± 5.0
Final weight	259.0 ± 16.1^{bc}	295.1 ± 11.6^{a}	251.3 ± 22.3^{c}	277.1 ± 13.8^{ab}	270.5 ± 5.4^{bc}	261.1 ± 17.0^{bc}
Weight increment	3.9 ± 0.6^{b}	4.8 ± 0.4^{a}	3.8 ± 0.3^{b}	4.2 ± 0.5^{b}	4.2 ± 0.1^{b}	4.0 ± 0.2^{b}
Fat around the kidney	0.88 ± 0.27^{b}	1.45 ± 0.41^{a}	0.91 ± 0.4^{b}	1.28 ± 0.24^{ab}	1.02 ± 0.39^{ab}	0.90 ± 0.23^{b}

Source: From Kwon, D.Y. et al. 2006. *Biofactors* 26: 245–258.

body weight and burning body fat (Kwak et al. 2012). Also, it has been largely indicated that *doenjang* is more effective to antiobesity than unfermented soybeans through various animal and clinical tests. Ingesting *doenjang* is more effective to reduce body weight than ingesting substitution foods (casein) or other soybean processed foods (*gochujnag* or *cheonggukjang*) (Kwon et al. 2006) (Table 12.8). It is due to the fact that the isoflavones, which are nonglycosides generated during the fermentation process of *doenjang* according to increases in the period of such fermentation, are increased, and this affects the result positively. As ingesting *doenjang* in a high fat dietary animal model exhibits more decreases in accumulating visceral fats and fatty cells than that of ingesting unfermented soybeans (Kwak et al. 2012), it shows the same results in clinical studies (Cha et al. 2012, Jung et al. 2014).

In a test of ingesting *doenjang* for overweight and fat adults who represent BMI more than 23 kg/m^2 where *doenjang* pills are applied by 9.9 g/day (about 40 g of raw *doenjang*) for 12 weeks while their daily diet levels and activities are maintained, the body weight and body fat rate are significantly decreased compared to that of the control group (Table 12.9). It is the same amount as three bowls of *doenjang* soup, which is similar to Japanese *miso* soup and is usually consumed daily by Koreans . That is, the content of isoflavones in a bowl of *doenjang* soup (about 13.3 g of raw *doenjang*) is about 20–30 mg/day (containing 8.57 mg aglycones) (Cha et al. 2012). Thus, it reveals that there is a high possibility of preventing arteriosclerosis based on the fact that ingesting *doenjang* for a long period of time decreases visceral fat.

12.3.6.1.6 Immune Improvement

Cytokine is a water-soluble protein generated in the cells of immune and nonimmune systems and plays an important role in controlling immune responses through increasing or inhibiting the growth, differentiation, proliferation, and activation of the cells of an immune system. An immune control substance (Fraction of the Korean Fermented Soybean Paste; KFSP) is not found in steamed soybeans but found in *doenjang* (Kim et al. 2014). This substance in traditional *doenjang* shows four to ten times higher immune activation levels than in other regular *doenjang* and Japanese *doenjang, miso,* respectively (Park 2009). KFSP in traditional *doenjang*

Table 12.9 Changes in Body Weight, Composition, and Abdominal Fat Area Measurements at the 0-week and 12-week in This Study

	Doenjang Group (n = 26)			*Placebo Group (n = 25)*				
Parameters	*0-wk*	*12-wk*	*Change*	*0-wk*	*12-wk*	*Change*	*Absolute Group Difference*[a]	*P-value*[b]
Body weight (kg)	70.2 ± 1.8[c]	69.4 ± 1.8	−0.8**	67.8 ± 1.7	67.6 ± 1.8	−0.3	0.55 ± 0.4	<0.001
Body fat mass (kg)	22.1 ± 1.0	21.4 ± 0.9	−0.7**	22.1 ± 0.9	21.8 ± 0.9	−0.4*	0.31 ± 0.3	<0.001
Body fat (%)	31.7 ± 1.2	31.1 ± 1.6	−0.6**	32.6 ± 0.9	32.2 ± 0.9	−0.4	0.17 ± 0.3	0.007
Total fat (cm^2)	333.1 ± 3.5	248.8 ± 10.5	−84.3***	327.9 ± 38.8	253.6 ± 12.3	−74.4 *	9.9 ± 35.6	0.788
Visceral fat (cm^2)	74.4 ± 4.8	65.9 ± 3.6	−8.6***	65.8 ± 4.0	65.3 ± 3.4	−0.60	7.9 ± 3.7	0.041
Subcutaneous fat (cm^2)	258.6 ± 23.7	182.9 ± 9.7	−75.7**	262.1 ± 39.3	188.3 ± 10.8	−73.8 *	1.9 ± 38.7	0.960
VSR	0.35 ± 0.03	0.39 ± 0.03	0.04 *	0.31 ± 0.03	0.37 ± 0.02	0.06***	0.01 ± 0.02	0.447

Source: From Cha, Y.S. et al. 2012. *Nutrition Research Practice* 6: 520–526.

[a] Values in this column represent differences between the mean changed scores of the *doenjang* group and those of the placebo group; 95% CIs in parentheses.
[b] *p* values derived from the repeated measurement analysis (per protocol) after adjusting for age, gender, and BMI.
[c] Values are expressed as means ± SE. WHR, waist–to-hip ratio; VSR, visceral to subcutaneous ratio.

$^*p < 0.05$, $^{**}p < 0.01$, $^{***}p < 0.001$: *p*-values indicate significant differences in the variables between 0-week and 12-week, which were evaluated by paired t-test.

exhibits stability in thermal treatment, which is implemented at 100°C for 30 min, and which makes possible to expect the same effect in the daily ingesting of *doenjang* soup. The immune control substance in an animal mouse model increases B lymphocyte proliferation particularly and represents an increase in generating cytokine of the macrophage and B lymphocyte. That is, traditional *doenjang* increases the generation of TNF-liferation particularly and represents an increase of generating cytokine of the macrophage and B lymphocyte. That is, traditional *Doenjang* increases the generation of TNF-α, IL-12, and IL-6 in the peritonea cell of the mouse and reinforces its immune function through more increases in generating the IFN-γ of lymphocyte and activating natural killer (NK) cells (Lee et al. 1997). Also, there is a report that it improves and prevents allergies by decreasing the generation of IgE inhibitors, which are generated by antigens (Jang et al. 2008).

12.4 Gochujang

Gochujang uses a special type of *meju* as a major raw ingredient mixed with a large amount of red pepper powder, which is a hot-flavored spice, different from other fermented soybean products. In particular, *gochujang* uses a peculiar production method that mixes different materials for fermenting and maturing based on a solution of glucoses obtained from grain starches including rice. *Gochujang* is a flavored paste type spice and represents a balanced taste of hot, sweet, sour, and salty flavors. Also, it is a legendary and traditional fermented food in Korea that cannot be found in other countries even in similar styles (Figures 12.12 and 12.13).

Gochujang has been used in various foods as a spice source and the demand for *gochujang* has increased in accordance with recent preferences for hot-flavored tastes (Shin et al. 2012).

12.4.1 History

As one of major ingredients in *gochujang* is red pepper, *gochujang* has been made since the introduction of the red pepper in Korea as a popular flavor spice. It is estimated that the red

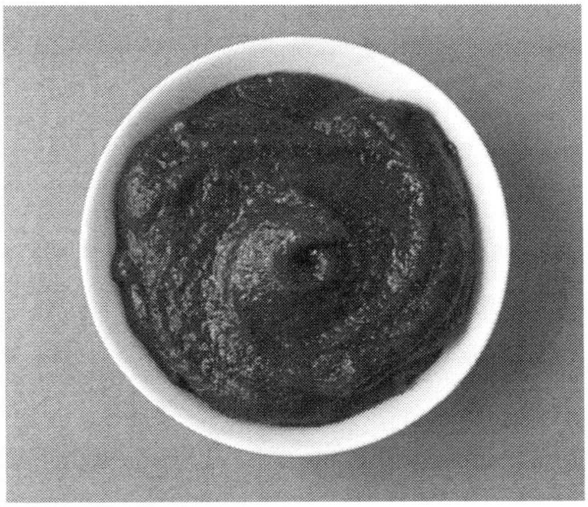

Figure 12.12 ***Gochujang*** **(traditional).**

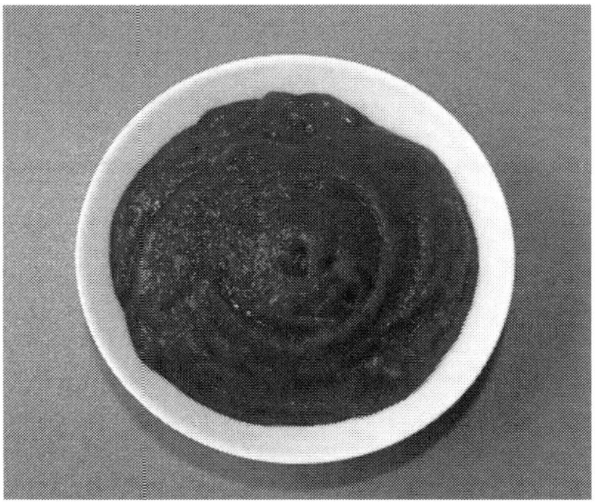

Figure 12.13 *Gochujang* (commercial).

pepper was first introduced at the end of the sixteenth century or the early seventeenth century from China or Portugal and Poland through the south routes but some researchers estimated that it was introduced long before those periods in what is called the *Goryeo* period in the tenth century (Kwon et al. 2011a). Therefore, the use of *gochujang* in Korean dietary life is estimated since that period. Thus, according to literature and research it is estimated that the red pepper, which is native to South America, was introduced to Korea through Europe and *gochujang* was also introduced by Korean around this period as the red pepper was used as a raw fermentation material.

A culture of serving side dishes was settled in Korea from pre-Biblical times, with the consumption of grains as a main dish and fermented soybean products used as spice sources in order to cover the plain taste of grains. In particular, with the introduction of the red pepper, which is a representative hot-flavored taste, this pepper can be used as a type of powder including its combined and fermented types. Before the introduction of the red pepper in Korea, various hot-flavored spices, such as green onion, garlic, ginger, mustard, and so on, were used in Korean cuisine (Kim 1999). After the introduction of the red pepper, it was balanced with other spices and contributed to opening a new era of flavored spices.

12.4.2 Preparation and Culinary Process

The most important raw material in producing *gochujang* is *meju* for *gochujang*. Although there are some differences in making *meju* for *gochujang* according to regions and the times, it is made of soybeans with some additives like grains, usually nonglutinous rice, by the mixture ratio of 6:4 (Shin et al. 2012). Then, the mixture is to be steamed and shaped for fermenting (Figure 12.14). Here, microorganisms proliferated under appropriate natural conditions play a major role in fermenting *meju* for *gochujang*.

Gochujang has been produced using traditional and industrial processes and the major differences in these processes is the use of *meju* for *gochujang* (Park et al. 1995, Shin et al. 2012). The traditional method uses the *meju* and the industrial process fully manages the fermentation processes using pure bacilli where flour is used as starch material. In general, the production process of traditional *gochujang* is presented in Figure 12.15. Savory and sweet tastes are generated during the

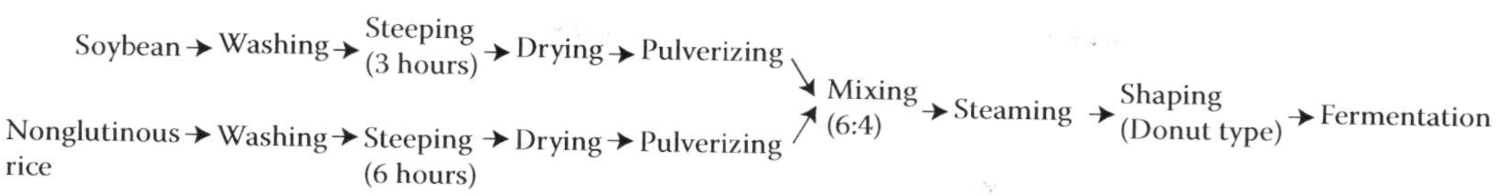

Figure 12.14 Process of making *meju* for *gochujang*. (From Kwon, D.Y. et al. 2009. *Nutrition* 25:790–799; Shin, D.H. et al. 2012. *Public Health Education* 10–133.)

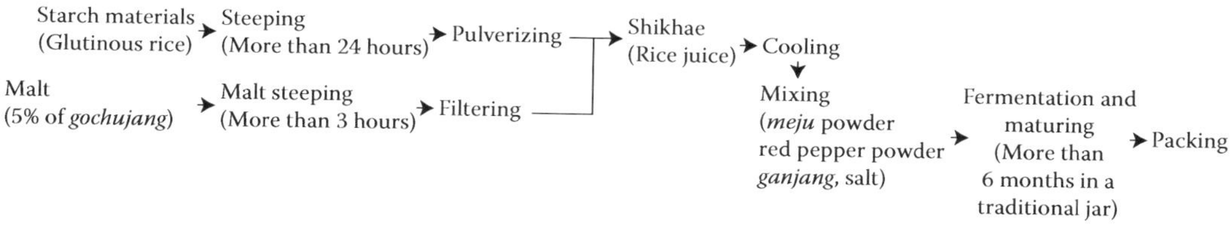

Figure 12.15 General process of producing traditional *gochujang*.

decomposition of soybean proteins and starches in its fermentation process and that leads to present the peculiar flavor in *gochujang* through harmonizing such tastes and the hot-flavored tastes of red pepper. *Gochujang* has been used as a flavor spice in Korean cuisine and is largely used in different pot stews. In addition, it is used to make *ssamjang* by mixing it with *doenjang*. Moreover, it is used as a seasoning of the *bulgogi*, which is a Korean traditional food. It can also become a popular spice for Mexicans, Spaniards, and Italians who prefer hot-flavored tastes. *Gochujang* is known to those in the world who like hot-flavored tastes.

12.4.3 Socioeconomy

Gochujang has been presented as an important element in Korean cuisine over several hundred years ago together with other fermented soybean products. In particular, its hot-flavored taste opens a new era of tastes. In recent years, the daily personal consumption of *gochujang* in Korea is about 6.4 g and the annual gross production reaches 149 thousand tons. Also, the annual values of shipments are about 319 billion won ($1 = 1100 won) and the value of exports is about 17.93 million dollars (Ministry of Food and Drug Safety 2012). The exports are targeted to Japan, China, and Europe and the amount of export has been increasing every year. Producing *gochujang* was first implemented as a family business and has now developed to a large-scale. Also, both traditional and industrial products are released to markets. The products of small and medium scale businesses contribute to improve incomes of famers who cultivate soybeans.

12.4.4 Microbiology and Food Safety

Raw materials of *gochujang* are red pepper powder, rice, *meju* powder, and salt, and various microorganisms are presented in these materials. In the natural fermentation, some bacilli from the air are also presented (Kwon et al. 2009). In the case of industrially produced *gochujang*, although the microorganisms inoculated by starters contribute to its major fermentation, the microorganisms that existed in the unpasteurized main raw and extra materials are also rolled in a different way. The number of general bacilli in *gochujang* is about 10^7–10^8/g. The frequency of detecting separated bacilli in traditional *gochujang* is presented by the order of *B. velegensis* > *B. amyloliquefaciens* > *B. subtilis* and halophilic bacilli are determined by the order of *B. liqueformis* > *B. subtilis* > *B. velegensis* > *B. amyloliqueformis*. In addition, a genus of *Oceanobacillus* is detected (Nam et al. 2012). In the case of the factory made *gochujang, B. subtilis* is a dominant bacillus. In enzymes, the detection frequency is presented by *Zygosaccharomyces* > *Candida lactis*. Also, the highest frequency of halophilic is presented by *Zygorouxii*. As the factory made products are sterilized, there are no detections of enzymes. In molds, a genus of *Aspergillus* is a dominant one and other bacilli including genera of *Penicillium* and *Rhizopus*, which are found in *meju*, are also presented (Kim et al. 2013). However, proliferations in molds can be allowed on surfaces at a limited level because anaerobic fermentation is processed in the fermentation of *gochujang*.

As *gochujang* shows lower protein contents compared with other fermented soybean products, the content of biogenic amine represents a low level of about 1.5–27 mg/kg (Kim et al. 2011a,b). Also, the aflatoxin content is presented by 0.04–2.46 μg/kg and lower than the legal level of 15 μg/kg. Based on the results of several experiments, it has been known that the amount of aflatoxin is decreased as *meju* is dried in the sun. In addition, the methylcarbonate content shows a very low level of 0.56 ppb average.

12.4.5 Nutritional Composition and Functional Properties

Regarding the general ingredients in 100 g of *gochujang*, they are 44.6 g of moisture, 4.9 g of protein, 1.1 g of lipid, 8.2 g of ash, 43.8 g of carbohydrate, 40 mg of calcium, 3.164 mg of sodium, and 2.445 μg of beta-carotene (RDA2011). Also, capsaicin is included as a peculiar ingredient in which the content of capsaicin in the traditional Korea's red pepper is about 200~300 mg% and will be presented in *gochujang* according to the amount of red pepper (Choi 2004).

Functionalities in *gochujang* have been indicated as antiobesity, anticancer, antitumor, and antihypertension effects. A spoonful (18 g/L serving) of *gochujang* has about 30 kcal (about 160 kcal/100 g) (The Korean Nutrition Society 2009). Fermentation extracts generated by combining different ingredients, which are obtained by the fermentation of red pepper, soybeans, and starch, play a role in biological functions. Clinical researches on *gochujang* are on antiobesity, dyslipidemia, and antistress.

12.4.5.1 Anticancer and Antitumor Effects

Fermentation and maturation processes carried out by mixing *meju* and red pepper powder are very important in making *gochujang* (Park and Oh 1995). Recently, it has been reported that increases in the period of time for fermenting *gochujang* exhibit higher effects on preventing cancer and the *gochujang* produced by traditional methods represents better anticancer effects than factory made products. The traditional product generates more anticancer substances during its maturation period than the factory made product and that increases such effects.

In addition, it is reported that in all clinical studies the garlic soup with added *gochujang* shows strong anticancer activations for all cancer cells including stomach cancer (MKN45), colon cancer (HCT116), and lung cancer cells (NCI-H460) and excellent anticancer effects based on experiments using an MTT assay method. In particular, the anticancer effect of *gochujang* on stomach cancer (MKN45) cells shows the highest level (Song et al. 2008) (Figure 12.16).

In antitumor effects of *gochujang* in an animal model, the tumor weight of the control group decreased by 6.0 g in which tumor cells (PBS, phosphate-buffered saline) are implanted after transplanting sarcoma-180 tumor cells to the hypoderm of a mouse (Park et al. 2001). Whereas,

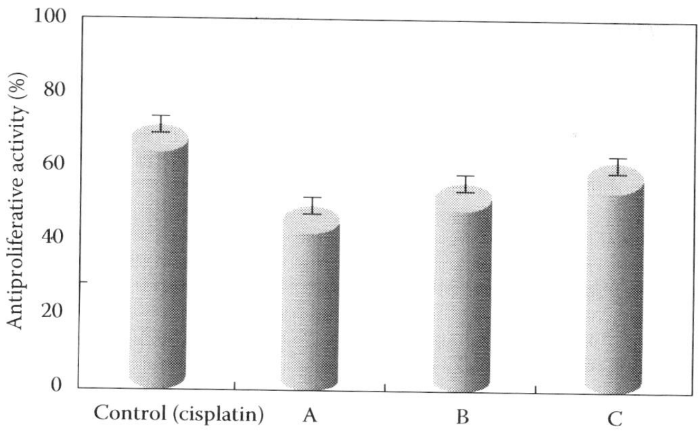

Control group: Cisplatin 25 ppm, A: Factory made *gochujang*,
B: Raw garlic (100 ppm) added *gochujang*, C: Garlic soup (100 ppm) added *gochujang*

Figure 12.16 Comparison of the inhibition of proliferation effects in *gochujang* extracts.

the tumor weight in the group with fermented *gochujang* is 3.3 g. Also, the inhibition effects on generating tumors in the groups of applying fermented and unfermented *gochujang* are presented by 45% and 17% respectively. In the case of the factory made product, the effect is determined by 23% (Park et al. 2001) (Table 12.10). Anticancer experiments using a living body represent the same results where the fermentation process of *gochujang* becomes an important factor in such anticancer effects in considering the fact that the fermented *gochujang* shows 2–3 times higher anticancer activation levels than the unfermented *gochujang*. In the tumor metastatic inhibition effects in *gochujang*, the numbers of tumors that are metastasized to the lung after applying colon 26-M3.1 metastatic cancer cells in mouse models for the control group and the group with red pepper powder are 318 and 308 (an inhibition rate of 3%), respectively. However, in the metastatic

Table 12.10 Inhibition Effects of the Methanol Extracts in *Gochujang* and Red Pepper Powder on Generating Tumors in Sarcoma-180 Cancer Cell Implanted Balb/c Mouse Models

Sample	*Tumor Weight (g)*	*Inhibition Rate (%)*
Sarcoma-180 cancer cell (A) + PBS (control group)	6.0 ± 0.1^{a}	–
(A) + traditional *gochujang* (0 day fermentation)	50 ± 0.9^{ab}	17
(A) + traditional *gochujang* (6 months fermentation)	6.0 ± 0.1^{c}	45
(A) + factory made *gochujang*	$4.5 + 0.1^{bc}$	23
(A) + red pepper powder	$4.7 + 0.3^{b}$	22

Source: From Park, K. et al. 2001. *Journal of Food Science Nutrition* 6: 181–191.

Note: Significant differences in a–c Duncan's multiple range tests ($p < 0.05$).

inhibition effects of cancer cells in the traditional *gochujang*, which is fermented for 6 months, the number of tumors is 52 (an inhibition rate of 79%). It shows the highest inhibition effect (Cheng-Bi et al. 2002), that is, the fermented *gochujang* represents higher cancer cell metastatic inhibition effects than the unfermented product. It reveals that the fermentation extracts, which are generated or transformed during the fermentation process of *gochujang*, play an important role in inhibiting tumor metastasis.

12.4.5.2 Antiobesity and Glycemic Control Effects

The capsaicinoid and isoflavone included in *gochujang* affect antiobesity functions through facilitating the lipid metabolism in the human body (Cha et al. 2012). Also, these are effective to reduce body weight due to specific compounds in *gochujang*, or isoflavones, capsaicin, and capsioids. In addition, red pepper powder and extra materials generate some fermentation extracts and this contributes to control energy and glucose metabolism and to reduce both fat cell sizes and fat accumulations. Moreover, although red pepper powder contributes to partly reduce body fat accumulations and to decompose fat based on capsaicin and dietary fiber, *gochujang* represents higher biological activation levels than that of red pepper powder.

In particular, the capsaicin included in red pepper powder facilitates the secretion of adrenalin by stimulating the spinal cord and this activates metabolism. Then, the capsaicin decomposes not only glycogen accumulated in the liver, but also the fat cells in order to use them as energy (Choo 2000, Koo et al. 2008, Soh et al. 2008). The hot-flavored taste, capsaicin, reduces body fat through increasing the β-adrenergic activity, which is a brown adipose tissue, and inhibits the activation of acetyl CoA carboxylase that is a restraint enzyme in a composition process of fatty acids existed in the liver. Thus, it increases the activation of lipoprotein lipase in fatty tissues and inhibits accumulations of body fat. In addition, the degree of fermentation in *gochujang* affects antiobesity effects (Table 12.11). The group ingesting *gochujang*, which is fermented for 6 months, shows more decreases in body weight than the group consuming red pepper and nonfermented *gochujang*. The antiobesity effect is presented only by fermentation of *gochujang* (Rhee et al. 2003).

In animal experiments, the diet of fermented traditional *gochujang* represents effects on reducing body weight and improving cholesterol metabolism, while other groups ingesting unfermented *gochujang* and red pepper powder show no large decreasing effects (Joo 2000).

Table 12.11 Effect of *Gochujang* in High-Fat Dietary Mouse Model (for 21 days) on the Bodyweight

	Normal	*High Fat*	*Gochujang (Before)*	*Gochujang (6-month Fermentation)*	*Red Pepper*
Initial weight (g)	199.9 ± 7.5	198.0 ± 6.4	200.7 ± 9.6	199.9 ± 9.7	199.9 ± 2.7
Final weight (g)	333.8 ± 0.5[b]	382.8 ± 1.4[a]	362.6 ± 2.5	354.5 ± 0.1[c]	376.5 ± 5.1[a]
Increment (g/day)	4.4 ± 0.2[d]	6.4 ± 0.1[a]	5.8 ± 0.4[b]	5.6 ± 0.5[c]	6.2 ± 0.3[ab]

Source: From Rhee, S. et al. 2003. *Journal of Korean Society Food Science Nutrition* 32: 882–886.

[a–d] Means significantly difference by Duncan on the bodyweight ($p < 0.05$).

Table 12.12 Changes in Internal Organ Weights and Fat Tissues in Mouse Models by Applying Capsaicin and *Gochujang* Diets

Internal Organ Weight? (g/100 g Weight)	*Normal Group*	*High-Fat Diet*	*High-Fat Diet + Capsaicin*	*High-Fat Diet + Gochujang*
Liver	4.19 ± 0.09^{b}	4.42 ± 0.11^{a}	4.36 ± 0.11^{ab}	4.27 ± 0.05^{bc}
Spleen	0.23 ± 0.02^{ns}	0.23 ± 0.02	0.22 ± 0.02	0.21 ± 0.02
Kidney	1.02 ± 0.08^{ns}	1.02 ± 0.06	0.99 ± 0.04	1.01 ± 0.01
Epididymal adipose tissue	0.88 ± 0.14^{d}	1.67 ± 0.19^{a}	1.35 ± 0.11^{b}	1.19 ± 0.08^{c}
Tissues around the kidney	1.02 ± 0.04^{d}	1.69 ± 0.01^{a}	1.39 ± 0.07^{b}	1.26 ± 0.06^{c}

Source: From Choo, J. and H. Shin. 1999. *Korean Journal of Nutrition* 32: 533–539.

[a–d] Means significantly difference by Duncan's multiple range test ($p < 0.05$).

According to whether the fermentation of *gochujang* is applied, it becomes an important variable in decreasing body weight and fat tissues (Choo and Shin 1999) (Table 12.12). In addition, it is possible to estimate increases in its synergy effects on antiobesity in red pepper powder itself through the mutual interaction between the isoflavones, which are nonglycosides of the *meju* included in *gochujang*, and the capsaicin in the red pepper powder in addition to the *gochujang* extracts (Kim 2004).

In recent years, an experiment of ingesting *gochujang* pills of 32 g/day over 12 weeks for overweight and obese adults shows that it improves both the visceral fat area and the rate between visceral fat and subcutaneous fat significantly compared with that of the group with placebos, and agrees with the animal experiments mentioned above (Cha et al. 2013) (Figures 12.17 and 12.18). In addition, the combination between the red pepper included in *gochujang* and the fermented soybeans (5% of *gochujang* powder) represents an improvement in insulin sensitivity, a decrease in insulin resistance, and an increase in blood glucose homeostasis in diabetes rats, which have a 90% pancreatectomized peripheral insulin resistance, and improves the glucose tolerance through increasing the insulin sensitivity due to decreases in body fat cells (Kwon et al. 2009). That is, the activation of capsaicin, which is the major component of *gochujang*, increases the secretion of catecholamine in the adrenal medulla through activating the sympathetic nervous system and this leads to improved energy and lipid metabolism (Diepvens et al. 2007). Also, it reveals that ingesting *gochujang* for a long period of time prevents and improves coronary artery diseases through controlling obesity and blood sugar levels.

12.4.5.3 Serum Lipid Improvement Effect

In rats that are introduced to obesity through a high fat diet, ingesting fermented *gochujang* exhibits effects on improving lipids by decreasing serum TG and TC significantly. In particular, in more decreases in the serum TG content of traditional *gochujang* than that of industrial *gochujang*, the extracts generated during the fermentation of *gochujang* play an important role in the results

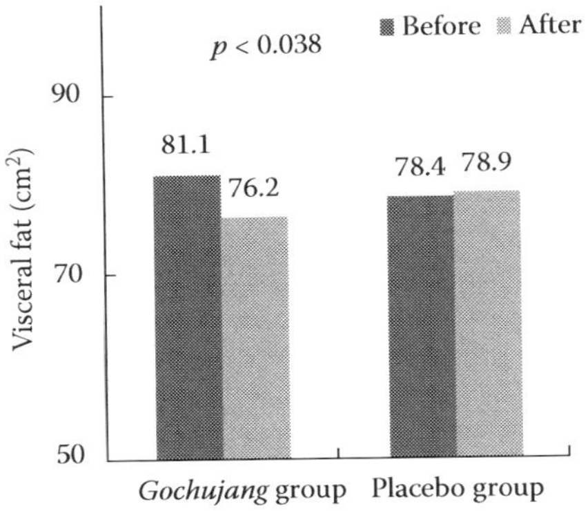

Figure 12.17 Changes in visceral fat. (From Cha, Y.S. et al. 2013. *Nutrition Metabolism (London)* 10:1.)

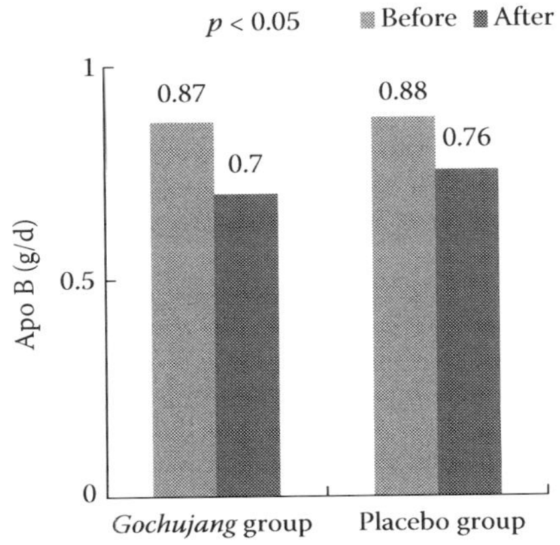

Figure 12.18 Changes Apo B. (From Cha, Y.S. et al. 2013. *Nutrition Metabolism (London)* 10:1.)

(Choo and Shin 1999). Also, the fermented *gochujang* diet positively affects lipid metabolism because of decreasing serum TG and TC contents and ingesting *gochujang* pills for 12 weeks decreases serum TC and LDL-C levels lipids through the feces (Lim et al. 2014). In addition, in adults who show hyperlipidemia ingesting *gochujang* significantly compared with that of the group with placebos and this agrees with the results of animal *experiments* (Im 2013). Ingesting such *gochujang* pills (32.0 g/day) in overweight female adults who represent BMI more than 23 kg/m^2 also decreases serum TC and LDL-C levels (Kim et al. 2010a). It is considered that the isoflavones of the *meju* included in *gochujang* contribute to improve lipids.

12.4.5.4 Stress Control and Relief (Stabilizing the Autonomic Nervous System)

The autonomic nervous system plays a role in automatically controlling the human body. It is divided into two different systems; sympathetic and parasympathetic nervous systems. The sympathetic nervous system covers responses such as fighting or running away and the parasympathetic nervous system shows a role in digesting or sleeping. In a normal state, these two nervous systems are balanced and maintain the homeostasis in a human body through facilitating or inhibiting responses in each internal organ. Autonomic nervous diseases in the cardiovascular system degrade the quality of life in patients by causing tachycardia, exercise intolerance, myocardiac infarction, and left ventricular systolic and diastolic dysfunctions (Singh et al.1998), and increase dangers in coronary artery diseases due to inappropriate controls in heart autonomic nerves (Liao et al. 2002). There is a close relation in the heart rate variability (HRV), autonomic nervous system (ANS), and stress. That is, continuous stresses decrease regulation capabilities in the human body and degrade functions of the autonomic nervous system.

As functions of the autonomic nervous system are degraded, the responsibility and adaptability of the human body for external stimuli are significantly decreased. It can be verified in decreasing such HRV. In tests for inspecting the autonomic nervous system, changes in HRV for Valsalva maneuver, changing body postures, and inspiratory and expiratory periods in repeated deep breathing and in blood pressure for standing up and for grasping power are to be measured to evaluate the functions of the sympathetic and parasympathetic nervous systems (Nguewa et al. 2011). In recent years, there are some positive effects of ingesting *gochujang* in hyperlipidemia patients on easing stresses and improving such autonomic nervous system functions through reducing the difference in inspiratory and expiratory periods in repeated deep breathing (Table 12.13) (Im 2013). It reveals that ingesting *gochujang* for a long period of time improves or stabilizes the autonomic nervous system through easing and controlling stresses leading to the prevention and reduction of coronary artery diseases.

Table 12.13 Autonomic Nervous Functions (Deep Breathing) in *Gochujang* and Placebo Groups for 0 and 12 weeks in the Study

	Gochujang Group (n = 13)			*Placebo Group (n = 13)*			
	0 week	*12 week*	*p-Value*[a]	*0 week*	*12 week*	*p-Value*[a]	*p-Value*[b]
Breathing	0.2 ± 0.3	0.0 ± 0.0	0.008**	0.1 ± 0.2	0.2 ± 0.4	0.387	0.027*
ECG	0.4 ± 0.4	0.3 ± 0.5	0.613	0.4 ± 0.4	0.5 ± 0.5	0.613	0.470
Valsalva	0.3 ± 0.4	0.4 ± 0.4	0.570	0.3 ± 0.4	0.6 ± 0.5	0.022*	0.340
Upright	0.2 ± 0.2	0.1 ± 0.2	0.337	0.0 ± 0.1	0.1 ± 0.2	0.337	0.192
Handgrip	0.0 ± 0.0	0.0 ± 0.0	–	0.0 ± 0.0	0.0 ± 0.0	–	–
T_score	1.1 ± 0.8	0.8 ± 0.7	0.279	0.8 ± 0.6	1.4 ± 1.0	0.073	0.035*

Source: From Im, J.H. 2013. The effect of *Kochujang* pills on blood lipid profiles in hyperlipidemia subjects: A 12 weeks, randomized, double-blind, placebo-controlled clinical trial. MS thesis, Chonbuk National University, Joenju (Korea).

Note: Abnormal = 1, borderline = 0.5, normal = 0.

Note: All values are presented as mean ± SD

[a] Analyzed by paired t-test.
[b] Independent-test, *$P < 0.05$, **$P < 0.01$.

12.5 Ssamjang

Ssamjang is a mixture of *deonjang, cheonggukjang,* and *gochujang*. Sometimes it is mixed with sesame oil and some other spices like red pepper. The main usage of *ssamjang* is as a wrapp with salad like vegetables and some meat, mostly pork. The general pictures are as shown in Figures 12.19 and 12.20.

12.6 Ganjang

Ganjang is one of the representative fermented soybean foods of Korea and has been known as soy sauce throughout the world. In the Orient, *ganjang* has long been used as both seasoning and flavoring in different foods in a number of countries. Amino acids and peptides that are generated by decomposing soybeans by microorganisms represent savory flavors and are used for seasoning

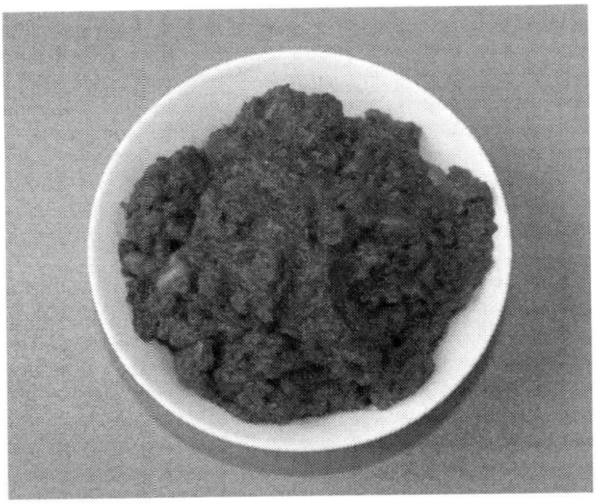

Figure 12.19 ***Ssamjang*** **(traditional).**

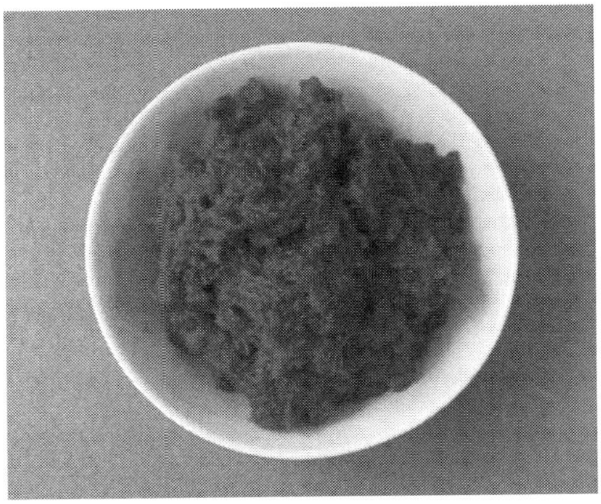

Figure 12.20 ***Ssamjang*** **(commercial).**

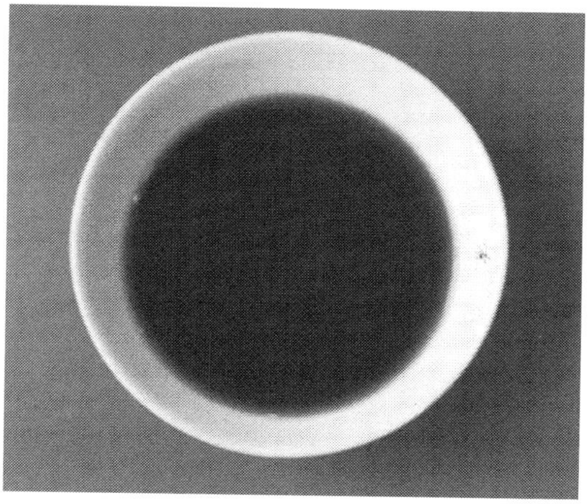

Figure 12.21 ***Ganjang* (traditional).**

foods using the salty taste of *ganjang*. *Ganjang* can be produced using improved methods, which apply a purely fermented process with molds using soybeans and flour, and traditional methods, which use *meju*. As Korea's traditional *ganjang* uses naturally fermented *meju* (see Korearally fermented *doenjang*), a complex fermentation process in which molds, bacilli, and enzymes contribute to the fermentation is used. Thus, there are large differences in ingredients and flavors between the improved and the traditional products. The improved products, factory made *ganjang*, are widely used across the world. However, the traditional *ganjang* has still been selling in limited fashion, due to its deep tastes and flavors (Figures 12.21 and 12.22).

The history of the *ganjang* goes back to the birth of Christ. Since then, *ganjang* has been largely consumed in the Orient, in particular, Japan, China, and Korea. The traditional *ganjang* shows a relatively simple process. Soybeans are steamed and mashed to make the shape of *meju*. Then, the *meju* is naturally fermented for 2–3 months and dried. The dried *meju* is steeped in salt water (about 18%–20%) in order to mature it. The maturing is continued over 4–6 months and the liquid part of the *meju* steeped in salt water is separated. This is a type of traditional *ganjang*. In the early

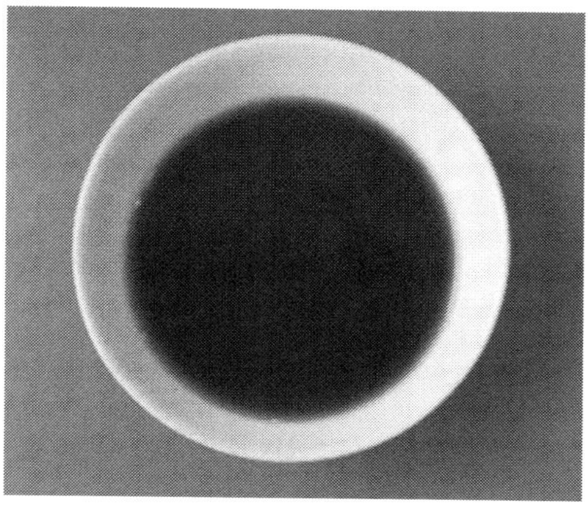

Figure 12.22 ***Ganjang* (commercial).**

state of separating the liquid part, it shows a bright brown color and changes to a dark brown color over time (caramelization). In general, it can be used as a particular seasoning even after storing it for several decades.

12.7 Conclusion

Soybean is globally placed next to rice, wheat, and corn in terms of importance as a food resource, and has been utilized as an important nutrition source in particular for supplementing animal proteins in Asian countries including Korea, China, and Japan. The people of these countries have long eaten various fermented soybean foods. In recent years consumption of soybeans as fermented products has been significantly increasing as scientific research confirms that the products show some functionalities. While some countries utilized the soybean as a source of oil and animal feed, there are a variety of soybean applications as food resources today. In addition, the scientific community is paying attention to functional substances created by fermentation. The functionalities of fermented foods have been well-known throughout the world and many countries are advertising the excellence of their traditional fermented foods in combination with their own dietary culture. Another advantage is the probiotic role of microorganisms involved in fermentation processes. Researchers have actively studied the intestinal role of microorganisms that are used for safety-guaranteed fermented foods. We expect that future research will reveal several positive roles of some components and the microorganisms. It is important to broadly study various fermented foods, including fermented soybean products, in all the countries of the world, to unveil their functionalities, and to propose ways to improve them. We believe that such research activities will highly increase the possibility of promoting new industries and contribute to improving the fitness of human beings across the world.

References

Back, H.I. 2009. Effects of *Chungkookjang* supplementation on obesity and atherosclerosis indices in overweight/obese subjects 12 weeks, randomized, double-blind, placebo controlled clinical trial. MS thesis, Chonbuk National University, Jeonju (Korea).

Back, H.I., S.R. Kim, J.A. Yang, M.G. Kim, S.W. Chae, and Y.S. Cha. 2011. Effects of *Chungkookjang* supplementation on obesity and atherosclerotic indices in overweight/obese subjects: A 12-week, randomized, double-blind, placebo-controlled clinical trial. *Journal of Medicinal Food* 14: 532–537.

Baek, J.G., S.M. Shim, D.Y. Kwon, H.K. Choi, C.H. Lee, and Y.S. Kim. 2010. Metabolite profiling of *Cheonggukjang*, a fermented soybean paste, inoculated with various *Bacillus* strains during fermentation. *Bioscience Biotechnology Biochemistry* 74: 1860–1868.

Banaszkilwicz, T. 2011. Nutritional value of soybean meal, in *Soybean and Nutrition*, Ed. El-Shemy H.A, Intech 1–20.

Burkitt, D.P. 1971. Epidemiology of cancer of colon and rectum. *Cancer* 28: 3–13.

Cha, I.H., Y.K. Lee, Y. Gyun, K.K. Kim, and Y.W. Choi. 1999. Influence of Traditional foods on the survival of *Escherichia coli* O157. *Journal Agricultural Technology and Development Institute* 9: 1–5.

Cha, Y.S., S.R. Kim, J.A. Yang, H.I. Back, M.G. Kim, S.J. Jung, W.O. Song, and S.W. Chae. 2013. *Kochujang*, fermented soybean-based red pepper paste, decreases visceral fat and improves blood lipid profiles in overweight adults. *Nutrition Metabolism (London)* 10:1.

Cha, Y.S., J.A.Yang, H.I. Back, S.R. Kim, M.G. Kim, S.J. Jung, W.O. Song, and S.W. Chae. 2012.Visceral fat and body weight are reduced in overweight adults by the supplementation of *Doenjang*, a fermented soybean paste. *Nutrition Research Practice* 6: 520–526.

Chang, J., Y. Shim, S. Kim, K. Chee, and S. Cha. 2005. Fibrinolytic and immunostimulating activities of *Bacillus* spp. strains isolated from *Chungkukjang. Korean Journal Food Science Technology* 37: 255–260.

Cheng-Bi., C.S. Oh, D. Lee, S. Ham. 2002. Effect of the biological activities of ethanol extract from Korean traditional *Kochujang* added with sea tangle *(Laminaria longissima). Korean Journal Food Preservation* 9: 1–7.

Cho, J. 1980. *Study on Korean Fermented Foods. Keejeon yeongusa* 48–90. Korea.

Cho, T., G. Han, K.N. Bahn, Y. Son, M. Jang, C. Lee, S. Kim, D. Kim, and S. Kim. 2006. Evaluation of biogenic amines in Korean commercial fermented foods. *Korean Journal of Food Science Technology* 38: 730–737.

Choi, G., S. Lim, and J. Choi. 1998. Antioxidant and nitrile scavenging effect of soybean, *meju* and *doenjang. Korean Journal Life Science* 8: 473–478.

Choi, H. 2004. *Fermentation and Food Science of Kimchi. Hyoil Book* 382–383. Korea.

Choi, J., S.H. Kwon, K.Y. Park, B.P. Yu, N.D. Kim, J.H. Jung, and H.Y. Chung. 2010. The anti-inflammatory action of fermented soybean products in kidney of high-fat-fed rats. *Journal of Medicinal Food* 14: 232–239.

Choi, S.H., M.H. Lee, S.K. Lee, and M.J. Oh. 1995. Microflora and enzyme activity of conventional *meju* and isolation of useful mould. *Journal of Agricultural Science,* Chungnam National University, Korea 22: 188–197.

Choo, J. 2000. Anti-obesity effects of *kochujang* in rats fed on a high fat diet. *Korean Journal of Nutrition* 33: 787–793.

Choo, J. and H. Shin. 1999. Body-fat suppressive effects of capsaicin through ß-adrenergic stimulation in rats fed a high-fat diet. *Korean Journal of Nutrition* 32: 533–539.

Chung, D.H., H.C. Lee, S.K. Shim, B.Y. Han. 2006. Soybean fermented foods. *Hong Ik Jae,* 910–918, Korea, CRC Press.

Devi, M.K., M. Gondi, G. Sakthivelu, P. Giridhar, T. Rajasekaran, and G.A. Ravishankar. 2009. Functional attributes of soybean seeds and products, with reference to isoflavone content and antioxidant activity. *Food Chemistry* 114: 771–776.

Diepvens, K., K. Westerterp, and M.S. Plantenga. 2007. Obesity and thermogenesis related to the consumption of caffeine, ephedrine, capsaicin, and green tea. *American Journal of Physiology-Regulatory Integrative and Comparative Physiology* 292: 77–85.

Forsythe, W. A., 3rd. 1995. Soy protein, thyroid regulation and cholesterol metabolism. *Journal of Nutrition* 125: 619–623.

Hahm, J.H., T.Y. Lee, J.S. Lee, C. Park, M. H. Sung, and H. Poo. 2004. Antitumor effect of poly-glutamic acid by modulating cytokine production and NK cell activity. *International Meeting of the Federation of Korean Microbiological Societies* 21–22. Korea.

Hong, M.S. 1715. *Sallimgyeongje (Korean translation), Min Moon Go. Seoul.* CRC Press.

Im, J.H. 2013. The effect of *Kochujang*pills on blood lipids profiles in hyperlipidemia subjects: A 12 weeks, randomized, double-blind, placebo-controlled clinical trial. MS thesis, Chonbuk National University, Joenju (Korea).

Inoguchi, S., Y. Ohashi, A. Narai-Kanayama, K. Aso, T. Nakagaki, and T.Fujisawa. 2012. Effects of non-fermented and fermented soybean milk intake on faecal microbiota and faecal metabolites in humans. *International Journal of Food Sciences and Nutrition* 63: 402–410.

Jang, I.H., M.J. Ahn, and H.J. Chae. 2004. Manufacturing method for traditional *Doenjang* and screening of high fibrin clotting inhibitory samples. *Journal of Applied Biological Chemistry* 47: 149–153.

Jang, S., K. Kim, S. Kang. 2008. Effects of PGA-LM on CD4+CD25+foxp3+ Treg cell activation in isolated CD4+ T cells in NC/Nga mice. *Korean Journal Microbiology Biotechnology* 36: 160–169.

Joo, J.J. 2000. Anti-obesity effects of *Kochujang* in rats fed on a high fat diet. *The Korean of Nutrition* 33: 787–793.

Jung, J.H., S.G. Kang, Y.S. Kim, and H.J. Chung. 1990. Degradation of phytic acid in *Chungkookjang* fermented with phytase-producing bacteria. *Korean Journal Applied Microbiology Biotechnology* 18: 423–428.

Jung, K.O., S.Y. Park, and K.Y. Park. 2006. Longer aging time increases the anticancer and antimetastatic properties of *doenjang. Nutrition* 22: 539–545.

Jung, S.J., S.H. Park, E.K. Choi, B.H. Cho, Y.S. Cha, Y.K. Kim, M.G. Kim et al. Chae. 2014. Beneficial effects of Korean traditional diets in hypertensive and type 2 diabetic patients. *Journal of Medicinal Food* 17: 161–171.

Kim, D.H., S.H. Kim, S.W. Kwon, Lee, J.K., and S.B. Hong. 2013. Fungal diversity of rice straw for *meju* fermentation. *Journal of Microbiology and Biotechnology* 23: 1654–1663.

Kim, D.M., S.H. Chung, and H.S. Chun. 2011b. Multiplex PCR assay for the detection of aflatoxigenic and non-aflatoxigenic fungi in meju, a Korean fermented soybean food starter. *Food Microbiology* 28: 1402–1408.

Kim, H.L., T.S. Lee, B.S. Noh, and J.S. Park. 1999. Characteristics of the stored Samjangs with different *Doenjangs*. *Korean Journal of Food Science Technology* 31: 36–44.

Kim, H.S., J.Y. Yoon, and S.R. Lee. 1994. Effect of cooking and processing on the phytate content and protein digestibility of soybean. *Korean Journal Food Science Technology* 2: 603–608.

Kim, J. 2004. Antiobestic and cancer preventive effects of Kochujang. MS thesis. Busan University, Busan, Korea.

Kim, J., M. Kang, and T. Kwon. 2003. Antidiabetic effect of soybean and Chunkukjang. *Korean Soybean Digest* 20: 44–52.

Kim, J.H., Y. Jia, J.G. Lee, B. Nam, J.H. Lee, K.S. Shin, B.S. Hurh, Y.H. Choi, and S.J. Lee. 2014. Hypolipidemic and antiinflammation activities of fermented soybean fibers from meju in C57BL/6 J mice. *Phytotherapy Research* Mar 12. doi: 10.1002/ptr.5134.

Kim, J.Y., O.Y. Kim, H.J. Yoo, T.I. Kim, W.H. Kim, Y.D. Yoon, and J.H. Lee. 2006. Effects of fiber supplements on functional constipation. *Korean Journal Nutrition* 39: 35–43.

Kim, K.Y. and Y.T. Hahm. 2002. Recent studies about physiological functions of *Chungkkokjang* and Functional enhancement with genetic engineering. *The Institute of Molecular Biology and Genetic* 16: 1–18.

Kim, M.J. 2009. Effect of *Cheonggukjang* powder on the large bowel function in rats with Loperamide induced constipation. MS thesis, Kyungpook National University, Daegu, Korea.

Kim, S. 1998. New trends of studying on potential activities of *Deonjang* fibrinolytic activity. *Korean Soybean Digest* 15: 8–15.

Kim, S.H., J.L. Yang, and Y.S. Song. 1999. Physiological functions of *Chongkukjang*. *Food Industry and Nutrition* 4: 40–46.

Kim, S.H., J.Y. Yang, K.H. Lee, K.H. Oh, G.M. Kim, J.M. Kim, D.J. Paik, S.M. Hong, and J.H. Youn. 2009. *Bacillus subtilis*—Specific poly-g-glutamic acid regulates development pathways of naive CD41 T cells through antigen-presenting cell-dependent and -independent mechanisms. *International Immunology* 21: 977–990.

Kim, T.W., Y.H. Kim, S.E. Kim, J.H. Lee, C.S. Park, and H.Y. Kim. 2010b. Identification and distribution of *Bacillus* species in *doenjang* by whole-cell protein patterns and 16S rRNA gene sequence analysis. *Journal of Microbiology Biotechnology* 20: 1210–1214.

Kim, W., K. Choi, Y. Kim, H. Park, J. Choi, Y. Lee, H. Oh, Kwon, I., and S. Lee. 1996. Purification and characterization of fibrinolytic enzyme produced from *Bacillus* sp. Strain CK-11–4 screened from *Chungkook-Jang*. *Applied and Environmental Microbiology* 62: 2482–2488.

Kim, Y., Y.J. Park, S.O. Yang, S.H. Kim, S. Cho, Y.S. Kim, D.Y. Kwon, Y.S. Cha, S.W. Chae, H.K. Choi. 2010a. Hypoxanthine levels in human urine serve as a screening indicator for the plasma total cholesterol and low-density lipoprotein modulation activities of fermented red pepper paste. *Nutrition Research* 30: 455–461.

Kim, Y.G. 1999. Studies on the chemical composition and proper ties of tradition al *kochujang* at *Sunchang* region. MS thesis, *Chonbuk* National University, Jeonju (Korea).

Kim, Y.S., M.C. Kim, S.W. Kwon, S.J. Kim, I.C. Park, J.O. Ka, and H.Y. Weon. 2011a. Analyses of bacterial communities in *meju*, a Korean traditional fermented soybean bricks, by cultivation-based and pyrosequencing methods. *Journal of Microbiology* 49: 340–348.

Koh, J. 2006. Effects *Cheonggukjang* added *Phellinus linteus* on lipid metabolism in hyperlipidemic rats. *Journal Korean Society Food Science Nutrition* 35: 301–308.

Koo, B., S.H. Seong, D.Y. Kown, H.S, and Y.S. Cha. 2008. Fermented *Kochujang* supplement shows antiobesity effects by controlling lipid metabolism in C57BL/6 J mice fed high fat diet. *Food Science and Biotechnology* 17: 336–342.

Kwak, C.S., M.Y. Kim, and S.A. Kim, and M.S. Lee. 2002. Cytotoxicity on human cancer cells and anti-tumorigenesis of *Chungkookjang*, a fermented soybean product, in DMBA-treated rats. *The Korean of Nutrition* 39: 346–356.

Kwak, C.S., S. Park, and K.Y. Song. 2012. *Doenjang*, a fermented soybean paste, decreased visceral fat accumulation and adipocyte size in rats fed with high fat diet more effectively than nonfermented soybeans. *Journal of Medicinal Food* 15: 1–9.

Kwon, D.Y., J.S. Jang, J.E. Lee, Y.S. Kim, D. W. Shin, and S. Park. 2006. The Isoflavonoid aglycone-rich fractions of *Chungkookjang*, fermented unsalted soybeans, enhance insulin signaling and peroxisome proliferator-activated receptor-activity in vitro. *Biofactors* 26: 245–258.

Kwon, D.Y., S.M. Hong, I.S. Ahan, Y.S., Kim, D.W. Shin, and S.M. Park. 2009. *Kochujang*, a Korean fermented red pepper plus soybean paste, improves glucose homeostasis in 90% pancreatectomized diabetic rats. *Nutrition* 25: 790–799.

Kwon, D.Y., J.W. Daily III, H.J. Kim, and S.M. Park. 2010. Antidiabetic effects of fermented soybean products on type 2 diabetes. *Nutrition Research* 30:130ri.

Kwon, D.Y., K.R. Chung, H.J. Yang, and D.J. Jang. 2011a. *The Story of Kochu (Redpepper)*. 121–190, Hyoilbooks, ISBN: 978-89-8489-303-0, Seoul, Korea.

Kwon, D.Y., H.J. Yang, M.J. Kim, H.J. Kang, H.J. Kim, K.C. Ha, H.I. Back et al. 2011b. Influence of the *Chungkookjang* on histamine-induced wheal and flare skin response: A randomized, double-blind, placebo controlled trial. *BMC Complementary Alternative of Medicine* 11 2011 Dec 5;11:125. doi: 10.1186/1472-6882-11-125.

Kwon, S., K. Lee, K. Im, S. Kim, and K. Park. 2006. Weight reduction and lipid lowering effects of Korean traditional soybean fermented products. *Journal of Korean Society Food Science Nutrition* 35: 1194–1199.

Lae, P. 2005. The effect of fermented soybean powder on improvement of constipating patients receiving maintenance hemo dialysis. MS thesis, Kyung Buk National University, Daegu, Korea.

Lee, H., M.J. Chang, and S.H. Kim. 2010. Effects of poly-gamma-glutamic acid on serum and brain concentrations of glutamate and GABA in diet-induced obese rats. *Nutrition Research Practice* 4: 23–29.

Lee, H.A. and J.H. Kim. 2012. Isolation of *Bacillus amyloliquefaciens* strains with antifungal activities from Meju. *Preventive Nutrition and Food Science* 17: 64–70.

Lee, H.J. and E.H. Hwang. 1997. Effects of alginic acid, cellulose and pectin level on bowel function in rats. *Korean Journal Nutrition* 30: 465–477.

Lee, I. and J. Lee. 2002. Effects of dietary supplementation of Korean soybean paste (Deonjang) on the lipid metabolism in rats fed a high fat and/or a high cholesterol diet. *Journal Korean Public Health Association* 28: 282–305.

Lee, J., C. Cho, H. Kim, J. Kim, J.Y. Kim, D.S. Kee, and H.B. Kim. 2001. Antioxidant activity of substances extracted by alcohol from *Chungkookjang* powder. *Korean Journal Microbiology* 37: 177–181.

Lee, J.O., S.D. Ha, A.J. Kim, C.S. Yuh, I.S. Bang, and S.H. Park. 2005. Industrial application and physiological functional of *Chungkukjang*. *Journal Food Science and Industry* 38: 69–78.

Lee, M.N. 2012. Analyses of aflatoxin biosynthesis gene cluster in *Aspergillus oryzae/flavus* complex strains. MS thesis, Korea University, Seoul, Korea.

Lee, N.R., S.M. Lee, K.S. Cho, S.Y. Jeong, D.Y. Hwang, D.S. Kim, C.O. Hong, and H. J. Son. 2014. Improved production of poly-γ-glutamic acid by *Bacillus subtilis* D7 isolated from *Doenjang*, a Korean traditional fermented food, and its antioxidant activity. *Applied Biochemistry and Biotechnology* 173: 918–932.

Lee, S.H., M.Y. Yoo, and D.B. Shin. 2011. Determination of biogenic amines in *Cheonggukjang* using ultra high pressure liquid chromatography coupled with mass spectrometry. *Food Science and Biotechnology* 20: 123–129.

Lee, Y.W., J.D. Kim, J.Z. Zheng, and K.H. Row. 2007. Comparisons of isoflavones from Korean and Chinese soybean and processed products. *Biochemical Engineering Journal* 36: 49–53.

Liao, D.P., M. Carnethon, G.W. Evans, W.E. Cascio, and G. Heiss. 2002. Lower heart rate variability is associated with the development of coronary heart disease in individuals with diabetes. The Atherosclerosis Risk in Communities (ARIC) Study. *Diabetes* 51: 3524–3531.

Lim, J.H., E.S. Jung, E.K. Choi, D.Y. Jeong, S.W. Jo, J.H. Jin, J.M. Lee, B.H. Park, and S.W. Chae. 2014. Supplementation with *Aspergillus oryzae*-fermented *Gochujang* lowers serum cholesterol in subjects with hyperlipidemia. *Clinical Nutrition* Jun 9. pii: S0261-5614(14)00158-7. doi: 10.1016/j.clnu.2014.05.013. [Epub ahead of print].

Lim, J.S., C.H. Jang, I.A. Lee, H.J. Lee, C.H. Kim, J.H. Park, C.S. Kwon, D.Y. Lim, J.K. Hwang, Y.H. and J.S. Kim 2009. Biotransformation of free isoflavones by *Bacillus* species isolated from traditional *Cheonggukjnag*. *Food Science Biotechnology* 18: 1046–1050.

Ministry of Food and Drug Safety. 2012. Statistical annual report of Food and Food additive. Ministry of Food and Drug Safety. p89. Koreahttp://www.mfds.go.kr/index.do?mid=690&cd=&cmd=v&seq=15989.

Nam, Y.D., Park, S.L., and S.I. Lim. 2012. Microbial composition of the Korean traditional food "kochujang" analyzed by a massive sequencing technique. *Journal of Food Science* 77: 250–256.

Nguewa, J.L., E. Sobngwi, E. Wawo, M. Azabji-Kenfack, M. Dehayem, E. Ngassam, and J.C. Mbanya. 2011. Cardiac autonomic neuropathy: Characteristics and associated factors in a group of patients with type 2 diabetes. *Diabetes and Metabolism* 37: 43.

Okamoto, A., H. Hanagata, Y. Kawamura, and F. Yanagida. 1995. Antihypertensive substances in fermented soybean and *natto*. *Plant Foods for Human Nutrition* 47: 39–47.

Park, J.M. and H.I. Oh. 1995.Changes in microflora and enzyme activities of traditional *Kochujang meju* during fermentation. *Korean Journal of Food Science Technology* 27: 56–62.

Park, J.M., S.S. Lee, and H.H. Oh. 1995. Changes in chemical characteristics of traditional Kochujang Mejuduring fermentation. *Korean Journal Food and Nutrition* 8: 184–191.

Park, K., K. Kong, K. Jung, and S. Rhee. 2001. Inhibitory effect of *kochujang* extracts on the tumor formation and lung metastasis in mice. *Journal of Food Science Nutrition* 6: 181–191.

Park, K.Y. 2009. Science and Functionality of fermented soybean products. *Korea Jang Cooperation* 105–130, CRC Press, Korea.

Park, S., H. Lee, and K. Kang. 1998. A study on the effect of oligosaccharides on growth of intestinal bacteria. *Korean Journal Dairy Science* 10.

RDA. 2011. *Food Composition Table* (8th ed). Seoul, Republic of Korea, The Korean Nutrition Society.

Rhee, S., K. Kong, K. Jung, and K. Park. 2003. Decreasing effect of *Kochujang* on body weight and lipid levels of adipose tissues and serum in rats fed a high fat diet. *Journal of Korean Society Food Science Nutrition* 32: 882–886.

Ryu, B., K. Sugiyama, J.S. Kim, M.H. Park, and G. Moo. 2007. Studies on physiological and functional properties of *Susijang* fermented soybean paste. *Journal Korean Society Food Science Nutrition* 36: 317–142.

Shurtleff, W. and A. Aoyagi. 2012. History of Natto and its relatives. *Extensively Annotated Biblography and Source book*. Japan.http://books.google.co.kr/books?id=53cqYOK4l98C&pg=PA369&dq=bacillus+natto,+sawamura,1985,+B.+natto&hl=ko&sa=X&ei=u1aqU-C6DI3EkwWE3YDYAg&ved=0CB0Q6AEwAA#v=onepage&q=bacillus%20natto%2C%20sawamura%2C1985%2C%20B.%20natto&f=false.

Shin, D.H. 2011. Utilization of soybean as food stuffs in Korea. In *Soybean and Nutrition*. Ed. H.A. El-Shemy. *Intech Inpress* 81–110.

Shin, D.H., D.Y. Kwon, Y.S. Kim, and D.Y. Jeong. 2012. Science and technology of Korean *Gochujang*. *Public Health Education* 10–133.

Shin, S.K., J.H. Kwon, M. Jeon, J. Choi, and M.S. Choi. 2011. Supplementation of *Cheonggukjang* and Red Ginseng *Cheonggukjang* can improve plasma lipid profile and fasting blood glucose concentration in subjects with impaired fasting glucose. *Journal of Medicinal Food* 14: 108–113.

Singh, J.P., M.G. Larson, H. Tsuji, J.C. Evans, C.J. O'Donnell, and D. Levy. 1998. Reduced heart rate variability and new-onset hypertension insights into pathogenesis of hypertension: The Framingham Heart Study. *Hypertension* 32: 293–297.

Soh, J.R., D.H. Shin, D.Y. Kwon, and Y.S. Cha. 2008. Effect of *Cheonggukjang* supplementation upon hepatic acyl-CoA synthase, carnitine palmitoyltransferase I, acyl-CoA oxidase and uncoupling protein 2 mRNA levels in C57BL/6 J mice fed with high fat diet. *Genes and Nutrition* 2: 365–369.

Son, M. 1995. Anticancer effect of doenjang and its mechanisms in mice. MS thesis, Pusan National University, Busan, Korea.

Song, H., Y. Kim, and K. Lee. 2008. Antioxidant and anticancer activities of traditional Kochujang added with garlic porridge. *Journal of Life Science* 18: 1140–1146.
Sung, M.H., C. Park, C.J. Kim, H. Poo, K. Soda, and M. Ashiuchi. 2005. Natural and edible biopolymer poly-gamma-glutamic acid: Synthesis, production, and applications. *Chemical Record* 5: 352–366.
The Korean Nutrition Society. 2009. *Food Values*. Han Aha Ruem p. 482. Korea.
Tiisala, S., M.I. Majuri, O. Carpen, and R. Renkonen. 1994. Genistein enhances the ICAM-mediated adhesion by inducing the expression of ICAM-1 and its counter-receptors. *Biochemistry Biophysics Research Community* 203: 443–449.
Tolhurst, G., H. Heffron, Y.S. Lam, H.E. Parker, A.M. Habib, E. Diakogiannaki, J. Cameron, J. Grosse, F. Reimann, and F.M. Gribble. 2012. Short-chain fatty acids stimulate glucagon-like peptide-1 secretion via the g-protein-coupled receptor FFAR2. *Diabetes* 61: 364–371.
Velichkovskii, B.T. 2001. Free radical oxidation as a link of early and prolonged adaptation to environmental factors. *Vestnik Rossiiskoi Akademii Meditsinskikh Nauk* 6: 45–52.
Wei, H., L. Wei, F. Frenkel, R. Brown, and S. AMS. 1993. Inhibition of tumor promoter-induced hydrogen peroxide formation *in vitro* and *in vivo* by genistein. *Nutrition Cancer* 20: 1–8.
Wu, W.J. and A. Yong. 2011. Improved menaquinone (Vitamin K_2) production in *cheonggukjang* by optimization of the fermentation conditions. *Food Science and Biotechnology* 20: 1585–1591.
Yang, B. 2000. Hypolipidemic effect of extracts of soybean paste containing mycelia of mushrooms in hyperlipidemic rats. *Korean Journal Microbiology and Biotechnology* 28: 228–232.
Yang, J., S. Lee, and Y. Song. 2003. Improving effect of powders of cooked soybean and *Chungkukjang* on blood pressure and lipid metabolism in spontaneously hypertensive rats. *Journal Korean Society Food Science Nutrition* 32: 899–905.

Chapter 13

Health Benefits of *Natto*

Toshirou Nagai

Contents

13.1 Introduction

Natto is an unsalted fermented soybean food produced and consumed mainly in Japan (Figure 13.1; Nagai and Tamang 2010).

A Gram-positive rod-shaped *Bacillus* strain was isolated from *natto* and named *Bacillus natto* (Sawamura 1906). Later, *B. natto* was included in *Bacillus subtilis* in Bergey's *Manual of Determinative Bacteriology*, 8th edition, because of the biochemical and bacteriological similarities between them (Gibson and Gordon 1974). DNA–DNA hybridization and phylogenic analyses of *Bacillus* strains strongly supported the fact that *Bacillus* strains isolated from *natto* or *natto* starters were *B. subtilis* (Seki et al. 1975, Tamang et al. 2002, Kubo et al. 2011). Industrial strains of *B. subtilis* used for producing *natto* are, however, often called *B. subtilis* (*natto*) to distinguish

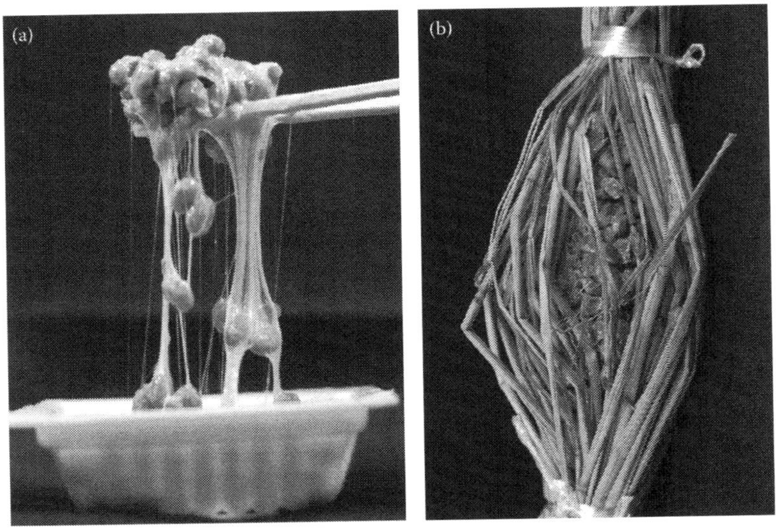

Figure 13.1 ***Natto*****. (a) The most popular type of *natto*, served in a white polystyrene box. The strings are a viscous polymer of PGA. (b) The traditional form of *natto*. These days the rice straw is sterilized and the *natto* is sold as a souvenir.**

them from the typical strains of *B. subtilis*, which cannot produce *natto*. *B. subtilis* (*natto*) is also distinguishable from *B. subtilis* by its requirement for biotin (Kida et al. 1956). Interestingly, the type strain of *B. subtilis* has no plasmids or insertion sequences, as found in *B. subtilis* (*natto*) strains (Tanaka and Koshikawa 1977, Hara et al. 1981, Nagai et al. 2000, Kimura and Itoh 2007). Other important differences are: *natto* is characterized by an ammonia odor, short-chain fatty acids (Ikeda and Tsuno 1984, Kanno et al. 1984), and a highly viscous polymer composed of poly-γ-glutamic acid (PGA) and levan (fructose polymer) (Fujii 1963). The viscosity of *natto* is due to PGA and is an important determinant of the quality of *natto* (Figure 13.1a).

The process of *natto* fermentation is very simple: cleaned soybeans are soaked in water, boiled, inoculated with spores of *B. subtilis* (*natto*), and incubated (Figure 13.2).

Until a century ago, *natto* was produced by wrapping boiled soybeans in bags made of rice straw, which *B. subtilis* (*natto*) inhabits (Figure 13.1b). The rice straw served as both the source

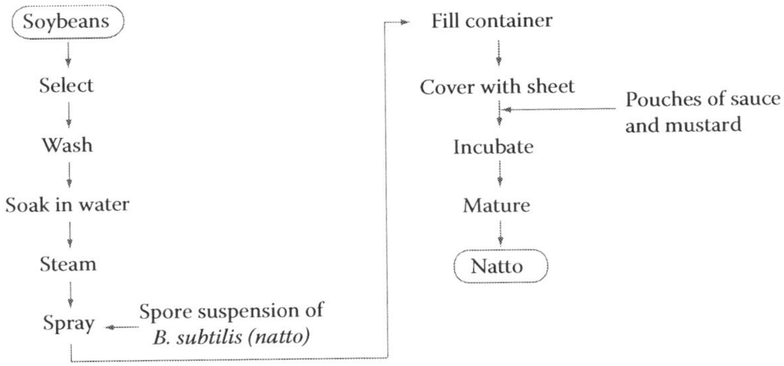

Figure 13.2 Process of *natto* production.

of inoculum and the storage container. With the discovery of *B. subtilis* (*natto*), this method was abandoned for reasons of hygiene, and polystyrene boxes are now used (Figure 13.1a). *Natto* is usually eaten raw (one 30–50 g package per meal) with cooked rice and soy sauce or seasonings. It is also used in sushi, Chinese fried rice, spaghetti, snacks, and so on.

The Japanese have eaten *natto* for over a thousand years without any harm to health. This indicates that both *natto* and *B. subtilis* (*natto*) are safe. In addition, most of the medical effects of *natto*, passed down in folklore or proverbs for hundreds of years, have been supported by scientific analyses or investigations, as described below.

13.2 Nutritional Aspects of *Natto*

Soybean is rich in proteins, earning it the sobriquet "meat from the field." Boiled soybeans (water content, 63.5%) contain 16.0% protein, whereas beef shoulder (water content, 66.3%) contains 20.2%. *Natto* inherits this nutritional advantage. *B. subtilis* (*natto*) produces proteases (Akimoto et al. 1990, Nakamura et al. 1992), which digest the proteins to peptides or amino acids (Figure 13.3; Ohta et al. 1964).

This explains the easy digestibility of *natto*. However, after consuming the sugars, *B. subtilis* (*natto*) dissimilates the amino acids and releases ammonia via deamination. So although longer fermentation facilitates the digestion of proteins, the release of ammonia impacts the eating quality of the *natto*.

Experiments using rats showed that the digestion–absorption rate of soybean nitrogen increased after fermentation by *B. subtilis* (*natto*) from 81.0% to 83.6% (Miura 1959). Over 79 days, rats gained 166.4 g on dried and boiled soybeans but 180.6 g on *natto*. There were no differences in serum

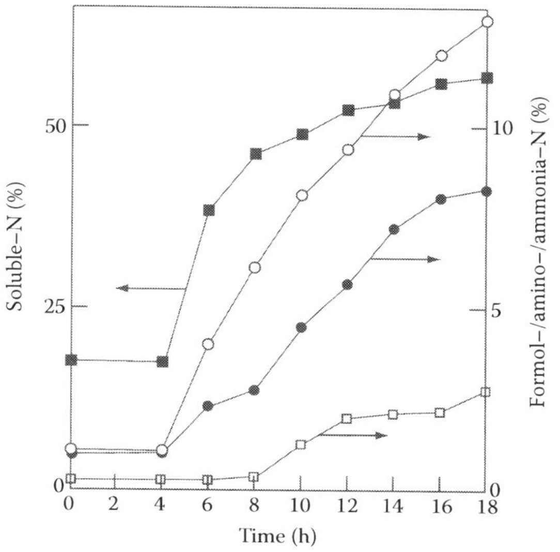

Figure 13.3 Digestion of proteins during *natto* fermentation. Ratios of soluble N content (■), formol N (from amino acids and oligopeptides) content (○), amino N content (●), and ammonia N content (□) to total N content in soybeans. Arrows indicates the *y*-axis. (From Ohta, T. et al. 1964. *Report of the Food Research Institute* 18: 46–52 [In Japanese].)

biochemical measures. The digestion–absorption rates of soybeans after fermentation increased from 71% to 81% of crude protein and from 73% to 82% of crude fat, and although the content of carbohydrate decreased from 20 to 15 g/100 g, the digestion–absorption rate dropped from 98% to only 97% (Fujii 1953). These reports suggest the nutritional superiority of *natto* over that of boiled soybeans. In the other research, in contrast, *natto* had a slightly lower digestion–absorption rate of protein and net efficiency of energy utilization than boiled soybeans, and products made from soy milk had higher values (Table 13.1) (Science and Technology Agency of Japan 1979).

In addition, *natto* was not always nutritionally superior to boiled soybeans, as measured by apparent absorption rates of nitrogen and fat in humans and by growth efficiency and protein efficiency in rats (Arimoto and Tamura 1964). So it could be concluded that fermentation by *B. subtilis* (*natto*) does not contribute greatly to the effective utilization of nutrients in soybeans by humans.

An advantage of *B. subtilis* (*natto*) proteases is the decomposition of a major allergenic protein, *Gly m* Bd 30 K, in soybeans. Although the protein was detected in unfermented soybean foods (soy milk, *tofu*, *yuba* [soy milk skin]), it was not detected in fermented soybean foods (*natto*, *miso*, soysauce) (Tsuji et al. 1995), and was degraded during fermentation (Yamanishi et al. 1995). Although the degradation of allergens does not actively promote human health, it reduces the risk of allergies caused by soy proteins. However, several cases of *natto*-induced late-onset anaphylaxis have been reported in Japan (Inomata et al. 2004, Matsubayashi et al. 2010, Horimukai et al. 2011). The causal agents of the anaphylaxis were found to be two proteins in the *natto* extract: allergens to the patient were not detected in either the soybean itself or in the suspension of *B. subtilis* (*natto*) cells (Inomata et al. 2004). It should be emphasized that the late-onset anaphylaxis induced by *natto* is a very, very rare disease.

Table 13.1 Digestion–Absorption Rates of Protein (Nitrogen) and Fat and Net Efficiency of Energy Utilization on Japanese Soybean Foods

	Protein (%)	*Fat (%)*	*Energy (%, net)*
Soybean (boiled)	92.0	90.1	85.3
Natto	90.1	92.7	82.5
Tofu	96.6	96.4	93.4
Abura-age	90.7	98.1	87.6
Nama-age	96.6	98.3	91.1
Kori-dofu	92.9	93.8	88.3
Yuba	100	100	98.5
Kinako	78.1	86.8	78.8

Source: Science and Technology Agency of Japan. 1979. *Research Report on the Revision of the Standard Table of Food Composition in Japan*. Tokyo: Science and Technology Agency of Japan [In Japanese, translated title].

Note: *Tofu*, coagulated soy milk; *Abura-age*, fried sliced *tofu*; *Nama-age*, fried *tofu*; *Kori-dofu*, frozen and dehydrated *tofu*; *Yuba*, soy milk skin; *Kinako*, flour of roasted soybeans. Contents of protein were based on the contents of total N determined by the Kjeldahl method.

B. subtilis (*natto*) consumes most oligosaccharides in soybeans and decreases glucose and fructose to near 0% after 18 h fermentation (Kanno et al. 1982). Levansucrase produces levan, a fructose polymer, from the fructose monomers. Although soybean oligosaccharides favor intestinal microflora, *B. subtilis* (*natto*) greatly decreases this advantage. Instead, however, *B. subtilis* (*natto*) itself has probiotic effects, as described below.

During soaking, soybeans absorb about 1.2 times their weight of water, halving the contents of most nutrients (Table 13.2). In addition, about 2% of the solids content is lost to the water (Ohta et al. 1964). Therefore, soaking time should be kept to a minimum. The most prominent change during fermentation is an increase in the content of vitamin K, which is produced by *B. subtilis* (*natto*). Vitamin K is discussed below.

13.3 Functional Aspects of *Natto*

Soybean contains many kinds of functional components: metals, dietary fibers, lectins, phytate, saponins, isoflavones, unsaturated fatty acids, vitamins, polyphenols, and so on (Science and Technology Agency of Japan 1979, Cabrera-Orozco et al. 2013). Two oligosaccharides, stachyose and raffinose, enhance the growth of bifidobacteria in human intestines, but are consumed by *B. subtilis* (*natto*) during fermentation (Kanno et al. 1982). *B. subtilis* (*natto*) improves intestinal microflora in other ways, as described in Section 13.3.3.

13.3.1 Nattokinase

Natto can digest insoluble fibrin (Sumi et al. 1987). The enzyme responsible was named nattokinase, after *natto* and urokinase. Thus, *natto* might supply a thrombolytic enzyme. Commercial thrombolytic enzymes (streptokinase, urokinase, tissue plasminogen activator, etc.) are used to treat thrombotic diseases, but are expensive, have a short shelf-life, or have undesirable side effects. On the other hand, *natto* is a very cheap and safe food. If it could achieve thrombolysis *in vivo*, or activate the built-in fibrinolytic system in humans, it could bring huge benefits.

Nattokinase is a serine protease of the subtilisin family, with a molecular weight of 28 kDa and 257 amino acid residues (Fujita et al. 1993). It is stable at pH 7–12 and below 60°C. Its N-terminal amino acid sequence is identical to that of elastase, a protease which digests the elastin that supports collagen fibers and that is also produced in *natto* (Muramatsu et al. 1994, Sumi et al. 1999).

The nattokinase activity of 1 g of *natto* is equivalent to the fibrinolytic activity of 40 CU of plasmin or 1600 IU of urokinase (typical quantities used in treatment). When healthy adult volunteers ate 200 g (about 4 times the usual maximum in Japan) of *natto* at breakfast, activation of the fibrinolytic system, shortening of euglobulin lysis time, and enhancement of euglobulin fibrinolytic activity in plasma were observed after 2–4 h (Sumi et al. 1990). Purified nattokinase (1.3 g taken after meals 3 times a day) increased the amount of degradation products from fibrin/fibrinogen in serum, tissue plasminogen activator, and euglobulin fibrinolytic activity (Sumi et al. 1990). All these changes indicate that nattokinase can activate the fibrinolytic system in humans when ingested. Intravenously injected nattokinase proteolyzed chemically-induced thrombosis in rats (Fujita et al. 1995). However, such treatment is difficult to apply in humans.

In addition to nattokinase, *natto* has at least three pro-urokinase activators that differ from nattokinase in molecular weight and in the strength of their activity (Sumi et al. 1996). Oral administration of dried *natto* with a high level of the pro-urokinase activators enhanced plasma

Table 13.2 Nutritional Composition per 100 g of Boiled Soybeans, *Natto* and Raw Soybeans

	Boiled Soybeans	*Natto*	*Raw Soybeans*
Energy (kcal)	180	200	417
Water (g)	63.5	59.5	12.5
Protein (g)	16.0	16.5	35.3
Lipid (g)	9.0	10.0	19.0
Carbohydrate (g)	9.7	12.1	28.2
Ash (g)	1.8	1.9	5.0
Minerals			
Sodium (mg)	1	2	1
Potassium (mg)	570	660	1900
Calcium (mg)	70	90	240
Magnesium (mg)	110	100	220
Phosphorus (mg)	190	190	580
Iron (mg)	2.0	3.3	9.4
Zinc (mg)	2.0	1.9	3.2
Copper (mg)	0.24	0.61	0.98
Vitamins			
A, retinol (μg)	(0)	(0)	(0)
A, α-carotene (μg)	0	–	0
A, β-carotene (μg)	3	–	6
A, cryptoxanthin (μg)	0	–	0
D (μg)	(0)	(0)	(0)
E, α-tocopherol (mg)	0.8	0.5	1.8
E, β-tocopherol (mg)	0.3	0.2	0.7
E, γ-tocopherol (mg)	6.0	5.9	14.4
E, δ-tocopherol (mg)	3.4	3.3	8.2
K (μg)	7	600	18
B_1 (mg)	0.22	0.07	0.83
B_2 (mg)	0.09	0.56	0.30
Niacin (mg)	0.5	1.1	2.2
B_6 (mg)	0.11	0.24	0.53
B_{12} (μg)	(0)	Tr	0
Folate (μg)	39	120	230
Pantothenic acid (mg)	0.29	3.60	1.52
C (mg)	Tr	Tr	Tr

Table 13.2 (*Continued*) Nutritional Composition per 100 g of Boiled Soybeans, *Natto* and Raw Soybeans

	Boiled Soybeans	*Natto*	*Raw Soybeans*
Fatty acids			
Saturated (g)	1.22	1.47	2.59
Monounsaturated (g)	1.73	1.90	3.66
Polyunsaturated (g)	4.93	5.39	10.41
Cholesterol			
Cholesterol (mg)	(Tr)	Tr	Tr
Dietary fibers			
Soluble (g)	0.9	2.3	1.8
Insoluble (g)	6.1	4.4	15.3

Source: Ministry of Education, Culture, Sports, Science and Technology. 2010. *Standard Tables of Food Composition in Japan: Food Composition Database.* http://fooddb.jp/
Note: –, not determined; (), estimated; Tr, trace.

fibrinolysis (Sumi et al. 1996). The factors were also found to be serine proteases, and nattokinase could activate pro-urokinase (Sumi et al. 1992). Nattokinase and the pro-urokinase activators catalyze various reactions (Figure 13.4).

Following the discovery of nattokinase, nattokinase-rich *natto* products, supplements, and food additives have been developed (Kiuchi and Suzuki 1991, Takaoka 2003). *B. subtilis* (*natto*) strain NN-1, which had previously been reported to produce high levels of PGA and protease, was also found to produce more nattokinase than other commercial strains (Kiuchi and Suzuki 1991, Nagai et al. 1994). Higher-producing strains may yet be found.

13.3.2 Antibiotic Activity

B. subtilis (*natto*) has antibiotic or antagonistic activities against some microorganisms. Early researchers focused on its effects on human-pathogenic bacteria because of rampant infection in Japan at that time. In the first attempt at a cure by the administration of *natto*, a patient infected with *Salmonella* Paratyphi B that could not be eradicated by drugs was fed *natto* and *B. subtilis* (*natto*) together; and the bacteria were not detected in his feces after the 4th day (*B. subtilis* [*natto*] alone was not sufficient) (Eguchi and Kumashiro 1931). *B. subtilis* (*natto*) and its culture filtrate had antibacterial activity against *Salmonella* Paratyphi A and B (Matsumura 1934b). The activity was lost by heating. *B. subtilis* (*natto*) injected intraperitoneally with Paratyphi A, Paratyphi B, or *Salmonella enterica* var. *enterica* serovar. Typhi into mice did not prevent death (Matsumura 1934c), but injected 24–48 h before the target pathogens did prevent death, indicating that it took time to show antagonistic activity. Antagonism against *S. enterica* var. *enterica* serovar. Typhi was confirmed (Saito 1938). It did not have *in vivo* antagonistic effects on *Escherichia coli* or *Shigella dysenteriae*. Dead cells and culture filtrate of *B. subtilis* (*natto*) had no *in vivo* inhibitory activity against target pathogens. Although oral administration of *B. subtilis* (*natto*) protected mice from death caused by *S. dysenteriae*, the *S. dysenteriae* remained in the intestines and continued to be detected in the feces (Arima 1937). *B. subtilis* (*natto*) inhibited the *in vitro* growth of

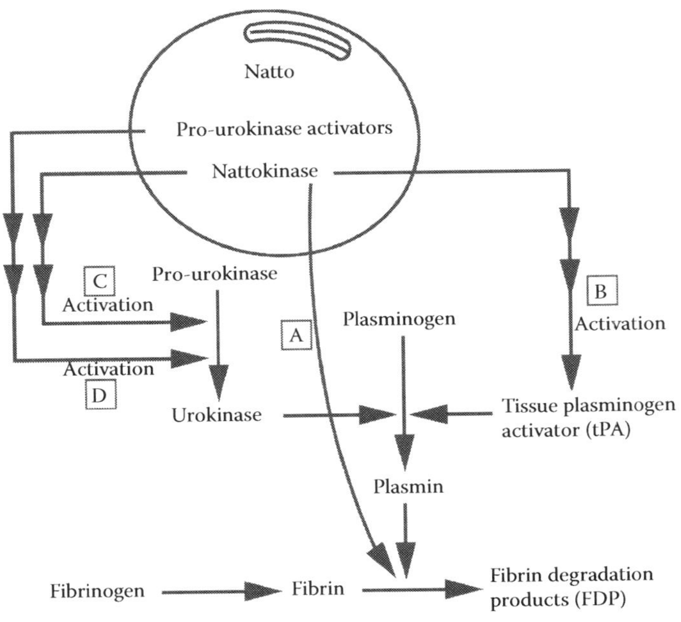

Figure 13.4 Fibrinolysis activities in *natto*. (A) *In vitro* digestion of fibrin (Sumi et al. 1987) or *in vivo* direct hydrolysis of fibrin in a vessel after intravenous injection (Fujita et al. 1995). (B) Activation of tissue plasminogen activator by nattokinase (Sumi et al. 1990). (C) Activation of pro-urokinase by nattokinase (Sumi et al. 1992). (D) Activation of pro-urokinase by pro-urokinase activators (Sumi et al. 1996). Double arrowheads indicate unknown pathways. (From Nagai, T. 2014. *Handbook of Indigenous Foods Involving Alkaline Fermentation*, Boca Raton, FL, USA: CRC Press, pp. 355–359.)

E. coli, *Salmonella pullorum*, *Salmonella typhimurium*, *Clostridium perfringens*, and *Fusobacterium necrophorum*, which had been isolated from humans and animals, depending on strain and dose (Kanoe et al. 1982). Fluctuations in antagonism might depend on the strains of *B. subtilis* (*natto*) and pathogens tested and on experimental conditions. A mouthwash using culture extract of *B. subtilis* (*natto*), which is commercially supplied, showed a high cure rate for periodontitis of 83% (Tsubura 2012). One-month rinse by the mouthwash could reduce the swelling of gums and drive out microorganisms in plaque from periodontitis patients.

B. subtilis (*natto*) also inhibits the growth of fungi and yeasts. Rubbed in directly or as an ointment, it cured patients of ringworm caused by *Trichophyton* fungus (Senbon 1940). Culture filtrate inhibited the growth of *Candida albicans*, dependent on target stain (Ozawa et al. 1979). The presence of *B. subtilis* (*natto*) in a continuous-flow culture system decreased the viable counts of cocultured *C. albicans*. Extracts from *natto* also inhibited an *Aspergillus* fungus, *Saccharomyces cerevisiae*, and a blue mold (Sumi 1997). The intraperitoneal or intravenous injection of *B. subtilis* (*natto*) cells did not harm test mice or rabbits (Matsumura 1934a). This result indicates its safety, even if it enters blood vessels.

An antibiotic compound produced by *B. subtilis* (*natto*) was identified as dipicolinic acid (Figure 13.5), which inhibited the growth of a variety of microorganisms, including fungi and yeasts, at concentrations ranging from 0.03% to 1.2% (Udo 1936).

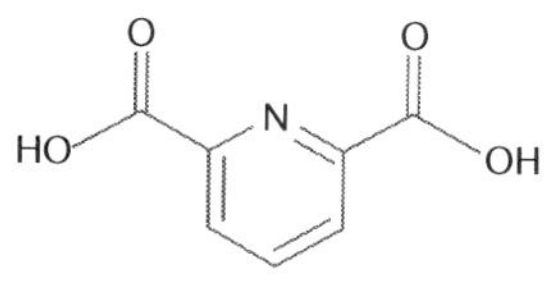

Figure 13.5 Dipicolinic acid.

Dipicolinic acid at around 1% inhibited the growth of *B. subtilis* (*natto*) itself. Dipicolinic acid is localized in spores; it was present in commercial *natto* at 6–48 mg/100 g and in *B. subtilis* (*natto*) cells at 500–3600 mg/100 g (Sumi and Ohosugi 1999).

13.3.3 Probiotics

The traditional treatment of gastrointestinal upsets by *natto* indicates that the Japanese have empirically recognized the probiotic effects of *natto* for a long time. The treatment of domestic animals with *natto* is now under investigation as a replacement for antibiotics (Kimura 1979). The administration of *B. subtilis* (*natto*) resulted in body weight gain and disease resistance in chickens (Ebata et al. 1960, Kimura 1979) and swine (Kimura 1979, Saka 2008), and in improvement of milk production in cows (Sun et al. 2013). Although the mechanisms may vary, the probiotic effect of *B. subtilis* (*natto*) might be summarized boldly from many investigations as follows: in the intestines, it favors the growth of "good" bacteria (*Bifidobacterium* and *Lactobacillus*) and suppresses the growth of "bad" bacteria (*Clostridium*, Enterobacteriaceae, and *Streptococcus*) (Murata et al. 1977, Ozawa et al. 1981, Tsuchihashi et al. 1986, Isshiki and Onozaki 1992, Maruta et al. 1996a,b, Saka 2008). Oral administration of *B. subtilis* (*natto*) or *natto* to human adults increased *Bifidobacterium* counts in feces (Terada et al. 1999, Mitsui et al. 2006) and decreased counts of lecithinase-positive clostridia (Terada et al. 1999). Although *B. subtilis* C-3102 spores decreased the number of Enterobacteriaceae and the contents of ammonia and putrefactive products in feces, exceptions were also observed (Suzuki et al. 2004). The spores did not affect the number of lactic acid bacteria. The results depend on experimental conditions (including age and sex of subjects, the region of the intestine, diet, and microflora before the experiments).

There were no significant probiotic effects from either boiled soybeans or soybeans in which the oligosaccharides were enzymatically digested (to mimic the degradation of oligosaccharides in *natto*; Kanno et al. 1982), indicating that the *B. subtilis* (*natto*) cells, or fermentation by the bacteria, or products produced by the bacteria (e.g., antibiotics) are essential for probiotic effects (Isshiki and Onozaki 1992, Mitsui et al. 2006, Takemura et al. 2009). As spores and cells of *B. subtilis* (*natto*) find it difficult to germinate and grow in the intestines (Murata et al. 1977, Hisanaga et al. 1978, Hisanaga 1980), it is unlikely that the bacteria produce bioactive agents there. The fluid from the spores or from germinated or lysed cells might instead promote the intestinal microflora. On the other hand, Ozawa et al. (1981) reported increased recovery of *B. subtilis* (*natto*) administered to pigs, indicating multiplication of the bacteria in the digestive organs. Hosoi et al. (1999) observed that the growth of *Lactobacillus murinus* was enhanced by intact spores of *B. subtilis* (*natto*), but not by autoclaved ones, and they thought that the germination or growth of *B. subtilis* (*natto*) in the intestines might be important for probiotic effects (Hosoi et al. 1999). The mechanisms by which *B. subtilis* (*natto*) exerts its probiotic effects, including the behavior of spores or living cells in the digestive system, remain to be elucidated but antibiotic production by the bacteria could be responsible.

13.3.4 Immunomodulating Activity

Prior inoculation of hosts with *B. subtilis* (*natto*) cells can avoid death due to pathogenic bacteria. This phenomenon, named nonspecific immunity, was investigated using mice and *Staphylococcus aureus*. Ohkuro et al. (1974) injected live *B. subtilis* (*natto*) cells, dead cells, or dead *Staph. aureus* cells intraperitoneally into mice before administering live *Staph. aureus* cells. The dead *Staph. aureus* cells promoted resistance as expected. In addition, the live *B. subtilis* (*natto*) cells conferred resistance, but the resistance waned as the period between inoculation and challenge increased. The peak of the nonspecific immunity was around 1–3 days after inoculation (Komatsuzaki et al. 1978). Dead *B. subtilis* (*natto*) cells were effective only 3 days before the challenge. The effectiveness of the nonspecific immunity conferred by *B. subtilis* (*natto*) depended on the strain, but not on whether the cells were vegetative or spores (Komatsuzaki et al. 1976, 1979, Ohkuro et al. 1980).

Although *B. subtilis* (*natto*) produces antibiotics, the antibiotics are not responsible for the nonspecific immunity, because *B. subtilis* (*natto*) did not inhibit the growth of *Staph. aureus* in a mixed culture (Komatsuzaki et al. 1978). The nonspecific immunity was ascribed to an increase in the number of phagocytes (neutrophils), stimulated by *B. subtilis* (*natto*) (Suzuki 1975). Some enzymes might additionally be involved (Komatsuzaki et al. 1976, 1979).

Several research groups have reported stimulation of the immune system by *B. subtilis* (*natto*). It induced the production of interferon type II in mice after intravenous injection: the active fraction was not identified, but there seemed to be a variety of molecules localized on the surface of the cells of *B. subtilis* (*natto*) or contained in the cells (Sato 1980). The active fraction also enhanced the induction of interferon type I (Sato 1980). Heat-treated and formalin-treated *Bacillus* cells implanted with target lymphoma cells increased the natural killer (NK) activity of mice spleen cells against the lymphoma, and they increased the production of antibodies against sheep red blood cells (Hamajima et al. 1983). Oral administration of *natto* also increased frequencies and activities of NK cells from Peyer's patches of murine intestines, but not from spleens (Kobayashi et al. 2013). Chickens fed a diet with *B. subtilis* (*natto*) cells showed increased production of antibodies against sheep red blood cells after injection of the antigen, owing to the postulated stimulation of lymphoid organs in the intestinal tract by the bacteria or a substance originating from them (Inooka and Kimura 1983). *B. subtilis* (*natto*) cells induced the secretion of cytokines, IL (interleukin)-6 and IL-8, by epithelial-like human colon carcinoma Caco-2 cells (Hosoi et al. 2003). Autoclaved cells and spores of *B. subtilis* (*natto*) and mucilage produced by *B. subtilis* (*natto*) induced production of IL-12 p40 and TNF (tumor necrosis factor)-α by murine macrophages (J744.1 and RAW264.7, respectively). The active fraction was identified as levan, a polysaccharide in the mucilage of *natto* (Xu et al. 2006). Orally administered levan decreased both IgE and IL-4 levels of mice; this result indicates the possibility of the suppression of allergic diseases. *B. subtilis* (*natto*) TTCC865 cells (vegetative cells, spores, or disrupted cells) induced IL-12 p40 production by a mouse J774.1 macrophage-like cell line (Kawane 2007). *B. subtilis* (*natto*) also reduced inflammation and IgE production and increased IgG2a and INF(interferon)-γ production in model mice with atopic dermatitis. An orally administered encapsulated extract of products of *B. subtilis* (*natto*) increased NK cell activity in peripheral blood mononuclear cells in50% of tested healthy adult rats (Takeda et al. 2005). These results show that the oral administration of the bacteria or their products can enhance immunological activities in animals, as well as humans.

An epidemiological study on the relationship of maternal intake of foods during pregnancy and occurrence of infant eczema showed that frequent intake of *natto* might reduce the occurrence in 6-month-old infants (Ozawa et al. 2014). The authors thought that *natto* could cause improvement of the intestinal environments (see Section 13.3.3) and immune regulation in the mothers' bodies, resulting in the decrease of eczema in the infants. However, the details remain to be elucidated.

13.3.5 Antitumor Activity

B. subtilis (*natto*) KMD 1126 had antitumor activity against Ehrlich carcinoma cells (Kameda et al. 1968). The carcinoma cells were implanted into the groins of mice and 2 days later *B. subtilis* (*natto*) cells were injected there. The weight of the challenged tumors decreased remarkably in comparison with the control tumors. The antitumor activity of the *B. subtilis* (*natto*) cells might be due to cooperation among surfactins (Figure 13.6), protease, and an unknown acidic substance (Kameda et al. 1971, 1972, 1978).

Whereas all the control mice implanted intraperitoneally with tumor cells alone died within 16 days, 65% of the mice implanted with both tumor cells and *B. subtilis* (*natto*) cells survived for 35 days (Hamajima et al. 1983). The *in vivo* antitumor activity of the bacteria was effective only at the early stage of carcinogenesis. A hexane extract of *natto* inhibited the tumor-promoting activity of phorbol acetate *in vitro* as measured by a dye-transfer method (Takahashi et al. 1995). Cultured cells treated with the tumor promoter showed reduced dye transfer through gap junctions, but the extract recovered the dye transfer. The activity was ascribed to straight-chain saturated hydrocarbons with 30–32 carbons, of which C_{31} (hentriacontane) had the strongest activity. How the hydrocarbons are produced remains unclear. That soybeans and *Bacillus* cells do not contain the hydrocarbons may indicate that the fermentation of soybeans by *B. subtilis* (*natto*) or the growth conditions of the bacteria are essential to their production. One package of *natto* is enough to give an effective concentration of the hydrocarbons in the blood to prevent the promotion of cancers, if the hydrocarbons are absorbed effectively into the blood (Takahashi et al. 1995).

13.3.6 Vitamin K

Vitamin K-dependent proteins are important regulators of health; these include blood coagulation factors (II or prothrombin, VII, IX, and X), blood coagulation inhibitors (proteins C and S), Ca^{2+}-binding protein of bone matrix (osteocalcin), matrix Gla protein, and growth arrest-specific gene 6 product (Vermeer 2012). Vitamin K_1 (phylloquinone) is derived from plants and vitamin K_2 (menaquinone) from bacteria. *B. subtilis* (*natto*) produces vitamin K_2 with 7 isoprene units as its side chain (menaquinone-7, MK-7). *Natto* contains 8.6 μg/g MK-7 and very small amounts of vitamin K_1, MK-4,-5,-6, and -8 (Sakano et al. 1988)—6.2 μg/g (Ikeda 1992) or 6.0 μg/g (Table 13.2). The vitamin K_1 in *natto* is derived from the soybeans. Although most vitamin K (including MK-7) is hydrophobic, vitamin K_2 from *natto* is water soluble (Ikeda 1992). Almost all of the vitamin K_2 in *natto* occurs in the water outside of the beans and bacterial cells (Figure 13.7). The vitamin K_1 remains in the soybeans and is not extracted into the water.

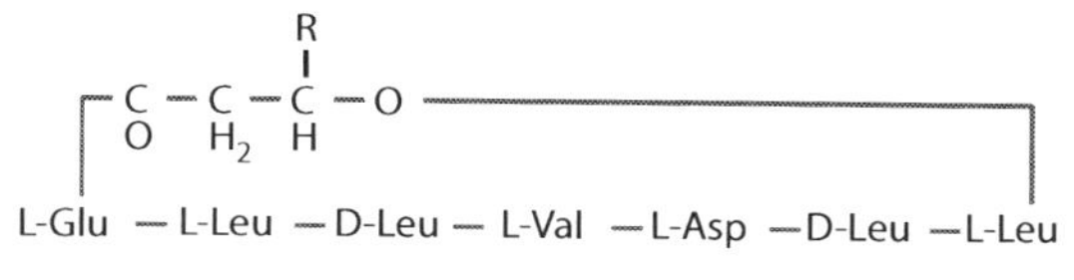

Figure 13.6 Basic structure of surfactins. R = hydrocarbon moiety.

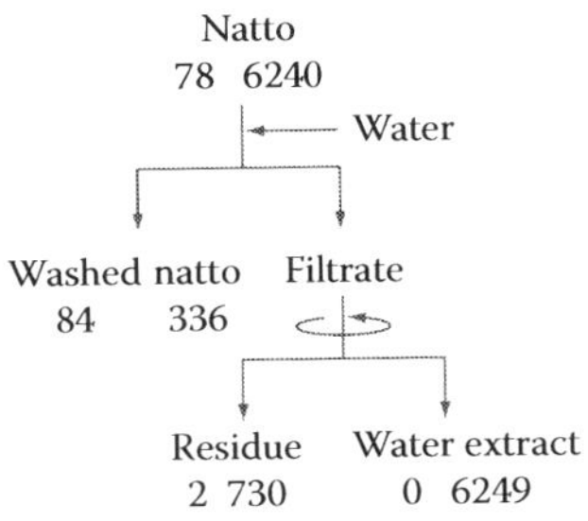

Figure 13.7 Fractionation of vitamin K in *natto*. Left-hand number of each pair, vitamin K_1; right-hand number, vitamin K_2(ng/g). The washed *natto* was strained through gauze and the water was centrifuged to obtain the residue and extract fractions. (From Ikeda, H. 1992. *Journal of Home Economics of Japan* 43: 643–648 [In Japanese].)

Glycopeptides surround MK-7 molecules produced by *B. subtilis* (*natto*) to form water-soluble mixed micelles of 100 kDa (Ikeda and Doi 1990, Ikeda 1992). The glycopeptides, called vitamin-K_2-binding factor, are 2 kDa, and are composed mainly of acidic amino acids (Glu and Asp) and hydrophobic amino acids (Leu and Val). The water solubility conferred by the glycopeptides seems to favor the uptake of vitamin K into the body. Vitamin K-deficiency bleeding (VKDB) is contracted suddenly by apparently healthy infants, especially breast-fed infants, at a rate of 1 in 1500. VKDB causes intracranial bleeding and the death rate is high. Since VKDB leaves serious after-effects in patients who survive, prevention by injection or oral administration of vitamin K to infants is crucial. One of the causes of VKDB is a low concentration of vitamin K in breast milk. The mean vitamin K concentration in breast milk from *natto*-fed mothers was 20.4 μg/mL, 3.5 times that in the control (5.9 μg/mL) (Ryo and Baba 1981, Ryo 1982). Activities of blood coagulation factors (determined by hepaplastin tests) were 46.6 HPT% in infants fed milk from *natto*-fed mothers but 40.0 HPT% in control infants. Oral administration of *natto* to mothers increased both levels. The placentas of *natto*-fed mothers also contained 10 times more MK-7 than those of the controls (Hiraike et al. 1986). However, the placental permeability of vitamin K is very low, and umbilical cord blood contains less vitamin K than the serum of the mother, so the transport of vitamin K administered orally to the mother via the blood to the fetus is not effective (Shirahata 1987).

Although *natto* is suitable as a source of vitamin K, *natto* along with green vegetables (cabbage, spinach, broccoli) or *Chlorella* is contraindicated for persons who are treated with warfarin, an anticoagulant, as vitamin K and warfarin are mutually antagonistic. Ten patients who had undergone cardiac valve replacement had increased thrombo-test (TT) values (indicating an increase in blood coagulating activity) despite adequate control by oral administration of warfarin: average TT values before and after the abnormal increase were 17% (range, 12%–29%) and 50% (32%–100%), respectively. The patients were found to have eaten *natto*, and one patient with a TT value of 100%, who had eaten *natto* every day, suffered cerebral infarction (Kudo et al. 1978, Kudo 1990). After the patients stopped eating *natto*, their TT values declined to normal within a few days in all but two patients. To investigate, a healthy doctor received warfarin and then *natto*. The warfarin decreased his TT values to 40%. Within 24 h and despite continuous administration of warfarin, his TT value then increased to 86%. TT values in rabbits given warfarin were also increased by powdered *B. subtilis* (*natto*). Two new oral anticoagulants, rivaroxaban and dabigatran, which are not affected by vitamin K, are now available (Phillips and Ansell 2010) to take the place of warfarin.

13.3.7 Isoflavones

Although isoflavones in soybeans have estrogenic, antitumor, and antioxidant activities, too high an intake might harm health, especially when an isoflavone supplement is taken every day. The effect of isoflavones on human health remains inconclusive, but the Food Safety Commission in Japan (2006) recommends a maximum average daily intake of aglycones over the long term of 70–75 mg/day, although it also says that isoflavones have no significant influence on health, even when taken in excess. The median intake by the Japanese over 15 years old is 18 mg/day. Although soy isoflavones have both positive and negative effects, the safety of soybean products has long been known.

Among isoflavones, soybeans contain aglycones (daidzein and genistein), glycosides (daidzin and genistin), and malonyl glycosides (Figure 13.8).

Bacteria in the intestines convert the glycosides into aglycones, which are absorbed into the body. Soaking has no effect on the isoflavone composition in soybeans, but steaming and fermentation by *B. subtilis* (*natto*) change it. After steaming, almost all malonyl glycosides are degraded to glycosides. In turn, 42% of the glycosides are succinylated by *B. subtilis* (*natto*) (Toda et al. 1999, Shimakage et al. 2006). The succinylated isoflavones are also biologically active (Toda et al. 1999). Almost all isoflavones in soybeans remain in the soybeans during fermentation, and the amount in the drainage from the soaking and steaming processes is negligible: about 0.4% of the total is lost. In contrast, a different type of *natto*, *hikiwari-natto* (broken *natto*), loses 9.8% of its isoflavones in dust when the soybeans are broken before soaking (Shimakage et al. 2006).

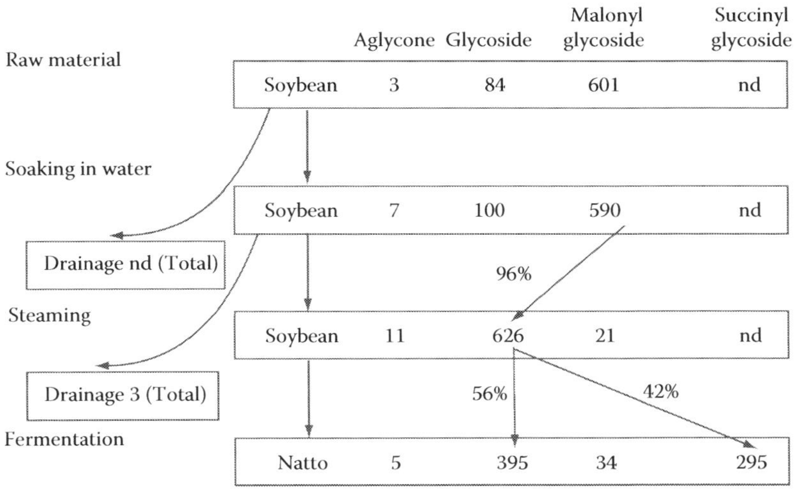

Figure 13.8 Changes in isoflavone contents of soybeans (initial 100 g dry weight) and *natto*. Numbers show contents of isoflavones in μmol. Percentages show conversion rates. nd, not detected. (From Shimakage, A. et al. 2006. *Nippon Shokuhin Kagaku Kogaku Kaishi* 53: 185–188 [In Japanese].)

13.3.8 Angiotensin I-Converting Enzyme Inhibitor

Blood pressure rise in spontaneously hypertensive rats was suppressed by the administration of *natto* or *natto* juice, but not by boiled soybeans (Hayashi et al. 1976). The suppression was canceled when the *natto* was first extracted with ethanol (but not ether). The blood pressure rise was suppressed also by administration of boiled soybeans with the ethanol extract or of boiled soybeans with spores of *B. subtilis* (*natto*). The ethanol-soluble substance was not identified, and the mechanisms of the suppression were not elucidated, but the substance might be an ACE inhibitor.

In the renin–angiotensin system, the ACE cleaves angiotensin I to produce angiotensin II, which is a hypertensive hormone. The ACE also decomposes a hypotensive peptide, bradykinin. Hence, substances or foods which inhibit the ACE *in vivo* would be expected to lower blood pressure in persons with hypertension. Strong ACE-inhibitory activities were detected in 50 samples of *natto*, soybean, other soybean products, shellfish, teas, fruits, and black wheat (Suzuki et al. 1983). The ACE-inhibitory activity of soybean was higher than that of *natto*. The inhibitors were heat-stable substances with low molecular weights (the heat stability of the inhibitor in *natto* was not tested). In 31 fermented foods, *natto* had a comparatively high ACE-inhibitory activity (Okamoto et al. 1995a). About 80% of the ACE-inhibitory activity of *natto* occurred in the viscous material, from which three fractions were partially purified (Okamoto et al. 1995b). Fraction 1, a water extract of the viscous material, seemed to consist of serine protease and an unknown inhibitor, both of which were heat labile and of high molecular weight. Fractions 2 and 3 were an ethanol extract of the supernatant and the precipitate after centrifugation of the viscous material, respectively. Both contained heat-stable ACE inhibitors with low molecular weights (Fraction 2, 780 Da; Fraction 3, 200 Da). However, their modes of ACE inhibition were different. The ratio of ACE-inhibitory activities in the three fractions was roughly 65:35:5. The inhibitors have not been identified yet.

Raw soybeans show ACE-inhibitory activity, which is increased by soaking and decreased by steaming (Ibe et al. 2006). Inoculation of steamed soybeans with *B. subtilis* (*natto*) increases the ACE-inhibitory activity for 16–20 h and then decreases it. Two ACE inhibitors, with molecular weights of 592 and 507 Da, were separated from a methanol extract of *natto* by gel filtration chromatography (Ibe et al. 2009). The inhibitors seemed to be different from inhibitors previously reported. The difference might be due to the solvent used. Oral administration of the 592-Da inhibitor at 1 mg/kg body weight moderately decreased blood pressure of spontaneously hypertensive rats. These results indicate the possibility of pharmaceutical uses of *natto*. However, the ACE inhibitors remain to be identified.

13.3.9 Saponins

Saponins in soybeans, often referred as soyasaponins, have foaming properties and a harsh taste. Although other types of saponins are hemolytic, soyasaponins have a very low degree of hemolysis and no acute toxicity. Moreover, they can inhibit lipid oxidation. Soyasaponins are classified into three groups depending on aglycones (or sapogenols).

Total contents of soyasaponins measured in soybeans (three samples from Japan and three from overseas) and *natto* (one sample from a Japanese market) were 0.278% (0.247%–0.326%) and 0.246% (dry weight basis), respectively (Kitagawa et al. 1984). Thus, fermentation did not seem to affect the total content or composition of soyasaponins, although changes in the composition during fermentation were not monitored in detail. The effects of soyasaponins in *natto* on human health were not investigated directly, but the results of an enormous amount of studies on their functions provide an overview (Yoshiki et al. 1998).

13.3.10 Polyamines

Polyamines (putrescine, spermidine, and spermine), which are synthesized in cells, have an important role in the growth and differentiation of cells (Yatin 2002). Their synthesis decreases with age, but they can be supplemented in food (Soda et al. 2009). Soybeans are rich in polyamines, although fermentation by *B. subtilis* (*natto*) degrades them (putrescine, 470 to 110 nmol/g; spermidine, 1430 to 190–680 nmol/g; spermine, 340 to 41 nmol/g) (Okamoto et al. 1997). Long-term intake of synthesized polyamines increased the concentration of polyamines in mouse blood, but not short-term intake (Soda et al. 2009). Intake of *natto* for 2 months also elevated the concentration of spermine, but not spermidine, in human blood. Older people tend to increase their blood polyamine content more effectively than younger people from polyamine-rich foods (Soda et al. 2009).

13.4 Conclusion

Natto, a food product made by the fermentation of soybeans by *B. subtilis* (*natto*), is produced and consumed mainly in Japan, where it has been eaten for over a thousand years without adverse effects. Soybeans contain various bioactive components with medicinal effects. All except oligosaccharides are retained in *natto*. In addition, *B. subtilis* (*natto*) produces other bioactive compounds, notably nattokinase, antibiotics, vitamin K, immunomodulating substances, antitumor substances, and unknown factors that benefit the intestinal microflora. Owing to its high vitamin K content, *natto* is contraindicated for cardiac patients treated with warfarin. The proteolytic activity of *B. subtilis* (*natto*) has long been held to improve the digestibility of soybeans, yet experiments show that the digestibility and absorption of proteins in *natto* is not always higher than those in boiled soybeans. The many experiments and analyses using humans, test animals, and cultured cells show that *natto* has health-promoting effects. Although people other than the Japanese have started to discover *natto*, its odor of ammonia, and branched short-chain fatty acids pose a barrier to its adoption as a common foodstuff around the world.

References

Akimoto, T., Yamada, S., and Matsumoto, I. 1990. The relation between protease and γ-glutamyl transpeptidase activities and qualities of natto. *Nippon Shokuhin Kogyo Gakkaishi* 37: 872–877 [In Japanese].

Arima, S. 1937. Experimental study of antagonistic action of *Bacillus "natto"* towards dysentery *Bacillus*. Part II. Antagonistic action of *Bacillus "natto"* towards Shiga dysentery *Bacillus* in vivo. *Bulletin of the Naval Medical Association* 26: 398–419 [In Japanese].

Arimoto, K. and Tamura, E. 1964. Studies on the nutrition of natto. *Annual Report of the National Institute of Nutrition* S37: 36–54 [In Japanese, translated title].

Cabrera-Orozco, A., Jiménez-Martínez, C., and Dávila-Ortiz, G. 2013. Soybean: Non-nutritional factors and their biological functionality. In H.A. El-Shemy (Ed.), *Soybean: Bio-Active Compounds*, Rijeka, Croatia: InTechin, pp. 387–410. http://www.intechopen.com/contact.html

Ebata, N., Matui, K., and Uno, R. 1960. The efficaciousness of *Bacillus natto*. Science Report of the Faculty of Liberal Arts and Education, Gifu University. *Natural Science* 2: 384–387 [In Japanese].

Eguchi, Y. and Kumashiro, N. 1931. A cured case of Paratyphoid B bacilli-career by eating of natto (first report). *Bulletin of the Naval Medical Association* 20: 245–247 [In Japanese].

Food Safety Commission of Japan. 2006. Q & A on soybeans and soybean isoflavones. http://www.fsc.go.jp/sonota/daizu_isoflavone.html [In Japanese, translated title].

Fujii, H. 1963. On the formation of mucilage by *Bacillus natto*. Part III. Chemical constituents of mucilage in natto. (1). *Nippon Nogeikagaku Kaishi (Journal of the Agricultural Chemical Society of Japan)* 37: 407–411 [In Japanese].

Fujii, M. 1953. Studies on the Japanese foods. Report 11. On the digestibility and absorption rate of legumes (II). *Hukuoka Acta Medica: Hukuoka-igaku-zassi* 44: 374–381 [In Japanese].

Fujita, M., Nomura, K., Hong, K., Ito, Y., Asada, A., and Nishimuro, S. 1993. Purification and characterization of a strong fibrinolytic enzyme (nattokinase) in the vegetable cheese natto, a popular soybean fermented food in Japan. *Biochemical and Biophysical Research Communications* 197: 1340–1347.

Fujita, M., Hong, K., Ito, Y., Fujii, R., Kariya, K., and Nishimuro, S. 1995. Thrombolytic effect of nattokinase on a chemically induced thrombosis model in rat. *Biological and Pharmaceutical Bulletin* 18: 1387–1391.

Gibson, T. and Gordon, R. 1974. Genus I. *Bacillus* Cohn 1872. In R. Buchanan and N. Gibbons (Eds.), *Bergey's Manual of Determinative Bacteriology*, 8th ed., Baltimore: The Williams & Wilkins Company, pp. 529–550.

Hamajima, K., Yamada, S., Okuda, K., and Tadokoro, I. 1983. Immunoregulatory effects of so-called *Bacillus natto*. *Yokohama Medical Journal* 34: 139–142 [In Japanese].

Hara, T., Aumayr, A., and Ueda, S. 1981. Characterization of plasmid deoxyribonucleic acid in *Bacillus natto*: Evidence for plasmid-linked PGA production. *Journal of General and Applied Microbiology* 27: 299–305.

Hayashi, U., Nagao, K., Tosa, Y., and Yoshioka, Y. 1976. Experimental studies on the nutritive value of "natto" VIII. Relationship between food containing "natto" and the blood pressure of SHR. *Bulletin of Teikoku-Gakuen* 2: 9–17 [In Japanese].

Hiraike, H., Kimura, M., and Itokawa, Y. 1986. Measurement of K vitamins in human placenta by high-performance liquid chromatography with fluorometric detection. *Nippon Eiseigaku Zasshi (Japanese Journal of Hygiene)* 41: 764–768 [In Japanese].

Hisanaga, S. 1980. Studies on the germination of genus *Bacillus* spores in the rabbit's and canine intestines. *Journal of Nagoya City University Medical Association* 30: 456–469 [In Japanese].

Hisanaga, S., Mase, M., Mizuno, A., Hayakawa, Y., Ohkubo, T., and Hachisuka, Y. 1978. Germination of *Bacillus natto* spores in the canine intestine. *Japanese Journal of Bacteriology (Nippon Saikingaku Zasshi)* 33: 689–696 [In Japanese].

Horimukai, K., Nakatani, K., Yoshida, K., Tsumura, Y., Futamura, M., Narita, M., and Ohya, Y. 2011. Late-onset anaphylaxis after ingestion of *Bacillus subtilis*-fermented soybeans (natto) which could increase its allergenicity gradually with time; a case report of 7-year old boy. *Japanese Journal of Pediatrics* 64: 1659–1662.

Hosoi, T., Ametani, A., Kiuchi, K., and Kaminogawa, S. 1999. Changes in fecal microflora induced by intubation of mice with *Bacillus subtilis* (*natto*) spores are dependent upon dietary components. *Canadian Journal of Microbiology* 45: 59–66.

Hosoi, T., Hirose, R., Saegusa, S., Ametani, A., Kiuchi, K., and Kaminogawa, S. 2003. Cytokine responses of human intestinal epithelial-like Caco-2 cells to the nonpathogenic bacterium *Bacillus subtilis* (*natto*). *International Journal of Food Microbiology* 82: 255–264.

Ibe, S., Yoshida, K., and Kumada, K. 2006. Angiotensin I-converting enzyme inhibitory activity of natto, a traditional Japanese fermented food. *Nippon Shokuhin Kagaku Kogaku Kaishi* 53: 189–192 [In Japanese].

Ibe, S., Yoshida, K., Kumada, K., Tsurushiin, S., Furusho, T., and Otobe, K. 2009. Antihypertensive effects of natto, a traditional Japanese fermented food, in spontaneously hypertensive rats. *Food Science and Technology Research* 15: 199–202.

Ikeda, H. 1992. A water soluble vitamin K_2 complex in natto. *Journal of Home Economics of Japan* 43: 643–648 [In Japanese].

Ikeda, H. and Doi, Y. 1990. A vitamin-K_2-binding factor secreted from *Bacillus subtilis*. *European Journal of Biochemistry* 192: 219–224.

Ikeda, H. and Tsuno, S. 1984. The componential changes during the manufacturing process of natto (Part 1) On the amino nitrogen, ammonia nitrogen, carbohydrates and vitamin B_2. *Journal of Food Science, Kyoto Women's University* 39: 19–24 [In Japanese].

Inomata, N., Osuna, H., and Ikezawa, Z. 2004. Late-onset anaphylaxis to *Bacillus natto*-fermented soybeans (natto). *Journal of Allergy and Clinical Immunology* 113: 998–1000.

Inooka, S. and Kimura, M. 1983. The effect of *Bacillus natto* in feed on the sheep red blood cell antibody response in chickens. *Avian Diseases* 27: 1086–1089.

Isshiki, S. and Onozaki, H. 1992. Effects of natto and steamed soybeans on intestinal microflora in rats. *Journal of Sugiyama Jogakuen University (Part. 1)* 23: 273–283 [In Japanese].

Kameda, Y., Kanatomo, S., Kameda, Y., and Saito. Y. 1968. A contact antitumor activity of *Bacillus natto* on solid type Ehrlich carcinoma cells. *Chemical and Pharmaceutical Bulletin* 16: 186–187.

Kameda, Y., Kanatomo, S., Matsui, K., Nakabayashi, T., Ueno, K., Nagai, S., and Ohki, K. 1978. Antitumor activity of *Bacillus natto*. VI. Analysis of cytolytic activity on Ehrlich ascites carcinoma cells in the culture medium of *Bacillus natto* KMD 1126. *Yakugaku Zasshi* 98: 1432–1435 [In Japanese].

Kameda, Y., Matsui, K., Kato, H., Yamada, T., and Sagai, H. 1972. Antitumor activity of *Bacillus natto*. III. Isolation and characterization of a cytolytic substance on Ehrlich ascites carcinoma cells in the culture medium of Bacillus natto KMD 1126. *Chemical and Pharmaceutical Bulletin* 20: 1551–1557.

Kameda, Y., Sagai, H., Kamada, T., Kanatomo, S., and Matsui, K. 1971. Antitumor activity of *Bacillus natto*. II. Formation of cytolytic substances on Ehrlich ascites carcinoma in *Bacillus natto* KMD 1126. *Chemical and Pharmaceutical Bulletin* 19: 2572–2578.

Kanno, A., Takamatsu, H., Takano, N., and Akimoto, T. 1982. Change of saccharides in soybeans during manufacturing of natto (Studies on natto Part I), *Nippon Shokuhin Kogyo Gakkaishi* 29: 105–110 [In Japanese].

Kanno, A., Takamatsu, H., and Takano, N. 1984. Determination of several volatile components produced by *Bacillus natto* in commercial "natto" (Studies on "natto" Part II). *Nippon Shokuhin Kogyo Gakkaishi* 31: 587–595 [In Japanese].

Kanoe, M., Kido, M., Komatsu, T., and Toda, M. 1982. Growth inhibitory effect of *Bacillus natto* on several microorganisms of animal pathogen. *Bulletin of the Faculty of Agriculture, Yamaguchi University* 33: 1–24 [In Japanese].

Kawane, M., 2007. Development of *Bacillus subtilis* (*natto*) controlling immune function. *Shokuhin to Gijutsu* 433: 11–17 [In Japanese, translated title].

Kida, S., Hashida, W., and Teramoto, S. 1956. Nutritional studies on natto and *B. natto*. I. nutritional requirement of *B. natto*. *Journal of Fermentation Technology (Hakko Kogaku Zasshi)* 34: 542–546 [In Japanese].

Kimura, K. and Itoh, Y. 2007. Determination and characterization of IS*4Bsu1*-insertion loci and identification of a new insertion sequence element of the IS*256* family in a natto starter. *Bioscience, Biotechnology, and Biochemistry* 71: 2458–2464.

Kimura, M. 1979. Effect of a feed-additive, *Bacillus natto* (BN strain) product, on economic performances of animals and poultry. *Animal-Husbandry* 33: 31–36 [In Japanese, translated title].

Kitagawa, I., Yoshikawa, M., Hayashi, T., and Taniyama, T. 1984. Quantitative determination of soyasaponins in soybeans of various origins and soybean products by means of high performance liquid chromatography. *Yakugaku Zasshi* 104: 275–279 [In Japanese].

Kiuchi, K. and Suzuki, H. 1991. The current state on development of natto containing a high activity of nattokinase. *Food Science*, 33(6): 85–89 [In Japanese, translated title].

Kobayashi, R., Arikawa, K., Ichikawa, K., Taguchi, C., Utsunomiya, T., Iijima, M., Uchiyama, T. et al. 2013. Traditional Japanese fermented food natto enhances NK cell activity in intestine. *International Journal of Oral-Medical Sciences* 12: 90–94.

Komatsuzaki, T., Ohkuro, I., Kohno, T., and Ito, S. 1976. Virulence and lipase of *Bacillus natto*. *Medicine and Biology* 93: 403–406 [In Japanese].

Komatsuzaki, T., Ohkuro, I., Kawashima, M., and Ito, S. 1978. Non-specific immunity within a short time after pretreatment with natto bacilli. *Medicine and Biology* 97: 459–463 [In Japanese].

Komatsuzaki, T., Ohkuro, I., Kawashima, M., and Kuriyama, S. 1979. The difference in unspecifically immunizing effects among strains of natto bacilli. *Medicine and Biology* 99: 343–345 [In Japanese].

Kubo, Y., Rooney, A.P., Tsukakoshi, Y., Nakagawa, R., Hasegawa, H., and Kimura, K. 2011. Phylogenetic analysis of *Bacillus subtilis* strains applicable to natto (fermented soybean) production. *Applied and Environmental Microbiology* 77: 6463–6469.

Kudo, T. 1990. Warfarin antagonism of natto and increase in serum vitamin K by intake of natto. *Artery* 17: 189–201.

Kudo, T., Uchibori, Y., Atsumi, K., Numao, Y., Kawamorita, H., Miura, I., Sidara, M., Kitamura, N., Ishii, K., and Hashimoto, A. 1978. Warfarin antagonist of natto. *Heart* 10: 595–598 [In Japanese].

Maruta, K., Miyazaki, H., Masuda, S., Takahashi, M., Marubashi, T., Tadano, Y., and Takahashi, H. 1996a. Exclusion of intestinal pathogens by continuous feeding with *Bacillus subtilis* C-3102 and its influence on the intestinal microflora in broilers. *Animal Science and Technology (Japan)* 67: 273–280.

Maruta, K., Miyazaki, H., Tadano, Y., Masuda, S., Suzuki, A., Takahashi, H., and Takahashi, M. 1996b. Effects of *Bacillus subtilis* C-3102 intake on fecal flora of sows and on diarrhea and mortality rate of their piglets. *Animal Science and Technology (Japan)* 67: 403–409.

Matsubayashi, R., Matsubayashi, T., Yokota, T., Ohro, Y., Fujita, N., Nakashima, Y., Takeda, S., and Enoki, H. 2010. Pediatric late-onset anaphylaxis caused by natto (fermented soybeans). *Pediatrics International* 52: 657–658.

Matsumura, T. 1934a. Experimentelle Studien zur Bekämpfung der Bakterienträger mittels der antagonistischen Wirkung anderer Bakterien. Teil I. Untersuchung von Bacillus natto. Versuche in Reagenzgläsern. *Mitteilungen aus der Medizinischen Akademie zu Kioto* 12: 38–52 [In Japanese].

Matsumura, T. 1934b. Experimentelle Studien zur Bekämpfung der Bakterienträger mittels der antagonistischen Wirkung anderer Bakterien. Teil II. Versuche über die antagonistische Wirkung des Natto-Bazillus gegen die Typhusbazillengruppe. Versuche in Reagenzgläsern. *Mitteilungen aus der Medizinischen Akademie zu Kioto* 12: 53–89 [In Japanese].

Matsumura, T. 1934c. Experimentelle Studien zur Bekämpfung der Bakterienträger mittels der antagonistischen Wirkung anderer Bakterien. Teil III. Versuche über die antagonistische Wirkung des Natto-Bazillus gegen die Typhusbazillengruppe im Tierkörper. Versuche in Reagenzgläsern. *Mitteilungen aus der Medizinischen Akademie zu Kioto* 12: 1185–1210 [In Japanese].

Ministry of Education, Culture, Sports, Science and Technology. 2010. Standard tables of food composition in Japan: Food Composition Database. http://fooddb.jp/

Mitsui, N., Kajimoto, O., Tsukahara, M., Murasawa, H., Tamura, M., Nishimura, A., Kajimoto, Y., and Benno, Y. 2006.Effect of natto including *Bacillus subtilis* K-2 (spore) on defecation and fecal microbiota, and safety of excessive ingestion in healthy volunteers. *Japanese Pharmacology and Therapeutics* 34: 135–148 [In Japanese].

Miura, T. 1959. Influence of natto and miso on growth and nitrogen metabolism in rats. Part I. Influence of natto and miso on growth and nitrogen metabolism in normal rats. *Journal of Japan Pediatric Society* 63: 2241–2248 [In Japanese].

Muramatsu, K., Kanai, Y., Kimura, N., Miura, N., Yoshida, K., and Kiuchi, K. 1994. Production of natto with high elastase activity. *Nippon Shokuhin Kagaku Kogaku Kaishi* 41: 123–128 [In Japanese].

Murata, H., Yaguchi, H. Sano, H., and Namioka, S., 1977. Effect of administration of *Bacillus natto* upon weanling piglets. *Journal of the Japan Veterinary Medical Association* 30: 645–649 [In Japanese].

Nagai, T. 2014. Fibrinolytic activity. In P.K. Sarkar, and M.J.R.Nout (Eds.), *Handbook of Indigenous Foods Involving Alkaline Fermentation*. Boca Raton, FL, USA: CRC Press, pp. 355–359.

Nagai, T., Nishimura, K., Suzuki, H., Banba, Y., Sasaki, H., and Kiuchi, K. 1994. Isolation and characterization of a *Bacillus subtilis* strain producing natto with strong umami-taste and high viscosity. *Nippon Shokuhin Kogyo Gakkaishi* 41: 123–128 [In Japanese].

Nagai, T. and Tamang J.P. 2010. Fermented legumes: Soybeans and non-soybean products. InJ.P. Tamang and K.K. Kailasapathy (Eds.), *Frermented Foods and Beverages of the World*. Boca Raton, FL, USA: CRC Press, pp.191–224.

Nagai, T., Tran, L., Inatsu,Y., and Itoh, Y. 2000. A new IS*4* family Insertion Sequence, IS*4Bsu1*, Responsible for genetic instability of poly-γ-glutamic acid production in *Bacillus subtilis*. *Journal of Bacteriology* 182: 2387–2392.

Nakamura, T., Yamagata, Y., and Ichishima, E. 1992. Nucleotide sequence of the subtilisin NAT gene, aprN; of *Bacillus subtilis* (*natto*). *Bioscience, Biotechnology, and Biochemistry* 56: 1869–1871.

Ohkuro, I., Suzuki, K., Ito, S., and Komatsuzaki, T. 1974. Resistance of mice pretreated with "*Bacillus natto*" to lethal challenge with *Staphylococcus. aureus. Medicine and Biology* 89: 35–40 [In Japanese].
Ohkuro, I., Komatsuzaki, T., Kuriyama, S., and Kawashima, M. 1980. Non-specifically immunizing effects of vegetative cells and spores of natto bacilli. *Medicine and Biology* 100: 351–355 [In Japanese].
Ohta, T., Ebine, H., Nakano, M., Hieda, H., and Sasaki, H. 1964. Manufacturing new-type fermented soybean food product employing *Bacillus natto*. Part 1. Investigation on the manufacturing on a laboratory scale. *Report of the Food Research Institute* 18: 46–52 [In Japanese].
Okamoto, A., Hanagata, H., Matsumoto, E., Kawamura, Y., Koizumi, Y., and Yanagida, F. 1995a. Angiotensin I converting enzyme inhibitory activities of various fermented foods. *Bioscience, Biotechnology, and Biochemistry* 59: 1147–1149.
Okamoto, A., Hanagata, H., Kawamura, Y., and Yanagida, F. 1995b. Anti-hypertensive substances in fermented soybean, natto. *Plant Foods for Human Nutrition* 47: 39–47.
Okamoto, A., Sugi, E., Koizumi, Y., Yanagida, F., and Udaka, S. 1997. Polyamine content of ordinary foodstuffs and various fermented foods. *Bioscience, Biotechnology, and Biochemistry* 61: 1582–1584.
Ozawa, N., Shimojo, N., Suzuki, Y., Ochiai, S., Nakano, T., Morita, Y., Inoue, Y., Arima, T., Suzuki, S., and Kohno, Y. 2014. Maternal intake of natto, a Japan's traditional fermented soybean food, during pregnancy and the risk of eczema in Japanese babies. *Allergology International* 63: 261–266.
Ozawa, K., Yabu-uchi, K., Yamanaka, K., Yamashita, Y., Ueba, K., and Miwatani, T., 1979. Antagonistic effects of *Bacillus natto* and *Streptococcus faecalis* on growth of *Candida albicans. Microbiology and Immunology* 23: 1147–1156.
Ozawa, K., Yokota, H., Kimura, M., and Mitsuoka, T. 1981. Effects of administration of *Bacillus subtilis* strain BN on intestinal flora of weanling piglets. *Japanese Journal of Veterinary Science* 43: 771–775.
Phillips, K.W. and Ansell, J. 2010. The clinical implications of new oral anticoagulants: Will the potential advantages be achieved? *Thrombosis and Haemostasis* 103: 34–39.
Ryo, S. 1982. Vitamin K in diets and breast milk. *Perinatal Medicine (Shusanki Igaku)* 12: 1101–1106.
Ryo, S. and Baba, K. 1981. Studies on the effect of postpartum administration of natto to mothers on the content of vitamin K in breast milk. *Perinatal Medicine (Shusanki Igaku)* 11: 1191–1195.
Saito, T. 1938. Antagonism action of *Bacillus subtilis* (*natto*) against *S. enterica* var *enterica* serovar Typhi. *Acta Medica Hokkaidonensia* 16: 82–92 [In Japanese, translated title].
Saka, N. 2008. Effects of natto that gives to health of piglets. *All About Swine* 33: 15–19 [In Japanese].
Sakano, T., Notsumoto, S., Nagaoka, T., Morimoto, A., Fujimoto, K., Masuda, S., Suzuki, Y. et al. 1988. Measurement of K vitamins in food by high-performance liquid chromatography with fluorometric detection. *Vitamins (Japan)* 62: 393–398 [In Japanese].
Sato, T. 1980. Studies on induction of interferon by "*Bacillus natto*". *Journal of Tokyo Medical College* 38: 815–826 [In Japanese].
Sawamura, S. 1906. On the micro-organisms of natto. *Bulletin of College of Agriculture, Tokyo Imperial University* 7: 107–110.
Science and Technology Agency of Japan. 1979. *Research Report on the Revision of the Standard Table of Food Composition in Japan*. Tokyo: Science and Technology Agency of Japan [In Japanese, translated title].
Seki, T., Oshima, T., and Oshima, Y. 1975. Taxonomic study of *Bacillus* by deoxyribonucleic acid-deoxyribonucleic acid hybridization and interspecific transformation. *International Journal of Systematic Bacteriology* 25: 258–270.
Senbon, S. 1940. Anwendung des Bazillus natto zur Therapie gegen Trichophytia. *Journal of the Medical Association of Formosa* 39: 14–17 [In Japanese].
Shimakage, A., Shinbo, M., Yamada, S., and Ito, H. 2006. Changes in isoflavone content in soybeans during the manufacturing processes of tubu-natto and hikiwari-natto. *Nippon Shokuhin Kagaku Kogaku Kaishi* 53: 185–188 [In Japanese].
Shirahata, A. 1987. Vitamin K. *Blood and Vessel* 18: 181–194. [In Japanese].
Soda, K., Kano, Y., Sakuragi, M., Takao, K., Lefor A., and Konishi, F. 2009. Long-term oral polyamine intake increases blood polyamine concentrations. *Journal of Nutritional Science and Vitaminology* 55: 361–366.
Sumi, H., 1997. A miracle soybean food natto—Thrombolytic and antibacterial (O-157) activities. *Dempun to Shokuhin* 22: 9–11 [In Japanese].

Sumi, H., Hamada, H., Tsushima, H., Mihara, H., and Muraki, H. 1987. A novel fibrinolytic enzyme (nattokinase) in the vegetable cheese natto; a typical and popular soybean food in the Japanese diet. *Experientia* 43: 1110–1111.

Sumi, H., Hamada, H., Nakanishi, K., and Hiratani, H. 1990. Enhancement of the fibrinolytic activity in plasma by oral administration of nattokinase. *Acta Haematologica* 84: 139–143.

Sumi, H., Taya, N., Nakajima, N., and Hiratani, H. 1992. Structure and fibrinolytic properties of nattokinase. *Fibrinolysis* 6 (Supplement 2): 86.

Sumi, H., Banba, T., and Kishimoto, N. 1996. Strong pro-urokinase activators proved in Japanese soybean cheese natto. *Nippon Shokuhin Kagaku Kogaku Kaishi* 43: 1124–1127 [In Japanese].

Sumi, H. and Ohosugi, T. 1999. Anti-bacterial component dipicolic acid measured in natto and natto bacilli. *Journal of the Agricultural Chemical Society of Japan* 73: 1289–1291 [In Japanese].

Sumi, H., Yoshikawa, M., Baba, T., Matsuda, K., and Kubota, H. 1999. Elastase activity in natto, and its relation to nattokinase. *Journal of the Agricultural Chemical Society of Japan* 73: 1187–1190 [In Japanese].

Sun, P., Wang, J.Q., and Deng, L.F. 2013. Effects of *Bacillus subtilis natto* on milk production, rumen fermentation and ruminal microbiome of dairy cows. *Animal* 7: 216–222.

Suzuki, K. 1975. Analysis of protective effects of pretreatment with "*Bacillus natto*" on mice to lethal challenge with *Staphylococcu. aureus. The Journal of Tokyo Medical College* 33: 311–327 [In Japanese].

Suzuki, T., Ishikawa, N., and Meguro, H. 1983. Angiotensin I-converting enzyme inhibiting activity in foods (Studies on vasodepressive components in foods. Part I). *Nippon Nōgeikagaku Kaishi* 57: 1143–1146 [In Japanese].

Suzuki, H., Watabe, J., Takeuchi, H., Tadano, Y., Masuda, S., and Maruta, K. 2004. Effect of *Bacillus subtilis* C-3102 intakes on the composition and metabolic activity of fecal microflora of humans. *Journal of Intestinal Microbiology* 18: 93–99.

Takahashi, C., Kikuchi, N., Katou, N., Miki, T., Yanagida, F., and Umeda, M. 1995. Possible anti-tumor-promoting activity of components in Japanese soybean fermented food, natto: Effect on gap junctional intercellular communication. *Carcinogenesis* 16: 471–476.

Takaoka, S. 2003. Function and market trend of NSK (extract containing a high activity of nattokinase from culture broth of *Bacillus natto*). *New Food Industry* 45(8): 25–30 [In Japanese, translated title].

Takeda, K., Ohshiro, T., Ohshiro, T., and Okumura, K. 2005. Enhancement of natural killer cell activity by supplementation of extract of metabolic products of *Bacillus subtilis* AK (EMBSAK). *Japanese Journal of Complementary and Alternative Medicine* 2: 127–133 [In Japanese].

Takemura, H., Shioya, N., Komori, Y., and Tho, Y. 2009. Effect of fermented soybeans containing *Bacillus subtilis* MC1 on defecation, fecal properties and fecal microflora of healthy female volunteers. *Journal of Urban Living and Health Association* 53: 11–18.

Tamang, J.P., Thapa, S., Dewan, S., Jojima, Y., Fudou, R., and Yamanaka, S. 2002. Phylogenetic analysis of *Bacillus* strains isolated from fermented soybean foods of Asia: *Kinema, chungkokjang* and *natto*. *Journal of Hill Research* 15(2): 56–62.

Tanaka T. and Koshikawa, T. 1977. Isolation and characterization of four types of plasmids from *Bacillus subtilis* (*natto*). *Journal of Bacteriology* 131: 699–701.

Terada, A., Yamamoto, M., and Yoshimura, E. 1999. Effect of the fermented soybean product "natto" on the composition and metabolic activity of the human fecal flora. *Japanese Journal of Food Microbiology* 16: 221–230.

Toda, T., Uesugi, T., Hirai, K., Nukaya, H., Tsuji, K., and Ishida, H. 1999. New 6-*O*-acyl isoflavone glycosides from soybeans fermented with *Bacillus subtilis* (*natto*). I. 6-*O*-Succinylated isoflavone glycosides and their preventive effects on bone loss in ovariectomized rats fed a calcium-deficient diet. *Biological and Pharmaceutical Bulletin* 22: 1193–1201.

Tsubura, S. 2012. Anti-periodontitis effect of *Bacillus subtilis* (*natto*). *Shigaku (Odontology)* 99: 160–164 [In Japanese, translated title].

Tsuchihashi, N., Watanabe, T., Shimizu, K., and Takai, Y. 1986. Effect of living cells of *Bacillus* on rats. *Bulletin of Chiba College of Health Science* 5(1): 3–8 [In Japanese].

Tsuji, H., Okada, N., Yamanishi, R., Bando, N., Kimoto, M., and Ogawa, T. 1995. Measurement of *Gly m* Bd 30 K, a major soybean allergen, in soybean products by a sandwich enzyme-linked immunosorbent assay. *Bioscience, Biotechnology, and Biochemistry* 59:150–151.

Udo, S. 1936. Composition of natto (1) dipicolic acid in natto and its activity. *Journal of the Agricultural Chemistry Society of Japan* 12: 386–394. [In Japanese, translated title].

Vermeer, C. 2012. Vitamin K: the effect on health beyond coagulation—An overview. *Food and Nutrition Research* 56: 5329—DOI: 10.3402/fnr.v56i0.5329. http://www.foodandnutritionresearch.net/index.php/fnr/article/view/5329.

Xu, Q., Yajima, T., Li, W., Saito, K., Ohshima, Y., and Yoshikai, Y. 2006. Levan (β-2, 6-fructan), a major fraction of fermented soybean mucilage, displays immunostimulating properties via toll-like receptor 4 signaling: induction of interleukin-12 production and suppression of T-helper type 2 response and immunoglobulin E production. *Clinical and Experimental Allergy* 36: 94–101.

Yamanishi, R. Huang, T., Tsuji, H., Bando, N., and Ogawa, T. 1995. Reduction of the soybean allergenicity by the fermentation with *Bacillus natto*. *Food Science and Technology International* 1:14–17.

Yatin, F. 2002. Polyamines in living organisms. *Journal of Cell and Molecular Biology* 1: 57–67.

Yoshiki, Y., Kudou, S., and Okubo, K. 1998. Relationship between chemical structures and biological activities of triterpenoid saponins from soybean. *Bioscience, Biotechnology, and Biochemistry* 62: 2291–2299.

Chapter 14

Health Benefits of Functional Proteins in Fermented Foods

Amit Kumar Rai and Kumaraswamy Jeyaram

Contents

14.1 Introduction

Fermentation has wide application in a broad range of food substrates and today there is an array of fermented food products in the market labeled as having health-promoting properties. Health benefits of fermented foods can be due to live organisms (probiotic), compounds produced by the fermenting microorganisms (peptides, exopolysaccharides, etc.), and bioactive compounds formed by hydrolysis of food components (free polyphenols and peptides) during fermentation (Haque and Chand 2008, Cho et al. 2011). The World Health Organization has estimated that by 2020, heart disease and stroke will surpass infectious diseases to become the leading cause of death and disability across the globe (Lopez and Murray 1998). Research findings have confirmed that several food components and dietary habits can prevent or even reduce the risk of several diseases (Groziak and Miller 2000, He and Chen 2013). With the increased incidence of cardiovascular diseases, the production of fermented foods enriched with bioactive components (peptides, isoflavones, etc.) has become increasingly important in the development of functional foods.

Fermentation has shown to improve the health benefits of various foods such as fermented soybean (Gibbs et al. 2004, Zhang et al. 2006), fermented milk (Ashar and Chand 2004, LeBlanc et al. 2004), fermented fish and meat (Jung et al. 2005, Peralta et al. 2005, Jemil et al. 2014), and fermented cereal products (Coda et al. 2012). Worldwide researchers are focusing more on health benefits of different fermented foods by identifying and characterizing the bioactive components formed during fermentation, and by determining their effect and mechanism on body physiology. Currently, with the support of exclusive research in the area of health benefits of fermented foods, many fermented products (*calpis, evolus, festivo, natto, douchi,* etc.) are marketed globally as functional foods, nutraceuticals, or health foods (Haque and Chand 2008). The advantage of fermented foods in the treatment of diseases is that they do not exhibit any side effects and the fermented products are very economical in comparison to many synthetic drugs available in the market.

Research in the last two decades has shown that many functional proteins and peptides in fermented foods exhibit specific biological activities beyond their nutritional role (FitzGerald et al. 2004, Hartmann and Meisel 2007, Haque and Chand 2008). The functional properties are due to enzymes (fibrinolytic enzymes) (Mine et al. 2005) or peptides (bacteriocin) produced by the starter culture (Leelavatcharamas et al. 2011) or due to the peptide formed by hydrolysis of food protein (Hartmann and Meisel 2007). Usually, bioactive peptides correspond to cryptic sequences from native proteins in the unfermented food, which are released mainly through hydrolysis by microbial enzymes during fermentation or digestive enzymes after consumption. This chapter focuses on therapeutic enzymes and various bioactive peptides associated with protein-rich fermented foods.

14.2 Protein-Based Bioactive Compounds in Fermented Foods

Protein-rich fermented foods are becoming very popular in recent past due to their bioactive components. The bioactive components are either produced by the starter (enzymes, peptides) or by hydrolysis of food proteins (peptides) (Hartmann and Meisel 2007, Haque and Chand 2008, Wang et al. 2009). In this chapter, the functional protein molecules in fermented foods have been categorized into enzymes and bioactive peptides.

14.2.1 Enzymes

Many enzymes are involved during fermentation process, which generally hydrolyses or transform the food components. As enzymes are specific biological catalysts they are one of the most desirable agents for the treatment of metabolic diseases. Enzymes produced from microbial sources apart from fermented foods have shown to possess desirable therapeutic attributes, which includes superoxide dismutase (antioxidant and anti-inflammatory), streptokinase (anticoagulant), and lipase (lipids hydrolysis) (Sabu 2003). Most of these enzymes present in fermented foods are produced by microorganisms. These enzymes have not been associated with toxicity and are considered intrinsically safe for application in food industry. The enzymes produced by starter culture during fermentation are associated with hydrolysis of complex biomolecules into their monomeric form (e.g., proteases, carbohydrate-degrading enzymes, lipases, etc.), degradation of antinutrional factors (phytase), degradation of bound polyphenols to free form (β-glucosidase), and enzymes having health benefits (fibrinolytic enzymes). Among them, fibrinolytic enzymes have been reported in several protein-rich fermented foods for its usefulness in thrombolytic therapy (Mine et al. 2005). Fibrinolytic enzymes have also been produced by *Bacillus* sp. and lactic acid bacteria (LAB) isolated from various fermented foods (Wang et al. 2006, 2009). Oral administrations of purified enzyme or along with fermented foods are one of the potential tools for the management of heart diseases.

14.2.2 Bioactive Peptides

Peptides are specific fragments of protein formed by hydrolysis, which have a positive impact on body functions and may ultimately influence the health beyond their nutritional role. These peptides are inactive when they are encrypted in parent proteins, but once released during hydrolysis, they may act as physiological modulators with hormone-like activity. The size of the peptide formed by hydrolysis may range from 2 to 20 amino acids and the activity is dependent on its size, amino acid content, and their composition. Some of the peptides are multifunctional and can exert more than one of the functional properties (Saito et al. 2000). Once absorbed in the small intestine these bioactive peptides exert beneficial effect on the various systems of the body such as the nervous system, cardiovascular, endocrine, and the immune system. Depending on the sequence of amino acid, peptides exhibit various biological activities such as antioxidant (Erdmann et al. 2008, Sabeena et al. 2010, Perna et al. 2013), antimicrobial (Haque and Chand 2008, Meira et al. 2012), immunomodulatory (Vinderola et al. 2007, Qian et al. 2011), antithrombic (Erdmann et al. 2008), hypocholesterimic (Nagaoka et al. 1992, Hartmann and Meisel 2007), and antihypertensive properties (Chen et al. 2010, Phelan and Kerins 2011). Bioactive peptides and biological properties of selected protein-rich fermented foods are shown in Table 14.1.

These bioactive peptides are formed by: (i) hydrolysis of food protein by gastrointestinal enzymes, (ii) through hydrolysis by proteolytic enzymes derived from microorganisms and plant, and (iii) through hydrolysis by proteolytic microorganisms during fermentation. Apart from peptides formed by hydrolysis of food protein, there are some peptides produced by the starter culture (LAB and *Bacillus* spp.) having health benefits. Several products (*calpis, evolus*) are commercially available with bioactive peptide, which has been experimentally and clinically proven for their specific health benefits.

14.3 Health Benefits of Proteinaceous Bioactive Components

Protein-rich fermented foods are becoming very popular in the recent past for the prevention of various cardiovascular diseases. The protein-based bioactive components exhibit their biological properties by specifically hydrolyzing specific proteins (fibrinolytic enzymes), inhibiting certain metabolic enzyme (angiotensin-converting enzymes [ACE]), and inducing physiological modulators with hormone-like activity (Sumi et al. 1987, Matar et al. 1997, Hartmann and Meisel 2007, Singh et al. 2014). Some of the most studied health benefits of the protein-rich fermented foods are shown in Figure 14.1.

In this section, we discuss the health benefits of fibrinolytic enzymes and bioactive peptides in various protein-rich fermented foods.

Table 14.1 Health Benefits of Bioactive Peptides in Different Fermented Foods

Fermented Food	*Country*	*Microbial Strain*	*Functional Properties*	*Reference*
Natto	Japan	*B. subtilis*	ACE inhibitory	Gibbs et al. (2004)
Kumis	Colombia	Yeast	ACE inhibitory	Chaves-López et al. (2012)
Fermented milk	China	*Lb. delbrueckii*	ACE-inhibitory, antioxidant, immunomodulatory	Qian et al. (2011)
Douchi	China	*Aspergillus, Mucor*	ACE inhibitory	Zhang et al. (2006), Wang et al. (2007)
Sheep milk yogurt	Greece	*Lactobacillus* sp.	ACE inhibitory	Papadimilriou et al. (2007)
Dahi	India	LAB, *Lactobacillus* sp.	ACE inhibitory	Ashar and Chand (2004)
Kefir	Russia	Yeast and LAB	Antimutagenic, antioxidant	Liu et al. (2005)
Sour milk	Japan	*Lb. helveticus* CP790, *Saccharomyces cerevisiae*	ACE inhibitory	Nakamura et al. (1995)
Fermented sodium caseinate	Ireland	*Lb. acidophilus*	Antimicrobial	Hayes e al. (2006)
Fresco cheese	Mexico	*Ent. faecium*	ACE inhibitory	Torres-Llanez et al. (2011)
Fermented fish	Japan	*Aspergillus oryzae*	Antioxidant	Giri et al. (2011)

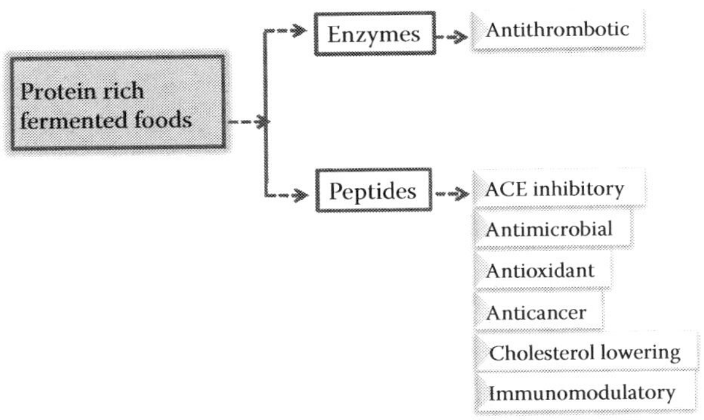

Figure 14.1 Heath benefits of proteinaceous bioactive compounds in fermented foods.

14.3.1 Antithrombic Properties

Fermented foods are the potential source of fibrinolytic enzymes, which are useful in thrombolytic therapy to prevent rapidly emerging cardiovascular diseases in the modern world. More than 20 enzymes are produced by the human body to assist blood clotting, while only one is involved in the breakdown of the blood clot called "plasmin" (Mine et al. 2005). The balance between anti-coagulation and blood coagulation is affected by various factors such as aging, genetic defect, sedentary life style, improper fat consumption, poor diet, toxin accumulation, and pathogen attack. Imbalance in the circulatory system leads to fibrin accumulation in the blood vessels, slows down blood flow, and increases blood viscosity contributing to the elevation of blood pressure, which leads to myocardial infarction and other cardiovascular diseases.

To prevent thrombosis, daily intake of fibrinolytic enzymes from fermented food sources is recommended. Fibrinolytic enzymes with high specificity toward fibrin in fermented foods are preferred by therapeutic industries because of its lesser side effects and allergic reactions. *Nattokinase* produced by *Bacillus subtilis* subsp. *natto* is the origin of this fibrinolytic activity in fermented soybean *natto*. Sumi et al. (1990) demonstrated that oral administrations of this nattokinase enhance systemic fibrinolytic activity in a rat model without any allergic reactions. Further, Fujita et al. (1995) demonstrated that nattokinase could pass through the intestinal track by showing its availability in plasma and simultaneous degradation of fibrinogen after intraduodenal administration of nattokinase to rats. Subsequently, various fermented foods were reported with fibrinolytic activity namely *hawaizar* (Indian fermented soybean), *chungkookjang* (Korean fermented soybean product), *douchi* (Chinese fermented soybean), *jeotgal* (Korean fermented fish), and *tempe* (Indonesian fermented soybean) (Mine et al. 2005, Singh et al. 2014). In most of the studies, fermented soybean and fish products were found to be a potential source of fibrinolytic enzymes (Kotb 2012). In fermented soybean *Bacillus* spp. used for fermentation were found to be responsible for the fibrinolytic activity, but in the case of fermented fish products it is mostly of endogenous origin (Singh et al. 2014). Fibrinolytic enzymes *myulchikinase* reported from Korean pickled anchovy (Jeong et al. 2004) and *katsuwokinase* from Japanese *skipjack shiokara* (Sumi et al. 1995) showed similar amino acid sequences to endogenous trypsin of starfish and dogfish, respectively, used as raw materials for fermentation.

If a fibrinolytic enzyme is produced by food-grade microorganisms isolated from fermented food, it can be directly consumed daily for the prevention of cardiovascular diseases (Mine et al. 2005, Singh et al. 2014). Bacteria of the genus *Bacillus* mostly *B. subtilis* and *Bacillus amyloliquefaciens* isolated from fermented soybean products have been demonstrated as the origin of fibrinolytic activity by earlier researchers (Peng et al. 2003, Zeng et al. 2013). Recently, Chang et al. (2012) purified and characterized fibrinolytic enzymes from red bean fermented by *B. subtilis*. Montriwong et al. (2012) isolated novel fibrinolytic enzymes from *Virgibacillus halodenitrificans* SK1-3-7 isolated from fish sauce fermentation. Kim et al. (1997) purified and characterized novel fibrinolytic enzymes from *Bacillus* sp. KA38 isolated from *jeotgal*, a fermented fish of Korea.

Fifty-four traditional fermented foods collected from different states of Northeast India were screened for fibrinolytic activity (Table 14.2).

Among these, protein-rich fermented foods (Figure 14.2) particularly fermented soybean products (*tungrymbai, hawaizar, peru, perumb, akhani, bekang*) and fermented fish products (*ngari, shedal, tungtap, hentak*) had fibrinolytic activity. Fibrin zymogram pattern generated from these fermented foods also showed microbial origin of fibrinolytic activity in fermented soybean products and endogenous origin in fish products (Singh et al. 2014). Several fibrinolytic *Bacillus* spp. and LAB from these traditional fermented foods have been characterized. LAB with fibrinolytic

Table 14.2 Fibrinolytic Fermented Foods of Northeast India and Its Associated Microorganisms

Local Name[a]	*Place of Collection*		*pH*	*Fibrinolyti Activity*[b] *(KPU/g)*	*F/C ratio*[c]	*Associated Fibrinolytic Microbes*
1. Fermented Soybean Products						
Tungrymbai	Shillong	Meghalaya	8.10 ± 0.10	36.74 ± 3.34	2.09 ± 0.74	*B. subtilis, B. amyloliquefaciens, Vag. carniphilus*
Hawaijar	Imphal	Manipur	8.17 ± 0.13	15.86 ± 10.85	3.8 ± 0.21	*B. subtilis, B. amyloliquefaciens, Proteus mirabilis*
Peru	Itanagar	Arunachal Pradesh	7.17 ± 0.09	34.23 ± 0.83	0.55 ± 0.10	*B. subtilis, B. amyloliquefaciens, Vag. lutrae, Pediococcus acidilactici, Ent. faecalis*
Perumb	Itanagar Pashighat	Arunachal Pradesh	7.14 ± 0.13	48.43 ± 10.02	0.83 ± 0.37	*B. subtilis, B. cereus, Vag. carniphilus Ent. faecalis, Ent. gallinarum, Staphylococcus sciuri*
Akhoni	Dimahpur	Nagaland	7.47 ± 0.97	30.89 ± 2.50	2.18 ± 1.08	*B. subtilis, P. mirabilis*
Bekang	Aizawl	Mizoram	7.39 ± 0.09	26.72 ± 1.67	0.75 ± 0.14	*B. subtilis, B. amyloliquefaciens, P. mirabilis*
2. Fermented Fish Products						
2.1 Fermented Fish, Hilsa (Tenualosa ilisha, Hamilton)						
Lona ilish	Guwahati	Assam	5.35 ± 0.14	13.36 ± 3.34	0.80 ± 0.15	ND[d]
Lona ilish	Agartala	Tripura	5.44 ± 0.19	2.50 ± 0.83	0.70 ± 0.20	ND
Iliha ngari	Guwahati	Assam	5.28 ± 0.12	2.50 ± 2.50	0.70 ± 0.42	ND
2.2 Fermented Fish (Puntius sophore, Hamilton)						
Ngari	Imphal	Manipur	6.09 ± 0.20	43.02 ± 1.67	0.18 ± 0.04	ND
Shedal	Jorhat	Assam	6.82 ± 0.79	52.62 ± 5.84	0.27 ± 0.05	ND

Shedal	Guwahati	Assam	6.48 ± 0.35	116.06 ± 4.17	1.19 ± 0.09	ND
Shedal	Silchar	Assam	6.75 ± 0.30	131.09 ± 4.10	1.29 ± 0.04	ND
Shedal/Berma	Agartala	Assam	6.46 ± 0.22	123.58 ± 5.01	0.90 ± 0.19	ND
Ngawum	Aizawl	Mizoram	6.31 ± 0.30	76.82 ± 6.68	2.00 ± 0.42	ND
Tungtap	Shillong	Meghalaya	6.40 ± 0.22	74.31 ± 4.17	0.75 ± 0.05	ND
2.3 Fermented Fish (Raw Material used for Fermentation is not Yet Identified)						
Shedal	Silchar	Assam	7.63 ± 0.40	34.23 ± 4.17	1.5 ± 0.58	ND
Ngawum	Aizawl	Mizoram	8.18 ± 0.09	27.55 ± 2.50	1.65 ± 0.88	ND
2.4 Fermented Small Fish/Shrimp Paste (Mixture of Different Fish Species)						
Hentak	Imphal	Manipur	6.14 ± 0.31	59.28 ± 5.84	1.4 ± 0.55	Debaromyces fabryi
Dang-pui-thu	Aizawl	Meghalaya	7.35 ± 0.06	33.40 ± 5.01	0.65 ± 0.31	*B. subtilis, Staphylococcus simulans, Streptomyces* sp.
Ngapi	Imphal	Manipur	6.70 ± 0.13	17.53 ± 2.50	1.10 ± 0.32	*B. subtilis, B. amyloliquefaciens, Bacillus licheniformis*
3. Fermented Meat (Pork Fat)						
Sa'um	Aizawl	Mizoram	6.42 ± 0.55	13.32 ± 3.80	0.70 ± 0.37	*P. mirabilis, E. faecium*

Source: From Singh, T. A. et al. 2014. *Food Research International* 55: 356–62.

[a] Name indicated here to identify the difference in the indigenous process of preparation and place of collection even though some of them have the same vernacular name.
[b] Fibrinolytic activity measured by spectrophotometric assay using plasmin as standard. KPU is kilo units of plasmin equivalent.
[c] Mean of five samples reading of fibrinolytic to caseinolytic activity.
[d] ND means fibrinolytic colonies were not detected during fibrin plate assay.

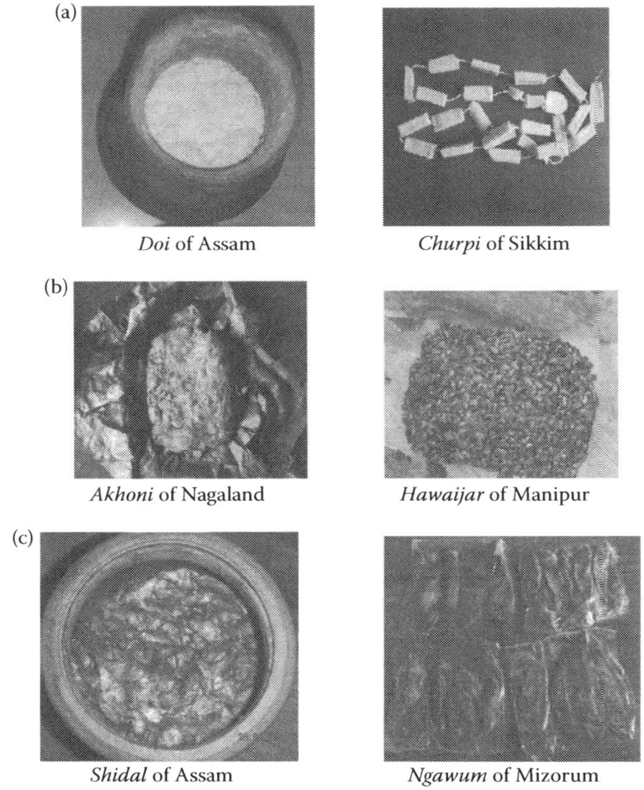

Figure 14.2 Examples of protein-rich fermented foods of Northeast India. (a) Fermented milk products. (b) Fermented soybean products. (c) Fermented fish products.

activity in the fermented foods included *Vagococcus carniphilus*, *Vagococcus lutrae*, *Enterococcus faecalis*, *Enterococcus faecium*, *Enterococcus gallinarum*, and *Pediococcus acidilactici*. *B. subtilis* strain MH10B5 (MTCC 5481) isolated from *hawaijar*, a traditional fermented soybean food of Manipur, India (Jeyaram et al. 2008) with high fibrinolytic activity and superior fermentative parameters were selected for fermented soybean production (Figure 14.3) with fibrinolytic activity of 5000 Kilo plasmin units/kg. Fermented foods rich in fibrinolytic enzymes can be a potential weapon for the treatment of cardiovascular diseases (Mine et al. 2005).

14.3.2 ACE-Inhibitory Properties

Hypertension is the main cause of several risk factors such as heart failure, stroke, coronary heart disease, and myocardial infarction. A decrease in blood pressure by 5 mmHg has been equated with 16% decrease in cardiovascular diseases (FitzGerald et al. 2004). As various side effects such as hypotension, increased potassium level, cough, reduced renal function angioedema, and skin rashes are associated with the use of synthetic drugs, ACE-inhibitory peptides derived from food protein are gaining much importance for treating hypertension (Hartmann and Meisel 2007,

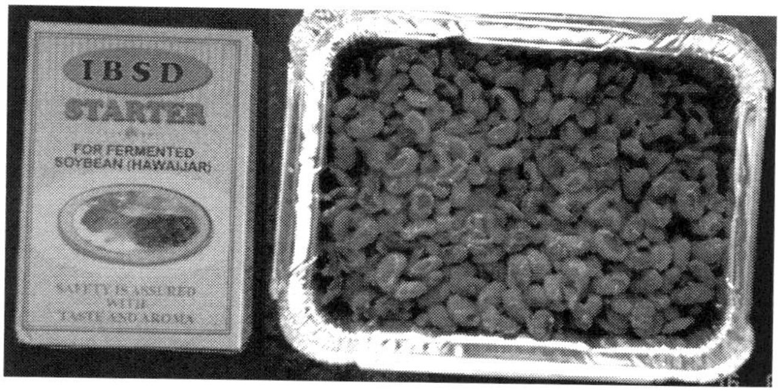

Figure 14.3 Fibrinolytic-fermented soybean food produced by *B. subtilis* strain MH10B5 (MTCC 5481).

Haque and Chand 2008). Antihypertensive peptides are one of the most studied bioactive peptides in the case of fermented foods, which depend on proteolytic properties of the starter. These peptides inhibit ACE, which is a key enzyme responsible for the conversion of angiotensin I to angiotensin II, a strong vasoconstrictor. Angiotensin II causes vasoconstriction, reabsorption of water and sodium ions, which affects the electrolyte balance, volume, and pressure of blood. Inhibition of ACE by peptides is considered to be the first line of therapy for the treatment of hypertension.

ACE-inhibitory properties have been studied in various fermented milk products such as fermented sour milk (Nakamura et al. 1995), *dahi* (Ashar and Chand 2004), *kefir* (Quiros et al. 2005), *koumiss*, fermented mare milk (Chen et al. 2010), sheep milk yogurt (Papadimitriou et al. 2007), fermented camel milk (Moslehishad et al. 2013), and fermented goat milk (Minervini et al. 2009). In the case of cheese products, *in vitro* ACE-inhibitory properties has also been reported in water-soluble extracts of Cheddar, Blue, Norvegia, Jarlsberg (Stepaniak et al. 2001), Gouda, Edam, Emmental, Camembert (Saito et al. 2000), and Swiss cheeses (Meyer et al. 2009).

Various fermented milk products are available commercially such as *calpis* (sour milk in Japan) and *festivo* (fermented milk in Finland). Quiros et al. (2007) have purified and identified several novel ACE-inhibitory peptides in milk fermented with *Ent. faecalis* strains, which were isolated from raw milk. Antihypertensive properties of fermented milk products have also been proven by various animal studies (Nakamura et al. 1995, Sipola et al. 2002) and clinical trials (Hata et al. 1996, Seppo et al. 2002, 2003). Calpis, fermented sour milk containing two potent tripeptides VPP and IPP, has shown hypotensive effect in spontaneously hypertensive rats (Nakamura et al. 1995) and in human subjects (Hata et al. 1996). Nakamura et al. (1996) also showed a decrease in the activity of tissue ACE upon feeding sour milk in spontaneously hypertensive rats. Fermented milk with *Lactobacillus helveticus* reduces elevated blood pressure in subjects with normal high blood pressure as well as mild hypertension without any adverse effect (Aihara et al. 2005). Recently, milk fermented with *Lactococcus lactis* NRRL B50571 and NRRLB-50572 showed similar hypotensive properties in comparison to captopril (40 mg/kg of body weight) in spontaneously hypertensive rats (Rodríguez-Figueroa et al. 2013).

Apart from milk products, fermented soybean products have also been found to possess antihypertensive properties such as *douchi* (Zhang et al. 2006), *sufu* (Iwamik and Buki 1986), *natto* (Okamoto et al. 1995), *tempe* (Gibbs et al. 2004), and soy sauce (Kinoshita et al. 1993). Consumption of fermented soybean foods has generated much interest because of the fact that their consumption lowers the risk of cardiovascular diseases (Liu and Pan 2011). Peptide- including amino acids Ala, Phe, and His showing ACE-inhibitory properties have been isolated from soybeans fermented by *B. natto* and *chunggugjang* fermented with *B. subtilis* (Korhonen and Pihlanto 2003). Fractionated whey from soy milk fermented with probiotics, *Lactobacillus casei, Lactobacillus acidophilus, Lactobacillus bulgaricus, Streptococcus thermophilus,* and *Bifidobacterium longum* exhibit good antihypertensive property (Tsai et al. 2006). Rho et al. (2009) have purified and identified ACE-inhibitory peptides from fermented soybean. The purified peptide (Leu-Val-Gln-Gly-Ser) showed 66-fold higher activities in comparison to fermented soybean extract. Recently, Jakubczyk et al. (2013) showed the impact of fermentation by *Lactobacillus plantarum* 299 V on the formation of ACE-inhibitory peptides from pea protein. In the case of sourdough fermentation 14 different peptides with ACE-inhibitory activity were identified in lactic-acid-fermented white wheat, whole wheat, and rye flour (Rizzello et al. 2008)

Fermented fish and shrimp in many Asian countries have also been studied for the activity of ACE-inhibitory peptides. Okamoto et al. (1995) reported ACE-inhibitory properties in fermented fish sauce prepared from salmon, sardine, and anchovy. Je et al. (2005a) have purified and characterized ACE-inhibitory peptide from the sauce of fermented blue mussel. The purified peptide on oral administration was able to significantly reduce blood pressure in spontaneous hypertensive rats (Je et al. 2005a). Similarly, ACE-inhibitory peptides are also reported in fermented oyster sauce (Je et al. 2005b), fermented anchovy sauce (Ichimura et al. 2003), fermented sardine sauce (Ichimura et al. 2003), and fermented botino sauce (Ichimura et al. 2003). Further, clinical studies for antihypertensive properties are required in the case of fermented fish and soybean products.

14.3.3 Antimicrobial Properties

Antimicrobial activity in fermented foods is mainly due to organic acids and antimicrobial peptides (bacteriocin). The synergistic activity of naturally occurring peptides, peptides produced by the fermenting microflora, and peptides formed by hydrolysis of dietary protein during fermentation gives the overall antimicrobial properties of peptides in fermented foods. Antimicrobial peptides (<10 kDa; 3–50 amino acids) produced by microorganisms find potential application in food preservation and medicine (Cleveland et al. 2001). Bacteriocins produced by LAB are low molecular weight, ribosomally synthesized peptides that possess antimicrobial activity toward closely related Gram-positive and Gram-negative bacteria (Vuyst and Leroy 2007). Several bacteriocins produced by LAB having application in food industry have been purified and characterized (Leelavatcharamas et al. 2011, Einatsson and Lauzon 1995, Vuyst and Leroy 2007). Bacteriocin-producing starter cultures have been applied to obtain a desired population in sourdough fermentation, antilisterial effect in fermented sausages, and anticlostridial effects in cheese (Leroy and De Vuyst 1999, Leroy et al. 2006, Vuyst and Leroy 2007).

Another group of peptide having antibacterial properties is those that are produced by hydrolysis of food protein by the starter culture. Casein on hydrolysis during milk fermentation is a promising source of antimicrobial peptides. Antimicrobial peptides are derived by hydrolysis of α_{S1}-casein, α_{S2}-casein, β-casein, and κ-casein in various fermented milk products using LAB (Haque and Chand 2008, Meira et al. 2012). They act against different pathogenic Gram-negative (*Escherichia, Helicobacter,* and *Salmonella*) and Gram-positive bacteria (*Listeria* and *Staphylococcus*), yeasts, and filamentous fungi (Haque and Chand 2008). Hayes et al. (2006) have also reported that antimicrobial peptides are produced by fermentation of milk casein by LAB. They purified three peptides produced on fermentation of sodium caseinate by *Lb. acidophilus* DPC6026 showing antibacterial properties against pathogenic strains *Enterobacter sakazakii* ATCC 12868 and *E. coli* DPC5063. Earlier, Minervini et al. (2003) have reported an antimicrobial peptide corresponding to β-casein f (184–210) by hydrolysis of sodium caseinate with proteases of *Lb. helveticus* PR4. This peptide exhibited a broad spectrum of antibacterial activity against pathogens such as *Staphylococcus aureus, Enterobacter faecium, Yersinia enterocolitica,* and *Salmonella* spp. (Rizzello et al. 2005). The mechanism of action of antibacterial peptide formed by the hydrolysis of food proteins includes disruption of microbial membrane, leading to ion and metabolic leakage, disruption of membrane-coupled respiration, depolarization, and finally cell death (Phadke et al. 2005). *Tempe* has also been reported to exhibit antibacterial activity against selected Gram-positive bacteria (Kobayasi et al. 1992, Kiers et al. 2002). Protein extract of fish meat fermented with *B. subtilis* A26 showed antibacterial activity against Gram-positive bacteria such as *Bacillus cereus, Ent. faecalis, Staph. aureus,* and *Micrococcus luteus* (Jemil et al. 2014).

LAB isolated from various foods such as fermented milk (Todorov et al. 2007, Powell et al. 2007), fermented vegetables (Jiang et al. 2012, Hu et al. 2013), and fermented meat and fish products (Pringsulaka et al. 2012) have shown to possess ability to produce antimicrobial peptides (bacteriocin). *B. subtilis* SC-8 isolated from Korean fermented soybean (Yeo et al. 2012) and *B. amyloliquefaciens* isolated from Thai shrimp paste (Kaewklom et al. 2013) have shown to exhibit antibacterial properties against *B. cereus* group and *Listeria monocytogenes*, respectively. The future of antimicrobial peptides in fermented foods looks promising not only as nutraceuticals or natural drug in pharmaceutical industry but also as a preservative in food industry.

14.3.4 Antioxidant Properties

Free radicals can result in cellular damage, which can give rise to several diseases such as cancer, diabetic, arthrosclerosis, and arthritis (Halliwell 1994). Peptides are emerging as potential antioxidants in recent years in various protein-rich fermented foods. The antioxidant activity of the peptides in fermented foods can be attributed due to their ability to scavenge free radicals, metal ion chelating property, and due to their ability to inhibit lipid peroxidation. As the use of artificial antioxidants has been prohibited in some countries due to their potential risk to human health (Kahl and Kappus 1993), antioxidant peptides has gained much attention across the globe. Antioxidant peptides have been reported in milk products such as yogurt (Kudoh et al. 2001, Sabeena et al. 2010, Perna et al. 2013), cheese (Meira et al. 2012), and *kefir* (Liu et al. 2005). Researchers across the globe have purified and characterized several antioxidant peptides from fermented milk products (Qian et al. 2011, Meira et al. 2012). Kudoh et al. (2001) have purified an antioxidant peptide derived from κ-casein (ARHPHPHLSFM) from milk fermented with *Lactobacillus delbrueckii* subsp. *bulgaris* IFO13953.

Peptides showing antioxidant properties are generally rich in aromatic and/or hydrophobic amino acids and histidine (Sarmadi and Ismail 2010). Antioxidant properties of peptides are affected by peptide linkage and peptide conformation (Erdmann et al. 2008). Antioxidant activity has also been reported in a number of fermented fishery products such as fermented blue mussels (Jung et al. 2005), fish sauces (Harada et al. 2003), fermented mussel sauce (Rajapakse et al. 2005), fermented shrimp paste (Peralta et al. 2005), and Thai fermented shrimp and krill products such as *jaloo, koong-sam,* and *kapi* (Faithong et al. 2010). Peralta et al. (2008) have reported that antioxidant activity of Philippine salt-fermented shrimp paste increased with prolonged fermentation time, in comparison to normal fermentation time in their previous study (Peralta et al. 2005). Traditional Thai fermented shrimp and krill products showed antioxidant activity against DPPH and ABTS free radicals. Recently, protein extract of different fish meat (*sardinella, zebra blenny, goby, ray*) fermented with *B. subtilis* A26 showed stronger antioxidant activity (Jemil et al. 2014).

Antioxidant peptides are also reported in Sourdough fermentation of cereal flours by LAB (Coda et al. 2012). The study showed that the radical-scavenging activity of water/salt-soluble extracts prepared from fermented sourdoughs was significantly higher than that of chemically acidified doughs and the highest activity was found for whole wheat, spelt, rye, and *kamut* sourdoughs (Coda et al. 2012). They concluded that the antioxidant properties were due to peptides formed on proteolysis of native cereal proteins by LAB. Fermented food enriched with antioxidant peptides can be a better alternative to synthetic antioxidant for the reduction of oxidative stress-related diseases.

14.3.5 Immunomodulatory Properties

Peptides derived from food protein can enhance the immune system by lymphocyte proliferation, antibody synthesis, cytokine regulation, and by enhancing natural killer cell activity. Feeding mice with fermented milk have resulted in increases in various immune responses such as IgA-producing cells, macrophage activity, and specific antibody responses during infections (Perdigon et al. 1999). LeBlanc et al. (2002) reported that mice administered with three peptidic fractions from milk fermented with *Lb. helveticus* significantly increased IgA-producing cell count and reduced fibrosarcoma size. In another study, LeBlanc et al. (2004) have reported that peptides released on hydrolysis by *Lb. helveticus* induced a protective humoral immune response against an *E. coli* O157:H7 infection in mice. Oral administration of nonbacterial fraction of milk fermented with *Lb. helveticus* R389 containing bioactive peptides modulated the gut mucosal immune response (Vinderola et al. 2007). In a recent study, Qian et al. (2011) reported that peptidic fraction of milk fermented with *Lb. delbrueckii* subsp. *bulgaricus* LB340 displayed good immunomodulatory properties. In the case of peptides from milk protein, immunomodulatory properties is either due to stimulation of vitality of lymphocytes and promoted proliferation (derived from κ- and β-casein) or due to inhibition of lymphocyte activity and reduced proliferation (derived from α-casein) (Sutas et al. 1996).

Matar et al. (2001) showed that milk fermented with a *Lb. helveticus* strain fed to mice for 3 days significantly increased the numbers of IgA-secreting cells in their intestinal mucosa, compared with control mice fed with similar milk incubated with a nonproteolytic variant of the same strain. As there was immunostimulatory effect of fermented milk with proteolytic variant, the effect was attributed to peptides released from the casein fraction. Wagar et al. (2009) have reported immunomodulatory properties of fermented soy and dairy milk prepared with pure and mixed culture of *Strep. thermophilus* ST5, *B. longum* R0175, and *Lb. helveticus* R0052. Metabolites, especially peptides, formed during food fermentation can have a positive impact on the immune system and research on a wide range of fermented foods is needed.

14.3.6 Anticancer Properties

Cancer is the second leading cause of mortality worldwide and 90%–95% cancer cases are attributed to environment and life style (Anand et al. 2008). Several studies have shown that several food components in fermented foods could lower the risk of cancer (Chen et al. 2007, Yasuda et al. 2010). In the last few years, peptides derived from food proteins have shown to possess anticancer properties by preventing the different stages of cancer (De Mejia and Dia 2010). Several fermented foods and LAB in fermented foods have also been reported for their cancer protective effects (Lee et al. 2004) but studies on the mechanism of their effect is still at its preliminary phase. Goat milk fermented with *Lb. plantarum* and *Lactobacillus paracasei* showed decrease viability of HeLa cells with increasing concentration of goat milk hydrolysate (Nandhini and Palaniswamy 2013).

Balansky et al. (1999) have reported inhibitory effect of dried milk fermented with selected *Lb. bulgaricus* strain on carcinogenesis induced by 1,2-dimethyl hydrazine in rats. Even the LAB isolated from fermented foods have shown to reduce the risk of certain cancers (Tuo et al. 2010). A recent study demonstrated differential antiproliferative properties of 12 different cow milk cheeses in HL-60 cells, which was used as a cancer model (Yasuda et al. 2010). Similar antiproliferative activities were also observed in the case of 11 goat milk cheeses in HL-60 cells (Yasuda et al. 2012). Peptide fractions isolated from anchovy sauce showed strong anticancer activity, as they possessed strong antiproliferative activity against U937 by inducing apoptosis (Lee et al. 2004). The peptide fraction having antiproliferative activity was found to be composed of Ala and Phe, and its molecular weight was estimated to be 440.9 Da.

Kefir, a traditional fermented milk product, and yogurt showed higher antiproliferative effects on human breast cancer cells in comparison to unfermented milk (Chen et al. 2007). In their study peptide content and capillary electrophoresis analyses showed that *kefir*-mediated milk fermentation led to an increase in peptide concentration and a change in peptide profiles, which might be responsible for anticancer properties. Cell-free fraction of *kefir* has also shown to induce cell-cycle arrest and apoptosis in HTLV-1-negative malignant T-lymphocytes (Maalouf et al. 2011) and apoptosis of gastric cancer cells SGC7901 *in vitro.*

14.3.7 Cholesterol-Lowering Properties

Hypercholesterolemia is a significant risk factor in the development of cardiovascular diseases, which is one of the major causes of death in various countries. Consumption of whey proteins (Zhang and Beynen 1993, Nagaoka et al. 1992), soy proteins (Hori et al. 2001), and fish proteins has been reported to have hypocholesterolemic properties, but the exact mechanism behind the action of these protein or peptides derived on fermentation is not identified. Ataie-Jafari et al. (2009) have studied the effect of consumption of probiotic yogurt on serum cholesterol level in mild to moderate hypercholesterolemic subjects and found that consumption of probiotic yogurt resulted in significant ($p < 0.05$) decrease in serum total cholesterol during the clinical trials. Yogurt prepared from buffalo milk and soy milk also showed reduction in plasma total cholesterol level in rats fed on a cholesterol-enriched diet (AbdEl-Gawad et al. 2005).

Soy protein has been reported for its higher hypocholesterolemic activity compared with casein (Nagaoka et al. 1999), whereas soy protein hydrolysates showed higher hypocholesterolemic activity in comparison to soy proteins (Anderson et al. 1995, Nagaoka et al. 1999). *Natto* (*B. subtilis*) has shown to reduce plasma cholesterol and triglyceride levels in hypercholesterolemic rats (Iwai et al. 2002). Feeding *tempe, Rhizopus oligosporus*-fermented soybean, to rats has also shown to exhibit hypocholesterolemic effect (Guermani et al. 1993). In a recent study, feeding fermented soy milk to rats fed a high cholesterol diet, reduced plasma cholesterol level significantly (Kobayashi et al. 2012). The study reported a significant decrease in the expression of SREBP-2, a cholesterol synthesis-related gene, but significant increase in the expression of CYP7a1, a cholesterol catabolism-related gene. Protein-rich fermented foods have been studied for lowering blood cholesterol and triglyceride levels but future studies on the molecular mechanism of the peptide/protein need to be explored.

14.4 Conclusion

Protein-rich fermented foods beyond their nutritional role exhibit a wide range of biological activities that positively influence the functions of specific organs. The research in the area of bioactive peptides from fermented foods is only at its beginning and many novel peptides with physiological effects will be discovered in the future. Apart from ACE-inhibitory properties of milk products, physiological properties of other important fermented foods have not been proven by animal models and long-term human trials. Animal studies and clinical trials using sufficient number of subjects need to be carried out to decide the dose of specific peptides. The protein-rich traditional fermented foods of developing countries are not yet explored for their bioactive peptides. Studies on these unpopular protein-rich fermented foods will lead to the discovery of novel bioactive peptides. Moreover, molecular mechanism for the action of many known bioactive peptides in fermented foods needs to be studied for their application in food and pharmaceutical industries. Owing to increase in research in the area of fermented functional foods, there is now considerable consumer awareness on the effect of ingesting such foods in relation to health promotion and disease prevention. The advances in the area of fermented foods coupled with advances in biotechnology promise to revolutionize the future of fermented foods as nutraceutical and functional foods for the prevention and treatment of various diseases.

References

Abdel-Gawad, I., E. M. Ei-Sayad, S. A. Hafez, H. M. El-Zeine, and F. A. Saleh. 2005. The hypocholesterolaemic effect of milk yoghurt and soy-yoghurt containing bifidobacteria in rats fed on a cholesterol-enriched diet. *International Dairy Research* 15: 37–44.

Aihara, K., O. Kajimoto, H. Hirata, R. Takahashi, and Y. Nakamura. 2005. Effect of powdered fermented milk with *Lactobacillus helveticus* on subjects with high-normal blood pressure or mild hypertension. *Journal of American College of Nutrition* 24: 257–65.

Anand, P., A. B. Kunnumakara, C. Sundaram, K. B. Harikumar, S. T. Tharakan, O. S. Lai, B. Sung, and B. B. Aggarwal. 2008. Cancer is a preventing disease that requires major lifestyle changes. *Pharmaceutical Research* 25: 2097–2116.

Anderson, J. W., B. M. Johnstone, and M. E. Cook-Newell. 1995. Meta-analysis of the effects of soy protein intake on serum lipids. *New England Journal of Medicine* 333: 276–282.

Ashar, M. N. and R. Chand. 2004. Fermented milk containing ACE inhibitory peptides reduces blood pressure in middle aged hypertensive subjects. *Milchwissenschaft* 59: 363–366.

Ataie-Jafari, A., B. Larijani, M. H. Alavi, and F. Tahbaz. 2009. Cholesterol-lowering effect of probiotic yogurt in comparison with ordinary yogurt in mildly to moderately hypercholesterolemic subjects. *Annals of Nutrition and Metabolism* 54: 22–27.

Balansky, R., B. Gyosheva, G. Ganchev, Z. Mircheva, S. Minkova, and G. Georgiev. 1999. Inhibitory effects of freeze-dried milk fermented by selected *Lactobacillus bulgaricus* strains on carcinogenesis induced by 1,2-dimethylhydrazine in rats and by diethylnitrosamine in hamsters. *Cancer Letters* 147: 125–137.

Chang, C. T., P. M. Wang, Y. F. Hung, and Y. C. Chung. 2012. Purification and biochemical properties of a fibrinolytic enzyme from *Bacillus subtilis*—fermented red bean. *Food Chemistry* 133: 1611–1617.

Chaves-López, C., R. Tofalo, A. Serio, A. Paparella, G. Sacchetti, and G. Suzzi. 2012. Yeasts from Colombian kumis as source of peptides with angiotensin I converting enzyme (ACE) inhibitory activity in milk. *International Journal of Food Microbiology* 159: 39–46.

Chen, C., H. M. Chan, and S. Kubow. 2007. Kefir extracts suppress *in vitro* proliferation of estrogen-dependent human breast cancer cells but not normal mammary epithelial cells. *Journal of Medicinal Food* 10: 416–22.

Chen, Y., Z. Wang, X. Chen, Y. Liu, H. Zhang, and T. Sun. 2010. Identification of angiotensin I-converting enzyme inhibitory peptides from koumiss, a traditional fermented mare's milk. *Journal of Dairy Science* 93: 884–92.

Cho, K. M., J. H. Lee, H. D. Yun, B. Y. Ahn, H. Kim, and W. T. Seo. 2011. Changes of phytochemical constituents (isoflavones, flavanols, and phenolic acids) during cheonggukjang soybeans fermentation using potential probiotics Bacillus subtilis CS90. *Journal of Food Composition and Analysis* 24: 402–410.

Cleveland, J., T. J. Montville, I. F. Nes, and M. L. Chikindas. 2001. Bacteriocins: Safe, natural antimicrobials for food preservation. *International Journal of Food Microbiology* 71: 1–20.

Coda, R., C. G. Rizzello, D. Pinto, and M. Gobbetti. 2012. Selected lactic acid bacteria synthesize antioxidant peptides during sourdough fermentation of cereal flours. *Applied and Environmental Microbiology* 78: 1087–96.

De Mejia, E. G. and V. P. Dia. 2010. The role of nutraceutical proteins and peptides in apoptosis, angiogenesis, and metastasis of cancer cells. *Cancer Metastasis* 29: 511–528.

Einatsson, H. and H. L. Lauzon. 1995. Biopreservation of brined shrimp (*Pandalus borealis*) by bacteriocin of lactic acid bacteria. *Applied and Environmental Microbiology* 61: 669–676.

Erdmann, K., B. W. Y. Cheung, and H. Schroder. 2008. The possible role of food derived bioactive peptides in reducing the risk of cardiovascular diseases. *Journal of Nutritional Biochemistry* 19: 643–654.

Faithong, N., S. Benjakul, S. Phatcharat, and W. Binsan. 2010. Chemical composition and antioxidative activity of Thai traditional fermented shrimp and krill products *Food Chemistry* 119: 133–140.

FitzGerald, R. J., B. A. Murray, and D. J. Walsh. 2004. Hypotensive peptides from milk protein. *Journal of Nutrition* 34: 9805–9885.

Fujita, M., K. Hong, and Y. Ito. 1995. Transport of nattokinase across the rat intestinal tract. *Biological Pharmacological Bulletin* 18: 1194–1196.

Gibbs, B. F., A. Zougman, R. Masse, and C. Mulligan. 2004. Production and characterization of bioactive peptides from soy hydrolysate and soy-fermented food. *Food Research International* 37: 123–131.

Giri A., K. Osako, A. Okamoto, E. Okazaki, and T. Ohshima. 2011. Antioxidative properties of aqueous and aroma extracts of squid *miso* prepared with *Aspergillus oryzae*-inoculated *koji*. *Food Research International* 44: 317–325.

Groziak, S. M. and G. D. Miller. 2000. Natural bioactive substances in milk and colostrum: Effects on the arterial blood pressure system. *British Journal of Nutrition* 84: S119–S125.

Guermani, L., C. Villaume, H. M. Bau, J. P. Nicolas, and L. Mejean. 1993. Modification of soyprotein hypocholesterolemic effect after fermentation by *Rhizopus oligosporus* spT3. *Sciences des Aliments* 13: 317–324.

Halliwell, B. 1994. Free radicals, antioxidants, and human disease: Curiosity, cause, or consequence? *Lancet* 344: 721–724.

Haque, E. and R. Chand. 2008. Antihypertensive and antimicrobial bioactive peptides from milk protein. *European Food Research Technology* 227: 7–15.

Harada, K., C. Okano, H. Kadoguchi, Y. Okubo, M. Ando, S. Kitao, and Y. Tamura. 2003. Peroxyl radical scavenging capability of fish sauces measured by the chemiluminescence method. *International Journal of Molecular Medicine* 12: 621–625.

Hartmann, R. and H. Meisel. 2007. Food-derived peptides with biological activity: From research to food applications. *Current Opinion in Biotechnology* 18: 163–169.

Hata, Y., M. Yamamoto, M. Ohni, K. Nakajima, Y. Nakamura, and T. Takano. 1996. A placebo-controlled study of the effect of sour milk on blood pressure in hypertensive subjects. *American Journal of Clinical Nutrition* 64: 767–771.

He, F. J. and J. Q. Chen. 2013. Consumption of soybean, soy foods, soy isoflavones and breast cancer incidence: Differences between Chinese women and women in Western countries and possible mechanisms. *Food Science and Human Wellness* 2: 146–161.

Hayes, M., R. P. Ross, G. F. Fitzgerald, C. Hill, and C. Stanton. 2006. Casein-Derived Antimicrobial peptides generated by *Lactobacillus acidophilus* DPC6026. *Applied and Environmental Microbiology* 72: 2260–2264.

Hori, G., M. F. Wang, Y. C. Chan et al. 2001. Soy protein hydrolysate with bound phospholipids reduces serum cholesterol level in hypercholesterolemic adult male volunteers. *Bioscience Biotechnology and Biochemistry* 65: 72–78.

Hu, M., H. Zhao, C. Zhang, J. Yu, and Z. Lu. 2013. Purification and characterization of plantaricin 163, a novel bacteriocin produced by *Lactobacillus plantarum* 163 isolated from traditional Chinese fermented vegetables. *Journal of Agriculture and Food Chemistry* 61: 11676–82.

Ichimura, T., J. Hu, D. O. Aita, and S. Maruyama. 2003. Angiotensin I-converting enzyme inhibitory activity and insulin secretion stimulative activity of fermented fish sauce. *Journal of Bioscience and Bioengineering* 96: 496–499.

Iwai, K., N. Nakaya, Y. Kawasaki, and H. Matsue. 2002. Antioxidant function of Natto, a kind of fermented soybean: Effect of LDL oxidation and lipid metabolism in cholesterol fed rats. *Journal of Agriculture and Food Chemistry* 50: 3597–3610.

Iwamik, S. K. and F. Buki. 1986. Involvement of post-digestion hydropholic peptides in plasma cholesterol-lowing effect of dietary plant proteins. *Agricultural and Biological Chemistry* 50: 1217–1222.

Jakubczyk, A., M. Karas, B. Baranaik, and M. Pietrzak. 2013. The impact of fermentation and *in vitro* digestion on formation of angiotensin converting enzyme (ACE) inhibitory peptides from pea protein. *Food Chemistry* 141: 3774–3780.

Je, J. Y., P. J. Park, H. G. Byun, Jung, W. K., and S. K. Kim. 2005a. Angiotensin I converting enzyme (ACE) inhibitory peptide derived from the sauce of fermented blue mussel. *Mytilus edulis. Bioresource Technology* 6: 1624–1629.

Je, J. Y., J. Y. Park, W. K. Jung, Park, P. J., and S. K. Kim. 2005b. Isolation of angiotensin I converting enzyme (ACE) inhibitor from fermented oyster sauce, *Crassostrea gigas. Food Chemistry* 90: 809–814.

Jemil, I., M. Jridi, R. Nasri et al. 2014. Functional, antioxidant and antibacterial properties of protein hydrolysates prepared from fish meat fermented by *Bacillus subtilis* A26. *Process Biochemistry* 49: 963–972.

Jeong, Y., W. S. Yang, K. H. Kim., K. T. Chung, W. H. Joo, J. H. Kim, D. E. Kim, and J. U. Park. 2004. Purification of a fibrinolytic enzyme (*myulchikinase*) from pickled anchovy and its cytotoxicity to the tumor cell lines. *Biotechnology Letters* 26: 393–97.

Jeyaram, K., W. M. Singh, T. Premarani, A. R. Devi, K. S. Chanu, N. C. Talukdar, and M. R. Singh. 2008. Molecular identification of dominant microflora associated with Hawaijar—A traditional fermented soybean (Glycine max (L.)) food of Manipur, India. *International Journal of Food Microbiology* 122: 259–268.

Jiang, J., B. Shi, D. Zhu, Q. Cai, Y. Chen, J. Li, K. Qi, and M. Zhang. 2012. Characterization of a novel bacteriocin produced by *Lactobacillus sakei* LSJ618 isolated from traditional Chinese fermented radish. *Food Control* 23: 338–44.

Jung, W., N. Rajapakse, and S. Kim. 2005. Antioxidative activity of a low molecular weight peptide derived from the sauce of fermented blue mussel, *Mytilus edulis* European. *Food Research and Technology* 220: 535–539.

Kaewklom, S., S. Lumlert, W. Kraikul, and R. Aunpad. 2013. Control of *Listeria monocytogenes* on sliced bologna sausage using a novel bacteriocin, amysin, produced by *Bacillus amyloliquefaciens* isolated from Thai shrimp paste (Kapi). *Food Control* 32: 552–57.

Kahl, R. and H. Kappus, 1993. Toxicology of the synthetic antioxidant BHA and BHT in comparison with the natural antioxidant vitamin E. *ZLebensmUntersForsch* 196: 329–38.

Kiers, J. L., M. J. R. Nout, F. M. Rombouts, M. J. A. Nabuurs, and J. Van der Meulen. 2002. Inhibition of adhesion of enterotoxic *Escherichia coli* K88 by soya bean tempe. *Letters of Applied Microbiology* 35: 311–315.

Kim, H. K., G. T. Kim, D. K. Kim et al. 1997. Purification and characterization of a novel fibrinolytic enzyme from *Bacillus* sp. KA38 originated from fermented fish. *Journal of Fermentation and Bioengineering* 84: 307–312.

Kinoshita, E., J. Yamakashi, and M. Kikuchi. 1993. Purification and identification of an angiotensin I-converting enzyme inhibitor from soy sauce. *Bioscience Biotechnology and Biochemistry* 57: 1107–1110.

Kobayashi, M., R. Hirahata, E. Shintaro, and F. Mitsuru. 2012. Hypocholesterolemic effects of lactic acid-fermented soymilk on rats fed a high cholesterol diet. *Nutrients* 4: 1304–1316.

Korhonen, H. and A. Pihlanto. 2003. Food-derived bioactive peptides—Opportunities for designing future foods. *Current Pharmaceutical Design* 9: 1297–1308.

Kotb, E. 2012. Fibrinolytic bacterial enzymes with thrombolytic activity. *Fibrinolytic Bacterial Enzymes with Thrombolytic Activity*. Berlin Heidelberg: Springer, pp. 1–74.

Kudoh, Y., S. Matsuda, K. Igoshi, and T. Oki. 2001. Antioxidant peptides from milk fermented with *Lactobacillus delbrueckii* ssp bulgaris IFO13953. *Journal of Japanese Society of Food Science and Technology* 48: 44–50.

LeBlanc, J., I. Fliss, and C. Matar. 2004. Induction of a humoral immune response following an Escherichia coli O157:H7 infection with an immunomodulatory peptidic fraction derived from *Lactobacillus helveticus* -fermented milk. *Clinical and Diagnostic Laboratory Immunology* 11: 1171–1181.

LeBlanc, J. G., C. Matar, J. C. Valdéz, J. LeBlanc, and G. Perdigón. 2002. Immunomodulating effects of peptidic fractions issued from milk fermented with *Lactobacillus helveticus*. *Journal of Dairy Science* 85: 2733–2742.

Lee, Y. G., K. W. Lee, J. Y. Kim, K. H. Kim, and H. J. Lee. 2004. Induction of apoptosisina human lymphoma cell line by hydrophobic peptide fraction separated from anchovy sauce. *BioFactors* 21: 63–67.

Leelavatcharamas, V., N. Arbsuwan, J. Apiraksakorn, P. Laopaiboon, and M. Kishida. 2011. Thermotolerant bacteriocin-producing lactic acid bacteria isolated from Thai local fermented foods and their bacteriocin productivity. *Biocontrol Science* 16: 33–40.

Leroy, F., T. DeWinter, T. Adriany, P. Neysens, and L. DeVuyst. 2006. Sugars relevant for sourdough fermentation stimulate growth of and bacteriocin production by Lactobacillus amylovorus DCE471. *International Journal of Food Microbiology* 112: 102–111.

Leroy, F. and L. De Vuyst, 1999. Temperature and pH conditions that prevail during the fermentation of sausages are optimal for production of the antilisterial bacteriocin sakacin K. *Applied and Environmental Microbiology* 65: 974–981.

Liu, C. F. and T. M. Pan. 2011. Beneficial effects of bioactive peptides derived from soybean on human health and their production by genetic engineering, soybean and health, Hany El-Shemy (Ed.), ISBN: 978-953-307-535-8, InTech, DOI: 10.5772/18678. Available from: http://www.intechopen.com/books/soybean-and-health/beneficial-effects-of-bioactive-peptides-derived-from-soybean-on-human-health-and-their-production-b-health-and-their-production-b

Liu, J. R., M. J. Chen, and C. W. Lin. 2005. Antimutagenic and antioxidant properties of milk-kefir and soymilk-kefir. *Journal of Agriculture and Food Chemistry* 53: 2467–2474.

Lopez, A. D. and C. C. Murray. 1998. The global burden of disease 1990–2020. *Nature Medicine* 4: 1241–43.

Maalouf, K., E. Baydoun, and S. Rizk. 2011. Kefir induces cell-cycle arrest and apoptosis in HTLV-1-negative malignant T-lymphocytes. *Cancer Management and Research* 3: 39–47.

Matar, C., S. S. Nadathur, A. T. Bakalinsky, and J. Goulet. 1997. Antimutagenic effects of milk fermented by *Lactobacillus helveticus* L89 and a protease-deficient derivative. *Journal of Dairy Science* 80: 1965–1970.

Matar, C., J. C. Valdez, M. Medina, M. Rachid, and G. Perdigo. 2001. Immunomodulating effects of milks fermented by *Lactobacillus helveticus* and its non-proteolytic variant. *Journal of Dairy Research* 68: 601–609.

Meira, S. M. M., D. J. Daroit, V. E. Helfer et al. 2012. Bioactive peptides in water soluble extract of ovine cheese from southern Brazil and Uruguay. *Food Research International* 48: 322–329.

Meyer, J., U. Butikofer, B. Walther, D. Wechsler, and R. Sieber. 2009. Hot topic: Changes in angiotensin-converting enzyme inhibition and concentration of the teripeptides Val-Pro-Pro and Ile-Pro-Pro during ripening of different Swiss cheese varieties. *Journal of Dairy Science* 92: 826–836.

Mine, Y., A. H. K. Wong, and B. Jiang. 2005. Fibrinolytic enzymes in Asian traditional fermented foods. *Food Research International* 38: 243–250.

Minervini, F., F. Algaron, G. C. Rizello, P. F. Fox, V. Monnet, and M. Gobbetti. 2003. Angiotensin I-converting-enzyme-inhibitory and antibacterial peptides from *Lactobacillus helveticus* PR4 proteinase-hydrolyzed caseins of milk from six species. *Applied and Environmental Microbiology* 69: 5297–5305.

Minervini, F., M. T. Bilanca, S. Siragusa, M. Gobbetti, and F. Caponio. 2009. Fermented goat milk produced with selected multiple starters as a potentially functional foods. *Food Microbiology* 26: 559–564.

Montriwong, A., S. Kaewphuak, S. Rodtong, and S. Roytrakul. 2012. Novel fibrinolytic enzymes from *Virgibacillus halodenitrificans* SK1-3-7 isolated from fish sauce fermentation. *Process Biochemistry* 47: 2379–2387.

Moslehishad, M., M. R. Ehsani, and M. Salami. 2013. The comparative assessment of ACE-inhibitory and antioxidant activities of peptide fractions obtained from fermented camel and bovine milk by *Lactobacillus rhamnosus* PTCC1637. *International Dairy Research* 29: 82–87.

Nagaoka, S., Y. Kanamaru, T. Kojima, and T. Kuwata, 1992. Comparative studies on serum cholesterol lowering action of whey protein and soybean protein in rats. *Bioscience Biotechnology and Biochemistry* 56: 1484–1485.

Nagaoka, S., K. Miwa, M. Eto, Y. Kuzuya, G. Hori, and K. Yamamoto. 1999. Soy protein peptic hydrolysate with bound phospholipids decreases micellar solubility and cholesterol adsorption in rats and caco-2 cells. *Journal of Nutrition* 129: 1725–1730.

Nakamura, Y., O. Masuda, and T. Takano. 1996. Decrease of tissue angiotensin I-converting enzyme activity upon feeding sour milk in spontaneously hypertensive rats. *Bioscience Biotechnology and Biochemistry* 60: 488–489.

Nakamura, Y., Yamamoto, N., K. Sakai, A. Okubo, Yamazaki, S., and T. Takano. 1995. Purification and characterization of angiotensin I-converting enzyme inhibitors from sour milk. *Journal of Dairy Science* 78: 777–783.

Nandhini, B. and M. Palaniswamy. 2013. Anticancer effect of goat milk fermented by *Lactobacillus plantarum* and *Lactobacillus paracasei*. *International Journal of Pharmacy and Pharmaceutical Sciences* 5: 898–901.

Okamoto, A., H. Hanagata, E. Matsumoto, Y. Kawamura, Y. Koizumi, and F. Yanagida. 1995. Angiotensin I converting enzyme inhibitory activities of various fermented foods. *Bioscience Biotechnology and Biochemistry* 59: 1147–1149.

Papadimitriou, C. G., A. Vafopoulou-Mastrojiannaki, S. V. Silva, A. M. Gomes, F. X. Malcata, and E. Alichanidis. 2007. Identification of peptides in traditional and probiotic sheep milk yoghurt with angiotensin I-converting enzyme (ACE)-inhibitory activity. *Food Chemistry* 105: 647–656.

Peng, Y., Q. Huang, R. Zhang, and Y. Zhang. 2003. Purification and characterization of a fibrinolytic enzyme produced by *Bacillus amyloliquefaciens* DC-4 screened from *douchi*, a traditional Chinese soybean food. *Comparative Biochemistry and Physiology-B Biochemistry and Molecular Biology* 134: 45–52.

Peralta, E., H. Hatate, D. Watanabe, D. Kawabe, H. Murata, Y. Hama, and R. Tanaka. 2005. Antioxidative activity of Philippine salt-fermented shrimp paste and variation of its contents during fermentation. *Journal of Oleo Science* 54: 553–558.

Peralta, E. M., H. Hatate, D. Kawabe, R. Kuwahara, S. Wakamatsu, T. Yuki, and H. Murata. 2008. Improving antioxidant activity and nutritional components of Philippine salt-fermented shrimp paste through prolonged fermentation. *Food Chemistry* 111: 72–77.

Perdigon, G., E. Vintini, S. Alvarez, M. Medina, and M. Medici. 1999. Study of the possible mechanisms involved in the mucosal immune system activation by lactic acid bacteria. *Journal of Dairy Science* 82: 1108–1114.

Perna, A., I. Intaglietta, A. Simonetti, and E. Gambacorta. 2013. Effect of genetic type and casein halotype on antioxidant activity of yogurts during storage. *Journal of Dairy Science* 96: 1–7.

Phadke, S. M., B. Deslouches, S. E. Hileman, R. C. Montelaro, H. C. Wiesenfeld, and T. A. Mietzner. 2005. Antimicrobial peptides in mucosal secretions: The importance of local secretions in mitigating infection. *Journal of Nutrition* 135: 1289–1293.

Phelan, M. and D. Kerins. 2011. The potential role of milk derived peptides in cardiovascular diseases. *Food and Function* 2: 153–167.

Powell, J. E., R. C. Witthuhn, S. D. Todorov, and L. M. T. Dicks. 2007. Characterization of bacteriocin ST8KF produced by a kefir isolate Lactobacillus plantarum ST8KF. *International Dairy Journal* 17: 190–98.

Pringsulaka, O., N. Thongngam, N. Suwannasai, W. Atthakor, K. Pothivejkul, and A. Rangsiruji. 2012. Partial characterisation of bacteriocins produced by lactic acid bacteria isolated from Thai fermented meat and fish products. *Food Control* 23: 547–551.

Qian, B., M. Xing, L. Cui, Y. Deng, Y. Xu, M. Huang, and S. Zhang. 2011. Antioxidant, antihypertensive, and immunomodulatory activities of peptide fraction from fermented skim milk with *Lactobacillus delbrueckii* ssp *bulgaricus* LB340. *Journal of Dairy Research* 78: 72–79.

Quiros, A., B. Hernandez-Ledesma, M. Ramos, L. Amigo, and I. Recio. 2005. Angiotensin-converting enzyme inhibitory activity of peptides derived from *caprine kefir*. *Journal of Dairy Science* 88: 3480–3487.

Quiros, A., M. Ramos, B. Muguerza, M. Delgado, M. Miguel, A. Alexaindre, and I. Recio. 2007. Identification of novel antihypertensive peptides in milk fermented with *Enterococcus faecalis*. *International Dairy Journal* 17: 33–41.

Rajapakse, N., E. Mendis, W. K. Jung, J. Y. Je, and S. K. Kim. 2005. Purification of a radical scavenging peptide from fermented mussel sauce and its antioxidant properties. *Food Research International* 38: 175–182.

Rho, S. J., J. S. Lee, Y. L. Chung, Y. W. Kim, and H. G. Lee. 2009. Purification and identification of an angiotensing I-converting enzyme inhibitory peptide from fermented soybean extract. *Process Biochemistry* 44: 490–493.

Rizzello, C. G., A. Cassone, R. D. Cagno, and M. Gobbetti. 2008. Synthesis of angiotensin I-converting enzyme (ACE)-inhibitory peptides and γ-aminobutyric acid (GABA) during sourdough fermentation by selected lactic acid bacteria. *Journal of Agriculture and Food Chemistry* 56: 6936–6943.

Rizzello, C. G., I. Losito, M. Gobbetti, T. Carbonara, M. D. De Bari, and P. G. Zambonin. 2005. Antibacterial activities of peptides from the water-soluble extracts of Italian cheese varieties. *Journal of Dairy Science* 88: 2348–2360.

Rodríguez-Figueroa, J. C., A. F. González-Córdova, H. Astiazaran-García, A. Hernández-endoza, and B. Vallejo-Cordoba. 2013. Antihypertensive and hypolipidemic effect of milk fermented by specific *Lactococcus lactis* strains. *Journal of Dairy Science* 7: 4094–4099.

Sabeena, F. K. H., C. P. Baron, N. S. Nielsen, and C. Jacobsen. 2010. Antioxidant activity of yoghurt peptides:Part1-in vitro assays and evaluation in ω-3 enriched milk. *Food Chemistry* 123: 1081–1089.

Sabu, A. 2003. Sources, properties and applications of microbial therapeutic enzymes. *Indian Journal of Biotechnology* 2: 334–341.

Sarmadi, B.H. and A. Ismail. 2010. Antioxidative peptides from food proteins: A review. *Peptides* 31: 1949–1956.

Saito, T., T. Nakamura, H. Kitazawa, Y. Kawai, and T. Itoh. 2000. Isolation and structural analysis of antihypertensive peptides that exist naturally in Gouda cheese. *Journal of Dairy Cheese* 83: 1434–1440.

Seppo, L., T. Jauhiainen, T. Poussa, and R. Korpela. 2003. A fermented milk high in bioactive peptides has a blood pressure-lowering effect in hypertensive subjects. *American Journal of Clinical Nutrition* 77: 326–330.

Seppo, L., O. Kerojoki, T. Suomalainen, and R. Korpela. 2002. The effect of a Lactobacillus helveticus LBK-16 H fermented milk on hypertension—A pilot study on humans. *Milchwissen* 57: 124–127.

Singh, T. A., K. R. Devi, G. Ahmed, and K. Jeyaram. 2014. Microbial and endogenous origin of fibrinolytic activity in traditional fermented foods of Northeast India. *Food Research International* 55: 356–362.

Sipola, M., P. Finckenberg, R. Korpela, H. Vapaatalo, and M. Nurminen. 2002. Effect of long-term intake of milk products on blood pressure in hypertensive rats. *Journal of Dairy Research* 69: 103–111.

Stepaniak, L., L. Jedrychowski, B. Wroblewska, and T. Sorhaug. 2001. Immunoreactivity and Inhibition of angiotensin-I converting enzyme and lactococcal oligopeptidase by peptides from cheese. *Italian Journal of Food Science* 13: 373–381.

Sumi, H., H. Hamada, K. Nakanishi, and H. Hiratani. 1990. Enhancement of the fibrinolytic activity in plasma by oral administration of nattokinase. *Acta Haematologica* 84: 139–143.

Sumi, H., H. Hamada, H. Tsushima, H. Mihara, and H. Muraki. 1987. A novel fibrinolytic enzyme (nattokinase) in the vegetable cheese natto; a typical and popular soybean food in the Japanese diet. *Experientia* 43: 1110–1111.

Sumi, H., N. Nakajima, and C. Yatagai. 1995. A unique strong fibrinolytic enzyme (*katsuwokinase*) in skipjack *'shiokara'*, a Japanese traditional fermented food. *Comparative Biochemistry and Physiology—B Biochemistry and Molecular Biology* 112: 543–547.

Sutas, Y., E. Soppi, H. Korhonen, E. L. Syvaoja, M. Saxelin, T. Rokka, and E. Isolauri. 1996. Suppression of lymphocyte proliferation *in vitro* by bovine caseins hydrolyzed with *Lactobacillus casei* GG-derived enzymes. *Journal of Allergy and Clinical Immunology* 98: 216–224.

Todorov, S. D., H. Nyati, M. Meincken, and L. M. T. Dicks. 2007. Partial characterization of bacteriocin AMA-K, produced by Lactobacillus plantarum AMA-K isolated from naturally fermented milk from Zimbabwe. *Food Control* 18: 656–664.

Torres-Llanez, M. J., A. F. González-Córdova, A. Hernandez-Mendoza, H. S. Garcia, and B. Vallejo-Cordoba. 2011. Angiotensin-converting enzyme inhibitory activity in Mexican Fresco cheese. *Journal of Dairy Science* 94: 3794–3800.

Tsai, J. S., Y. S. Lin, B. S. Pan, and T. J. Chen. 2006. Antihypertensive peptides and g-aminobutyric acid from prozyme 6 facilitated lactic acid bacteria fermentation of soymilk. *Process Biochemistry* 41: 1282–1288.

Tuo, Y. F., L. W. Zhang, H. X. Yi, Y. C. Zhang, W. Q. Zhang, X. Han, M. Du, Y. H. Jiao, and S. M. Wang. 2010. Antiproliferative effect of wild *Lactobacillus* strains isolated from fermented foods on HT-29 cells. *Journal of Dairy Science* 93: 2362–2366.

Vinderola, G., C. Matar, and G. Perdigon. 2007. Milk fermented with *Lactobacillus helveticus* R389 and its non bacterial fraction confer enhanced protection against *Salmonella enteritidis* serovar *typhimurium* infection in mice. *Immunobiology* 212: 107–118.

Vuyst, L. D. and E. Leroy. 2007. Bacteriocin from lactic acid bacteria: Production, purification, and food applications. *Journal of Molecular Microbiology and Biotechnology* 13: 194–199.

Wagar, L. E., C. P. Champagne, N. D. Buckley, Y. Raymond, and J. M. Green-Johnson. 2009. Immunomodulatory properties of fermented soy and dairy milks prepared with lactic acid bacteria. *Journal of Food Science* 74: M423–M430.

Wang, C. T., B. P. Ji, B. Li et al. 2006. Purification and characterization of a fibrinolytic enzyme of *Bacillus subtilis* DC33, isolated from Chinese traditional *Douchi*. *The Journal of Industrial Microbiology and Biotechnology* 33: 750–758.

Wang, L. J., D. Li, L. Zou, X. D. Chen, Y. Q. Cheng, K. Yamaki, and L. T. Li. 2007. Antioxidative activity of *douchi* (a Chinese traditional salt-fermented soybean food) extracts during its processing. *International Journal of Food Properties* 10: 1–12.

Wang, C., M. Du, D. Zeng, F. Kong, G. Zu, and Y. Feng. 2009. Purification and characterization of nattokinase from *Bacillus subtilis* Natto B-12. *Journal of Agricultural and Food Chemistry* 57: 9722–9729.

Wergedahl, H., B. Liaset, O. A. Gudbrandsen, E. Lied, M. Espe, Z. Muna, S. Mork, and R. K. Berge. 2004. Fish protein hydrolysate reduces plasma total cholesterol, increases the proportion of HDL cholesterol, and lowers acyl-CoA cholesterol acyltransferase activity in liver of Zucker rats. *Journal of Nutrition* 134: 1320–1327.

Yasuda, S., H. Kuwata, K. Kawamoto et al. 2012. Effect of highly lipolyzed goat cheese on HL-60 human leukemia cells: Antiproliferative activity and induction of apoptotic DNA damage. *Journal of Dairy Science* 95: 2248–2260.

Yasuda, S., N. Ohkura, K. Suzuki, M. Yamasaki, K. Nishiyama, H. Kobayashi, Y. Hoshi, Y. Kadooka, K. Igoshi. 2010. Effects of highly ripened cheeses on HL-60 human leukemia cells: Antiproliferative activity and induction of apoptotic DNA damage. *Journal of Dairy Science* 93: 1393–1400.

Yeo, I. C., N. K. Lee, and Y. T. Hahm. 2012. Genome sequencing of *Bacillus subtilis* SC-8, antagonistic to the *Bacillus cereus* group, isolated from traditional Korean fermented-soybean food. *Journal of Bacteriology* 194: 536–537.

Zeng, W., W. Li, L. Shu, J. Yi, G. Chen, and Z. Liang. 2013. Non-sterilized fermentative co-production of poly (γ-glutamic acid) and fibrinolytic enzyme by a thermophilic *Bacillus subtilis* GXA-28. *Bioresource Technology* 142: 697–700.

Zhang, J. H., E. Tatsumi, C. H. Ding, and L. T. Li. 2006. Angiotensin I-converting enzyme inhibitory peptides in douchi, a Chinese traditional fermented soybean product. *Food Chemistry* 98: 551–557.

Zhang, X. and A. C. Beynan. 1993. Lowering effect of dietary milk–whey protein v casein on plasma and liver cholesterol concentration in rats. *British Journal of Nutrition* 70: 139–146.

Chapter 15

Health Benefits of Fermented Fish

Sanath Kumar H. and Binaya Bhusan Nayak

Contents

15.1 Introduction

Fermentation is a traditional method of preserving fish practiced for thousands of years throughout the world. In the absence of other modern methods of preserving highly perishable seafood, fermentation was the method of choice to preserve fish landed in large quantities during times of glut (FAO 1971). Preservation by fermentation made fish available throughout the year, often at prices cheaper than fresh fish. Fermentation of fish is an easy and low-cost method of extending the shelf life of otherwise highly perishable fish. Gradually, fermented fish products became part of the regular diet in countries where people developed a penchant for the characteristic flavor and taste of fermented fish products. Several different types of fermented fish or shellfish are historically associated with different countries, particularly in Asia. Examples are *nam pla* of Thailand, *budu* of Malaysia, *patis* of Philippines, and *nuoc mam* of Vietnam (VanVeen 1965, Steinkraus 1996, 2002, Sanchez 2008), *pissala* of France and *garos* of Greece (Beddows 1985), *hentak, ngari,* and *tungtap* of India (Thapa et al. 2004, Tamang et al. 2012), *jeotgal* or *jeot* of Korea (Guan et al. 2011), *pla som* of Thailand (Saithong et al. 2010), *shiokara* of Japan (Fujii et al.

1999), *surströmming* of Sweden (Kobayashi et al. 2000); sundried or smoked fish products of India, Nepal, and Bhutan such as *gnuchi, sidra*, and *sukuti* (Thapa et al. 2006), and dried and preserved fish products of India such as *bordia, karati,* and *lashim* (Thapa et al. 2007). Fermented products such as sauces and pastes are rich sources of proteins, vitamins, essential amino acids, and minerals to the people of Southeast Asian countries, whose diets are predominantly cereal based (Amano 1962, Curtis 2009). Fermentation of fish occurs principally by endogenous autolytic enzymes such as pepsin and trypsin and to a lesser extent by the associated microflora depending on the method of fermentation (Cutting and Bakken 1957). In most cases, fermentation of fish occurs in the presence of added salt which removes moisture by osmosis. In general, fermented fish contain >15% salt, but the salt content can be as high as 20%–25% in some products (TPI 1982, Berkel et al. 2004). The biological process underlying the production of fish sauce or paste is very simple requiring no scientific intervention. The traditional processes of fermentation are well established and yield products of uniform quality and taste. In the presence of salt, the activities of the spoilage microorganisms will completely cease, but the endogenous autolytic enzymes of fish start decomposing the fish tissues. Protracted hydrolysis of proteins, lipids, and carbohydrates result in the formation of products which impart distinct aroma and taste. When bacteria are involved in the fermentation process, organic acids such as acetic acid and lactic acid are formed (Fujii et al. 1999, Steinkraus 2002). Fish sauces and pastes are the examples of fermentation products derived by employing the endogenous enzymes of fish. The enzyme groups in the fish gut are composed of pepsin, trypsin, carboxypeptidases, amylases, and lipases (Lovell 1988), which start acting on the fish tissue immediately after the death of the fish. The tissue protein hydrolysis by the endogenous enzyme activity of fish can vary greatly in different species of fish depending on the types of enzymes, rates of hydrolysis, and so on. As a consequence of this, the chemical composition of the final product of fermentation can also vary vastly depending on the fish species. For example, herbivorous fish produce large amounts of enzymes that degrade carbohydrates, while carnivorous fish produce enzymes that are predominantly proteolytic (Horn et al. 1986, Cockson and Bourne 1972, Hidalgo et al. 1999). Other factors such as the season, physiological state of fish, and the age can also influence the enzyme levels and their activities, which in turn may affect the characteristics of the fermented product.

15.2 Fish Sauces and Pastes of the World

Both fish sauces and pastes are produced by enzymatic degradation of fish proteins in the presence of high salt concentrations. In the case of fish sauce, the fish tissue is subjected to extensive liquefaction and the resultant fluid part is collected as the sauce. The paste products are prepared similar to sauces but the duration of fermentation is generally shorter and the final product includes solid parts of fish. Two types of fish pastes exist, ground pastes in which the fermented fish is ground or pounded into pastes (e.g., *belachan* of Malaysia) and unground paste (e.g., *shiokara* of Japan). Ground fish paste is produced by mixing fish or shrimp with salt followed by pounding or crushing to obtain a paste, which is subsequently sundried and stored in closed containers and allowed to mature (TPI 1982, Hajeb and Jinap 2012). Numerous traditional fish sauce and paste products exist in different Asian countries and some of the popular products are listed below (Table 15.1). Although in all fermented products the basic method involves the use of high amounts of salt, differences exist in the choice of raw materials, fish-to-salt ratio, duration of fermentation, and addition of other raw materials during the fermentation process. As a result, each fermented product has its own characteristic taste and flavor.

Table 15.1 Some Popular Fermented Fishery Products of Asia

Country	Fish Sauce	Fish Paste	Shrimp Paste
Bangladesh	–	–	*Nappi*
China	*Yu-lu*	*Yu-jiang*	*Shajiang*
Indonesia	*Kecap-ikan, Aekjeot*	*Trassi ikan*	*Trassi udang*
Japan	*Shottsuru, ishiru*	*Shiokara (shrimp/fish)*	
Philippines	*Patis*	*Bagoong*	*Bagoong, alamang, ainailan*
Cambodia	*Tuk trey*	*Pra hoc (fish)*	*Kapi*
Laos	*Nam pla*	*Pa daek*	
Korea	*Jeot-kuk*	–	*Saewoojeot*
Malaysia	*Budu*	–	*Belachan*
Myanmar	*Ngan-pya-ye*	*Ngapi*	*Ngapi seinsa*
Thailand	*Nam pla, budu, Thai pla*	*Pla ra*	*Kapi*
Vietnam	*Nuoc mam*	*Mam-chau, mam-mem*	*nam tom*
India	–	*Hentak, ngari, tungtap, Colombo cure*	

15.3 Fermented Fish Products of India

Most of the fermented fish consumption in India is limited to the northeastern Indian states of Tripura, Assam, Meghalaya, and Manipur. Some of the popular fermented fish products include *ngari* or *shidol*, *tungtap*, *sukuti*, and *lona ilish*. *Ngari* is a popular salt-free fermented product known by different names such as *shidol*, *hidol*, and *sepaa* in different states in the region. For *ngari* preparation, sundried *Puntius sophore* is briefly washed with water and allowed to drain overnight followed by manually pressing the fish to remove water, packing in oil smeared earthen pots, and packing the mouth of the pot with leaves and mud to make it airtight. The fish is allowed to ferment for at least 6 months and the fermented product is used mainly as a condiment (Jeyaram et al. 2009). The other popular fermented fish product of northeastern India is the *hentak*, which is a fermented paste prepared by a unique traditional method. For *hentak* preparation, dried fish (*Esomus danricus*) is powdered by pounding, followed by mixing with equal quantities of ground fresh petioles of *Alocasia macrorhiza* into a paste form, which is subsequently rolled into small balls and packed in earthen pots and allowed to ferment for 2 weeks. Since fish are fermented in the absence of salt, the process is uncontrolled and microorganisms play a major role in the fermentation process.

While *ngari* and *hentak* represent salt-free fermentation products of fish, *lona ilish* is a typical salt-fermented product of northeast India and Bangladesh. The raw material for *lona ilish* is the freshwater fish *Tenulosa ilisha*, previously known as *Hilsa ilisha*. Freshly caught fish is descaled, beheaded, and cut into diagonal steaks of 1.25–2.0 cm thickness, mixed with salt, and stored in bamboo baskets for 24–48 h. The fluid formed from the salted fish is allowed to drain out during this process (Majumdar et al. 2005). The steaks are packed tightly in tin vats over which boiled and cooled brine is poured until a layer is formed over the fish and the vats are closed airtight and allowed to ferment for 4–6 months (Majumdar and Basu 2010). Fermented fish are used as condiments in the preparation of versatile side dishes using vegetables and are eaten along with rice and bread. In the northeastern hilly region of India, fermented fish products such as the *shidol* are an integral part of tribal food culture and play a crucial role in supplementing the traditional diet of the tribal people with vital nutrients.

15.4 Nutritional Composition of Fish Sauces and Pastes

Nuoc mam, for example, is consumed in small quantities every day both as a cooking sauce and also as a dipping sauce (Saisithi et al. 1966, Beddows 1985). The fermentation is nonbacterial and hence the product is free from biological amines and bacterial metabolites, which may cause adverse effects when present in significant quantities. The salt content of *nuoc mam* is approximately 24%. The distinct aroma of *nuoc mam* is attributed to the amino acid composition of the sauce. *Nuoc mam* is prepared by mixing small fish with salt usually in 3:1 (fish:salt) (w/w) ratio in large clay tanks below the ground and allowing it to decompose for 6 months to 1 year. The liquid formed upon hydrolytic degradation of fish meat is collected, filtered, and stored in large containers and exposed to sun in a process of ripening for 2–12 weeks (Saisithi et al. 1966). A large amount of sludge is also produced during the process and the decomposition process is continued further. The sauce collected subsequently has lower qualities in terms of nutrient composition measured by the total nitrogen content, color, taste, or aroma and is classified into different grades based on the total nitrogen content, such as grade I (>20 g/L) or grade II (15–20 g/L) (Lopetcharat et al. 2001, Hjalmarsson et al. 2007). The characteristic umami taste of fish sauces is primarily due to the amino acids formed during fermentation. However, the chemical composition of fish sauces from different countries can vary. A comprehensive analysis of fish sauces from seven different Asian countries by Park et al. (2001) showed that the total amino acid content of the Vietnamese sauce was the highest followed by Japanese and Thai sauces, while the total amino acid content of fish sauces from Myanmar and Laos was significantly less. While the Vietnamese sauce contained high levels of glutamate, the Korean sauces were significantly lower in their glutamate content but were more enriched with amino acids such as glycine, valine, and proline, which are responsible for the characteristic sweet taste of Korean sauces compared with sauces from Vietnam or Japan (Park et al. 2001). The histidine content of sauces can vary depending on the type of fish used, whether marine or freshwater, with sauces from marine fish being rich in histidine. An analysis of the amino acid composition revealed that fish sauces from Vietnam, Thailand, and Japan were rich in alanine, valine, lysine, histidine, aspartate, and glutamate, but the levels of individual amino acids varied greatly among these sauces. In general, glutamic acid, lysine, and aspartic acid make up to 40% of the total amino acids. Since plant-based foods are deficient in lysine and methionine, consumption of fish sauce containing these will fulfill the amino acid requirements of people with a predominantly cereal-based diet. Nucleotides, uracil and uridine and hypoxanthine are also found in significant quantities, especially in sauces from Vietnam, Thailand, and Japan (Park et al. 2001). In addition, creatine and creatinine are also found but their relative proportions vary depending on the country. Thai fish sauce also contained 1–6 g/100 mL of sucrose. This study tried to categorize fish sauces from different countries based on their total amino acids, total nucleotides, bases, and creatinine as the "high content" group (Thailand, Vietnam, and Japan), "intermediate group" (China and Korea), and "low-content" group (Myanmar and Laos) (Park et al. 2001).

Typically, fish sauces have a pH of 5.3–6.7, salt content of 25%, total amino acid content of 2.9–7.7 g/mL, glutamic acid content of 0.38–1.32 g/100 mL, and organic acid content of 0.21–2.33 g/100 mL (Lopetcharat et al. 2001, Mizutani et al. 1992). However, the composition of fish sauces and pastes vary widely depending on the method of preparation, raw materials used, and so on. Fish sauces, which are subjected to higher degrees of protein hydrolysis or complete solubilization unlike fish pastes, are rich in free amino acids. Glutamic acid and aspartic acid are the predominant amino acids in both *nam pla* and *nuoc mam*, followed by alanine, valine, threonine, and lysine (Table 15.2).

Table 15.2 Free Amino Acid (mg/100 mL) Composition of Fish Sauces

Amino Acid	*Nam pla*	*Nuoc mam*
Aspartic acid	760	1150
Threonine	460	700
Serine	360	610
Glutamic acid	950	1370
Proline	230	330
Glycine	340	360
Alanine	700	1010
Valine	590	830
Cysteine	0	0
Methionine	230	270
Isoleucine	360	390
Leucine	450	490
Tyrosine	50	60
Phenyl alanine	310	420
Tryptophan	90	90
Lysine	890	1360
Histidine	320	460
Arginine	0	80

Source: From Ninomiya, K. 2002. *Food Review International* 18: 23–38; Yoshida, Y. 1998. *Food Reviews International* 14: 213–246.

15.5 Microflora of Fermented Fish

The indigenous microflora of fish and those introduced as contaminants at various stages of harvesting, handling, processing as well as through the salt used in fish fermentation constitute the initial flora of fish used in fermentation. However, majority of the bacteria initially found in fish are unable to survive in the high sodium chloride concentration and are gradually eliminated. Only halotolerant and halophilic bacteria continue to persist during the later stages of fermentation. Several studies have reported the presence of such bacteria in fermented fish products. For example, an analysis of 9-month old *nam pla* revealed the presence of *Bacillus* spp., *Coryneform* spp., *Streptococcus* spp., *Micrococcus* spp., and *Staphylococcus* spp. (Saisithi et al. 1966). Halophilic bacteria such as *Halococcus* and *Halobacterium* have also been isolated from *nam pla* (Thongthai and Suntinanalert 1991). The bacterial flora of shrimp paste *belacan* consists of *Bacillus* spp., *Pediococcus* spp., *Lactobacillus* spp., *Micrococcus* spp., *Sarcina* spp., *Clostridium* spp., *Brevibacterium* spp., *Flavobacterium* spp., and *Corynebacterium* spp. (Karim 1993). High salt-tolerant species were predominant in the product. Villar et al. (1985) found *Pediococcus halophilus* as the dominant bacterium in salted anchovies. Majumdar et al. (2008) reported *Bacillus licheniformis* and *Micrococcus kristinae* as the fermentation flora of *lona ilish* (salt-fermented Indian shad). Negasi (2013) reported isolation of *Tetragenococcus halophilus* as the dominant bacteria from maturing salt-fermented Indian mackerel. Bacteria such as *Bacillus* spp., *Pseudomonas* spp., *Micrococcus* spp., *Staphylococcus* spp., *Halococcus* spp., *Halobacterium salinarum,* and *H. cutirubrum* are known to produce proteolytic enzymes that enhance the digestion of fish tissues (Thongthai et al. 1992, Lopetcharat et al. 2001). Some strains of *Staphylococcus* spp. and *Bacillus* spp. produce compounds that may confer aroma and flavor to fermented fish products (Saisithi et al. 1966, Fukami et al. 2004). *Staphylococcus xylosus* has been found to improve the odor of fish sauce (Fukami et al. 2004).

Considerable information is available on the microbial composition of fermented fish products from India. Bacteria such as *Lactococcus plantarum* and *Lactobacillus plantarum, Bacillus subtilis, Bacillus pumilus, Micrococcus* spp., and the yeast *Candida* spp. have been isolated from *ngari* (Thapa et al. 2004). A similar bacterial and yeast composition has been reported in another traditional fermented fish product *hentak,* though different species of lactic acid bacteria such as *Lactobacillus fructosus* and *Lactobacillus amylophilus* were found to be predominant (Thapa et al. 2004). *Tungtap,* a traditional fermented fish product of Meghalaya in India, harbors *Lactobacillus coryniformis, Lactobacillus lactis, Lb. fructosus, Bacillus cereus, B. subtilis, Candida* spp., and *Saccharomycopsis* sp. (Thapa et al. 2004). Some of the important traditional smoked and sundried fish products of the Eastern Himalayan regions of Nepal and India such as *sukako maacha, gnuchi, sidra,* and *sukuti* have been reported to contain lactic acid bacteria *Lactococcus lactis* subsp. *cremoris, Lc. lactis* subsp. *lactis, Lb. plantarum, Leuconostoc mesenteroides, Enterococcus faecium, Enterococcus faecalis, Pediococcus pentosaceus,* and *Weissella confuse* with inhibitory activities against human pathogenic bacteria (Thapa et al. 2006). Lactic acid bacteria such as *Lb. lactis* subsp. *cremoris, Leuc. mesenteroides, Lb. plantarum* have been found to be predominant in *karati, bordia,* and *lashim,* all traditional salted and dried fish products of India's Northeastern state of Assam (Thapa et al. 2007). Lactic acid bacteria, some yeasts, and several species of *Bacillus* found in fermented products are known to produce compounds beneficial to human health, prevent pathogen colonization in the gut, enhance immune functions, and so on (Parvez et al. 2006). However, some of the microbes associated with high-salt fermented fish may not be culturable in regular microbiological media. While 16S rDNA-based DNA library will help in elucidating the diversity of fermentation flora, metagenomic library approach will allow isolation of genomic regions encoding the production of compounds responsible for various bioactivities of fermented fish products.

15.6 Beneficial Bacteria Isolated from Fermented Fish Products

Although there are few studies to indicate the health benefits from fermented fish by direct animal feeding experiments, there have been enough evidence of the health benefitting role of fermenting bacteria. The *Lactobacillus* group is reported to have been associated with many fermented fish foods such as *funazushi* (Japan), *jeotgal* (Korea), *hukuti mass* and *tungtap* (India), *pla som* and *som-fac* (Thailand), *narejushi* (Japan), *budu* (Malaysia), and *gajami sik-hae* (Korea). Lactobacilli have been known for bacteriocin production, which can inhibit pathogens. The metabolites of this group of bacteria, when consumed in foods, are known to have probiotic effects. In addition to *Lactobacilli,* Gram-positive bacteria also have antibacterial effects. A list of fish fermenting bacteria and their beneficial effects on humans, either demonstrated along with fish products or other foods, are summarized in Table 15.3.

Table 15.3 Health Beneficial Bacteria and Their Products Associated with Fermented Fish Products

Microbe and Associated Fermented Fish Product	*Health Benefits of the Prominent Flora*
Monascus purpureus in colored *Bagoong* (Angkak, red mold rice is used) (Pattanagul et al. 2007)	Hypolipidemic and antiatherogenic (Wei et al. 2003); cholesterol-lowering agent, monacolin K production (Wang et al. 1997), and anti-inflammation agent, monascin production (Lee et al. 2006)
Lactobacillus paracasei in *Funazushi* (Komatsuzaki et al. 2005) and in *som-fak,* a Thai low-salt fermented fish product (Paludan-Müller et al. 1999)	Bacteriocin production (Miao et al. 2014) and γ-aminobutyric acid (GABA) production (Komatsuzaki et al. 2005) (GABA-enriched food is good for depression, sleeplessness, and autonomic disorders) Inhibit the growth of many pathogenic microbes such as *Streptococcus mutans* (Chuang et al. 2011)
Lc. lactis in *Jeotgal*, a salt-fermented Korean fish product (Paludan-Müller et al. 1999; Lee et al. 2000), in *tungtap* (Thapa et al. 2004) and in *hukuti maas,* a fermented fish product from India (Kumar et al. 2014)	Lacticin NK24 bacteriocin against *Leuc. mesenteroides* (Lee and Paik 2001) Antibacterial effect against *Staphyloccus aureus* (Thapa et al. 2006) and *Listeria innocua* Anti*aeromonas* Bacteriocin (Kumar et al. 2014)
Weissella cibaria in *pla som* (Srionnual et al. 2007)	Weissellicin 110, a bacteriocin (Srionnual et al. 2007); able to inhibit the *in vitro* formation of *S. mutans* biofilm as well as the *in vivo* formation of oral biofilm (Kang et al. 2006b) Inhibitory effects on volatile sulfur compound production and *Fusobacterium nucleatum* proliferation (Kang et al. 2006a)
Lactobacillus reuteri in *pla som* (Saithong et al. 2010)	Inhibition of binding of *Helicobacter pylori* to the glycolipid receptors (Mukai et al. 2002)

(Continued)

Table 15.3 (*Continued*) Health Beneficial Bacteria and Their Products Associated with Fermented Fish Products

Microbe and Associated Fermented Fish Product	*Health Benefits of the Prominent Flora (References)*
Ped. pentosaceus in *Jeotgal* (Lee et al. 2014) and in *Plaasom*	Improves acute liver injury induced by D-galactosamine in rats (Lv et al. 2014); pediocin and pediocin K23-2-producing *Ped. pentosaceus* K23-2 (Shin et al. 2008)
Lb. plantarum from Budu ((Liasi et al. 2009; Saithong et al. 2010), in Funazushi (Nakamura et al. 2012) and in gajami sik-hae (Park et al. 2013)	The antibacterial agents produced by the isolates inhibited the growth of a range of Gram-positive and Gram-negative microorganisms (Paludan-Müller et al. 1999, Thapa et al. 2006, Saithong et al. 2010) Antimicrobial activities against *Listeria monocytogenes* (Nakamura et al. 2012) Inhibits adipogenesis (antiobesity properties) (Park et al. 2013)
Lactobacillus casei in *budu* (Liasi et al. 2009)	Inhibited the growth of a range of Gram-positive and Gram-negative microorganisms (Inoue et al. 2013)
T. halophilus in fish-*nukazuke* (Kuda et al. 2012) Fermented mackerel (Negasi, 2013)	Suppression of histamine accumulation in salt-fermented fish (Kuda et al. 2012)
Staph. xylosus in *Myeolchi-jeot* (Mah and Hwang 2009)	Inhibition of biogenic amine formation in a salted and fermented anchovy (Mah and Hwang 2009)
Lactobacillus pobuzihii in *tungtap* (India) (Rapsang et al. 2013)	Bacteriocin production (Rapsang et al. 2013)

15.7 Health Benefits of Fermented Fish Products

The availability of a nutritionally balanced diet is a major challenge in the contemporary world. Many health problems in the developing world, especially in newborns and children, are related to protein, vitamin, essential amino acid, and mineral deficiencies in the diet. Marasmus, for example, is an emaciation disorder in children less than 5 years of age due to the lack of protein and calories in diet, and this disease kills several million children every year (Müller and Krawinkel 2005). Another nutritional disease, Kwashiorkor, is a severe disorder in children as a result of protein-energy malnutrition (Schofield and Ashworth 1996). Lack of vitamins and minerals in the diet of children predisposes them to several nutritional diseases such as "beriberi" due to deficiency of vitamin B1 (thiamine), "osteoporosis" (brittle bones) due to lack of calcium and/or vitamin D, "rickets" due to vitamin D deficiency, "pellagra" due to niacin deficiency, and "scurvy" due to vitamin C deficiency (Baumgartner 2013). All these nutritional diseases can be overcome by supplementing the diet with the deficient nutrient. Fish sauces and pastes are good sources of dietary proteins in countries where much of the population cannot afford animal proteins in their diet every day or habituated to a traditional diet rich in carbohydrates and deficient in proteins (Steinkraus 2002). Though consumed in small quantities, fermented fish are a part of every meal and therefore play a very critical role in the nutrition and health of the people. The controlled enzymatic hydrolysis yields easily digestible simpler proteins, which makes fermented fish suitable for consumption by all age groups. Fermented fish, being rich in proteins, free amino acids, vitamins, and minerals, can be a good food supplement in regions of the world where malnutrition is prevalent (Steinkraus 2002). Fish sauces such as *nuoc mam* contain substantial quantities of essential minerals such as phosphorus and fluorine, and several vitamins such as vitamin C and other B-group vitamins such as folic acid, niacin, riboflavin, pantothenic acid, thiamine, vitamin B_6, and vitamin B_{12} (Wilaipun 1990). Therefore, a diet containing fermented fish can have profound positive effect on the gastrointestinal health of the consumers and help to overcome several nutritional disorders, especially in children. In addition, the easily digestible proteins and the availability of vitamins and essential amino acids will help patients with digestive disorders and can even help in preventing microbial infection of the gastrointestinal tract (Saisithi 1994). The amino acid content of fish sauces range from 7 to 10 g/100 mL and more than 70% of this is available in the free form and this vastly makes up for the deficiency of amino acids encountered in the predominantly vegetarian diet. Fermented fish such as pastes and sauces, though consumed in small quantities, are important dietary supplements and hence can aptly be called functional foods.

The health-promoting features of fermented foods such as wine, yoghurt, cheese, and so on have been scientifically proven (Steinkraus 1997). Fermented foods are now known to have antioxidant, antihypertensive, anticancer, immunostimulatory, and antidiabetic properties and are also known to alleviate neurodegenerative disorders. In addition, the fermentation process reduces the antinutritional factors in fresh food, concentrates proteins and vitamins and makes the food more digestible and easily absorbable. The positive health effects of other fish products such as fish protein hydrolysates are increasingly being explored and a number of studies have identified several health-promoting biological activities such as the antioxidant, anticoagulant, ACE inhibitory, anticancer, antidiabetic, immunomodulatory, antimicrobial, and antihypertensive activities (Harnedy and FitzGerald 2012). Although a number of shellfish sauces have been studied for their potential positive human benefits, scientific evidence on the health benefits of fermented fish products is very limited. For example, the oyster sauce prepared from *Mytilus edulis* reportedly contains peptides with antihypertensive and antioxidant activities (Je et al. 2005, Jung et al. 2006, Rajapakse et al. 2005). Natural antioxidants in food are known to be beneficial to health in several ways and more emphasis is being given to popularizing such foods. Antioxidants in foods lower the risk of age-related degenerative diseases, cancer, and cardiovascular diseases. According to Michihata (2003), the Japanese fish sauce *ishiru* contained 1.42–2.49 g/100 mL of total nitrogen, 14.81–27.33 g/100 mL salt, and 44.39–81.54 mmol/100 mL of total free amino acids. The major free amino acids in *ishiru* are alanine, glutamic acid, glycine, and lysine, followed by valine, leucine, and taurine. This fish sauce was found to have very strong antioxidant and radical scavenging activities. Fermented fish sauce rich in B-group vitamins can be effective in preventing megaloblastic anemia (Wongkhalaung 2004, Zaman et al. 2009).

Some of the traditional fermented foods are gradually entering the commercial market as functional foods or nutraceuticals. *Seacure* is a commercially available dried fish protein hydrolysate from the Pacific whiting (*Merluccius productus*) (Fitzgerald et al. 2005). This product is prepared by controlled fermentation of fresh fish using a proteolytic yeast strain *Hansenula* and is reported to contain 75–80% protein constituents in the form of peptides and free amino acids with glutamine being the major amino acid followed by asparagine and lysine, in addition to 6–10% fish oils (Fitzgerald et al. 2005). *Seacure* has been found to have biological functions in the form of gastrointestinal repair functions and could be an effective alternative to nonsteroidal anti-inflammatory drugs that have several side effects (Fitzgerald et al. 2005, Marchbank et al. 2008). Although glutamine in its single, dipeptide, or tripeptide form was vastly responsible for the biological activity of *seacure*, fatty acids and other unknown compounds may also contribute to the bioactivities of this product (Fitzgerald et al. 2005).

A peptide derived from anchovy sauce has been found to have apoptosis-inducing activities in human carcinoma cells and this function could be potentially useful in preventing the spread of cancer (Lee et al. 2003, 2004, Ngo et al. 2012). More than 70% of the amino acids in fish sauce are the free amino acids that are readily absorbed in the intestine. In addition, dipeptides, tripeptides, and oligopeptides are other easily digestible components of fish sauce. Some oligopeptides may function as bioactive molecules with antihypertensive and antioxidant properties. The health-promoting effects of fermented shellfish products are promising and have attracted scientific interest. A study has shown that the sauce obtained by fermentation of *Acetes chinensis* with *Lactobacillus fermentum* SM60 exhibited high angiotensin I-converting enzyme (ACE) inhibitory activity and thus could be beneficial in controlling hypertension and high blood pressure (Wang et al. 2008). A study has reported that fermented shrimp paste contains a neutral protease with fibrinolytic activities that can be useful in treating cardiovascular diseases (Wong and Mine 2004). Apart from fish and shellfish, the fermented seaweed reportedly contains polysaccharides that can be useful as anticoagulants (Pushpamali et al. 2008, De Zoysa et al. 2008). Alhough very few studies have been conducted on the health benefits of fermented fish products, they strongly suggest the beneficial roles of these products in the human diet make them valuable functional foods.

15.8 Conclusions

Fermented fish products are an integral part of diet in many countries of Southeast Asia and are important protein components of otherwise carbohydrate-rich diets. The chief constituents of fermented fish include hydrolyzed proteins, free amino acids, fatty acids, vitamins, and minerals. Fermented fish products are widely regarded as health foods, but scientific evidence on the health-promoting bioactive compounds in them is severely lacking. Therefore, more investigations are necessary to determine the health benefits of traditional fermented fish products, their bioactivities, and the beneficial aspects of consumption so that such products can also be recommended as therapeutic agents to treat chronic disorders such as gastrointestinal ailments, hypertension, cardiovascular diseases, or old-age-related debilitations.

References

Amano, K. 1962. The influence of fermentation on the nutritive value of fish with special reference to fermented fish products of Southeast Asia. In E. Heen and R. Kreuzer (Eds.), *Fish in Nutrition*. London: Fishing News (Books) Ltd, 180–200.

Baumgartner, M. R. 2013. Vitamin-responsive disorders: Cobalamin, folate, biotin, vitamins B1 and E. *Handbook of Clinical Neurology* 113: 1799–1810.

Beddows, C. G. 1985. Fermented fish and fish products. In B. J. B. Wood (Ed.), *Microbiology of Fermented Foods*, Vol. 2. London: Elsevier Applied Sciences, pp. 1–39.

Berkel, B. M., B. V. Boogaard, and C. Heijnen. 2004. Fermenting fish. In M. de Goffau-Markusse (Ed.), *Preservation of Fish and Meat*. The Netherlands: Agromisa Foundation, Wageningen, 54–63.

Chuang, L. C., C. S. Huang, L. W. Ou Yang, and S. Y. Lin. 2011. Probiotic *Lactobacillus paracasei* effect on cariogenic bacterial flora. *Clinical Oral Investigation* 15: 471–476.

Cockson, A. and D. Bourne. 1972. Enzymes in the digestive tract of two species of euryhaline fish. *Comparative Biochemistry and Physiology* A 41: 715–718.

Curtis R. I. 2009. Umami and the foods of classical antiquity. *American Journal of Clinical Nutrition* 90: 712S–718S.

Cutting, C. L. and K. Bakken. 1957. Fisheries products for tropical consumption. *FAO Fisheries Bulletin* 10: 1.

De Zoysa, M., C. Nikapitiya, Y-J. Jeon, Y. Jee, and J. Lee. 2008. Anticoagulant activity of sulfated polysaccharide isolated from fermented brown seaweed *Sargassum fulvellum*. *Journal of Applied Phycology* 20: 67–74.

FAO. 1971. Fermented fish products. In I. M. Mackie, R. Hardy, and G. Hobbs (Eds.), *FAO Fishery Report*, Rome: Food and Agricultural Organization, p. 54.

Fitzgerald, A. J., P. S. Rai, T. Marchbank, G. W. Taylor, S. Ghosh, B. W. Ritz, and R. J. Playford. 2005. Reparative properties of a commercial fish protein hydrolysate preparation. *Gut* 54: 775–781.

Fujii, T., Y. C. Wu, T. Suzuk, and B. Kimura. 1999. Production of organic acids by bacteria during the fermentation of squid *shiokara*. *Fisheries Science* 65: 671–672.

Fukami, K., M. Satomi, Y. Funatsu, K. I. Kawasaki, and S. Watabe. 2004. Characterization and distribution of *Staphylococcus* spp. implicated for improvement of fish sauce odor. *Fisheries Science* 70: 916–923.

Guan, L., K. H. Cho, and J. H. Lee. 2011. Analysis of the cultivable bacterial community in jeotgal, a Korean salted and fermented seafood, and identification of its dominant bacteria. *Food Microbiology* 28: 101–113.

Hajeb, P. and S. Jinap. 2012. Fermented shrimp products as source of Umami in Southeast Asia. *Journal of Nutrition and Food Science* S10: 6–17.

Harnedy, P. A. and R. J. Fitzgerald. 2012. Bioactive peptides from marine processing waste and shellfish: A review. *Journal of Functional Foods* 4: 6–24.

Hidalgo, M. C., E. Urea, and A. Sanz. 1999. Comparative study of digestive enzymes in fish with different nutritional habits: Proteolytic and amylase activities. *Aquaculture* 170: 267–283.

Hjalmarsson, G. H., J. W. Park, and Kristbergsson, K. 2007. Seasonal effects on the physicochemical characteristics of fish sauce made from capelin (*Mallotus villosus*). *Food Chemistry* 103: 495–504.

Horn, M. H., M. A. Neighbors, and S. N. Murray. 1986. Herbivore responses to a seasonally fluctuating food supply: growth potential of two temperate intertidal fishes based on the protein and energy assimilated from their macroalgal diets. *Journal of Experimental Marine Biology and Ecology* 103: 217–234.

Inoue, S., K. Suzuki-Utsunomiya, Y. Komori, A. Kamijo, I. Yumura, K. Tanabe, A. Miyawaki, and K. Koga. 2013. Fermentation of non-sterilized fish biomass with a mixed culture of film-forming yeasts and lactobacilli and its effect on innate and adaptive immunity in mice. *Journal of Bioscience and Bioengineering* 116: 682–687.

Je, J. Y., P. J. Park, H. G. Byun, W. K. Jung, and S. K. Kim. 2005. Angiotensin I converting enzyme (ACE) inhibitory peptide derived from the sauce of fermented blue mussel, *Mytilusedulis*. *Bioresource Technology* 96: 1624–1629.

Jeyaram, K., Th. A. Singh, W. Romi, A. R. Devi, M. W. Singh, H. Dayanidhi, N. R. Singh, and J. P. Tamang. 2009. Traditional fermented foods of Manipur. *Indian Journal of Traditional Knowledge* 8: 115–121.

Jung, K.-O., S.-Y. Park, and K.-Y Park. 2006. Longer aging time increases the anticancer and antimetastatic properties of *doenjang*. *Nutrition* 22: 539–545.

Kang, M. S., B. G. Kim, J. Chung, H. C. Lee, and J. S. Oh. 2006a. Inhibitory effect of *Weissellacibaria* isolates on the production of volatile sulphur compounds. *Journal of Clinical Periodontology* 33: 226–232.

Kang, M. S., J. Chung, S. M. Kim, K. H. Yang, and J. S. Oh. 2006b. Effect of *Weissella cibaria* isolates on the formation of *Streptococcus mutans* biofilm. *Caries Research* 40: 418–425.

Karim, M. I. A. 1993. Fermented fish products in Malaysia. In C. H. Lee, K. H. Steinkraus, and P. J. A. Reilly (Eds.), *Fish Fermentation Technology*. Tokyo: United Nations University Press, pp. 95–106.

Kobayashi, T., B. Kimura, and T. Fujii. 2000. Strictly anaerobic halophiles isolated from canned Swedish fermented herrings (Suströmming). *International Journal of Food Microbiology* 54: 81–89.

Komatsuzaki, N., J. Shima, S. Kawamoto, H. Momose, and T. Kimura. 2005. Production of γ-aminobutyric acid (GABA) by *Lactobacillus paracasei* isolated from traditional fermented foods. *Food Microbiology* 22: 497–504.

Kuda, T., Y. Izawa, S. Ishii, H. Takahashi, Y. Torido, and B. Kimura. 2012. Suppressive effect of *Tetragenococcus halophilus*, isolated from fish-nukazuke, on histamine accumulation in salted and fermented fish. *Food Chemistry* 130: 569–574.

Kumar, M., A. K. Jain, M. Ghosh, and A. Ganguli. 2014. Characterization and optimization of an anti-*Aeromonas* bacteriocin produced by *Lactococcus lactis* isolated from *Hukuti Maas*, an indigenous fermented fish product. *Journal of Food Processing and Preservation* 38: 935–947.

Lee, N. K., S. A. Jun, J. U. Ha, and H. D. Paik. 2000. Screening and characterization of bacteriocinogenic lactic acid bacteria from jeot-gal, a Korean fermented fish food. *Journal of Microbiology and Biotechnology* 10: 423–428.

Lee, N. K. and H. D. Paik 2001. Partial characterization of lacticin NK24, a newly identified bacteriocin of *Lactococcus lactis*, NK24 isolated from *Jeot-gal. Food Microbiology* 18:17–24.

Lee, Y. G., J. Y. Kim, K. W. Lee, K. H. Kim, and H. J. Lee. 2003. Peptides from anchovy sauce induce apoptosis in a human lymphoma cell (U937) through the increase of caspase-3 and -8 activities. *Annals of New York Academy of Science* 1010: 399–404.

Lee, Y. G., K. W. Lee, J. Y. Kim, K. H. Kim, and H. J. Lee. 2004. Induction of apoptosis in a human lymphoma cell line by hydrophobic peptide fraction separated from anchovy sauce. *Biofactors* 21: 63–67.

Lee, C. L., J. J. Wang, S. L. Kuo, and T. M. Pan. 2006. Monascus fermentation of dioscorea for increasing the production of cholesterol-lowering agent—Monacolin K and antiinflammation agent—Monascin. *Applied Microbiology and Biotechnology* 72: 1254–1262.

Lee, K. W., J. Y. Park, H. D. Sa, J. H. Jeong, D. E. Jin, H. J Heo, and J. H. Kim. 2014. Probiotic properties of *Pediococcus* strains isolated from *Jeotgals*, salted and fermented Korean sea-food. *Anaerobe* 26: 199–206.

Liasi, S. A., T. I. Azmi, M. D. Hassan, M. Shuhaimi, M. Rosfarizan, and A. B. Ariff. 2009. Antimicrobial activity and antibiotic sensitivity of three isolates of lactic acid bacteria from fermented fish product, Budu. *Malaysian Journal of Microbiology* 5: 33–37.

Lopetcharat, K., Y. J. Choi, J. W. Park, and M. A. Daeschel. 2001. Fish sauce products and manufacturing—A review. *Food Review International* 17: 65–88.

Lovell, T. 1988. Digestion and metabolism. In T. Lowell (Ed.), *Nutrition and Feeding of Fish*. New York: Chapman & Hall, pp. 73–92.

Lv, L. X., X. J. Hu, G. R. Qian, H. Zhang, H. F. Lu, B. W. Zheng, L. Jiang, and L. J. Li. 2014. Administration of *Lactobacillus salivarius* LI01 or *Pediococcus pentosaceus* LI05 improves acute liver injury induced by D-galactosamine in rats. *Applied Microbiology and Biotechnology* 98: 5619–5632.

Mah, J.-H. and H.-J. Hwang. 2009. Inhibition of biogenic amine formation in a salted and fermented anchovy by *Staphylococcus xylosus* as a protective culture. *Food Control* 20: 796–801.

Majumdar, R. K. and S. Basu. 2010. Characteristics of the traditional fermented fish product *Lona ilish* of Northeast India. *Indian Journal of Traditional Knowledge* 9: 453–458.

Majumdar, R. K., S. Basu, and R. Anandan. 2005. Biochemical and microbiological characteristics of salt fermented *Hilsa* (*Tenulosa ilisha*). *Fishery Technology* 42: 67–70.

Majumdar, R. K., B. B. Nayak, and S. Basu. 2008. Involvement of *Bacillus licheniformis* and *Micrococcus kristinae* during ripening of salt-fermented Indian Shad (*Tenualosa ilisha*). *Journal of Aquatic Food Product Technology* 17: 423–440.

Marchbank, T., J. K. Limdi, A. Mahmood, G. Elia, and R. J. Playford. 2008. Clinical trial: Protective effect of a commercial fish protein hydrolysate against indomethacin (NSAID)-induced small intestinal injury, *Aliment. Pharmacological Therapy* 28, 799–804.

Miao, J., H. Guo, Y. Ou, G. Liu, X. Fang, Z. Liao, C. Ke, Y. Chen, L. Zhao, and Y. Cao. 2014. Purification and characterization of bacteriocin F1, a novel bacteriocin produced by *Lactobacillus paracasei* subsp. *tolerans* FX-6 from Tibetan kefir, a traditional fermented milk from Tibet, China. *Food Control* 42: 48–53.

Michihata, T. 2003. Components of fish sauce *Ishiru* in Noto peninsula and its possibilities as a functional Food. *Foods & Food Ingredients Journal of Japan* 208: 1.

Mizutani, T., A. Kimizuka, K. Ruddle, N. Ishige. 1992. Chemical components of fermented fish products. *Journal of Food Composition and Analysis* 5: 152–159.

Mukai, T., T. Asasaka, E. Sato, K. Mori, M. Matsumoto, and H. Ohori. 2002. Inhibition of binding of *Helicobacter pylori* to the glycolipid receptors by probiotic *Lactobacillus reuteri*. *FEMS Immunology and Medical Microbiology* 32: 105–110.

Müller, O. and M. Krawinkel. 2005. Malnutrition and health in developing countries. *Canadian Medical Association Journal* 173: 279–86.

Nakamura, S., T. Kuda, C. An, T. Kanno, H. Takahashi, and B. Kimura. 2012. Inhibitory effects of *Leuconostoc mesenteroides* 1RM3 isolated from narezushi, a fermented fish with rice, on *Listeria monocytogenes* infection to Caco-2 cells and A/J mice. *Anaerobe* 18: 19–24.

Negasi, T. 2013. *Studies on salt-fermentation microflora of Indian Mackerel and their bioactivities*. Master's degree thesis. Central Institute of Fisheries Education, Mumbai, India, 110pp.

Ngo, D. H., T. S. Vo, D. N. Ngo, I. Wijesekara, and S. K. Kim. 2012. Biological activities and potential health benefits of bioactive peptides derived from marine organisms. *International Journal of Biological Macromolecules* 51(4): 378–383.

Ninomiya, K. 2002. Umami: A universal taste. *Food Review International* 18: 23–38.

Paludan-Müller, C., H. H. Huss, and L. Gram 1999. Characterization of lactic acid bacteria isolated from a Thai low-salt fermented fish product and the role of garlic as substrate for fermentation. *International Journal of Food Microbiology* 46: 219–229.

Park, J. E., S. H. Oh, and Y. S. Cha. 2013. *Lactobacillus plantarum* LG42 isolated from gajamisik-hae inhibits adipogenesis in 3T3-L1 adipocyte. *Biomedical Research International* 2013:1–7.

Park, J-N., Y. Fukumoto, E. Fujita, T. Tanaka, T. Washio, S. Otsuka, T. Shimizu, K. Watanabe K, and H. Abe. 2001. Chemical composition of fish sauces produced in Southeast and East Asian countries. *Journal of Food Composition and Analysis* 14: 113–125.

Parvez, S., K. A. Malik, S. Ah Kang, and H.-Y. Kim. 2006. Probiotics and their fermented food products are beneficial for health *Journal of Applied Microbiology* 100: 1171–1185.

Pushpamali, W. A., C. Nikapitiya, M. D. Zoysa, I. Whang, S. J. Kim, and J. Lee. 2008. Isolation and purification of an anticoagulant from fermented red seaweed *Lomentaria catenata*. *Carbohydrate Polymers* 73: 274–279.

Pattanagul, P., R. Pinthong, A. Phianmongkhol, and N. Leksawasdi. 2007. Review of angkak production (*Monascus purpureus*). *Chiang Mai Journal of Science* 34: 319–328.

Rajapakse, N., E. Mendis, K. Jung, J. Y. Je, and S. K. Kim. 2005. Purification of a radical scavenging peptide from fermented mussel sauce and its antioxidant properties. *Food Research International* 38: 175–182.

Rapsang, G., R. Kumar, and S. Joshi. 2013. Identification of *Lactobacillus pobuzihii* from tungtap: A traditionally fermented fish food, and analysis of its bacteriocinogenic potential. *African Journal of Biotechnology* 10: 12237–12243.

Saisithi, P. 1994. Traditional fermented fish: Fish sauce production. In A. M. Martin (Ed.), *Fisheries Processing: Biotechnological Applications*. London: Chapman & Hall, 111–129.

Saisithi, P., B. Kasemsarn, J. Liston, and A. M. Dollar. 1966. Microbiology and chemistry of fermented fish. *Journal of Food Science* 31: 105–110.

Saithong, P., W. Panthavee, M. Boonyaratanakornkit, and C. Sikkhamondhol. 2010. Use of a starter culture of lactic acid bacteria in *plaa-som*, a Thai fermented fish. *Journal of Bioscience and Bioengineering* 110: 553–557.

Sanchez, P. C. 2008. Philippine fermented foods. In P. C. Sanchez (Ed.), *Principles and Technology*. Diliman, Philippines: University of the Philippines Press, 405–435.

Schofield, C. and A. Ashworth. 1996. Why have mortality rates for severe malnutrition remained so high? *Bulletin World Health Organization* 74: 223–229.

Shin, M. S., S. K. Han, J. S. Ryu, K. S. Kim, and W. K. Lee. 2008. Isolation and partial characterization of a bacteriocin produced by *Pediococcuspentosaceus* K23-2 isolated from Kimchi. *Journal of Applied Microbiology* 105: 331–339.

Srionnual, S., F. Yanagida, L.-H. Lin, K.-N. Hsiao, and Y. Chen. 2007. Weissellicin 110, a newly discovered bacteriocin from *Weissellacibaria* 110, isolated from *plaa-som*, a fermented fish product from Thailand. *Applied and Environmental Microbiology* 73: 2247–2250.

Steinkraus, K. H. 1996. *Handbook of Indigenous Fermented Food*, 2nd ed. New York: Marcel Dekker, Inc.

Steinkraus, K. H. 1997. Classification of fermented foods: Worldwide review of household fermentation techniques. *Food Control* 8: 311–317.

Steinkrauss, K. H. 2002. Fermentations in world food processing. *Comprehensive Reviews in Food Science and Food Safety* 1: 23–32.

Tamang, J. P., N. Tamang, S. Thapa, S. Dewan, B. M. Tamang, H. Yonzan, A. K. Rai, R. Chettri, J. Chakrabarty, and N. Kharel. 2012. Microorganisms and nutritional value of ethnic fermented foods and alcoholic beverages of Northeast India. *Indian Journal of Traditional Knowledge* 11: 7–25.

Thapa, N., J. Pal, and J. P. Tamang, 2004. Microbial diversity in *ngari, hentak* and *tungtap,* fermented fish products of Northeast India. *World Journal of Microbiology and Biotechnology* 20: 599–607.

Thapa, N., J. Pal, and J. P. Tamang. 2006. Phenotypic identification and technological properties of lactic acid bacteria isolated from traditionally processed fish products of the Eastern Himalayas. *International Journal of Food Microbiology* 107: 33–38.

Thapa, N., J. Pal, and J. P. Tamang. 2007. Microbiological profile of dried fish products of Assam. *Indian Journal of Fisheries* 54: 121–125.

Thongthai, C. and P. Suntinanalert. 1991. Halophiles in Thai fish sauce *(nampla).* In F. Rodriguez-Valera (Ed.), *General and Applied Aspects of Halophilic Microorganisms.* New York: Plenum Press, pp. 381–388.

Thongthai, C., T. McGenity, J. P. Suntinanalert, and W. D. Grant. 1992. Isolation and characterization of an extremely halophilic archaeobacterium from traditionally fermented Thai fish sauce (*nampla*). *Letters in Applied Microbiology* 14: 111–114.

TPI (Tropical Products Institute). 1982. Fermented fish products: A review. In *Fish Handling, Preservation and Processing in the Tropics* Pt. 2. TPI, London, pp. 18–22.

VanVeen, A. G. 1965. Fermented and dried sea–food products in south East Asia. In G. Borgstrom (Ed.), *Fish as Food,* Vol 3. New York: Academic Press, pp. 227–250.

Villar, M., A. P. de Ruiz Holgado, J. J. Sanchez, R. E. Trucco, and G. Oliver. 1985. Isolation and characterization of *Pediococcus halophilus* from salted anchovies (*Engraulis anchoita*). *Applied and Environmental Microbiology* 49: 664–666.

Wang, J., Z. Lu, J. Chi, W. Wang, M. Su, W. Kou, P. Yu, L. Yu, L. Chen, J.-S. Zhu, and J. Chang. 1997. Multicenter clinical trial of the serum lipid-lowering effects of a *Monascus purpureus* (red yeast) rice preparation from traditional Chinese medicine. *Current Therapeutic Research* 58: 964–978.

Wang, Y-K., H-L. He, X-L. Chen, C-Y. Sun, Y-Z. Zhang, and B-C. Zhou. 2008. Production of novel angiotensin I-converting enzyme inhibitory peptides by fermentation of marine shrimp *Acetes chinensis* with *Lactobacillus fermentum* SM 605. *Applied Microbiology and Biotechnology* 79: 785–791.

Wei, W., C. Li, Y. Wang, H. Su, J. Zhu, and D. Kritchevsky. 2003. Hypolipidemic and anti-atherogenic effects of long-term cholestin (*Monascus purpureus*-fermented rice, red yeast rice) in cholesterol fed rabbits. *Journal of Nutrition and Biochemistry* 14: 314–318.

Wilaipun, P. 1990. Halophilic bacteria producing lipase in fish sauce. MS Thesis, Chulalongkom University, Bangkok, Thailand.

Wong, A. H. K. and Y. Mine. 2004. Novel fibrinolytic enzyme in fermented shrimp paste, a traditional Asian fermented seasoning. *Journal of Agricultural and Food Chemistry* 52: 980–986.

Wongkhalaung, C. 2004. Industrialization of Thai fish sauce (*Nam Pla*). In Steinkraus, K. H. (Ed.), *Industrialization of Indigenous Fermented Food,* New York: Marcel Decker, pp. 647–699.

Yoshida, Y. 1998. Umami taste and traditional seasonings. *Food Reviews International* 14: 213–246.

Zaman, M. Z., A. S. Abdulamir, F. A. Bakar, J. Selamat, and J. Bakar. 2009. A review: Microbiological, physicochemical and health impact of high level of biogenic amines in fish sauce. *American Journal of Applied Science* 6: 1199–1211.

Chapter 16

Wine: A Therapeutic Drink

Usha Rani M. and Anu Appaiah K. A.

Contents

16.1 Introduction

Multiple epidemiological studies suggest that daily moderate alcohol consumption (Thun et al. 1997, Doll et al. 2005), especially of wine (Renaud and de Lorgeril 1992) is associated with a reduction in all-cause mortality and has distinct health benefits. The term "French paradox" refers to the observation that while both the French and Americans have a diet high in saturated fats, smoke cigarettes, and exercise little—all risk factors for cardiovascular disease—the French have a significantly lower risk of cardiovascular disease than that of Americans: 36% compared with 75% (St. Leger et al. 1979). The difference in risk has been attributed to the consumption of alcohol and, in particular, red wine by the French. The French currently consume 53.9 L per capita of wine per year, while Americans only consume 8.5 L per year. This idea was established by St. Leger et al. (1979) who found an inverse relation between coronary heart disease mortality and wine consumption, with France having the lowest mortality. French authors have reported that according to a statistical report of the World Health Organization for the year of 1989, cardiovascular mortality in the population 35–64 years of age was much lower in France than in the similarly industrialized United States or United Kingdom in spite of the fact that the per capita consumption of alcoholic beverages in a year was the highest in France (corresponding to 15 liters of pure alcohol yearly). At the same time the other risk factors such as serum cholesterol level, average blood pressure, extent of smoking, and body mass index were similar in the age group studied. This phenomenon, the so-called French paradox is attributed to the high consumption of wine by the French. This presumption seems to be confirmed by the fact that the populations with the longest life expectancy—Cretan and Japanese people—regularly consume moderate amounts of alcohol, namely 20 and 28 g a day respectively; the former as wine, and the latter as beer (MacNeil 2001) (Table 16.1).

16.2 Molecules Involved in the Therapeutic Benefits of Wine

The therapeutic benefits derived from wine cannot be attributed to any one molecule or a single group of chemicals. Both the alcohol and the polyphenol components have been extensively studied and there is controversy over which component is more important (de Lorgeril et al. 2008, Bhagat and Anu-Appaiah 2011).

16.2.1 Phenols and Related Phenol (Phenyl) Derivatives

Phenols are a large and complex group of compounds of primary importance to the characteristics and quality of wine. Polyphenols constitute one of the most numerous and widely distributed groups of substances in the plant kingdom, with more than 8000 phenolic structures currently known (Paganga et al. 1999). Polyphenols are products of the secondary metabolism of plants and ubiquitous in all plant organs. They arise biogenetically from two main synthetic pathways: the shikimate and the acetate pathway. Natural polyphenols can range from simple molecules, such as phenolic acids, to highly polymerized compounds, such as tannins. They occur primarily in conjugated form, with one or more sugar residues linked to hydroxyl groups, although direct linkages of the sugar unit to an aromatic carbon atom also exist. Polyphenols can be divided into at least 10 different classes depending on their basic chemical structure. Flavonoids, which constitute the most important single group, can be further subdivided into 13 classes, with more than 4000 compounds described until 1990. Polyphenols are almost ubiquitous in plant foods

Table 16.1 List of Therapeutic Benefits of Fruits and Wine

Therapeutic Benefit	*Molecules Responsible/ Remarks*	*Commodity*	*References*
Anticarcinogenic (high consumption may increase the risk of certain cancers)	Phenolics—resveratrol Flavones, flavonols	Fruits and berries Wine Pomegranate	Seeram (2008) Prescott et al. (1999) Dhalawi et al. (2011)
Anti-inflammatory	Phenolics—resveratrol, anthocyanins	Wine Black raspberry wine	Stoclet et al. (2004) Jeong et al. (2010)
Antimicrobial, protection from diarrhea and dysentery	p-Coumaric acid (against Gram +ve), Other phenolics (against Gram −ve), Quercetin (inhibition of DNAgyrase), Epigallocatechin (disruption of cell membrane function)	Fruits—*Garcinia cowa* and *Garcinia pedunculata* Wine	Negi et al. (2008) Weisse et al. (1995)
Antimutagenic	Phenolics—flavonoids	Fruits—*Garcinia cowa* and *Garcinia pedunculata* Wine	Negi et al. (2010) Soleas et al. (1997)
Antioxidant	Phenolics—flavonoids, resveratrol Vitamins—A, C, and E	Fruits and berries Fruits—*Garcinia cowa and Garcinia pedunculata* Wine Fruit and berry wines	Wolfe et al. (2008) Negi et al. (2010) Rai et al. (2010) Heinonen et al. (1998) Lehtonen et al. (1999), German and Walzem (2000), Pinhero and Paliyath (2001), Yildirim (2006)
Antiplatelet aggregation	Phenolics—resveratrol, Flavonoids such as quercitin, catechin, epicatechin (enhance synthesis and release of nitric oxide by endo cells, induces vasodilation, and limits platelet adhesion)	Wine	Keli et al. (1994) Gupta and Triedi (2009)

(*Continued*)

Table 16.1 (*Continued*) List of Therapeutic Benefits of Fruits and Wine

Therapeutic Benefit	*Molecules Responsible/ Remarks*	*Commodity*	*References*
Anxiolytic effects	Phenolics	Wine	Paladini et al. (1999)
Digestive aid	Phenolics (activates release of saliva), Succinic acid (activates release of gastric juice), Ethanol (activates release of bile in intestine)	Wine	Jackson (2008)
Good for bones, lower risk of rip fracture	Phenolics—resveratrol (phytoestrogen effect), alcohol (enhanced Ca uptake)	Wine	Hoidrup et al. (1999) Ganry et al. (2000)
Nutritional value	Ethanol (calorific value), Minerals—K, Fe, etc. Vitamins—B1, B2, B12	Wine Fruit and berry wines	Rupasinghe and Clegg (2007) Teissèdre et al. (1996)
Prevent cardiovascular diseases, reduced incidence of heart attacks and mortality	Phenolics—resveratrol, flavonoids such as quercitin, ethanol, vitamins C and E, mineral selenium	Fruits Wine	Stoclet et al. (2004) Hertog et al. (1993), Knekt et al. (1996), Keil et al. (1998), Truelsen et al. (1998)
Prevent common cold	Phenolics (antiviral against Rhinovirus and Corona virus)	Wine	Takkouche et al. (2002)
Prevent eye diseases	Phenolics—resveratrol	Wine	Anonymous (www.indianwineacademy.com)
Prevent obesity	Phenolics—resveratrol (prevent immature fat cells from fully maturing)	Wine	Keli et al. (1994), Gupta and Sharma (2009)
Prevent secondary events of cerebral disease	Phenolics—flavonoids such as flavones	Fruits—sea buckthorn	Cheng et al. (1999)
Protect against Alzheimer's disease (heavy consumption is harmful).	Phenolics—resveratrol (promotes degradation of β peptides), Tannic acid (inhibit the formation and destabilize preexisting β amyloid fibrils), vitamins (protect neurons from β amyloid accumulation	Wine	Truelsen et al. (1998), Savaskan et al. (2003), Luchsinger et al. (2004), Marambaud et al. (2005)

Table 16.1 (*Continued*) List of Therapeutic Benefits of Fruits and Wine

Therapeutic Benefit	*Molecules Responsible/ Remarks*	*Commodity*	*References*
Protect brain of elderly, Protect against dementia	Phenolics	Wine	Orgogozo et al. (1997)
Protect kidney, fights the production and progression of renal diseases	Phenolics	Wine	Rodrigo and Rivera (2002) Bertelli et al. (1998)
Reduce incidence of metabolic syndrome X	Phenolics—resveratrol (hypoglycemic and hypolipidemic effects), element vanadium (antidiabetic)	Wine	Teissedre et al. (1996), Rosell et al. (2003), Su et al. (2006)
Reduced prevalence of goiter	Ethanol	Wine	Knudsen et al. (2001)
Reduce the risk of developing rheumatoid arthritis	Alcohol	Wine	Anonymous (www.indian wineacademy.com)
Safe for asthmatics (not for sulfite-sensitive patients)	Catechin	Wine	Halpern et al. (1985)

(vegetables, cereals, legumes, fruits, nuts, etc.) and beverages (wine, cider, beer, tea, cocoa, etc.) (Feher et al. 2007, Vaidya and Sharma 2009). Polyphenols are partially responsible for the sensory and nutritional qualities of plant foods. The astringency and bitterness of foods and beverages depends on the content of polyphenols (Rai et al. 2010). The polyphenols are mainly in the form of free polyphenols and bound forms (Gutiérrez et al. 2005). The bound forms are considered to be biologically inactive. During fermentation and maturation the majority of bound polyphenols are converted into free forms (Rani and Anu-Appaiah 2011, Rai and Anu-Appaiah 2014) (Table 16.2).

16.2.2 Classification and Bioavailability of Phenolics

Polyphenols are divided into several classes according to the number of phenol rings that they contain and according to the structural elements that bind these rings to one another. The main groups of polyphenols are: flavonoids, phenolic acids, phenolic alcohols, stilbenes, and lignans. The major phenolics found in wine are either members of the diphenylpropanoids (flavonoids) or phenylpropanoids (nonflavonoids).

Table 16.2 Main Classes of Phenolic Compounds in Higher Plants

Classes and Subclass	*Examples of Specific Compounds*
Nonflavanoids Compounds	
Phenolic acids	
Benzoic acids	Gallic acid; protocatechuic acid; *p*-Hydroxybenzoic acid
Hydroxycinnamic acid	Coumaric acid; caffeic acid; Ferulic acid; sinaptic acid
Hydrolyzable tannins	Pentagalloylglucose
Stilbenes	Resveratrol
Lignins	Secoisolariciresinol, matairesinol, Lariciresinol, pinoresinol
Flavonoid Compounds	
Flavonols	Kaempferol; quercetin; myricetin
Flavones	Apigenin; luteolin
Flavanones	Naringenin; hesperetins
Flavanols	Catechins; gallocatechins
Anthocyanidins	Pelargonidin; cyanidin; malvidin
Condensed tannins or proanthocyanidins	Trimeric procyanidin; prodelphinidin
Isoflavones	Daidzein; genistein; glycitein

Source: From Patil, M. M. and K. A. Anu-Appaiah. 2013. *Functional Food Science*. 110–119, Food Science Publisher, Dallas, TX, USA.

16.2.2.1 Flavonoids

Flavonoids share a common carbon skeleton of diphenyl propanes, two benzene rings joined by a linear three-carbon chain (Wulf and Nagel 1980). The central three-carbon chain may form a closed pyran ring with one of the benzene rings. Flavonoids are themselves divided into six subclasses, depending on the oxidation state of the central pyran ring: flavonols, flavones, flavanones, isoflavones, anthocyanidins, and flavanols (catechins and proanthocyanidins). The most common flavonoids in wine are flavonols, catechins (flavan-3-ols), and anthocyanins (red wines). Small amounts of flavan-3, 4-diols (leucoanthocyanins) also occur (Wulf and Nagel 1980).

16.2.2.2 Flavonols

Flavonols represent the most ubiquitous flavonoids in foods, with quercetin as the more representative compound. It is important to note that flavonols biosynthesis is stimulated by light, so they accumulate in the outer and aerial tissue of fruits (Merken and Beecher 2000). They exist in both the monomer and the polymer form (catechins and proanthocyanidins respectively). Unlike other classes of flavonoids, flavanols are not glycosylated in foods. The main representative flavanols in fruit are catechin and epicatechin, whereas gallocatechin, epigallocatechin, and epigallocatechin gallate are found especially in tea. Catechins are found in many fruits such as apricots (250 mg/kg fresh wt) and cherries (250 mg/kg fresh wt) (Arts et al. 2000a). Green tea (up to 800 mg/L), and chocolate (up to 600 mg/L), are by far the richest sources of catechins, which are also present in red wine (up to 300 mg/L) (Arts et al. 2000b).

16.2.2.3 Flavones

Flavones are much less common than flavonols in fruit and vegetables. The skin of fruits contains large quantities of polymethoxylated flavones. Flavones consist chiefly of glycosides of luteolin and apigenin. In human foods, flavanones are found in tomatoes and certain aromatic plants such as mint, but they are present in high concentrations only in citrus fruits. The main glycones are naringenin in grapefruit, hesperetin in oranges, and eriodictyol in lemons (Sartelet et al. 1996).

16.2.2.4 Flavanones

Flavanones are present in high concentrations only in citrus fruit. The main aglycones are narirutin in grapefruit, hesperidin in oranges, and neohesperidin in lemons (Gattuso et al. 2007). Orange juice contains 470–761 mg/L of hesperidin and 20–86 mg/L of narirutin. The solid parts of citrus fruit, in particular the white spongy portion (albedo) and the membranes separating the segments, have a very high flavanone content; this is the reason why the whole fruit may contain up to five times as much flavanone as a glass of orange juice (Holden et al. 2002).

16.2.2.5 Isoflavones

Isoflavones are contained almost exclusively in leguminous plants. Soya and its processed products represent the main source of isoflavones, and contain the three main molecules (genistein, daidzein, and glycitein) that occur as aglycones or, more often, as glucose-conjugate forms (Coward et al. 1998, Manach et al. 2005). Isoflavones are sensitive to heat and are often hydrolyzed to glycosides during industrial processing and storage, such as in the production of soya milk and wine (De Sanctis et al. 2012).

16.2.2.6 Anthocyanins

Anthocyanins are water-soluble pigments, responsible for most of the red, blue, and purple colors of fruits, vegetables, flowers, and other plant tissues or products (Clifford 2000). Anthocyanins are widely distributed in the human diet: they are found in red wine, certain varieties of cereals, and certain vegetables (cabbage, beans, onions, radishes), but they are most abundant especially in fruit. Food contents are generally proportional to color intensity and reach values up to 2–4 g/kg fresh wt. in blackcurrants or blackberries; the contents increase as the fruit ripens (Es-Safi et al. 2002). Anthocyanins are found mainly in the skin, except for some red fruits (cherries and strawberries) in which they also occur in the flesh. Wine contains up to 350 mg anthocyanins/L, and these anthocyanins are transformed into various complex structures as the wine ages (He et al. 2012).

16.2.2.7 Proanthocyanidins

Proanthocyanidins also known as condensed tannins, which are dimers, oligomers, and polymers of catechins. Proanthocyanidins are responsible for the astringent character of fruit (grapes, apples, berries, etc.) and beverages (wine, cider, tea, beer, etc.) and for the bitterness of chocolate (Santos-Buelga and Scalbert 2000). It is important to note that this astringency changes over the course of maturation and often disappears when the fruit reaches ripeness. Seed tannins are less polymerized than skin tannins—seed tannins contain up to 28 flavanol moieties, whereas skin tannins may possess up to 74 flavanol units. During wine aging, procyanidins slowly combine with monomeric flavonoids to generate polymers (tannins) from 8 to 14 units in length (He et al. 2008).

16.2.2.8 Phenolic Acids

These compounds could be divided into two classes: derivatives of benzoic acid and derivatives of cinnamic acid. Hydroxybenzoic acids are components of complex structures such as hydrolyzable tannins (Clifford 2000). Hydroxycinnamic acid is more common than hydroxybenzoic acids. These acids are rarely found in free forms and the bound forms and are glycosylated derivatives of esters of quinic acid, shikimic acid, and tartaric acid (Clifford 1999).

16.2.2.8.1 Hydroxybenzoic Acids

The hydroxybenzoic acids, such as gallic acid and protocatechuic acid, are found in very few plants eaten by humans; this is the reason why they are not currently considered to be of great nutritional interest. The content of hydroxybenzoic acids in edible plants is generally very low, except for certain red fruits, that is, blackberries which contain up to 270 mg/kg fresh wt. Raspberries contain up to 100 mg/kg fresh weight of protocatechuic acid (D'Archivio et al. 2007).

16.2.2.8.2 Hydroxycinnamic Acids

The hydroxycinnamic acids consist chiefly of coumaric, caffeic, and ferulic acid, that are rarely found in the free form (Manach et al. 2004). The bound forms are glycosylated derivatives or esters of quinic, shikimic, or tartaric acid. Caffeic and quinic acid combine to form chlorogenic acid, which is found in many types of fruits: blueberries contain 2 g hydroxycinnamic acids/kg fresh wt. Caffeic acid is the most abundant phenolic acid, representing between 75% and 100% of the total hydroxycinnamic acids contents in most fruits: kiwi contain up to 1 g caffeic acid/kg fresh wt. Hydroxycinnamic acids are present in all parts of fruit, although the highest concentrations are seen in the outer part of ripe fruit. The concentration decreases during the course of ripening, but the total quantity increases as the fruit increases in size.

16.2.2.9 Phenolic Alcohols

Tyrosol (4-hydroxyphenylethanol) and hydroxytyrosol (3,4-dihydroxyphenylethanol) are the main phenolic alcohols; they are contained mainly in extra virgin olive oil (40.2 and 3.8 mg/kg, respectively) (Servili et al. 2014). Tyrosol is also present in red and white wines and beer, while hydroxytyrosol is also found in red wine and is additionally produced *in vivo* after red wine ingestion. The concentration of total phenols in extra virgin olive oil has a mean value for commercial olive oil of approximately 180 mg/kg. The phenol concentration in olive oil depends on variety, climate, and area of growth, latitude, and ripeness of the olive. Despite the wide body of evidence linking the *in vitro* properties of olive oil phenolics with positive health outcomes, there are limited data on the absorption and excretion of these compounds (Stasiuk and Kozubek 2010). In part, this could be due to the low concentrations of such constituents and, accordingly, the difficulty in detecting the presumptively low concentrations of these compounds in biological systems.

16.2.2.10 Stilbenes

Low quantities of stilbenes are present in the human diet, and the main representative is resveratrol, mostly in glycosylated forms (Bertelli et al. 1998). It is produced by plants in response to infection by pathogens or to a variety of stress conditions. It has been detected in more than 70 plant species, including grapes, berries, and peanuts. The fresh skin of red grapes is particularly rich in resveratrol (50–100 g/kg net weight) which contributes to a relatively high concentration of resveratrol in red wine and grape juice (up to 7 mg aglycones/L and 15 mg glycosides/L in red wine) (Figure 16.1). Extensive data provide evidence for the anticarcinogenic effects of resveratrol (Bhat and Pezzuto 2002).

16.2.2.11 Lignans

Lignans are produced by oxidative dimerization of two phenylpropane units that are mostly present in nature in the free form, while their glycoside derivatives are only a minor form (MacRae and Towers 1984). Linseed represents the main dietary source, containing up to 3.7 g/kg dry wt. of secoisolariciresinol. Intestinal microflora metabolizes lignans to enterodiol and enterolactone. The low quantities of lignans normally contained in the human diet do not account for the concentrations of the metabolites enterodiol and enterolactone measured in plasma and urine (Adlercreutz and Mazur 1997). Thus, there are certainly other lignans of plant origin, precursors of enterodiol and enterolactone that have not been identified yet. The interest in lignans and their synthetic derivatives is growing because of their potential applications in cancer chemotherapy and various other pharmacological effects.

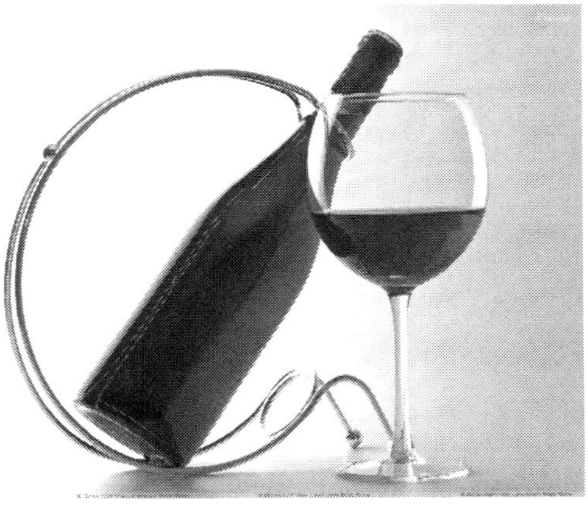

Figure 16.1 Red wine with all its therapeutic values.

16.2.3 Presence of Polyphenols in Fruits and Berries

Nutritional studies concerning examination of foods for their protective and disease preventing potential have established that fruits apart from grapes such as cranberries, sweet cherries, and blueberries, are an equal or sometimes better source of phenolics (Balasundram et al. 2006) (Table 16.3).

Table 16.3 Phenolics in Selected Fruits and Berries and Their Products (mg/kg)

Fruit/Berry	*Anthocyanins*	*Flavanols and Proanthocyanidins*	*Flavonols*	*Hydroxycinnamates*
Apple-juice	4–5	0–15 0–298	17–70 2.5	263–308 0.1–162
Bilberry juice	3450–4635	13–29	41–195	170–347
Blueberry	3970–4840	63–70	115–139	226–315
Blackcurrant juice	130–8100 24	205–374	133–157 36	104–167
Cherry, sweet, red	31–4500	20–63	10–23	100–1900
Cloudberry	7–15	2–6	34–90	90–128
Cranberry juice	460–1720	285	139–334	191
	18–512			
Grapes, red wine	72.5–765 0.6–385	1–160 0–500	13–25 10–55	5–19 4–13
Grapes, white wine	0 0	0 0–106	10–13.5	5.5 1–34
Orange juice			0–5	136–163
Peach canned	0–17.8	24.5–700	0–11.9	54–148
	0			11–29
Plum dried (prune)	19–76 0	140–600 0	5.7–27 42	500–900 1800
Raspberry, red	200–2200	4–480	6–39	3–35
Strawberry	202–790	9–184	7–174	14–69
Strawberry jam	4–22			11.4

Source: From Balasundram, N., K. Sundram, and S. Samman. 2006. *Food Chemistry* 99: 191–203.

16.2.4 Presence of Polyphenols in Wine

The majority of grape polyphenols are present in the skins and seeds, and the processing of grapes into wine has a greater effect on the total polyphenol content than does grape variety, although varietal and growing conditions influence the spectrum of polyphenols in the grapes (Halpern 2008). The degree to which flavonoids are extracted during wine production depends on many factors (Henick-Kling 1993). Extraction is ultimately limited by the amount present in the fruit. Traditional fermentation due to its longer maceration with the seeds and skins, extracts more phenolic compounds than carbonic maceration or thermovinification (Jackson 2008) (Figure 16.2). Flavonoid extraction is also markedly influenced by the pH, sulfur dioxide content, and ethanol content of the juice, as well as the temperature and duration of fermentation. During fruit and berry wine processing phenolic compounds undergo change and are effectively extracted into fruit and berry wines (Heinonen et al. 1998). They evaluated 44 different berry and fruit wines and liquors. The amount of total phenolics in the berry and fruit wines and liquors ranged from 91 to 1820 mg gallic acid equivalents per 100 g (mg GAE/100 g). Wines made of cherries (1080 mg GAE/L), red raspberries and black currants (1050 mg GAE/L), black currants and bilberries (average 1040 mg GAE/L), black currants and crowberries (1020 mg GAE/L), black and red currants (average 890 mg GAE/L), and black currants (average 870 mg GAE/L) contained the highest amounts of phenolic compounds (Heinonen et al. 1998). Yildirim (2006) evaluated the total phenolic content of fruit and berry wines and arranged them in the following order: Blackberry > Bilberry > Black Mulberry > Sour Cherry > Quince > Apple > Melon > Apricot. Vuorinen et al. (2000) estimated the total flavonoid content of different fruit and berry wines and found it to be in the range of 16.3–31.31 mg/L for red wines (Cabernet and Merlot varieties) and 10.4–34.5 mg/L for blackcurrant wines. Figure 16.3 shows compilation of total phenolic values of fruit and berry wines collected from different studies and clearly the fact that emerges is wines from blackcurrant, black and red currant, blueberry and elderberry seem better than grape wines like Cabernet and Merlot. Other wines from raspberry, cherry, blackcurrant and bilberry, blackcurrant and raspberry were also comparable to those of red wines. However, other fruits such as apple, plum, and peach showed lower level of phenolics (Satora et al. 2008, Anu-Appaiah 2010).

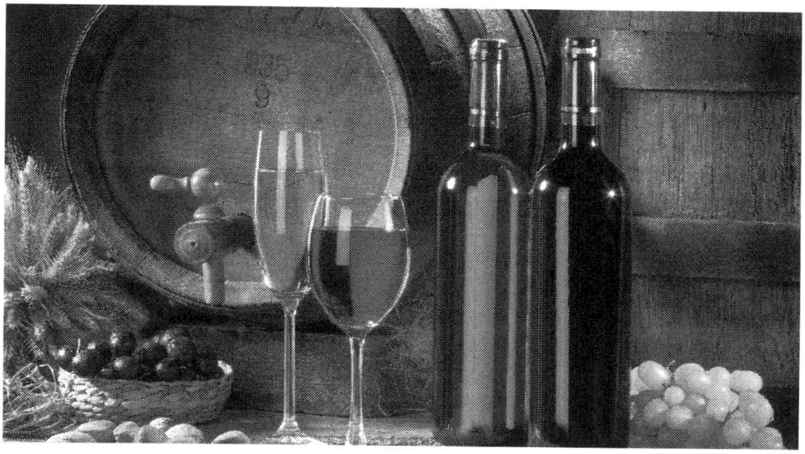

Figure 16.2 Ancient wine barrel with bottles of white and pink wine.

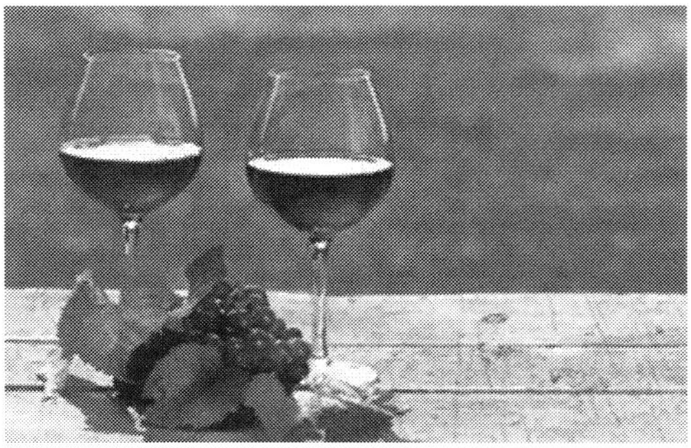

Figure 16.3 Red wine as served in the farm with the variety of grapes from which it is produced.

16.2.5 Therapeutic Benefits Due to Phenolics

Wine is known for its health-promoting values from ancient times. Recent research to understand its preventive features has led to the unravelling of some of the mechanisms of action.

16.2.5.1 Promotes Longevity

New research shows that red wine contains melatonin. Melatonin regulates the body clock, so drinking a glass of red wine before bed may help you sleep. Melatonin is also an antioxidant, which means it also has antiaging properties. Resveratrol has been shown to increase lifespan in animal studies (Corder et al. 2006).

16.2.5.2 Prevention against Cardiovascular Diseases

The most clearly established benefit of moderate alcohol consumption, notably wine, relates to nearly 30%–35% reduction in the death rate due to cardiovascular disease (Klatsky et al. 1974, Renaud and deLorgeril 1992, Klatsky et al. 2003). Studies have also demonstrated that daily consumption of alcohol significantly reduces the incidence of other forms of cardiovascular disease, such as hypertension (Keil et al. 1998), heart attack (Gaziano et al. 1999), stroke (Truelsen et al. 1998), and peripheral arterial disease (Camargo et al. 1997). Those who consume wine moderately live, on an average, 2.5–3.5 years longer than teetotalers, and considerably longer than heavy drinkers (Figure 16.4). Of the two principal forms, ethanol augments the presence of HDL3, whereas exercise increases the level of HDL2. Either form tends to remove cholesterol from the arteries, transferring it to the liver for metabolism. Another of alcohol's beneficial influence involves the disruption of events leading to clot formation. Some of the cardiovascular benefits are listed in Table 16.4.

In risk reduction of cardiac diseases due to vascular obstruction, the beneficial effect of the phenol components originating from wine may prevail via anticoagulant mechanisms. The polyphenols of wine inhibit platelet and macrophage cyclooxygenase and lipoxygenase enzyme activity, thus making the process of coagulation slower. Through their radical-scavenging, that is, antioxidant properties they inhibit the damage of endothelial prostacyclin and endothelium-dependent relaxation factor caused by lipid peroxidation. The polyphenols of red wine are probably synergists of tocopherol (Vitamin E) and ascorbic acid (Vitamin C), thus they inhibit lipid peroxidation

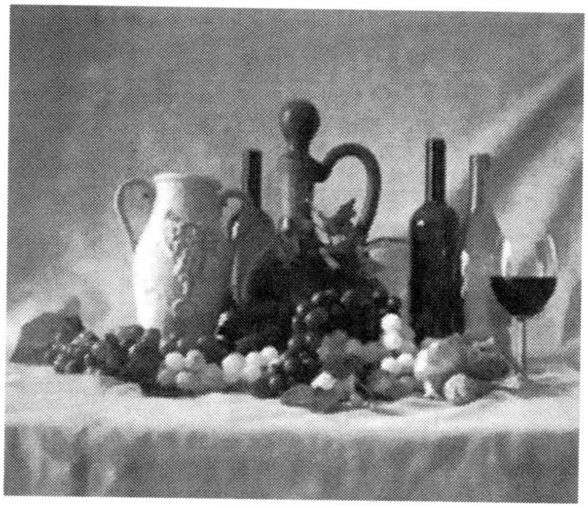

Figure 16.4 Old wine jars with wine exhibited during a wine festival.

(Feher et al. 2007). Red wine upregulates endothelial nitric oxide synthase (eNOS), a protective enzyme in the cardiovascular system (Wallerath et al. 2005).

The increase in eNOS in response to red wine involves several polyphenolic compounds with a major contribution from trans-resveratrol and lesser contributions from cinnamic and hydroxycinnamic acids, cyanidin, and some phenolic acids.

16.2.5.2.1 Hypertension

Polyphenols have vasorelaxing effects, which are associated with lower blood pressure (Carollo et al. 2007). Red wine, dealcoholized red wine, and grape juice consumption have lowered blood pressure in patients with coronary artery disease or hypertension (Jimenez et al. 2008, Papamichael et al. 2008).

16.2.5.2.2 Reduces the Risk of Diabetes

Research has shown that moderate levels of alcohol consumed with meals do not have a substantial impact on blood sugarlevels (Haimoto et al. 2009). A 2005 study presented to the American Diabetes Association suggests that moderate consumption may lower the risk of developing type 2 diabetes (Caimi et al. 2003, Koppes et al. 2005). Resveratrol activates nicotinamide adenine dinucleotide-dependent deacetylase SIRT1, a nuclear protein thought to mediate some of the beneficial metabolic effects of calorie-restriction. Diet-induced diabetic mice that were orally treated with resveratrol display enhanced muscle oxidative capacity, an effect that may account, at least in part, for the antidiabetic actions of resveratrol (Ramadori et al. 2009).

16.2.5.3 Reduces the Risk of Stroke

It is likely that the antioxidants present in wine prevent oxidative damage in the brain that is associated with the process of aging. The discovery that some wines contain hydroxytyrosol, a dopamine metabolite and potent antioxidant, suggest that wine constituents may modulate dopamine signaling in the brain (de la Torre et al. 2006).

Table 16.4 Therapeutic Benefits of Wine Polyphenols

Inhibition LDL Oxidation
Free radical scavenger
Metal ion chelator
Sparing of antioxidants (e.g., Vit E, carotenoids)
Increase or preserve paraoxonase activity
Inhibition SMC Proliferation and Vascular Hyperplasia
Cell cycle arrest
DNA strand breakage
Decrease cyclin A expression
Inhibition ICAM-1 and VCAM-1
Inhibition PDGF
Inhibition P13-K and p38-MAPK
Inhibition MMP9
Apoptosis
Inhibition platelet aggregation
Inhibition cyclo-oxygenase pathway
Inhibition thromboxane-2 synthesis
Potentiate prostacyclin
Increase phosphodiesterases (cAMP, cGMP)
Increase HDL
Increased apolipoproteins A-1 and A-2, C20:5 (omega-3)
Vasorelaxation
eNOS expression
NO release

Source: From Patil, M. M. and K. A. Anu-Appaiah. 2013. *Functional Food Science*. 110–119, Food Science Publisher, Dallas, TX, USA.

Note: eNOS: endothelial nitric oxide synthase; ICAM-1: intercellular adhesion molecule 1; MMP9: matrix metalloproteinase 9; P13-K: phosphatidylinositol 13-kinase; p38 MAPK: p28 mitogen-activated protein kinase; PDGF: platelet-derived growth factor; VCAM-1: vascular cell adhesion molecule 1.

16.2.5.4 Antioxidant Activity

The antioxidant and anticoagulant properties of wine may have a positive benefit in slowing the effects of age-related macular degeneration (AMD) that causes vision to decline as people age (Obisesan et al. 1998). An American study from the late 1990s showed that vision of moderate wine drinkers suffered less macular degeneration than nondrinkers. It was found that 4% of wine drinkers had AMD compared with 9% of people who drank no alcohol at all. Drinking wine was associated with decreased risk of AMD as shown below. The risk was decreased by 34% among those drinking wine, by 34% for those drinking beer and wine, and by 26% for those drinking wine and liquor (Simonetti et al. 1997, Obisesan et al. 1998).

Phenolic compounds in red grape wine have been shown to inhibit *in vitro* oxidation of human low-density lipoprotein (Kinsella et al. 1993, Leake 1998, Nigdikar et al. 1998, Kanner and Lapidot 2001). The antioxidant activity in one glass of red wine (150 mL) is equivalent to that found in: 12 glasses of white wine; 2 cups of tea; 5 apples; 5 (100 g) portions of onion; 3.5 glasses of black currant juice; 500 mL of beer; 7 glasses of orange juice; or 20 glasses of apple juice (Halpern 2008).

Fruits and berries contain a wide range of flavonoids and other phenolic compounds that possess antioxidant activity (Kahkonen et al. 1999). Oxygen radical absorbance capacity (ORAC) values of some fruits have been compiled in Table 16.5, which clearly shows that compared to red grapes, fruits like black and blue berries, choke berries, cranberries, sweet cherries, black and red currants, elderberries, raspberries, and strawberries show much higher ORAC activity and total phenolics. ORAC values are reported for hydrophilic-ORAC (H-ORAC), lipophilic-ORAC (L-ORAC), total-ORAC, and total phenolics (TP). H-ORAC, L-ORAC, and total-ORAC are reported in μmol of Trolox Equivalents per 100 g (μmol TE/100 g), while TP is reported in mg gallic acid equivalents per 100 g (mg GAE/100 g). The antioxidant activity of berries and the presence of a wide range of flavonoids have made berries an important source of nongrape wines (Joshi et al. 1999).

Antioxidant functions are associated with lowered DNA damage, diminished lipid peroxidation on inhibited malignant transformation, in vitro, further they are associated epidemiologically with lowered incidence of certain types of cancer and degenerative diseases such as ischemia heart disease and cataracts. Thus, along with total phenolic content, actual measurement of antioxidant activities can serve as a good yardstick for the assessment of the therapeutic values of fruit and berry wines (Rai et al. 2012).

Antioxidant potential can be measured by different assay systems like methyl linoleate (MeLo) oxidation, ferric reducing ability of plasma (FRAP) assay (Benzie and Strain 1996), and ORAC assay. Heinonen et al. (1998) compared antioxidant activity of different wines by MeLo oxidation method and showed that wine made of mixtures of blackcurrant and crowberries or bilberries were superior to red wines and equally active as α tocopherol in inhibiting hydroperoxide formation (Teixeira et al. 2013).

In another study total antioxidant capacity (TAC), expressed as ascorbic acid equivalents (AAE) in some fruit wines was determined using FRAP assay (Benzei and Strain 1996, Rupasinghe and Clegg 2007). The results of the study showed that the antioxidant activity of elderberry, blueberry, and blackcurrant were a little less than that of the control red wine. With respect to fruit wines especially berry wines, Heinonen et al. (1998) found that all the wines studied possess significant antioxidant activity but there was no strict correlation between the content of phenolic components and antioxidant activity. However, other workers have reported a strict positive correlation between polyphenols content and antioxidant effect (Abu-Amsha et al. 1996, Pinhero

Table 16.5 Oxygen Radical Absorbance Capacity (ORAC) of Selected Fruits

Fruits	*H-ORAC*	*L-ORAC*	*Total Phenolics*
	(μmol TE/100 g)	*(μmol TE/100 g)*	*(mg GAE/100 g)*
Apricot	1108	32	79
Blackberries	5245	103	660
Blueberries	6520	36	531
Cherries (sweet)	3348	17	339
Chokeberries	15,820	242	2010
Cranberries	9382	202	718
Black currants	10,060	84	1330
Red currants	3260	127	540
Elderberries	14,500	197	1950
Red grapes	1260	–	177
Orange	1785	34	337
Pear	2941	–	168
Plum	6241	17	367
Raspberries	4745	138	502
Strawberries	3541	36	368
Bananas	813	66	230
Mango	988	14	266
Peach	1781	50	148

Source: From Bhagwat, S., D. B. Haytowitz, and J. M. Holden. 2007. American Institute for Cancer Research Launch Conference, November 1–2, Washington, DC.

Note: H-ORAC = Hydrophilic-oxygen radical absorbance capacity; L-ORAC = lipophilic-oxygen radical absorbance capacity.

and Paliyath 2001, Rupasinghe and Clegg 2007). The contradictory results can be attributed to difference in evaluating the antioxidant function. Many fruits and berries contain significant amounts of anthocyanins compared to other flavonoids, markedly less flavan-3-ols and generally less hydroxycinnamic acids than grapes. According to Singleton (1972) anthocyanins respond poorly in the Folin-Ciocalteau assay, their response being 0.40 compared to the 1.00 and 0.99 responses of gallic acid and catechin, respectively. Therefore, the total phenolic content, that is, the reducing capacity of berry and fruit wines, does not accurately respond to the true antioxidant nature of their phenolic constituents. Grape wines, on the other hand, are especially rich in gallic acid and catechin. Moreover, the lack of correlation between the total phenolic content and the antioxidant activity of berry and fruit wines may also be explained in part by the wide range of raw materials differing significantly in their composition of phenolic compounds (Heinonen et al. 1998). Irrespective of the contradictory results, the presence of phenolics and the antioxidant capacity of fruit wines cannot be doubted. Since, each phenolic group differs with regard to its own antioxidant potency; these differences may result in variation in the antioxidant capacity of each wine (Gargi et al. 2009).

16.2.5.5 Wine Prevents Tooth Decay

Red wine, even nonalcoholic red wine, hardens the enamel to prevent tooth decay. Hardened enamel is more resistant to *Streptococcus mutans*, which is responsible for tooth decay. The polyphenols in red wine can also prevent gum disease, and even help to treat it by reducing inflammation in the gums (Yanagida et al. 2000).

16.2.5.6 Anticarcinogenic Activity

Many plant polyphenolic compounds have been shown to have cancer-preventing activities in laboratory studies (Lambert et al. 2005). For example, tea and tea preparations have been shown to inhibit tumorigenesis in a variety of animal models of carcinogenesis, involving organ sites such as the skin, lungs, oral cavity, esophagus, stomach, liver, pancreas, small intestine, colon, and prostate (Hertog et al. 1996). Several phenolics can limit or prevent cancer development through a diversity of effects, such as DNA repair, carcinogen detoxification, enhanced apoptosis (programmed cell death), and disrupted cell division (Hou 2003, Aggarwal et al. 2004). Wine has some interesting anticancer properties (Dahlaw et al. 2011). Red wine/extract may be a chemopreventive diet supplement in postmenopausal women with high risk of breast cancer; red wine was shown to be much more effective than white wine in suppression of aromatase (Mgbonyebi et al. 1998, Bertelli et al. 1999, Eng et al. 2002); this was demonstrated in different cell models, and in a model of transgenic mouse in which aromatase is overexpressed in the mammary tissue (Eng et al. 2001). Wine is also active versus other cancers or malignancies, for example, oral squamous carcinoma cell growth and proliferation (El Attar and Virji 1999). Data from several prospective studies confirmed that intake of (red) wine was associated with a reduced risk of lung cancer (Prescott et al. 1999, Ruano-Ravina et al. 2004). In contrast, increased consumption tends to increase the risk of certain cancers (Ebeler and Weber 1996). Quercetin has shown potent anticancer activity. Quercitin has been shown to inhibit the growth of cells derived from human and animal cancers, such as leukemia and Ehrlich ascites tumors, the estrogen receptor-positive breast carcinoma (MCF-7), squamous cell carcinoma of head and neck origin, gastric cancer and colon cancer, as well as human leukemia HL-60 cell in culture. Vang (2011) reported resveratrol to be active in normalizing HL-60 cells in culture back into normal cells. Quercetin has antiproliferative activity against breast and stomach cancer primary cultures.

Apoptosis, or programmed cell death, is an important physiological process in normal development (Subbaramaiah 1998, Elmore 2007) and induction of apoptosis is a highly desirable mode as a therapeutic strategy for cancer control (Thomasson et al. 1995, Bhouri et al. 2012). The major challenge in treating cancer is that many tumor cells carry mutations in key apoptotic genes such as p53, BCL family protein, or those affecting caspase signaling (Cregan et al. 2004).

16.2.6 Role of Alcohol in Wine

Excessive alcohol consumption, both acute and chronic, can have devastating effects on physical and mental wellbeing (Renaud et al. 2004). Alcohol is not necessary to have the catechins and other phenolics absorbed: dealcoholized wine is just as active as alcohol-rich wine (Donovan et al. 1999). Acute ingestion of red wine without alcohol led to higher flow-mediated dilation than ingestion of regular red wine in patients with coronary artery disease. The acute effect of red wine on endothelial function is different than its long-term effect, and should be attributed to constituents other than alcohol (Whelan et al. 2004). Low doses of alcohol (<10 g/day in a male Caucasian healthy adult) may not affect arterial blood pressure, higher doses do affect it and wipe out (Saunders 1987, Beevers and Maheswaran 1988, Fuchs 2005) any cardiovascular benefit of wine polyphenols.

16.2.6.1 Physiological Actions

One of the first physiological effects of alcohol consumption is a suppression of higher brain function; it quickly induces drowsiness (Stone 1980, Gurr 1996). This probably explains why taking a small amount of wine (90–180 mL) before bed often helps people, notably the elderly, suffering from insomnia (Kastenbaum 1982). Half a glass of wine provides the benefits of sleep induction, without causing agitation and sleep apnea—often associated with greater alcohol consumption. The effect on sleep may arise from alcohol facilitating the transmission of inhibitory γ-amino butyric acid (GABA), while suppressing the action of excitatory glutamate receptors (Thun et al. 1997, Haddad 2004). Another effect on brain function results from a reduction in hormonal secretion—notably vasopressin. As a consequence, urine production increases, producing the diuretic effect frequently associated with alcohol consumption.

To cash in on these benefits, one must drink wine with meals (Trevisan et al. 2001). Then, wine "works": if every North American drank 2 glasses of wine each day, cardiovascular disease, which accounts for almost 50% of deaths in this population, would be cut by 40%, and $40 billion could be saved annually (Goldberg 1995). Right from ancient times the medicinal and nutritional value of wine has been understood. Many of the mechanisms of action are yet to be understood (Takkouche et al. 2002). This has led to the development of a number of wines from various countries with varied process of cultivation, maceration, yeast used for fermentation, and aging processes. Further, scientific interest to study the lesser known regional wines from fruits and other berries has intensified.

16.3 Conclusion

Even though wine consists of less than 2% organic acids, phenolics, and mineral salts; they have a dramatic influence on sensory quality, and on the overall health of consumers. Humans ingest over 1 g/day of these types of polyphenolics by consuming various food products. But most of them are in the bound form (complex polyphenolics) and are not available to the biological systems. Fermentation is one of the modes to make them available. The presence of yeast and bacteria or other fungal organisms in wine has a definite impact on wine quality and flavor, and directly influences the metabolism of phenolics in wine. Many of the simpler phenolics produced during fermentation, along with the alcohols present in wine products, are associated with the beneficial effects of wine consumption on human health.

Atherosclerosis and heart disease are now associated with 50% of all mortality in the world today. Wine has been identified from ancient times to have a profound effect on the incidence of atherosclerosis and coronary heart disease in small mammals as well as in human studies.

In terms of the antioxidant phenolics present in wines, higher levels occur in red wines. Resveratrol is also present, especially in red wines but in much lower concentrations than others such as epicatechin. Each of these phenolics is at least 10–20 times more effective than vitamin E in protecting low-density lipoproteins against oxidation, and preventing the buildup of damaging cholesterol in arteries. Wine from ancient times has been associated with man in many forms, as a drink for relaxation, as a religious drink, and as an alcoholic drink. Only in recent times has it been recognized as a therapeutic drink in small and moderate quantities.

References

Abu-Amsha, R., K. D. Croft, I. B. Puddey, J. M. Proudfoot, and L. J. Beilin. 1996. Phenolic content of various beverages determines the extent of inhibition of human serum and low- density lipoprotein oxidation in vitro: Identification and mechanism of action of some cinnamic acid derivatives from red wine. *Clinical Science* 91: 449–458.

Adlercreutz, H. and W. Mazur. 1997. Phyto-oestrogens and Western diseases. *Annals of Medicine* 29: 95–120.

Aggarwal, B. B., A. Bhardwaj, R. S. Aggarwal, N. P. Seeram, and Y. Takada. 2004. Role of resveratrol in prevention and therapy of cancer: Preclinical and clinical studies. *Anticancer Research* 24(5A): 2783–2840.

Anu-Appaiah, K. A. 2010. *All about Fruit Wines*. Indian Grape processing Board, Ministry of Food Processing Industries (MOFPI), New Delhi.

Arts, I. C., B. van de Putte, and P. C. Hollman. 2000a. Catechin contents of foods commonly consumed in The Netherlands. Fruits, vegetables, staple foods, and processed foods. *Journal of Agriculture Food Chemistry* 48(5): 1746–1751.

Arts, I. C., B. van de Putte, and P. C. Hollman. 2000b. Catechin contents of foods commonly consumed in The Netherlands. Tea, wine, fruit juices, and chocolate milk. *Journal of Agriculture Food Chemistry* 48(5): 1752–1757.

Balasundram, N., K. Sundram, and S. Samman. 2006. Phenolic compounds in plants and agri-industrial by-products: Antioxidant activity, occurrence, and potential uses. *Food Chemistry* 99: 191–203.

Beevers, D. G. and R. Maheswaran. 1988. Does alcohol cause hypertension or pseudo-hypertension. *Proceedings of Nutritional Society* 47: 111–114.

Benzie, I. F. F. and J. J. Strain. 1996. The ferric reducing ability of plasma (FRAP) as a measure of antioxidant power: The FRAP assay. *Analytical Biochemistry* 239: 70–76.

Bertelli, A., A. A. E. Bertelli, A. Gozzini, and L. Giovannini. 1998. Plasma and tissue resveratrol concentrations and pharmacological activity. *Drugs Experimental and Clinical Research* 24: 133–138.

Bertelli, A. A., F. Ferrara, and G. Diana. 1999. Resveratrol, a natural stilbene in grapes and wine and fruit –honey wines. *Natural Product Radiance* 8(4): 345–355.

Bhagat, M. and K. A. Anu-Appaiah. 2011. Prospects of wine industry in India. *Indian Food Industry* 30(1): 20–26.

Bhagwat, S., D. B. Haytowitz, and J. M. Holden. 2007. American Institute for Cancer Research Launch Conference, November 1–2, Washington, DC.

Bhat, K. P. and J. M. Pezzuto. 2002. Cancer chemopreventive activity of resveratrol. *Annals of the New York Academy of Sciences* 957: 210–229.

Bhouri, W., J. Boubaker, I. Skandrani, K. Ghedira and L. C. Ghedira. 2012. Investigation of the apoptotic way induced by digallic acid in human lymphoblastoid TK6 cells. *Cancer Cell International*, 12: 26–33.

Caimi, G., C. Carollo, and R. Lo Presti. 2003. Diabetes mellitus: Oxidative stress and wine. *Current Medical Research and Opinion* 19: 581–586.

Camargo, C. A., M. J. Jr. Stampfer, R. J. Glynn, J. M. Gaziano, J. E. Manson, S. Z. Goldhaber, and C. H. Hennekens. 1997. Prospective study of moderate alcohol consumption and risk of peripheral arterial disease in US male physicians. *Circulation* 95: 577–580.

Carollo, C., R. Presti, and G. Caimi. 2007. Wine, diet, and arterial hypertension. *Angiology* 58: 92–96.

Cheng, K., Y. Kondo, and Suzuki. 1999. Inhibitory effects of total flavones of *Hippophae rhamnoides* L. on thrombosis from seed and pulp oils on atopic dermatitis. *Journal of Nutritional Biochemistry* 10(11): 622–630.

Clifford, M. N. 1999. Chlorogenic acids and other cinnamates—nature, occurrence and dietary burden. *Journal of Science and Food Agriculture* 79: 362–372.

Clifford, M. N. 2000. Anthocyanins—Nature, occurrence and dietary burden. *Journal of the Science of Food and Agriculture* 80(7): 1063–1072.

Clifford, M. N. and A. Scalbert. 2000. Ellagitannins—Occurrence in food, bioavailability and cancer prevention. *Journal Food Science Agriculture* 80: 1118–1125.

Cregan, S. P., V. L. Dawsonand, and R. S. Slack. 2004. Role of AIF in caspase-dependent and caspase-independent cell death. *Oncogene* 23: 2785–2796.

Corder, R., W. Mullen, N. Q. Khan, S. C. Marks, E. G. Wood, M. J. Carrier, and A. Crozier. 2006. Oenology: Red wine procyanidins and vascular health. *Nature* 444: 566.

Coward, L., M. Smith, M. Kirk, and S. Barnes. 1998. Chemical modification of isoflavones in soyfoods during cooking and processing. *American Journal of Clinical Nutrition* 68(Supplementary): 1486S–1491S.

D'Archivio, M., C. Filesi, R. Di Benedetto, R. Gargiulo, C. Giovannini, and R. Masella, 2007. Polyphenols, dietary sources and bioavailability. *Ann Ist super sAnItà* 43(4): 348–361.

de la Torre, R., M. I. Covas, M. A. Pujadas, M. Fito, and M. Farre. 2006. Is dopamine behind the health benefits of red wine? *European Journal of Nutrition* 45: 307–310.

DeSanctis, F., M. G. Silvestrini, R. Luneia, R. Botondi, A. Bellincontro, and F. Mencarelli. 2012. Postharvest dehydration of wine white grapes to increase genistein, daidzein and the main carotenoids. *Food Chemistry* 135(3): 1619–1625.

de Lorgeril, M., P. Salen, J. L. Martin, F. Boucher, and J. de Leiris. 2008. Interactions of wine drinking with omega-3 fatty acids in patients with coronary heart disease: A fish-like effect of moderate wine drinking. *American Heart Journal* 155: 175–181.

Dahlaw, I. H., N. Jordan-Mahy, M. R. Clench, and C. L. LeMaitre. 2011. Bioactive actions of pomegranate fruit extracts on leukemia cell lines in vitro hold promise for new therapeutic agents for leukemia. *Nutrition and Cancer* 1: 11–15.

Doll, R., R. Peto, J. Boreham, and I. Sutherland. 2005. Mortality in relation to alcohol consumption: A prospective study among male British doctors. *International Journal of Epidemiology* 34: 199–204.

Donovan, J. L., J. R. Bell, and S. Kasim-Karakas. 1999. Catechin is present as metabolites in human plasma after consumption of red wine. *Journal of Nutrition* 129: 1662–1668.

Ebeler, S. E. and M. A. Weber. 1996. Wine and cancer. In: *Wine in Context: Nutrition, Physiology, Policy, Proceedings of the Symposium on Wine and Health,* Waterhouse A. L. and J. M. Rantz, eds. American Society for Enology and Viticulture, C. A. Davis, 16–18.

El Attar, T. M. and A. S. Virji. 1999. Modulating effect of Resveratrol and quercetin on oral cancer growth and proliferation. *Anticancer Drugs* 10: 187–193.

Elmore, S. 2007. Apoptosis: A review of programmed cell death. *Toxicologic Pathology* 35(4): 495–516.

Eng, E. T., D. Williams, U. Mandava, N. Kirma, R. R. Tekmal, and S. Chen. 2001. Suppression of aromatase (estrogen synthetase) by red wine phytochemicals. *Breast Cancer Research Treatment.* 67: 133–146.

Eng, E. T., D. Williams, and U. Mandava. 2002. Anti-aromatase chemicals in red wine. *Annals of the New York Academy and Sciences* 963: 239–246.

Es-Safi, N. E., V. Cheynier, and M. Moutounet. 2002. Interactions between cyanidin 3-O-glucoside and furfural derivatives and their impact on food color changes. *Journal of Agriculture Food Chemistry* 50(20): 5586–5595.

Feher, J., G. Lengyel, and A. Lugasi. 2007. The cultural history of wine—theoretical background to wine therapy. *Central European Journal of Medicine* 2(4): 379–391.

Fuchs, F. D. 2005. Vascular effects of alcoholic beverages: Is it only alcohol that matters. *Hypertension* 45: 851–852.

Ganry, O., C. Baudoin, and P. Fardellone. 2000. Effect of alcohol intake on bone mineral density. *American Journal of Epidemiology* 151(8): 773–780.

Gao, C. and G. H. Fleet. 1988. The effects of temperature and pH on the ethanol tolerance of the wine yeasts, *Saccharomyces cerevisiae, Candida stellata* and *Kloeckera apiculata*. *Journal of Applied Bacteriology* 65: 405–410.

Gargi, D., N. Bharti, and G. Akanksha. 2009. Can fruit wines be considered as functional food?—An overview. *Natural Product Radiance* 8(4): 314–322.

Gaziano, J. M., C. H. Hennekens, S. L. Godfried, H. D. Sesso, R. J. Glynn, J. L. Breslow, and J. E. Buring. 1999. Type of alcoholic beverage and risk of myocardial infarction. *American Journal of Cardiology* 83: 52–57.

German, J. B. and R. L. Walzem. 2000. The health benefits of wine. *Annual Review of Nutrition* 20: 561–593.

Gindreau, E., E. Wailing, and A. Lonvaud-Funnel. 2001. Direct polymerase chain reaction detection of ropy *Pediococcus damnosus* strains in wine. *Journal of Applied Microbiology* 90: 535–542.

Goldberg, D. 1995. Does wine work? *Clinical Chemistry* 41: 14–16.

Gupta, J. K. and R. Sharma. 2009. Production technology and quality characteristics of mead and fruit–honey wines. *Natural Product Radiance* 8(4): 345–355.

Gupta, N. and S. Trivedi. 2009. Orange: Research analysis for wine studies. *International Journal of Biotechnology Applications* 1(2): 10–15.

Gurr, M. 1996. *Alcohol: Health Issues Related to Alcohol Consumption*. 2nd ed. ILSI Press: Washington, DC.

Gutiérrez, I. H., E. S. Lorenzo, and A.V. Espinosa. 2005. Phenolic composition and magnitude of copigmentation in young and shortly aged red wines made from the cultivars, Cabernet Sauvignon, Cencibel, and Syrah. *Food Chemistry* 92(2): 269–283.

Gattuso, G., D. Barreca, C. Gargiulli, U. Leuzzi, and C. Caristi. 2007. Flavonoid composition of citrus juices. *Molecules* 12: 1641–1673.

Haddad, J. J. 2004. Alcoholism and neuro-immune–endocrine interactions: Physiochemical aspects. *Biochemistry Biophysics Research Communication* 323: 361–371.

Haimoto, H., T. Sasakabe, H. Umegaki, and K. Wakai. 2009. Acute metabolic responses to a high-carbohydrate meal in outpatients with type 2 diabetes treated with a low-carbohydrate diet: A crossover meal tolerance study. *Nutrition and Metabolism* 6: 52.

Halpern, G. M. 2008. A celebration of wine: Wine is medicine. *Inflammopharmacology* 16: 240–244.

Halpern, G. M., M. E. Gershwin, and C. Ough. 1985. The effect of white wine upon pulmonary function of asthmatic subjects. *Annals of Allergy* 55: 686–690.

He, F., Q. Pan, Y., Shi, and C. Duan. 2008. Chemical synthesis of proanthocyanidins *in vitro* and their reactions in aging wines. *Molecules* 13: 3007–3032.

He, F., L. N. Mu, L. Q. Pan, J. Wang, M. J. Reeves, and C. Duan. 2012. Anthocyanins and their variation in red wines I. Monomeric anthocyanins and their color expression. *Molecules* 17(2): 1571–1601.

Heinonen, M., P. J. Lehtonen, and A. I. Hopia. 1998. Antioxidant activity of berry and fruit wines and liquors. *Journal of Agriculture Food Chemistry* 46: 25–31.

Henick-Kling, T. 1993. Malolactic fermentation. In: *Wine Microbiology and Biotechnology*, G. H. Fleet, ed. Harwood Academic, 289–326, Chur, Switzerland.

Hertog, M. G. L., P. C. H. Hollman, and B. Van de Putte. 1993. Content of potentially anticarcinogenic flavonoids of tea infusions, wines and fruit juices. *Journal of Agriculture Food Chemistry* 41: 1242–1246.

Hertog, M. G. L. and P. C. H. Hollman. 1996. Potential health effects of the dietary flavonol quercetin. *European Journal of Clinical Nutrition* 50: 63–71.

Holden, J. M., S. A. Bhagwat and K. Y. Patterson. 2002. Development of a multi-nutrient data quality evaluation system. *Journal of Food Composition and Analysis* 15(4):339–348.

Hoidrup, S., M. Gronbaek, and A. Gottschau. 1999. Alcohol intake, beverage preference, and risk of hip fracture in men and women, Copenhagen Centre for Prospective Population Studies. *American Journal of Epidemiology* 149: 993–1001.

Hou, D. X. 2003. Potential mechanism of cancer chemoprevention by anthocyanins. *Current Molecular Medicine* 3: 149–159.

Jackson R. S. 2008. *Wine Science: Principles and Applications*. 3rd Edition. Academic Press, 686–706, California.

Jeong, J., H. Junga, S. Leea, H. Leea, K. T. Hwanga, and T. Kimb. 2010. Anti-oxidant, anti-proliferative and anti-inflammatory activities of the extracts from black raspberry fruits and wine. *Food Chemistry* 123: 338–344

Jimenez, J. P., J. Serrano, M. Tabernero, S. Arranz, M. E. Diaz-Rubio, L. Garcia-Diz, I. Goni, and F. Saura-Calixto. 2008. Effects of grape antioxidant dietary fiber in cardiovascular disease risk factors. *Nutrition* 24: 646–653.

Joshi, V. K., D. K. Sandhu, and N. S. Thakur. 1999. Fruit based alcoholic beverages, In: *Biotechnology: Food Fermentation (Microbiology, Biochemistry and Technology)*. Vol. 2, Joshi V. K. and Pandey Ashok, ed. Educational Publishers & Distributors, 647–744, New Delhi.

Kahkonen, M. P., A. I. Hopia, H. J. Vuorela, J. Rauha, K. Pihlaja, T. S. Kujala, and M. Heinonen. 1999. Antioxidant activity of plant extracts containing phenolic compounds. *Journal of Agriculture Food Chemistry* 47: 3954–3962.

Kanner, J. and T. Lapidot. 2001. The stomach as a bioreactor: Dietary lipid peroxidation in the gastric fluid and the effects of plant derived antioxidants. *Free Radical Biology and Medicine* 31: 1388–1395.

Kastenbaum, R. 1982. Wine and the elderly person. In: *Proceedings of the Wine, Health and Society. A Symposium*, GRT Books, 87–95, Oakland, CA.

Keli, S. O., M. G. L. Hertog, E. J. M. Feskens, and D. Kromhout. 1994. Dietary flavonoids, antioxidant vitamins and the incidence of stroke: The Zutphen Study. *Archives of Internal Medicine* 154: 637–642.

Keil, U., A. Liese, B. Filipiak, J. D. Swales, and D. E. Grobbee. 1998. Alcohol, blood pressure and hypertension. *Novartis Found Symposium* 216: 125–144.

Kinsella, J. E., E. Frankel, J. B. German, and J. Kanner. 1993. Possible mechanisms for the protective role of antioxidants in wine and plant foods. *Food Technology* 47: 85–89.

Klatsky, A. L., G. D. Friedman, and A. B. Siegelaub. 1974. Alcohol consumption before myocardial infarction. Results from the KaiserPermanente epidemiologic study of myocardial infarction. *Annals of Internal Medicine* 81: 294–301.

Klatsky, A. L., G. D. Friedman, M. A. Armstrong, and H. Kipp. 2003. Wine, liquor, beer, and mortality. *American Journal of Epidemiology* 15: 585–595.

Knekt, P., R. Jarvinen, A. Reunanen, and J. Maatela. 1996. Flavonoid intake and coronary mortality in Finland: A cohort study. *British Medical Journal* 312: 478–481.

Knudsen, N., I. Bülow, P. Laurberg, H. Perrild, L. Ovesen, and T. Jorgensen. 2001. Alcohol consumption is associated with reduced prevalence of goitre and solitary thyroid nodules. *Clinical Endocrinology* 55: 41–46.

Koppes, L. L. J., J. M. Dekker, H. F. J. Hendriks, L. M. Bouter, and R. J. Heine. 2005. Moderate alcohol consumption lowers the risk of type 2 diabetes. *Diabetes Care* 28: 719–725.

Lambert, J. D., J. Hong, G. Y. Yang, J. Liao, and C. S. Yang. 2005. Inhibition of carcinogenesis by polyphenols: Evidence from laboratory investigations. *American Journal of Clinical Nutrition* 81(1 Suppl): 284S–291S.

Leake, D. S. 1998. Effects of flavonoids on the oxidation of low-density lipoproteins. In: *Flavonoids in Health and Disease*. Rice-Evans, C. A. and L. Packer, eds. 253–276, Dekker: New York.

Lehtonen, P. J., M. M. Rokka, A. I. Hopia, and I. M. Heinonen. 1999. HPLC determination of phenolic compounds in berry and fruit wines and liquers. *Wein- Wissenschaft Viticulture and Enological Sciences* 54: 33–38.

Luchsinger, J. A., M. X. Tang, M. Siddiqui, S. Shea, and R. Mayeux. 2004. Alcohol intake and risk of dementia. *Journal of American Geriatric Society* 52: 540–546.

MacRae, W. D., G. H. N. Towers. 1984. Biological activities of lignans. *Phytochemistry* 23(6): 1207–1220.

MacNeil, K. 2001. *The Wine Bible*. 170, Workman Publishing, NY.

Manach, C. and A. Scalbert, C. Morand, C. Remesy, and L. Jimenez. 2004. Polyphenols: Food sources and bioavailability. *American Journal of Clinical Nutrition* 79(5): 727–747.

Manach, C., G. Williamson, and C. Morand. 2005. Bioavailability and bioefficacy of polyphenols in humans. I. Review of 97 bioavailability studies. *American Journal of Clinical Nutrition* 81(1 Suppl): 230S–242S.

Marambaud, P., H. Zhao, and P. Davies. 2005. Resveratrol promotes clearance of Alzheimer's plasma after consumption of red wine. *Journal of Nutrition* 129: 1662–1668.

Merken, H. M. and G. R. Beecher. 2000. Measurement of food flavonoids by high performance liquid chromatography; a review. *Journal of Agriculture Food Chemistry* 48(3): 577–599.

Mgbonyebi, O. P., J. Russo, and I. H. Russo. 1998. Antiproliferative effect of synthetic resveratrol on human breast epithelial cells. *International Journal of Oncology* 12: 865–869.

Negi, P. S., G. K. Jayaprakasha, and B. S. Jena. 2008. Antibacterial activity of the extracts from the fruit rinds of *Garcinia cowa* and *Garcinia pedunculata* against food borne pathogens and spoilage bacteria. *LWT-Food Science and Technology* 41: 1857–1861.

Negi, P. S., G. K. Jayaprakasha, and B. S. Jena. 2010. Evaluation of antioxidant and antimutagenic activities of the extracts from the rinds of *Garcinia cowa*. *International Journal of Food Properties* 13: 1256–1265.

Nigdikar, S. V., N. R. Williams, B. A. Griffin, and A. N. Howard. 1998. Consumption of red wine polyphenols reduces the susceptibility of low-density lipoproteins to oxidation *in vivo*. *American Journal of Clinical Nutrition* 68: 258–265.

Obisesan, T. O., R. Hirsch, O. Kosoko, L. Carlson, and M. Parrott. 1998. Moderate wine consumption is associated with decreased odds of developing age-related macular degeneration in NHANES-1. *Journal of American Geriatric Society* 46: 1–7.

Orgogozo, J. M., J. F. Dartigues, and S. Lafont. 1997. Wine consumption and dementia in the elderly: A prospective community study in the Bordeaux area. *Review of Neurology (Paris)* 153: 185–192.

Paganga, G., N. Miller, and C. A. Rice-Evans. 1999. The polyphenol content of fruit and vegetables and their antioxidant activities. What does a serving constitute? *Free Radical Research* 30: 153–162.

Paladini, A. C., M. Marder, and H. Viola. 1999. Flavonoids and the CNS: From forgotten factor to potent anxiolytic compounds. *Journal of Pharmaceutical Pharmacology* 51: 519–526.

Palaskaa, I., E. Papathanasioua, and T. C. Theoharides. 2013. Use of polyphenols in periodontal inflammation. *European Journal of Pharmacology* 720: 77–83.

Papamichael, C. M., K. N. Karatzi, T. G. Papaioannou, E. N. Karatzis, P. Katsichti, V. Sideris, N. Zakopoulos, A. Zampelas, and J. P. Lekakis. 2008. Acute combined effects of olive oil and wine on pressure wave reflections: Another beneficial influence of the Mediterranean diet antioxidants? *Journal of Hypertension* 26: 223–229.

Patil, M. M. and K. A. Anu-Appaiah. 2013. Garcinia: Bioactive compounds and health benefit, In: *Functional Food Science*. Martirosyan, D. M. ed. Food Science Publisher, 110–119, Dallas, TX, USA.

Pinhero, R. G. and G. Paliyath. 2001. Antioxidant and calmodulin inhibitory activities of components in fruit wines and its biotechnological implications. *Food Biotechnology* 15(3): 179–192.

Prescott, E., M. Grønbaek, U. Becker, and T. I. Sørensen. 1999. Alcohol intake and the risk of lung cancer: Influence of type of alcoholic beverage. *American Journal of Epidemiology* 149: 463–470.

Rai, A. K., Maya Prakash, and K. A. Anu Appaiah. 2010. Production and evaluation of changes during fermentation of Garcinia (*Garcinia xanthochymus*) wine. *International Journal of Food Science and Technology* 45: 1330–1336.

Rai, A. K., M. Bhagat, and K. A. Anu-Appaiah. 2012. Wine fermentation: Microbial ecology and their influence on biochemical changes during fermentation. In: *Recent Advances in Microbiology* (Vol. 1), S. P. Tiwari, ed. Nova Science Publishers, 421–440, New York.

Rai, A. K. and K. A. Anu-Appaiah. 2014. Application of native yeast from Garcinia (*Garcinia xanthochumus*) for the preparation of fermented beverage: Changes in biochemical and antioxidant properties. *Food Bioscience* 5: 101–107.

Ramadori, G., L. Gautron, T. Fujikawa, R. Claudia, J. Vianna, K. Elmquist, and R. Coppari. 2009. Central administration of resveratrol improves diet-induced diabetes. *Endocrinology* 150: 5326–5333.

Rani, U. M. and K. A. Anu-Appaiah. 2011. *Gluconacetobacter hansenii* UAC09 mediated transformation of polyphenols and pectin of coffee cherry husk extract. *Food Chemistry* 130: 243–247.

Renaud, S. and M. de Lorgeril. 1992. Wine alcohol, platelets and the French paradox for coronary heart disease. *Lancet* 339: 1523–1526.

Renaud, S., D. Lanzmann-Petithory, R. Gueguen, and P. Conard. 2004. Alcohol and mortality from all causes. *Biological Research* 37: 183–187.

Rodrigo, R. and G. Rivera. 2002. Renal damage mediated by oxidative stress: A hypothesis of protective effects of red wine. *Free Radical Biology and Medicine* 33: 409–422.

Rosell, M., U. de Faire, and M. L. Hellenius. 2003. Low prevalence of the metabolic syndrome in wine drinkers—Is it the alcohol beverage or the lifestyle? *European Journal of Clinical Nutrition* 57: 227–234.

Ruano-Ravina, A., A. Figueiras, and J. M. Barros-Dios. 2004. Type of wine and risk of lung cancer: A case–control study in Spain. *Thorax* 59: 981–985.

Rupasinghe, H. P. V. and S. Clegg. 2007. Total antioxidant capacity, total phenolic content, mineral elements and histamine concentrations in wines of different fruit sources. *Journal of Food Composition and Analysis* 20: 133–137.

Santos-Buelga, C. and A. Scalbert. 2000. Proanthocyanidins and tannin-like compounds: Nature, occurrence, dietary intake and effects on nutrition and health. *Journal of the Science of Food and Agriculture* 80(7): 1094–1107.

Satora, P., P. Sroka, and T. Tarko. 2008. The profile of volatile compounds and polyphenols in wines produced from desert varieties of apples. *Food Chemistry* 111: 513–519.

Sartelet, H., S. Serghat, and A. Lobstein. 1996. Flavonoids extracted from fonio millet (*Digitaria exilis*) reveal potent antithyroid properties. *Nutrition* 12(2): 100–106.

Saunders, J. B. 1987. Alcohol: An important cause of hypertension. *British Medical Journal* 294: 1045–1046.

Savaskan, E., G. Olivieri, and F. Meier. 2003. Red wine ingredient resveratrol protects from beta-amyloid neurotoxicity. *Gerontology* 49: 380–383.

Seeram, N. P. 2008. Berry fruits for cancer prevention: Current status, and future prospects. *Journal of Agriculture Food Chemistry* 56(3): 630–635.

Servili, M., B. Sordini, S. Esposto, S. Urbani, G. Veneziani, I. Di Maio, R. Selvaggini, and A. Taticchi. 2014. Biological activities of phenolic compounds of extra virgin olive oil. *Antioxidants* 3: 1–23.

Simonetti, P., P. Pietta, and G. Testolin. 1997. Polyphenol content and total antioxidant potential of selected Italian wines. *Journal of Agriculture Food Chemistry* 45: 1152–1155.

Singleton, V. L. 1972. Effects on red wine quality of removing juice before fermentation to stimulate variation in berry size. *American Journal of Enology and Viticulture* 23: 106–113.

Soleas, G. J., E. P. Diamandis, and D. M. Goldberg. 1997. Wine as a biological fluid: History, production and role in disease prevention. *Journal of Clinical Lab Analysis* 11: 287–313.

Stasiuk, M. and A. Kozubek. 2010.Biological activity of phenolic lipids. *Cellular and Molecular Life Sciences* 67: 841–860.

St. Leger, A. S., A. L. Cochrane, and F. Moore. 1979. Factors associated with cardiac mortality in developed countries with particular reference to the consumption of wine. *Lancet* 12: 1017–1020.

Stoclet, J. C., T. Chataigneau, M. Ndiaye, M. H. Oak, J. E. Bedoui, M. Chataigneau and V. B. Schini-Kerth. 2004. Vascular protection by dietary polyphenols. *European Journal of Pharmacology* 500: 299–313.

Stone, B. M. 1980. Sleep and low doses of alcohol. *Electroencephalogr Clinical Neurophysiology* 48: 706–709.

Su, H. C., L. M. Hung, and J. K. Chen. 2006. Resveratrol, a red wine antioxidant, possesses an insulin-like effect in streptozotocin-induced diabetic rats. *American Journal of Physiology Endocrinology Metabolism* 290: 1339–1346.

Subbaramaiah, K., P. Michaluart, W. J. Chung, and A. J. Dannenberg. 1998. Resveratrol inhibits the expression of cyclooxygenase-2 in human mammary and oral epithelial cells. *Pharmaceutical Biology* 36(Suppl): 35–43.

Takkouche, B., C. Requeira-Mendez, R. Garcia-Closas, A. Figueiras, J. J. Gestal-Otero, and M. A. Hernan. 2002. Intake of wine, beer, and spirits and the risk of clinical common cold. *American Journal of Epidemiology* 155: 853–858.

Teissèdre, P. L., G. Cros, M. Krosniak, K. Portet, J. J. Serrano, and J. C. Cabanis. 1996. Contribution to wine in vanadium dietary intake: Geographical origin has a significant impact on wine vanadium levels. In: *Metal Ions in Biology and Medicine,* P. Collery, ed., John Libbey Eurotext, Vol. 4, 183–185, Paris.

Teixeira, J., A. Gaspar, E. M. Garrido, J. Garrido, and F. Borges. 2013. Hydroxycinnamic acid antioxidants: An electrochemical overview. *BioMedical Research International*: 1–11.

Thomasson, H. R., J. D. Beard, and T. K. Li. 1995. ADH2 gene polymorphism are determinants of alcohol pharmacokinetics. *Alcohol Clinical and Experimental Research* 19: 1494–1499.

Thun, M. J., R. Peto, A. D. Lopez, J. H. Monaco, S. J. Henley, Jr. C. W. Heath, and R. Doll. 1997. Alcohol consumption and mortality among middle-aged and elderly US adults. *New English Journal of Medicine* 337: 1705–1714.

Trevisan, M., E. Schisterman, and A. Menotti. 2001. Drinking pattern and mortality: The Italian Risk Factor and Life Expectancy pooling project. *Annals of Epidemiology* 11: 312–319.

Truelsen, T., M. Gronbaek, P. Schnohr, and G. Boysen. 1998. Intake of beer, wine, and spirits and risk of stroke: The Copenhagen city heart study. *Stroke* 29: 2467–2472.

Vaidya, D. and S. Sharma. 2009. Enzymatic treatment for juice extraction and preparation of preliminary evaluation of kiwifruits wine. *Natural Product Radiance* 8(4): 380–385.

Vang, O. 2011. What is new for an old molecule? Systematic review and recommendations on the use of resveratrol. *Public Library of Science One* 6(6): 19881.

Vuorinen, H., K. Mtt, and R. Trrnen. 2000. Content of the flavonols myricetin, quercetin, and kaempferol in Finnish berry wines. *Journal of Agriculture Food Chemistry* 48(7): 2675–2680.

Wallerath, T., H. Li, U. Godtel-Ambrust, P. M. Schwarz and U. Forstermann. 2005. A blend of polyphenolic compounds explains the stimulatory effect of red wine on human endothelial NO synthase. *Nitric Oxide* 12(2): 97–104.

Weisse, M. E., B. Eberly, and D.A. Person. 1995. Wine as a digestive aid: Comparative antimicrobial effects of bismuth salicylate and red and white wine. *Biomirror Journal* 311: 1657–1660.

Whelan, A. P., W. H. Sutherland, M. P. McCormick, D. J. Yeoman, D. J. de Jong, and M. J. Williams. 2004. Effects of white and red wine on endothelial function in subjects with coronary artery disease. *International Medical Journal* 34: 224–228.

Wolfe, K. L., X. Kang, X. He, M. Dong, Q. Zhang, and R. H. Liu. 2008. Cellular antioxidant activity of common fruits. *Journal Agriculture and Food Chemistry* 56(18): 8418–8426.

Wulf, L. and C. W. Nagel. 1980. Identification and changes of flavonoids in Merlot and Cabernet Sauvignon wines. *Journal of Food Science* 45: 479.

Yanagida, A., T. Kanda, M. Tanabe, F. Matsudaira, and J. G. O. Cordeiro. 2000. Inhibitory effects of apple polyphenols and related compounds on cariogenic factors of mutans Streptococci, *Journal of Agriculture Food Chemistry* 48: 5666–5671.

Yildirim, H. K. 2006. Evaluation of colour parameters and antioxidant activities of fruit wines. *International Journal of Food Science Nutrition* 57(1/2): 47–63.

Chapter 17

Antiallergic Properties of Fermented Foods

Adelene Song Ai Lian, Lionel In Lian Aun, Foo Hooi Ling, and Raha Abdul Rahim

Contents

17.1 Introduction

Allergy is a hypersensitivity disorder resulting from a person's immune system reacting toward a substance called an allergen. The major types of allergy include eczema (atopic dermatitis), food allergy, rhinitis, and asthma. The global prevalence of allergic diseases is increasing steadily with 30%–40% of the world population being affected by one or more allergic conditions (Pawankar et al. 2011). Allergic diseases can be caused by genetic factors as well as environmental factors such as pollution or climate changes. Allergies are most commonly diagnosed via a skin test or a blood test. A skin test involves introducing a series of tiny punctures to a patient's skin and introducing different suspected allergens to the prick sites. Signs of inflammation are then observed. Blood tests involve the measurement of IgE antibody levels in the blood. Current treatments for allergies include medications such as antihistamines, epinephrine, and steroids. Immunotherapy is also available for some forms of allergies. While immunotherapy provides a longer-lasting effect, it is also more expensive than typical pharmacotherapy. Allergies are a socioeconomic burden as antiallergic medication and hospitalization incur high costs. The quality of life is also significantly affected, a scenario most identified with by parents of children with allergic conditions. Apart from physical discomfort, allergies also affect the quality of sleep, social interactions, productivity in school or workplace, emotions, and everyday activities. Allergic disease is one of the most common causes of hospitalization and also of school and work absenteeism (Su et al. 1997).

17.2 Immunology of Allergy

Individuals often develop allergies when exposed to allergens such as pollen, dust mites, latex, insect venom, mold, animals, medications, and various food components (Schmid-Grendelmeier and Crameri 2001, Sicherer and Sampson 2013). The likelihood of allergic reactions occurring in a particular individual but not in others is not completely understood, but at present, is mostly attributed to three main reasons: (1) genetic predisposition factors; (2) environmental predisposition factors; and (3) combination of both genetic and environmental predisposition factors.

Our immune system generally reacts and defends ourselves against various biological and chemical threats through two separate, but interconnected systems. The first line of defense is called the innate immune system which consists of cells and proteins that are always present and ready to act. This system includes components such as mucosal epithelial barriers, natural killer cells, dendritic cells (DC), and phagocytic leukocytes (Janeway et al. 2001a). The second line of defense is termed the adaptive immune system which is a more specialized and potent form of immunity, and include the action of B-cells and T-cells. It is often called into action in circumstances where the innate immune defense is insufficiently effective or has been overcome.

17.2.1 Adaptive Immune Response

Our adaptive immune system is divided into two types of responses: (1) a cell-mediated response which involves the activation of phagocytes, cytotoxic T-lymphocytes (CTL), monocytes, macrophages, and natural killer (NK) cells; or (2) a humoral response which involves the activation of B-lymphocytes and effector granulocytes such as eosinophils, basophils, and mast cells

Table 17.1 Summary of Common Cytokines and Their Immunological Properties in Relation to Th1 and Th2 Responses

Cytokines	*Properties*
Th1 Bias	
Interleukin-2 (IL-2)	Promotes the growth, differentiation, and survival of $CD4^+$ T-helper cells
Interleukin-15 (IL-15)	Induces differentiation of Th0 cells to Th1 cells
Interleukin-12 (IL-12)	Augments NK cell function
Interleukin-18 (IL-18)	Promotes Th1 response by downregulating IL-4
Interferon-gamma (IFN-γ)	Augments IFN-γ signaling
Interferon-alpha (IFN-α)	
Th2 Bias	
Interleukin-4 (IL-4)	Promotes B-lymphocyte isotype switching to IgE
Interleukin-5 (IL-5)	Recruits granulocytes to site of inflammation
Interleukin-6 (IL-6)	Stimulates Th2 response via B-cell maturation
Interleukin-10 (IL-10)	Enhances B-cell survival and proliferation
Interleukin-13 (IL-13)	Inhibits synthesis of Th1 cytokines, particularly IFN-γ
Tumor necrosis alpha (TNF-α)	Recruits granulocytes to site of inflammation
	Recruit eosinophils to allergic inflammatory sites
	Induces Th2 type cytokines and chemokines

Source: From Deo, S. S. et al. 2010. *Lung India* 27(2): 66–71; Ngoc, P. L. et al. 2005. *Current Opinion in Allergy and Clinical Immunology* 5(2): 161–166.

(Alberts et al. 2002). The switching or choice our body makes between these two types of adaptive responses is highly dependent on the array of cross-regulatory cytokines being produced which may either favor a Th1 (cell-mediated) or Th2 (humoral-mediated) phenotypic response. A summary of common cytokines and their immunological properties in relation to Th1 and Th2 responses are listed in Table 17.1.

17.2.2 Immunology of Type-I Hypersensitivity Reactions

Hypersensitivity refers to a phenomenon where the immune system reacts toward intolerable or undesirable physiological conditions. These hypersensitivity reactions are further divided into five types (I–V) depending on their respective mediators and mechanism of action. Among these five types, type-I hypersensitivity is often referred to as immediate hypersensitivity or more commonly known as allergy. Our body can be exposed to nonself foreign substances either through inhalation, ingestion, injection, or direct physical contact routes. Upon exposure, these antigenic allergens which are foreign substances capable of triggering an allergic reaction are ingested via phagocytosis or receptor-mediated endocytosis by antigen-presenting cells (APC). APCs are found throughout our entire body, and include cells such as DC, macrophages, activated endothelial cells, and activated epithelial cells. These APCs then digest and complex ingested allergens to class

II major histocompatibility complex (MHC) molecules, and are presented on their cell surface in a process known as antigen presentation.

Upon antigen presentation, circulating $CD4^+$ T-helper cells harboring T-cell receptors (TCR) on their surface recognize these complexed antigens on APCs, and binds to them (Janeway et al. 2001b). Following this, $CD4^+$ T-helper cells will mature and stimulate the production of various cytokines which may either favor a Th1 or a Th2 response. A Th2 bias response is often the case during type-I hypersensitivity or allergic reactions, while a Th1 bias response is often observed when dealing with foreign pathogens such as bacterial infections, and noncommunicable diseases such as cancer (Romagnani 2006).

During the first exposure to an allergen, an individual is sensitized and produces allergen-specific immunoglobulin E (IgE). IgE is present in very minute amounts in our body, and is one of the five antibody isotypes responsible for triggering very potent inflammatory reactions as observed in most allergic diseases. The overproduction of this IgE then binds to high-affinity IgE receptors known as Fc epsilon RI (FcεRI) on various granulocytes, particularly mast cells which are found mostly in connective tissues, and blood circulating basophils.

When a sensitized individual comes in contact with a similar allergen (also known as second exposure), these allergens will immediately bind to antigenic sites on preformed allergen-specific IgE bound to mast cells and basophils during the first exposure. This causes the cross-linking of two or more IgE molecules which will then trigger the activation of granules within mast cells and basophils to release chemical effectors such as histamine, prostaglandin D_2, leukotriene $B_4/C_4/D_4/E_4$, and heparin into the surrounding tissue and the blood stream (Figure 17.1).

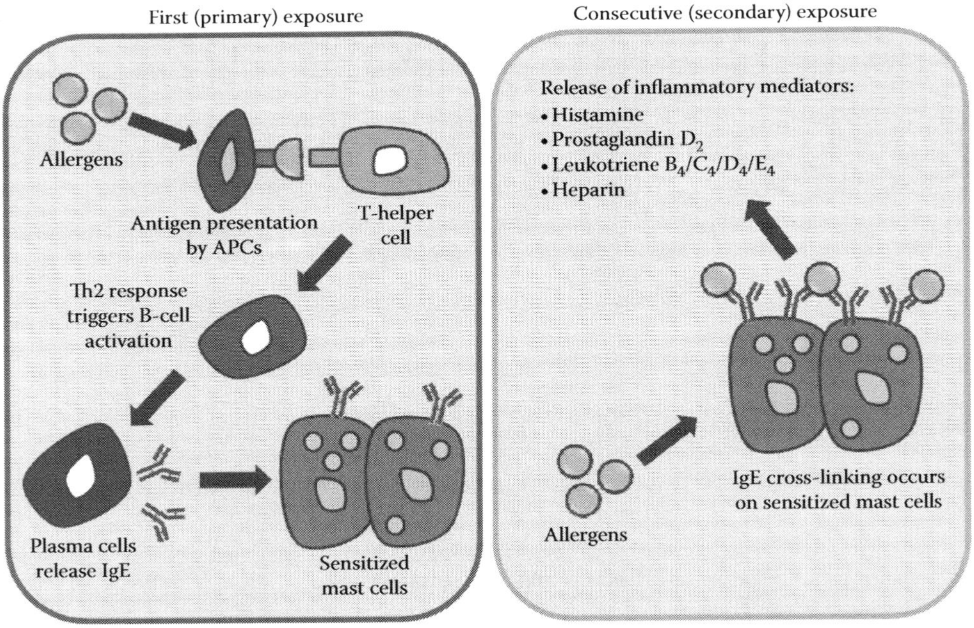

Figure 17.1 Overview of an allergic reaction following primary and secondary exposure toward an allergen.

17.2.3 Effector Molecules in Allergy

Chemical mediators such as histamines will bind to their respective G-coupled protein receptors (GPCR) which can be found on the surface of numerous types of cells throughout the body, resulting in increased capillary and vascular permeability (Kumar et al. 2012). An increase in blood vessel permeability causes fluid to escape into the surrounding tissue, leading to the clinical manifestation of allergic symptoms such as running nose, watery eyes, diarrhea, itchiness, vasodilatation, and bronchoconstriction which causes breathing difficulties and asthma. Prostaglandins on the other hand, are locally acting autocrine and paracrine chemical mediators which also bind to their respective GPCRs on various cell types such as smooth muscle endothelial cells. Increased levels of specific prostaglandins such as prostaglandin D_2, as well as leukotrienes such as leukotriene C_4 and D_4 are associated with inflammatory responses leading to the clinical manifestation of allergy including fever, pain, and constriction of the bronchi which causes difficulty in breathing, anaphylaxis, and even death. Another class of chemical mediators called heparins which are also released by activated mast cells, are naturally occurring, highly sulfated glycosaminoglycans. While heparin is well-known for its role as an anticoagulant, its presence also contributes significantly during allergic reactions. Heparin acts by initiating the production of the hormone bradykinin which in turn causes blood vessels to dilate or enlarge resulting in itchiness, rashes, and swelling manifestations (Oschatz et al. 2011).

17.2.4 Kinetics of Allergy

The immune kinetics of allergic clinical manifestations depends exclusively on the exposure cascade timeline toward the same allergen. During the initial or first exposure where sensitization of mast cells occurs, no clinical reactions are observed, and most individuals go about their daily lives without even realizing that they have been sensitized toward a particular allergen. This step is akin to a preparatory step for consecutive exposures, where sensitized mast cells act like bombs which are armed and ready to detonate at any given time. Development of chronic allergic manifestation occurs during the second or consecutive exposures where presensitized mast cells are activated to release all kinds of effector chemicals as mentioned previously (Nielsen et al. 2002). This typically happens within a short period of time of a few minutes to an hour after coming in contact with a similar allergen, hence the term immediate hypersensitivity.

17.3 Fermented Food with Antiallergic Effects

It has been more than a century since it has been known that the consumption of fermented food can be beneficial to health. However, it was only in the last decade or so that more and more studies have emerged to associate fermented food with the alleviation of allergy. To date, there have been many studies showing the benefits of various types of fermented food against common allergies as listed below.

17.3.1 Yoghurt and Fermented Milk

Studies have shown that long-term consumption of yoghurt in both young adults and senior citizens is associated with a decrease in allergic symptoms especially if given live-culture yoghurt (Van de Water et al. 1999). In infants, on the other hand, it was observed that milk whey supplemented with *Lactobacillus rhamnosus* could alleviate allergy symptoms such as atopic eczema and intestinal inflammation caused by food (cow's milk) allergy (Majamaa and Isolauri 1997). This was contributed by a significant decrease in fecal α_1-antitrypsin and TNF-α concentration. Lactic acid bacteria (LAB) in yoghurt are also known to enhance IFN-γ production, a cytokine which inhibits isotype switching of IgM to IgE (Peng et al. 2007). *Lactobacillus casei*, commonly found in yoghurt drinks like Vitagen (Malaysia Milk, Malaysia) and Yakult (Yakult Honsha, Japan) was also shown to increase IFN-γ production whilst inhibiting IL-4 and IL-5 secretion, resulting in significant suppression in IgE production when supplemented *in vitro* to splenocytes from ovalbumin-primed BALB/c mice (Shida et al. 1998). Heat-killed *Lb. casei* strain Shirota was also found to suppress the IgE and IgG_1 response in the food allergy model, suggesting possible use of this LAB in preventing food allergy (Shida et al. 2002).

In milk fermented with various LAB, it was also shown that LAB confers antiallergic effects on OVA/CFA-immunized mice by increasing the secretion ratio of IFN-γ/IL4 and decreasing the level of OVA-specific IgE (Peng et al. 2007). Nevertheless, immunomodulatory effects were strain specific with *Lactobacillus bulgaricus* Lb giving the best ratios (Peng et al. 2007). In another study, *Enterococcus faecium* T120 isolated from Mongolian fermented milk was shown to confer antiallergic effects on atopic dermatitis NC/NGA mice models (Hayashi et al. 2009). These mice spontaneously developed skin lesions when kept in dirty conventional conditions. Total IgE production was reduced while IL-12 and IFN-γ levels were increased. It was also elucidated that the bacteria strain acted on APCs to increase the production of IL-12, which in-turn increased the levels of IFN-γ. IFN-γ subsequently played a major role in controlling the production of IgE.

Dahi, or Indian yoghurt supplemented with probiotics (*Lactobacillus acidophilus* NCDC14, *Lb. casei* NCDC19 and *Lactococcus lactis biovar diacetylactis* NCDC-60) was shown to almost completely suppress total serum IgE increment in OVA-sensitized mice to basal levels (Jain et al. 2010). IgE levels of milk feeding treatment alone was insignificant compared with control allergic mice, while treatment with *dahi* cultured with *Lc. lactis biovar diacetylactis* alone was also not as effective in suppressing IgE levels, although the latter was still able to suppress IgE levels significantly (Jain et al. 2010). Th-1-specific cytokines (IFN-γ and IL-2) were also increased while Th-2-specific cytokines (IL-4 and IL-6) were decreased, possibly skewing the Th1/Th2 response to Th1 dominance.

17.3.2 Soy Sauce and Other Soybean Products

Soybeans and its products are one of the major allergenic foods worldwide. However, Gly mBD 30 k, a major soybean allergen was shown to be absent in fermented soy sauce products such as *miso*, soy sauce, and *natto* (Kataoka 2005). Soy sauce is a common seasoning used for cooking worldwide, especially in the East and in Southeast Asian countries. Soy sauce is made by the fermentation of soybean paste and roasted grains such as wheat by *Aspergillus oryzae* or *Aspergillus sojae*. It is known as a functional seasoning as it has been reported to have various biological activities including anticarcinogenic, antimicrobial, antioxidative, and antiallergic activities (Kataoka 2005). While grains are a common sauce of allergen, especially wheat, it was shown that the brewing process of Japanese soy sauce to the final product, *shoyu*, degraded all wheat allergens, thus making the final product allergen free (Kobayashi 2005). While the proteins of the raw material are totally degraded by microbial fermentation, the polysaccharide remains in the final product, termed *shoyu* polysaccharide (SPS). Extensive studies have been conducted on the antiallergic effects of SPS including clinical studies. It was shown that the inhibitory effects of SPS on hyaluronidase, implicated in allergic reactions, were as potent as disodium cromoglycate, an antiallergic medication. It was also found to suppress histamine release and had significant suppressive effect on passive cutaneous anaphylaxis reaction in the ears of mice. In double-blind, placebo-controlled clinical studies, SPS were found to improve the quality of life of patients with both perennial and seasonal allergic rhinitis. Symptoms such as sneezing, nasal stuffiness, and hindrance to daily life were reduced significantly. However, contrary to the animal studies, SPS treatment did not affect the levels of histamine, IgE, and Th1/Th2 in serum of patients tested in the clinical studies.

In another study, it was shown that levan, a fructose polymer produced by *Bacillus subtilis* during fermentation of soybean to *natto*, also had antiallergic effects. Levan from *natto* was shown to induce production of IL-12 and TNF-α by macrophages, subsequently significantly reducing the specific IgE and Th2 response in mice (Xu et al. 2005).

Cheonggukjang is another fermented soy bean product used in Korean cuisine, also fermented by *B. subtilis*, but with a longer fermentation time (Lee et al. 2014). *Cheonggukjang* was also shown to have an antiallergic effect against atopic dermatitis in mice, improving common allergic responses such as decreased ear thickness, dermis thickness, auricular lymph node, and infiltrating mast cells although *Cheonggukjang* treatment did not improve IgE levels nor epidermis thickness which remained constant (Lee et al. 2014).

17.3.3 Kefir

Kefir is a type of fermented milk drink popular in Russia, Europe, and Middle Eastern countries although its popularity has become worldwide due to its various benefits to health. *Kefir* is a mixture of live LAB and yeast cultures living on a substrate of dairy products. It produces cauliflower-like *kefir* grains during the fermentation process which have a slimy or gelatinous texture. *Kefir* has been shown to possess antimicrobial, antimycotic, antitumor, and antiinflammatory properties (Lee et al. 2007, Hong et al. 2010). Bulgarian peasants even credited their longevity to the frequent consumption of *kefir* (Gilliland 1990).

In 2006, a study was performed to analyze the antiallergic effects of *kefir* against asthma, based on studies performed on asthma mouse models (Lee et al. 2007). It was observed that *kefir* posed a new therapeutic potential for the treatment of allergic bronchial asthma as it was observed that *kefir* treatment administered orally significantly suppressed airway hyperresponsiveness (AHR) as well as inflammation of the airway. This is achieved by reducing the levels of IgE and Th2 cytokines, IL-4 and IL-13 released in the bronchoalveolar lavage fluid (BALF). Mucus production and tissue eosinophilia were similarly dramatically reduced. This study suggested *kefir* to be an effective treatment for airway inflammation and AHR, even more effective than zileuton, an antiasthmatic commercial drug.

In another study, it was shown that heat-inactivated *Lactobacillus kefiranofaciens* M1 isolated from *kefir* grains also had an antiallergic effect on ovalbumin sensitized BABL/c mice (Hong et al. 2010). This is achieved by inhibition of IgE production and overall skewing of Th1/Th2 balance toward Th1 dominance. *Cd2, Cd3, Cd28, Stat4*, and *Ifnr* were found to be upregulated with *Lb. kefiranofaciens* M1 treatment, while genes of the complement system and its components were downregulated. *Lb. kefiranofaciens* M1 showed promising potential for utilization in functional foods. A follow-up study by the same researchers also showed that heat-killed *Lb. kefirnofaciens* M1 had antiasthmatic effects on OVA-allergic mice by strong inhibition of the Th2 cytokines, proinflammatory cytokines, and Th17 cytokines in splenocytes and bronchoalveolar fluid (Hong et al. 2011), corresponding with earlier results by Lee et al. (2007).

17.3.4 Fermented Red Ginseng

Ginseng is an herbal medicine commonly used in East Asia including Korea, Japan, and China. It is from the family Araliaceae and genus *Panax*, of which strain *Panax ginseng* is from where the name originates. *Ginseng* is commercially categorized into fresh *ginseng*, white *ginseng*, and red *ginseng* (RG). Fresh *ginseng* is less than 4 years old and has not been dried in any way, white *ginseng* is 4–6 years old and has been peeled and dried while RG is older than 6 years and has been steamed (Jung et al. 2011). RG is the most pharmacologically active ginseng among the three, possibly owing to a chemical change in the ginsenosides during the steaming process. The active ingredient in ginseng is thought to be the ginsenosides where approximately 80 different types of ginsenosides have been identified (Lee et al. 2012).

Research has shown that both RG and fermented red *ginseng* (FRG) can increase the antiallergic effects in ovalbumin sensitized BALB/c mice with FRG being more effective (Lee et al. 2012). FRG has 38 and 50 times more Rh1 and Rh2 ginsenosides compared to RG. Rh1 and Rh2 were previously reported to alleviate inflammatory symptoms by reducing IgE levels. Total IgE and IgG_1 were significantly lowered in OVA-sensitized mice when the mice diet was supplemented with RG or FRG at 0.1% and 0.3%. OVA-specific IgE and IgG_1 were also significantly reduced especially in mice supplemented with 0.1% FRG. Concentrations of cytokines IL-5, TNF-α, and IL-4 associated with Th2 response which was elevated in OVA-sensitized mice were significantly reduced when the mice were treated with RG or FRG, with no significant difference between RG and FRG treatment. Furthermore, IFN-γ and IL-2, associated with Th1 response were increased thus shifting the Th2 response to be Th1 dominant. RG and FRG were also shown to decrease intestinal permeability which has been shown to increase with the increase of oral allergen (Lee et al. 2012).

In a clinical trial involving 59 patients experiencing allergic rhinitis problems (nasal congestion, runny nose, nasal itching, and sneezing) for at least 2 years, FRG was found to improve nasal congestion symptoms and improve the quality of life of the patients (Jung et al. 2011). Although total nasal symptom score (TNSS) was insignificant between treated group and placebo group, when symptoms were accessed separately, there was a significant difference in TNSS for nasal congestion over the period of 4 weeks. Furthermore, in the skin prick test, patients treated with FRG were observed to show a reduction in wheals and flares to histamine compared to the placebo group. Total IgE levels were also significantly increased between week 0 and 4 for the placebo group, which was not observed for the FRG-treated group. The study showed that FRG could potentially be used as an alternative treatment for allergic rhinitis without any adverse side effects.

17.3.5 Fermented Pickles

While *Ixeris dentata* (ID), an herbal Japanese medicine used for indigestion, pneumonia, hepatitis, and so on, inhibited systemic anaphylaxis in mice, *kimchi* prepared from fermented ID was more effective than nonfermented ID in inhibiting passive cutaneous anaphylaxis (PCA), scratching behaviors, and degranulation of RBL-2H3 cells, which is frequently used as a mast cell model (Park et al. 2008). Expression of TNF-α and IL-4 protein and IgE-antigen complex activation of NF-κB were also inhibited. Nitric oxide production (produced by macrophage activation in chronic allergic diseases) in RAW264.7 cells was also potently inhibited. In all cases, fermented ID was more potent than nonfermented ID (Park et al. 2008).

Kimchi prepared using *Ixeris sonchifolia* (IS), a bitter plant commonly cultivated and widespread in Korea, also was shown to possess antiallergic effects (Trinh et al. 2010). IS by itself was previously screened among other folk vegetables and was found to exhibit weak antiallergic effects.

However, when fermented to *kimchi*, its antiallergic effects increased. The main constituents in IS are luteolin and chlorogenic acid. In this study and previous studies, luteolin was found to be a potent inhibitor of passive cutaneous anaphylaxis induced by IgE as well as pruritic (itching) reactions. This was contributed by the expression inhibition of proinflammatory and allergic cytokines such as IL-4 and TNF-α, as well as inhibition of the NF-κB transcription factor. It was stipulated that fermentation of IS to *kimchi* by LAB (*Lb. brevis, Leuc. mesenteroides*) transformed glycosides or conjugates to the main constituents in IS, luteolin, and chlorogenic acid, significantly increasing their content and thereby increasing the antiallergic effects (Trinh et al. 2010).

Lactobacilli species isolated from *kimchi* were also found to modulate Th1/Th2 balance by producing a large amount of IL-12 and IFN-γ but less IL-4. Some strains were even more efficient than *Lb. rhamnosus* GG, a well-known reported probiotic with the ability to alleviate atopic dermatitis and food allergy (Won et al. 2011). This supports growing evidence that LAB isolated from plant sources has stronger health-promoting potential than milk-based LAB (Masuda et al. 2010, Won et al. 2011).

In a study by Masuda et al. (2010), 59 strains isolated from Japanese fermented vegetable pickles were screened for the ability to induce IL-12 and IFN-γ in mouse Peyer's patch (PP) cell culture. PP is lymphoid tissues in the small intestine which first encounters ingested foods and plays an important immunoregulatory role toward intestine microbes and food antigens. Of these 59 strains, *Pediococcus pentasaceus* Sn26 was found to be most effective in improving the Th1/Th2 balance and in the inhibition of OVA-specific IgE production and was selected for further testing (Masuda et al. 2010). It was demonstrated that Sn26 was able to induce production of IL-12, which then induced IFN-γ, thus decreasing IL-4 and IgE production. Furthermore, effects of oral administration of Sn26 against allergic diarrhea were examined. Sn26 was found to delay the onset of diarrhea by 2 weeks (control mice showed symptoms of diarrhea after 5 weeks) while also lowering the rate of diarrhea from 80% in control groups to only 35% in Sn26 treated groups at the end of the experiment (Masuda et al. 2010). The immunoregulatory effect of Sn26 is postulated to be due to the strength of the cell structure and cell wall since Sn26 was isolated from fermented vegetable pickles. LAB isolated from a plant source tend to possess more solid cell wall structures due to adaptation to severe growing conditions compared to LAB isolated from a dairy source.

Lactococcus lactis A17 isolated from Taiwanese fermented cabbage was also observed to produce high levels of IFN-γ when tested on human peripheral blood mononuclear cells (hPBMC), even higher than commercial *Lb. rhamnosus* GG (Mei et al. 2013). When tested on OVA-sensitized BALB/c mice, both live and heat killed *Lb. lactis* A17 administered orally showed potential prophylactic and therapeutic treatment of allergic disease suggesting that some intracellular or cell wall component is responsible for the immunomodulatory effect. Both total and specific IgE and specific IgG_1 levels were reduced in A17 treated groups, while OVA-specific IgG_2 levels were increased, showing a Th1 dominance over Th2 response (Mei et al. 2013). Correspondingly, Th1 cytokines were also increased while Th2 cytokines were decreased in A17 treated groups. In addition, mRNA expression of toll-like receptors (TLR-4) and nucleotide binding oligomerization domains (NOD-1 and NOD-2) associated with activation of the Th2 response were also suppressed significantly.

17.3.6 Fermented Fish Oil

Natural fish oil (NFO), rich with Omega-3 polyunsaturated fatty acids such as eicosapentaenoic acid (EPA) and docosahexaenoic acid (DHA), has been reported to have antiallergic effects including reducing sensitization to allergens and alleviation of symptoms of atopic dermatitis, eczema, and asthma (Han et al. 2012b). This is accounted to downregulation of proinflammatory cytokines and upregulation of antiinflammatory cytokines whilst upregulating regulatory T-cells (Tregs). Fermented fish oil (FFO), however, was found to have even greater antiallergic effects when tested on atopic dermatitis mice models (Han et al. 2012b). Itching was found to decrease after treatment with either NFO or FFO when a number of scratching mice was observed in a period of 10 min. However, FFO was more effective than NFO, although not as effective as treatment with commercial hydrocort cream. In addition, FFO and NFO-treated group showed significantly decreased IgE levels and histamine levels analyzed by ELISA, with FFO once again being more effective than NFO although not as effective as hydrocort cream treatment. Morphological observation of the spleen also showed that the NFO and FFO treatment reduced the size of enlarged spleens associated with allergic reactions to the smaller spleens observed in FFO treated groups. Finally, FFO was more effective than NFO in increasing Foxp3 expression and the number of $CD4^{+}CD25^{+}Foxp3^{+}$ Tregs more than twofold. This was postulated due to the chemical changes in FFO after fermentation, including a significant increase of EPA and DHA in FFO compared to NFO (Han et al. 2012b).

Interestingly, external application of fermented olive flounder fish oil (FOF) was also shown to alleviate inflammatory response in atopic dermatitis mouse models (Han et al. 2012a). Induced mice painted with FOF on their ears showed lowered IgE and histamine concentrations in their serum, comparable to the positive control, hydrocort treated group. Also, thymic stromal lymphopoietin (TSLP) produced in skin lesions of acute and chronic AD was inhibited significantly with FOF treatment. In addition, ear thickness and spleen size were reduced and both cytokines IFN-γ and IL-4 and transcription factors T-bet and GATA3 were also inhibited.

17.3.7 Alcoholic Beverages and Their By-Products

Sake is an alcoholic beverage of Japanese origin, typically fermented from rice and therefore sometimes called "rice wine." The main fermenter is *koji* or *Aspergillus oryzae*. However, over the brewing process, other fungus and LAB are also present. There are three types of *sake*, classified based on the method used to prepare the sake; *kimoto*, *yamahai-moto,* and *sokujo-moto* (Japan Sake and Shochu Makers Association 2011). *Kimoto* is the traditional method of *sake* preparation involving a long and tedious process. *Yamahai-moto* takes half the time with less laborious work by adjusting the fermentation conditions while *sokujo-moto* is the modern method of *sake* preparation involving the addition of commercial lactic acid which speeds up the fermentation process.

In a study involving LAB isolated from *kimoto*, it was found that *Leuc. mesenteroides* and *Lb. sakei* were able to suppress IgE-mediated hypersensitivity reaction significantly while *Lb. curvatus* did not (Masuda et al. 2012). Oral administration of the former two were found to reduce ear swelling of mice with hypersensitivity evoked by applying PiCl on the earlobes of the mice significantly. One *Lb. sakei* species LK-117 was most effective and was used for further testing on its ability to suppress development of AD-like skin lesions. Although total plasma IgE levels in Nc/Nga mice after sensitization was not significantly different between those treated with LK-117 and those untreated, total clinical scores of treated mice were significantly higher (Masuda et al. 2012). This observation demonstrates that LK-117 treatment was able to reduce symptoms of AD skin lesions independent of IgE levels.

There are a few studies showing antiallergic effects of fermented by-products of alcoholic beverages. For example, *sake* lees or *sake-kasu* is a by-product of *sake* production but can be used as a condiment for making other traditional Japanese food, although most is still discarded as industrial waste (Kawamoto et al. 2011). *Sake* lees fermented with *Lb. paracasei* and *Lb. brevis* was shown to prevent allergy rhinitis-like symptoms such as sneezing in OVA-sensitized mice. Interestingly, this prevention was independent of total and specific IgE levels as well as specific

IgG_1 and IgG_{2a} levels and was not modulated by Th1/Th2 cytokine response, unlike most antiallergic immunoregulatory responses (Kawamoto et al. 2011).

Shochu is another alcoholic Japanese distilled beverage typically produced from barley, sweet potato, rice, and so on. Fermented barley extract (FBE) prepared from *shochu* residue was reported to alleviate allergic rhinitis symptoms as well as suppress atopic dermatitis symptoms including development of AD-like skin lesions and scratching behavior by modulating cytokine production (Iguchi et al. 2009).

Grape pomace, which includes the skin and seed (usually discarded as a by-product of grapes used for wine making) was fermented with LAB and the antiallergic effect of fermented grape pomace (FG) was compared with nonfermented grape pomace (G) and the fermenting LAB, *Lb. plantarum* NB (NB) by itself (Kondo et al. 2011). Only FG showed a significant inhibitory effect on degranulation in RBL-2H3 cells. Total phenolic content which was highest in FG was contributed by the fermentation process and was found to be responsible for the inhibitory effect which explains why G or NB by itself was not as potent as FG.

17.3.8 Tea

There have been many health benefit reports of tea (*Camelia sinensis*) including antiallergic effects (Fujimura et al. 2002, 2008). These functional properties are usually contributed by the polyphenolic compounds and the catechins (Darvesh and Bishayee 2013). However, while teas are commonly classified to unfermented and fermented tea, the term "fermented" here is often a misnomer as it refers to an oxidation process as opposed to microbial fermentation. For example, green tea and white tea are unoxidized tea while *Oolong* tea is semioxidized and black tea is fully oxidized. There are however, few true microbial fermented teas including *Puerh* tea, *Fuzhuan* brick tea, *Kombucha,* and *Goishi* tea (Noguchi et al. 2008, Schillinger et al. 2010). Of these, there was only one report (to the best of our knowledge) on antiallergic effect which was on *Goishi* tea.

Goishi tea or *Goishi-cha* is a traditional Japanese tea with a slightly sour taste. There are two microbial fermentation steps involved in producing this tea; (1) aerobic fermentation using fungi, and (2) anaerobic fermentation using LAB. Interestingly, it is known as the "tea of legend" due to its efficiency in weight loss management as it improves lipid metabolism (Noguchi et al. 2008, Hirota et al. 2011). *Goishi* tea was shown to inhibit airway hyperresponsiveness (AHR), one of the important traits of bronchial asthma, in BALB/c mice sensitized with dust-mite, *Dermatophagoides farinae* (Derf) plus diesel exhaust particles (DEP) (Hirota et al. 2011). Eosinophils, neutrophils, and lymphocytes inflammatory cells of sensitized mice were markedly lowered when treated with *Goishi* tea compared to the untreated group. Furthermore, AHR was significantly inhibited while specific IgG_1 and IgE were lowered in *Goishi* treated mice. Goblet cells hyperplasia and eosinophilic infiltration was similarly lowered in *Goishi* treated mice based on histological stains. However, it should be noted that gallic acid, a component of tea leaves with known antiallergy properties also gave comparable results as *Goishi* treated mice (Kim et al. 2005). Therefore, it would seem that this antiallergic effect may not be contributed by microbial fermentation of the tea leaves and any tea with adequate amount of gallic acid may also show this antiallergic effect although more studies are needed to confirm this.

17.4 Immunoregulatory Mechanism of Probiotics in Allergy

While it is known that the microbes in fermented food which are mostly probiotic bacteria confer beneficial effects to the immune system, the precise mechanism is not entirely understood. While modulation of Th1/Th2 balance through regulation of cytokines is one of the mechanisms as described previously, the contributing factor or the property of these probiotics which contributes to this modulation remains unknown but many studies suggest that the cell wall plays an important role (Murosaki et al. 1998, Kato et al. 1999, Tejada-Simon et al. 1999).

Investigations carried out using mice models which were either fed with live viable cultures or injected with nonviable heat-killed cultures of *Lb. casei*, *Lb. plantarum*, and *Bifidobacteria* strains indicated that live cultures are potent downregulators of pro-Th2 cytokines while heat-killed cultures are potent upregulators of pro-Th1 cytokines (Murosaki et al. 1998, Kato et al. 1999, Tejada-Simon et al. 1999). This led to the conclusion that the integrity of the Gram-positive LAB cell wall and its cell wall components comprising phosphorylated polysaccharides, peptidoglycans, lipoteichoic acids, and glycolipid structures were crucial factors in determining cytokine induction properties by LAB (Bhakdi et al. 1991, Kitazawa et al. 1996). It was hypothesized that through the heat-killing process, these immunologically active cell wall components become more readily available and accessible as opposed to live cultures with intact and closely bound cell walls.

Over the years, studies employing purified LAB cell wall components revealed that these immunogenic molecules bind predominantly to leukocyte surface receptors such as toll-like receptors, endotoxin CD14 receptors, and type-I macrophage scavenger receptors (Dunne et al. 1994, Schwandner et al. 1999, Cross et al. 2001). Upon receptor binding, the production of specific cytokines is stimulated via two major cellular pathways: (1) the nuclear factor kappa-B (NF-κB) signaling pathway; and (2) the Janus kinase-signal transducer and activator of transcription (JAK-STAT) signaling pathway. These two pathways are in essence a family of kinase-activated transcription factors which regulate an array of genes encoding immune components including various cytokines (Miettinen et al. 2000).

Probiotics also modulate the intestinal microbiota by competing with pathogenic bacteria for nutrients and binding sites and also by releasing antimicrobial substances such as bacteriocin which inhibits the growth of other bacteria (Ouwehand 2007, Toh et al. 2012). Modulation of intestinal microbiota is important because it was observed that allergic infants have a different microbiota composition compared to healthy infants with the former having high levels of clostridia and lower levels of bifidobacteria. It was also observed that allergic infants had high levels of *Bifidobacter adolescentis* which is typical in an adult's microbiota in comparison with healthy infants whose microbiota are colonized mostly by *B. bifidum* (Ouwehand 2007).

In addition, probiotics improve the barrier function of intestinal mucosa, while regulating the function and expression of tight junction proteins and mucus secretion. This reduces the entry of antigens through the mucosa thereby decreasing exposure of the immune system to antigens (Ouwehand 2007). Tight junction proteins and the epithelial barrier integrity is also modulated by some short-chain fatty acids (SCFA) produced by probiotics (Toh et al. 2012). In addition, other SCFAs were reported to reduce inflammatory lesions in animal models of asthma and colitis (Maslowski et al. 2009).

17.5 Probiotic Therapy as Alternative Treatment for Allergy Management

One of the reasons of the rising of allergy prevalence is the reduced exposure of children to environmental microbes during the early stages of life. This has been attributed to change of lifestyle which includes improved hygiene, vaccinations, antibiotic usage, consumption of almost sterile food, reduced household size, and more. This is popularly known as the "hygiene hypothesis"

(Strachan 1989). In contrast, children who lived on farms were less likely to develop allergic diseases (Riedler et al. 2001). Some of the common methods currently used in treating or managing allergic diseases include feeding enzymatically hydrolyzed milk to infants with cow's milk allergy, total avoidance of food suspected to cause allergy, and use of chemical treatment such as antihistamine or steroid shots. However, based on the "hygiene hypothesis," it would seem feasible to use microbes to manage allergy.

Based on previous literature on the antiallergy effect of fermented food, it can be generally presumed that the causative factor of the benefits of fermented food is either the change of chemical composition of the food caused by fermentation or the presence of bacteria, with cytokine modulation being one of the most profound and well-understood effects of the latter (Figure 17.2).

The latter factor has been more extensively studied and there are many publications on the effect of probiotics on allergy. It is noteworthy to point out that the antiallergy effects are strain and species dependent and therefore, probiotic therapy should also be considered carefully based on the type of allergy and not be generalized (Tuomola et al. 2001). Probiotic therapy can be classified into two: (1) treatment, and (2) prevention which have been reviewed extensively by Toh et al. (2012) showing evidence performed in animal models as well as clinical trials. For treatment therapy, there were conflicting reports and it was difficult to come to a solid conclusion as there was too much variability in the way the trials were conducted including patient background and formulation of probiotic therapy. Furthermore, a long-term clinical trial studying the effects of long-term consumption of fermented milk containing *Lb. casei* in preschool children with allergic rhinitis and asthma showed that health status improved for children with allergic rhinitis but no significant effect was found on children with asthma (Giovannini et al. 2007). For preventive therapy, it was generally concluded that preventive probiotic treatment was most effective to a child when both prenatal and postnatal intervention was given to the mother and when the mother breastfed the child.

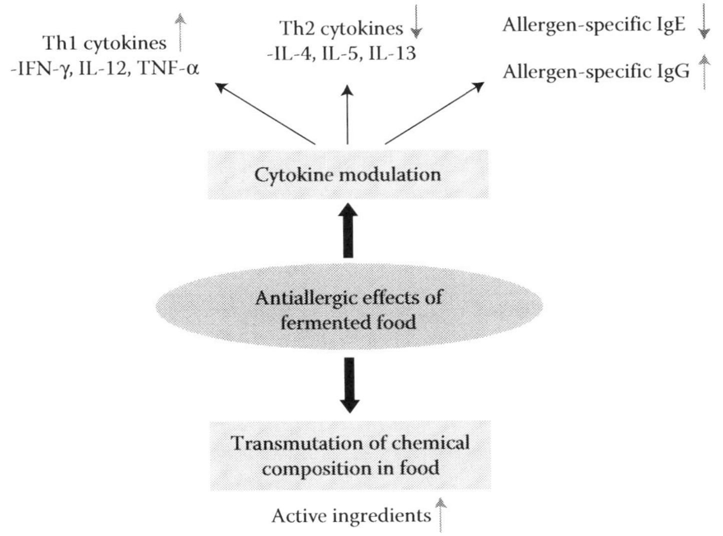

Figure 17.2 Ball-park figure on how fermented food imposes antiallergic effects.

Although many studies suggest the high potential of probiotic therapy to effectively treat allergy, there are still much areas which are unanswered and require further understanding. The biggest challenge faced is the high heterogeneity between studies. Most of these studies were performed using different bacterial strains or species and may not be widely applicable. Patient background including medical history and age were also significantly different; furthermore, studies proven in *in vitro* studies or animal models are often are not replicable in clinical studies. Finally, the understanding of the mechanism of action of these probiotics against allergy is still not fully understood. Therefore, there are still many unexplored areas in this research field but the studies which have been conducted so far show promising evidence of successfully using probiotics and fermented food to manage allergy, a much more natural and therefore acceptable alternative than current drug-driven treatments.

17.6 Conclusion

The trend of consumerism is moving toward natural and organic products due to the fear of negative long-term effects that processed food, chemicals, and drugs are imposing on our health. In view of this, the use of fermented food and probiotics to prevent or treat allergy is envisaged to be highly desirable, especially since research shows promising results pertaining to this. Apart from this natural aspect, use of fermented food and probiotics for allergy management also seems more affordable and cost-effective especially in terms of medication and hospitalization fees. Although the exact mechanism and function of how fermented food and probiotics help prevent or treat allergy as well as the extent of its effectiveness is still largely unknown, garnered research interest in this area is advancing, promising to unravel a better understanding and insight into this alternative treatment for allergy.

References

Alberts, B., A. Johnson, J. Lewis, M. Raff, K. Roberts, and P. Walter. 2002. The adaptive immune system. In *Molecular Biology of the Cell*, 4th edition. New York: Garland Science.

Bhakdi, S., T. Klonisch, P. Nuber, and W. Fischer. 1991. Stimulation of monokine production by lipoteichoic acids. *Infection and Immunity* 59: 4614–4620.

Cross, M. L., L. M. Stevenson, and H. S. Gill. 2001. Anti-allergy properties of fermented foods: An important immunoregulatory mechanism of lactic acid bacteria. *International Immunopharmacology* 1: 891–901.

Darvesh, A. S. and A. Bishayee. 2013. Chemopreventive and therapeutic potential of tea polyphenols in hepatocellular cancer. *Nutrition and Cancer* 65(3): 329–344.

Deo, S. S., K. J. Mistry, A. M. Kakade, and P. V. Niphadkar. 2010. Role played by Th2 type cytokines in IgE mediated allergy and asthma. *Lung India* 27(2): 66–71.

Dunne, D. W., D. Resnick, J. Greenberg, M. Krieger, and K. A. Joiner. 1994. The type I macrophage scavenger receptor binds to Gram positive bacteria and recognizes lipoteichoic acid. *Proceedings of the National Academy of Sciences USA* 91: 1863–1867.

Fujimura, Y., H. Tachibana, M. Maeda-Yamamoto, T. Miyase, M. Sano, and K. Yamada. 2002. Antiallergic tea catechin, (-)-epigallocathecin-3-O-(3-O-methyl)-gallate, suppresses FcepsilonRI expression in human basophil KU812 cells. *Journal of Agriculture and Food Chemistry* 50(20): 5729–5734.

Fujimura, Y., D. Umeda, K. Yamada, and H. Tachibana. 2008. The impact of 67 kDa laminin receptor on both cell-surface binding and anti-allergic effect of tea catechins. *Archives of Biochemistry and Biophysics* 476(2): 133–138.

Gilliland, S.E. 1990. Health and nutritional benefits from lactic acid bacteria. *FEMS Microbiology Reviews* 87: 175–188.

Giovannini, M., C. Agostoni, E. Riva, F. Salvini, A. Ruscitto, G. V. Zuccotti, G. Radaelli, and Felicita Study Group. 2007. A randomized prospective double-blind controlled trial on effects of long-term consumption of fermented milk containing *Lactobacillus casei* in pre-school children with allergic rhinitis and/or asthma. *Pediatric Research* 62(2): 215–220.

Han, S., G. Kang, Y. Ko, H. Kang, S. Moon, Y. Ann, and E. Yoo. 2012a. External application of fermented olive flounder (*Paralicthys olivaceus*) oil alleviates inflammatory responses in 2,4-dinitrochlorobenzene-induced atopic dermatitis mouse model. *Toxicology Research* 28(3): 159–164.

Han, S., G. Kang, Y. Ko, H. Kang, S. Moon, Y. Ann, and E. Yoo. 2012b. Fermented fish oil suppresses T helper 1/2 cell response in a mouse model of atopic dermatitis via generation of $CD4^{+}CD25^{+}Foxp3^{+}$ T cells. *BMC Immunology* 13: 44.

Hayashi, A., M. Kimura, Y. Nakamura, and H. Yasui. 2009. Anti-atopic dermatitis effects and the mechanism of lactic acid bacteria isolated from Mongolian fermented milk. *Journal of Dairy Research* 76: 158–164.

Hirota, R., N. R. Ngatu, M. Miyamura, H. Nakamura, and N. Suganuma. 2011. Goishi tea consumption inhibits airway hyperresponsiveness in BALB/c mice. *BMC Immunology* 12: 45.

Hong, W., Y. Chen, and M. Chen. 2010. The antiallergic effect of kefir *Lactobacilli*. *Journal of Food Science* 75(8): H244–253.

Hong W., Y. Chen, T. Dai, I. Huang, and M. Chen. 2011. Effect of heat-inactivated kefir-isolated *Lactobacillus kefiranofaciens* M1 on preventing an allergic airway response in mice. *Journal of Agriculture and Food Chemistry* 59: 9022–9031.

Iguchi, T., A. Kawata, T. Watanabe, T. K. Mazumder, and S. Tanabe. 2009. Fermented barley extract suppresses the development of atopic dermatitis-like skin lesions in NC/Nga mice, probably by inhibiting inflammatory cytokines. *Bioscience, Biotechnology and Biochemistry* 73(3): 489–493.

Jain, S., H. Yadav, P. R. Sinha, S. Kapila, Y. Naito, and F. Marotta. 2010. Anti-allergic effects of probiotic Dahi through modulation of the gut immune system. *The Turkish Journal of Gastroenterology* 21(3): 244–250.

Janeway, C. A. Jr., P. Travers, P. M. Walport, and M. J. Shlomchik, 2001a. The components of the immune system. In *Immunobiology: The Immune System in Health and Disease.* 5th edition. New York: Garland Science. Available from: http://www.ncbi.nlm.nih.gov/books/NBK27092/

Janeway, C. A. Jr., P. Travers, M. Walport, and M. J. Shlomchik. 2001b. Antigen recognition by T cells. In *Immunobiology: The Immune System in Health and Disease.* 5th edition. New York: Garland Science. Available from: http://www.ncbi.nlm.nih.gov/books/NBK27098/

Japan Sake and Shochu Makers Association. 2011. A comprehensive guide to Japanese sake. Japan Sake and Shochu Makers Association, Tokyo, Japan.

Jung, J., H. Kang, G. Ji, M. Park, W. Song, M. Kim, J. Kwon et al. 2011. Therapeutic effects of fermented red ginseng in allergic rhinitis: A randomized, double-blind, placebo-controlled study. *Allergy, Asthma and Immunology Research* 3(2): 103–110.

Kataoka, S. 2005. Functional effects of Japanese styled fermented soy sauce (shoyu) and its components. *Journal of Bioscience and Bioengineering* 100(3): 227–234.

Kato, I., K. Tanaka, and T. Yokokura. 1999. Lactic acid bacterium potently induces the production of interleukin-12 and interferon-γ by mouse splenocytes. *International Journal of Immunopharmacology* 21: 121–131.

Kawamoto, S., M. Kaneoke, K. Ohkouchi, Y. Amano, Y. Takaoka, K. Kume, T. Aki et al. 2011. Sake lees fermented with lactic acid bacteria prevents allergic rhinitis-like symptoms and IgE mediated basophil degranulation. *Bioscience Biotechnology Biochemistry* 75(1): 140–144.

Kim, S., C. Jun, K. Suk, B. Choi, H. Lim, S. Park, S. H. Lee, H. Shin, D. Kim, and T. Shin. 2005. Gallic acid inhibits histamine release and pro-inflammatory cytokine production in mast cells. *Toxicological Sciences* 91(1): 123–131.

Kitazawa, H., T. Itoh, Y. Tomioka, M. Mizugaki and T. Yamaguchi. 1996. Induction of IFN-gamma and IL-1 alpha production in macrophages stimulated with phosphopolysaccharide produced by *Lactococcus lactis* ssp. cremoris. *International Journal of Food Microbiology* 31: 99–106.

Kobayashi, M. 2005. Immunological functions of soy sauce: Hypoallergenicity and antiallergic activity of soy sauce. *Journal of Bioscience and Bioengineering* 100(2): 144–151.

Kondo, K., K. Nakamura, Y. Hamauzu, T. Kawahara, H. Sansawa, M. Suzuki, and H. Yasui. 2011. Inhibitory effect of fermented grape pomace on degranulation in RBL-2H3 cells and an analysis of its active ingredients. *Food Science and Technology Research* 17(3): 241–250.

Kumar, S., A. K. Verma, M. Das, and P. D. Dwivedi. 2012. Molecular mechanisms of IgE mediated food allergy. *International Immunopharmacology* 13: 432–439.

Lee, E., M. Song, H. Kwon, G. Ji, and M. Sung. 2012. Oral administration of fermented red ginseng suppressed ovalbumin-induced allergic responses in BALB/c mice. *Phytomedicine* 19: 896–903.

Lee, M., K. Ahn, O. Kwon, M. Kim, I. Lee, S. Oh, and H. Lee. 2007. Anti-inflammatory and anti-allergic effects of kefir in a mouse asthma model. *Immunobiology* 212: 647–654.

Lee, Y. J., J. E. Kim, M. H. Kwak, J. Go, D. S. Kim, H. J. Son, and D. Y. Hwang. 2014. Quantitative evaluation of the therapeutic effect of fermented soybean products containing high concentration of GABA on phtalic anhydride-induced atopic dermatitis in IL4/Luc/CNS-1 Tg mice. *International Journal of Molecular Medicine* 33(5): 1185–1194.

Majamaa, H. and E. Isolauri. 1997. Probiotics: a novel approach in the management of food allergy. *Journal of Allergy and Clinical Immunology* 99: 179–85.

Maslowski, K. M., A. T. Vieira, A. Ng, J. Kranich, F. Sierro, D. Yu, H. C. Schilter et al. 2009. Regulation of inflammatory responses by gut microbiota and chemoattractant receptor GPR43. *Nature* 461: 1282–1286.

Masuda, T., M. Kimura, S. Okada, and H. Yasui. 2010. *Pediococcus pentasaceus* Sn26 inhibits IgE production and the occurrence of ovalbumin-induced allergic diarrhea in mice. *Bioscience, Biotechnology and Biochemistry* 74(2): 329–335.

Masuda, Y., T. Takahashi, K. Yoshida, Y., Nishitani, M. Mizuno, and H. Mizoguchi. 2012. Anti-allergic effect of lactic acid bacteria isolated from seed mash used for brewing sake is not dependent on the total IgE levels. *Journal of Bioscience and Bioengineering* 114(3): 292–296.

Mei, H., Y. Liu, Y. Chiang, S. Chao, N. Mei, Y. Liu, and Y. Tsai. 2013. Immunomodulatory activity of *Lactococcus lactis* A17 from Taiwan fermented cabbage in OVA-sensitized BALB/c mice. *Evidence-based Complementary and Alternative Medicine* 2013: 287803

Miettinen, M., A. Lehtonen, I. Julkunen, and S. Matikainen. 2000. Lactobacilli and streptococci activate NF-κB and STAT signalling pathways in human macrophages. *Journal of Immunology* 164: 3733–3740.

Murosaki S., Y. Yamamoto, K. Ito, T. Inokuchi, H. Kusaka, H. Ikeda, and Y. Yoshikai. 1998. Heat killed *Lactobacillus plantarum* L-137 suppresses naturally fed antigen-specific IgE production by stimulation of IL-12 production in mice. *Journal of Allergy and Clinical Immunology* 102: 57–64.

Ngoc, P. L., D. R. Gold, A. O. Tzianabos, S. T. Weiss, and J. C. Celedón. 2005. Cytokines, allergy, and asthma. *Current Opinion in Allergy and Clinical Immunology* 5(2): 161–6.

Nielsen, G. D., J. S. Hansen, R. M. Lund, M. Bergqvist, S. T. Larsen, S. K. Clausen, P. Thygesen, and O. M. Poulsen. 2002. IgE-mediated asthma and rhinitis I: A role of allergen exposure. *Pharmacology and Toxicology* 90: 231–242.

Noguchi, A., Y. Hamauzu, and H. Yasui. 2008. Inhibitory effects of Goishi tea against influenza virus infection. *Food Science and Technology Research* 14(3): 277–284.

Oschatz, C., C. Maas, B. Lecher, T. Jansen, J. Björkqvist, T. Tradler, R. Sedlmeier et al. 2011. Mast cells increase vascular permeability by heparin-initiated bradykinin formation in vivo. Immunity 34(2): 258–268.

Ouwehand, A. C. 2007. Antiallergic effects of probiotics. *Journal of Nutrition.* 137(3): 794S–797S.

Park, E., J. Sung, H. Trinh, E. Bae, H. Yun, S. Hong, and D. Kim. 2008. Lactic acid bacterial fermentation increases the anti-allergic effects of *Ixeris dentata*. *Journal of Microbial Biotechnology* 18(2): 308–313.

Pawankar, R., G. W. Canonica, S. Holgate, and R. F. Lockey. 2011. *White Book of Allergy 2011–2012 Executive Summary*. World Allergy Organization, Wisconsin, USA.

Peng, S., J. Lin, and M. Lin. 2007. Anti-allergic effect of milk fermented with lactic acid bacteria in a murine animal model. *Journal of Agriculture and Food Chemistry* 55(13): 5092–5096.

Riedler, J., C. Braun-Fahrlander, W. Eder, M. Schreuer, M. Waser, S. Maisch, D. Carr, R. Schierl, D. Nowak and E. von Mutius. 2001. Exposure to farming in early life and development of asthma and allergy: A cross-sectional survey. *Lancet* 358: 1129–1133.

Romagnani, S. 2006. Regulation of the T cell response. *Clinical and Experimental Allergy* 36: 1357–1366.

Schillinger, U., L. Ban-Koffi, and C. M. A. P. Franz. 2010. Tea, coffee and cacao. In Fermented Foods and Beverages of the World. eds. JP Tamang and K Kailasapathy, New York: Taylor & Francis, CRC Press, pp. 354–357.

Schmid-Grendelmeier, P. and R. Crameri. 2001. Recombinant allergens for skin testing. *International Archieves of Allergy and Immunology* 125(2): 96–111.

Schwandner, R., R. Dziarski, H. Wesche, M. Rothe, and C. J., Kirschning. 1999. Peptidoglycan- and lipoteichoic acid-induced cell activation is mediated by Toll-like receptor 2. *The Journal of Biological Chemistry* 274: 1746–1749.

Shida, K., K. Makino, A. Morishita, K. Takamizawa, S. Hachimura, A. Ametani, T. Sato, Y. Kumagai, S. Habu, and S. Kaminogawa. 1998. Lactobacillus casei inhibit antigen induced IgE secretion through regulation of cytokine production in murine splenocyte cultures. *International Archives of Allergy and Immunology* 115: 278–87.

Shida, K., E. Takahashi, K. Iwadate, H. Yasui, T. Sato, S. Habu, S. Hachimura, and S. Kaminogowa. 2002. Lactobacillus casei Shirota suppreses serum immunoglobulin E and immunoglobulin G1 responses and systemic anaphylaxis in a food allergy model. Clinical and Experimental Allergy 32: 563–570.

Sicherer, S. H. and H. A. Sampson. 2013. Food allergy: Epidemiology, pathogenesis, diagnosis, and treatment. Clinical Review in Allergy and Immunology 133(2): 291–307.

Strachan, D.P. 1989. Hay fever, hygiene, and household size. *BMJ* 299: 1259–1260.

Su J. C., A. S. Kemp, G. A. Varigos, and T. M. Nolan. 1997. Atopic eczema: Its impact on the family and financial cost. *Archives of Disease in Childhood* 76: 159–162.

Tejada-Simon, M. V., Z. Ustunol, and J. J. Pestka. 1999. Ex vivo effects of lactobacilli, streptococci and bifidobacteria ingestion on cytokine and nitric oxide production in a murine model. *Journal of Food Protection* 62: 162–169.

Toh, Z. Q., A. Anzela, M. L. K. Tang, and P. V. Licciardi. 2012. Probiotic therapy as a novel approach for allergic diseases. *Frontiers in Pharmacology* 3: 171.

Trinh, H., E. Bae, Y. Hyun, Y. Jang, H. Yun, S. Hong, and D. Kim. 2010. Anti-allergic effects of fermented *Ixeris sonchifolia* and its constituents in mice. *Journal of Microbiol Biotechnology* 20(1): 217–223.

Tuomola, E., R. Crittenden, M. Playne, E. Isolauri, and S. Salminen. 2001. Quality assurance criteria for probiotic bacteria. *The American Journal of Clinical Nutrition* 73(Suppl. 2): 393S–398S.

Van de Water J., C. L. Keen, and M. E. Gershwin. 1999. The influence of chronic yogurt consumption on immunity. *Journal of Nutrition* 129(7 Suppl): 1492S–1495S.

Won, T. J., B. Kim, D. S. Song, Y. T. Lim, E. S. Oh, D. I. Lee, E. S. Park, H. Min, S. Park, and K. W. Hwang. 2011. Modulation of Th1/Th2 balance by *Lactobacillus* strains isolated from *kimchi* via stimulation of macrophage cell line J774A.1 *in vitro*. *Journal of Food Science* 76(2): H55–H61.

Xu, Q., T. Yajima, W. Li, K. Saito, Y. Ohshima, and Y. Yoshikai. 2005. Levan (b-2, 6-fructan), a major fraction of fermented soybean mucilage, displays immunostimulating properties via Toll-like receptor 4 signalling: induction of interleukin-12 production and suppression of T-helper type 2 response and immunoglobulin E production. *Clinical and Experimental Allergy* 36: 94–101.

Chapter 18

Antiallergenic Benefits of Fermented Foods

Swati B. Jadhav, Shweta Deshaware, and Rekha S. Singhal

Contents

18.1 Introduction

Allergies are one of the major immunological disorders of the modern world with more than 25% of the population in industrialized countries suffering from immunoglobulin E (IgE)-mediated allergies (Valenta 2002). According to a study released in 2013 by the Centre for Disease Control and Prevention, food allergies among children have increased approximately 50% between 1997 and 2011. The hygiene hypothesis provides a probable explanation for the rise in allergic occurrences. It suggests that small family sizes, increased cleanliness in urban societies, increased use of antibiotics, stable intestinal flora, and relative lack of microbial exposure, which play a role in building a mature immune system during the initial years of life, have resulted in an imbalance in Th1/Th2 cytokines which in turn have induced the development of allergic disorders (Flohr 2005).

18.2 Allergy and Allergens

18.2.1 Food Allergy and Allergens

Any abnormal clinical response associated with the ingestion of food is termed adverse food reaction. Adverse food reaction can be either food intolerances or food allergies based on the pathophysiological characteristics. Food intolerances may be due to inherent properties of the food (i.e., toxic contaminant and/or a pharmacologically active component) or characteristics of the host (i.e., metabolic disorders, idiosyncratic responses, and psychological disorders). They may not be reproducible and are often dose dependent. The majority of adverse reactions to food are due to food intolerances. A food allergy is an abnormal immunologic response to a food occurring in a susceptible host. A food allergy is not dose dependent and is reproducible each time the food is ingested (Sampson 1999, Nowak-Wegrzyn and Sampson 2006, Sicherer and Sampson 2009). A rare and violent reaction of the immune system toward food protein is called a food allergy. Food allergies are is a major challenge for the food industry due to their association with public health. An immunologically based adverse reaction shows response to dietary antigens which causes food allergies (Beyer and Teuber 2004). A group of eight major allergenic foods, commonly referred to as the "Big 8," comprises milk, egg, fish, soya, crustacean shellfish, tree nuts, peanuts, and wheat. The allergenic protein has a small antigenic determination region called the epitope which provokes the IgE-mediated allergenic response (Taylor and Hefle 2001). The allergen elicits an initial IgE antibody response. This results in a secondary IgE antibody response which signals an allergic reaction (Babu et al. 2001). Some of the common characteristics of food allergens are: they are water-soluble glycoproteins with molecular weight of 10–70 kDa, and they are relatively stable to heat, acid, and proteases.

The presence of immune-stimulatory factors in food may also contribute to such sensitization. For example, the major glycoprotein allergen from peanuts is Ara h 1 which is a seed storage protein from *Arachis hypogaea* (peanut). It is very stable and resistant to heat and digestive enzyme degradation and also acts as a Th2 adjuvant due to the expression of a glycan adduct (Cianferoni and Spergel 2009).

18.2.2 Mechanism of Food Allergy

Food allergies have a characteristic immunological mechanism which can be classified as follows:

1. IgE-mediated which are mediated by antibodies belonging to the immunoglobulin E (IgE) and are the best-characterized food allergy reactions.
2. Non-IgE-mediated (cell mediated), when the cell component of the immune system is responsible for the food allergy and mostly involves the gastrointestinal tract.

IgE-mediated classic food allergic reactions are immediate, reproducible, and readily diagnosed by detection of food-specific IgE. If oral tolerance of the food does not develop, it leads to the production of specific IgE antibodies. The allergic reactions are generated due to interactions of an allergen-specific IgE antibody with its high-affinity receptor (FcεRI) and low-affinity receptor (FcεRII). FcεRI are expressed on mast cells and basophils whereas FcεRII are present on macrophages, monocyte, lymphocytes, and platelets. The IgE linked to the FcεRI on binding a specific antigen causes receptor crosslinking and consequent release of mediators (Nowak-Wegrzyn and Sampson 2006, Sicherer and Sampson 2009). Basophils along with mast cells are also important in IgE-mediated acute reaction. Basophils spontaneously release high concentrations of histamine in the case of atopic dermatitis (AD) and food hypersensitivity, which normalizes after the offending food has been removed from the diet (Sampson et al. 1992, Babu et al. 2001). Histamines mainly cause an immediate reaction within a few minutes after contact with the allergen (Beyer and Teuber 2004). These reactions include vasodilation, tissue fluid exudation, smooth muscle contraction, and mucous secretion. Further, a late-phase response begins 4–6 h after contact with the allergen and continues for several days. The chemotactic mediators released cause selective recruitment of inflammatory cells, mainly eosinophils and neutrophils which infiltrate the tissue producing an inflammation lasting for a few days.

Non-IgE-mediated food allergies occur in the absence of a demonstrable food-specific IgE antibody in the skin or serum and are seen in a minority of immunologic reactions to food. These immune reactions depend on antibodies other than IgE, the immune complex of food and antibodies and cell-mediated immunity. An acute or chronic inflammation in the gastrointestinal tract where eosinophils and T cells seem to play a major role is the main characteristic of non-IgE-mediated food allergy (Yan and Shaffer 2009). Both these mechanisms are explained in Figure 18.1.

In general, during allergic reactions allergen sensitized Th2 cells secrete cytokines IL-4, IL-5, and IL-13, which recruit granular effector cells such as eosinophils, basophils, and mast cells to the site of allergic inflammation (Hamelmann and Gelfand 1999). These effector cells and cytophilic/reaginic IgE class antibodies promote the clinical manifestations of allergy and atopy. Moreover, IL-4 and IL-13 promote B lymphocyte immunoglobulin isotype switching to IgE (Punnonen et al. 1994) and help to increase circulating levels of total and allergen-specific IgE (Pene et al. 1988). Interferons, particularly interferon-gamma (IFN-γ), can downregulate IL-4 expression and reduce B-cell immunoglobulin isotype switching. Type I interferon (IFN-α) can act as an augmentative signal for IFN-γ production and promote Th1-type immune responses and reduce IgE production (Sinigaglia et al. 1999).

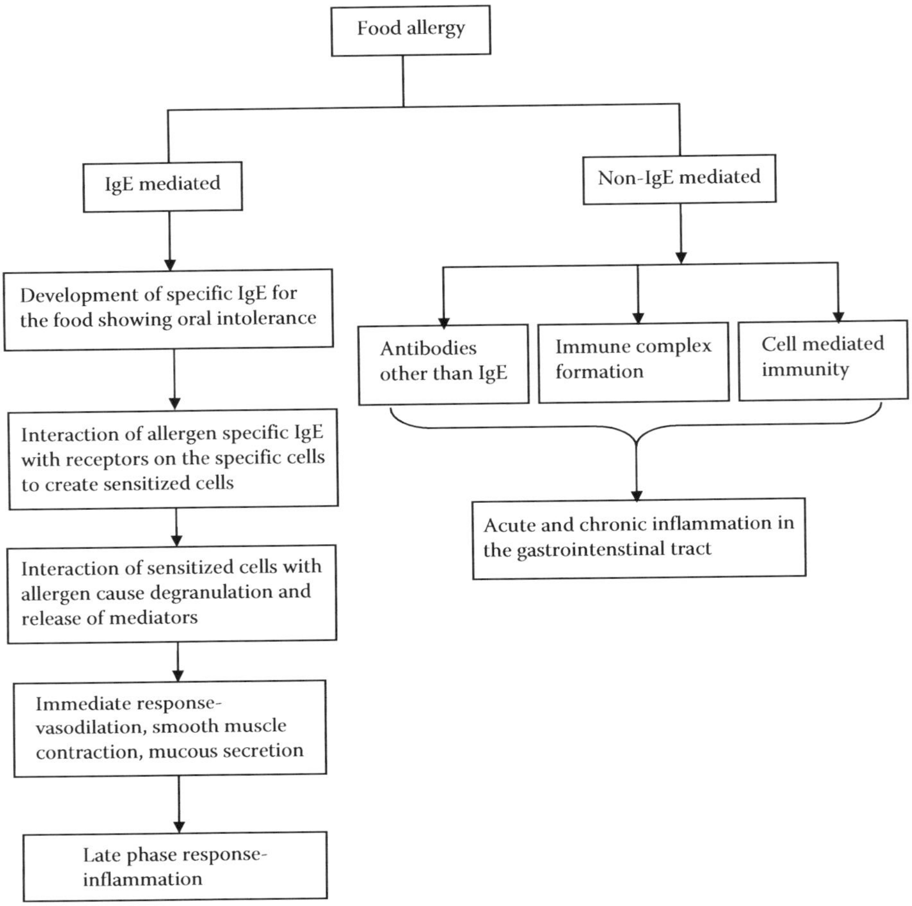

Figure 18.1 Mechanism of allergy. (Adapted from Ortolani, C. and E. A. Pastorello. 2006. *Best Practice and Research Clinical Gastroenterology* 20(3): 467–483.)

18.2.3 Treatment of Allergy

The treatment of allergy mainly comprises the complete removal of the allergen from the diet. This could create a nutritional deficiency which can be solved by giving vitamin and mineral supplements. The following approaches are used as a treatment or preventive measure for allergy (Yeung et al. 1998, Sampson 2001, Leung et al. 2004):

- Use of recombinant allergens engineered with modification of epitopes
- Use of allergen mixed with heat-killed listeria as an adjuvant
- Use of humanized monoclonal anti-IgE antibodies
- Acute food reaction therapy—use of antihistamine drugs
- Use of fermented food

18.3 Mechanism of Fighting Allergies

Methods by which allergic responses and symptoms can be immunologically alleviated are (Cross et al. 2001):

- Promote interferon expression
- Reduce allergen-stimulated production of proinflammatory cytokines IL-4 and IL-5
- Skewing the Th1/Th2 cytokine balance:
  - Upregulate Type 1 helper CD4+ T cells (Th1) response—Th1 cells inhibit IgE production by secreting IFN-γ.
- Downregulate Type 2 helper CD4+ cells—Th2 cells secrete cytokines such as IL-4, IL-5, IL-6, and IL-10, which promote production of IgE

18.3.1 Lactic Acid Bacteria: Potent Allergy Fighters

The cell wall of lactic acid bacteria (LAB) is made up of a complex mixture of phosphorylated polysaccharides and glycolipid structures (Kitazawa et al. 1996). The peptidoglycans (PG) and lipoteichoic acids (LTA) are predominant components in the cell wall. The cell wall is mainly immunologically active. There are many possible reasons by which LAB may show an antiallergenic property. These include the ability of LAB to enzymatically hydrolyze allergenic food molecules or to stabilize the gut mucosa sufficiently to reduce systemic uptake of food-borne allergens (Isolauri et al. 1993). The most accepted mechanism is that some LAB-containing fermented foods are able to promote deviation away from a proallergy phenotype via a mechanism of immunoregulation (Figure 18.2). The fermented foods or LAB have shown significant enhancement in the expression and secretion of both type I and type II interferons.

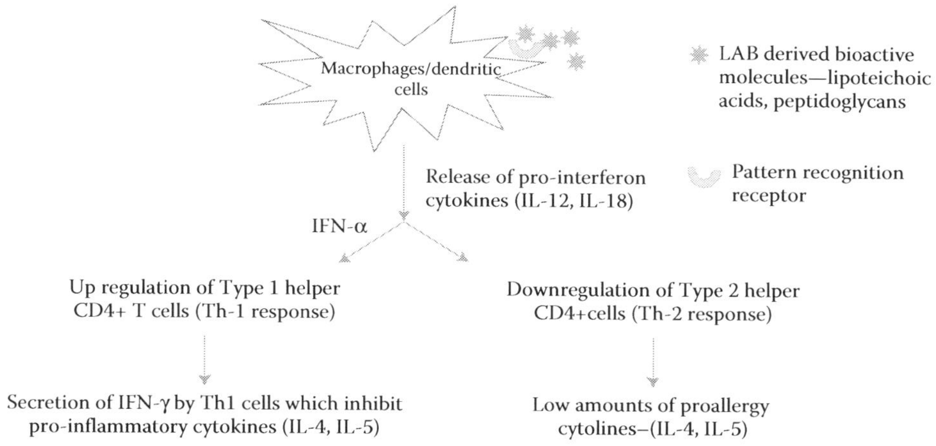

Figure 18.2 Immunoregulatory mechanism of LAB. (Adapted from Cross, M. L., L. M. Stevenson, and H. S. Gill. 2001. *International Immunopharmacology* 1: 891–901.)

18.3.2 Role of LAB in Preventing/Fighting Allergies

The phosphopolysaccharide of *Lactococcus lactis* has been shown to stimulate IFN-γ production by murine leukocytes *in vitro* (Kitazawa et al. 1996), whereas teichoic acid and muramyl dipeptide (a subfraction of peptidoglycan) have been shown to enhance IFN-γ production when added to cultures of mitogen-stimulated human mononuclear blood cells (Aattouri and Lemonnier 1997). Studies have indicated that Gram-positive cell wall components bind predominantly to leukocyte surface pattern recognition receptors, and are potent stimulators of monokine production. The antiallergenic properties of LAB in fermented food have been reported by Cross et al. (2001).

LAB in fermented food has health benefits and various strains of dietary LAB have been shown to benefit a number of host physiological responses including immune function (Macfarlane and Cummings 1999). Clinical symptoms of allergy in adults with atopic rhinitis or nasal allergies have been shown to be reduced by the long-term consumption of yogurt. It can further lower the serum levels of IgE, particularly among the elderly (Van de Water et al. 1999). In contrast, Wheeler et al. (1997) reported that yogurt supplemented with *Lactobacillus* show reduction of eosinophilia and increase in the production of IFN-γ as against no effect on atopy or immune parameters by normal yogurt. Various studies have indicated different strains of *Lactobacillus* and *Bifidobacteria* show promising effects of suppressing allergic responses in animal models and in human subjects (Matsuzaki et al. 1998, Ishida et al. 2003, Ohno et al. 2005, Morita et al. 2006). Preliminary studies on human subjects with high serum IgE levels and perennial allergic rhinitis who were given milk fermented with *Lactobacillus gasseri* for 28 days showed significant decline in serum IgE concentration and enhanced Th1 immune response (Morita et al. 2006).

18.4 Fermented Foods with Antiallergenic Properties

The nutritional and functional properties of a product can be improved by the process of fermentation. It is an interesting area of research which entails the ability to hydrolyze allergenic proteins of the food into smaller peptides. During the fermentation process, there is a change in the structure of epitopes of the allergenic protein which thereby lowers the immunoreactivity of the proteins. Moreover, the fermentation process improves the protein quality and digestibility due to partial degradation of complex stored proteins into more simple and soluble products and affects the nutritional quality of legumes (Shekib 1994). Many such fermented foods having antiallergenic potential are shown in Figure 18.3 and discussed below in detail.

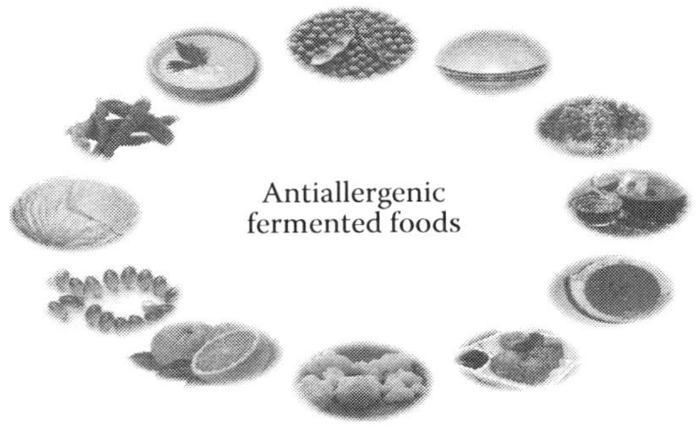

Figure 18.3 Antiallergenic fermented foods.

18.4.1 Soybeans

Soybean is one of the most important grains of the legume family and has essential economical and nutritional benefits. It is of low cost and has high nutritional quality which makes it beneficial for human consumption as well as animal feed. Currently, 33 IgE-binding allergenic proteins have been identified in soybean. A few of these proteins are known to cause the majority of allergenic responses. Hence, identification and purification of these proteins are important. The molecular mass of these proteins has been identified from 7 to 71 kDa (Wilson et al. 2005).

Many different technologies including soybean preparations by mutation, salting out, enzymatic degradation, and high pressure have been reported to enhance the reduction of soybean allergenic proteins (Ogawa et al. 2000, Penas et al. 2005). Among these technological approaches, fermentation is the best approach to decrease residual antigenicity of soybean proteins. The soybean allergen can be degraded using microbial proteolytic enzymes during fermentation. The fermentation of soybean gives different products such as soy sauce, *miso*, soybean ingredients, and feed-grade soybean meals (Hong et al. 2004, Kobayashi 2005, Yamanihi et al. 1995). Different soybean-based products have variations in their protein profile and immunogenicity.

18.4.1.1 Soy Containing Ingredients

Frias et al. (2008) detected and quantified soybean allergens, and reported on the production of hypoallergenic soy-containing ingredients by natural and induced fermentation with *Lactobacillus plantarum, Bacillus subtilis, Aspergillus oryzae*, and *Rhizopus oryzae*. The fermented cracked seeds and flour products contain proteins of low- and medium-range molecular weight. The aim of the fermentation was to remove or to reduce immunoreactivity of the proteins. The type of microorganism used during the fermentation process affects the immunoreactivity of proteins. Elimination of immunoreactive proteins by mold proteolysis was potentially weaker than bacterial proteolysis, which may be due to the slower growth rate of viable mold during the fermentation process. *B. subtilis, Lb. plantarum*, and natural fermentation showed the presence of peptide below 30 kDa, which is of smaller size and less intense immunoreactivity. *B. subtilis* reduced the immunoreactivity by more than 80%, whereas *Lb. plantarum* and natural fermentation showed greater than 90% of reduction in immunoreactivity. Fermentation can reduce or eliminate antigenic soybean proteins and also improve the nutritional value.

18.4.1.2 Soy Sauce

Many varieties of soy sauce (*shoyu*) are produced in Japan and other East Asian countries. Their characteristics depend on the various types and different ratios of raw materials used, the types of microorganisms employed, and the fermentation conditions (Kobayashi 2005). Although soy sauce is a traditional fermented seasoning of East Asian countries, it is available and used throughout the world. In Japanese soy sauce (*shoyu*), soybeans and wheat are the two main raw materials used. During fermentation of the soybeans, the proteins are completely degraded into peptides and amino acids by microbial proteolytic enzymes which help to eliminate the allergenic proteins present in the raw materials. The major soybean allergen, that is, Gly m Bd 30 K was also found to be degraded into peptides and amino acids (Kobayashi 2005). Another allergenic component of soy sauce is wheat which is also reported to be degraded in both salt-soluble and salt-insoluble fractions during the brewing processes between the raw materials and the final soy sauce.

However, enzymatic hydrolysis does not degrade the polysaccharides originating from the cell wall of soybeans. Hence, these polysaccharides are present in soy sauce after fermentation and termed *shoyu* polysaccharides (SPS). The purification and investigation of polysaccharides from soy sauce has been done by Kikuchi and Yokotsuka (1972). A large amount of galacturonic acid was found in soy sauce. Polysaccharides from either the dialysate or ethanol precipitate of raw soy sauce were obtained (Kobayashi et al. 2004). Hyaluronidase (mucopolysaccharide splitting enzyme) has been implicated in allergic reactions causing the migration of cancer cells, inflammation, and an increase in the permeability of the vascular system. The inhibitory effect of the SPS from raw soy sauce for this enzyme showed the same potency as the antiallergenic medicine disodium cromoglycate. Furthermore, SPS is also shown to inhibit histamine release from RBL-2H3 cells (Kobayashi et al. 2004). The inhibition of histamine release was reported to be concentration dependent, and was estimated to be about one-tenth that of ketotifen, an antiallergenic drug (Kanda et al. 1998). SPS is beneficial over ketotifen due to lower cytotoxicity of SPS (Kobayashi et al. 2004). Therefore, SPS from soy sauce would be safe and is expected to act as an antiallergenic seasoning for foods. Soy sauce generally contains about 1% (w/v) SPS and it shows potent antiallergenic activities, both *in vitro* and *in vivo*. A clinical study suggested an oral supplementation of SPS to be an effective intervention for patients with allergic rhinitis. Hence, soy sauce can be considered as a potentially promising seasoning for the treatment of allergic diseases through food due to its hypoallergenicity and antiallergenic activity (Kobayashi et al. 2005).

18.4.1.3 ImmuBalance

The probiotic, *ImmuBalance*™ (Nichimo Co., Ltd., Tokyo, Japan) is a proprietary *koji* fermentation product made by fermenting defatted soybeans with *A. oryzae* and LAB (*Pediococcus parvulus* and *Enterococcus faecium*) using a new Japanese fermentation technology. In many Japanese fermentation technologies, *koji* molds have traditionally been used to produce a number of foods such as *miso* (fermented soybean paste), *shoyu* (soy sauce) and *sake* (an alcoholic beverage) (Manabe et al. 1984). Consumption of fermented soy products is gaining attraction due to their antiallergenic properties. *ImmuBalance* is a unique product that not only contains heat-killed LAB, but also contains soybean oligofructose, bacterial metabolites (polysaccharides and peptides), and degraded metabolites (soybean polysaccharides, peptides, and amino acids) produced during fermentation. A cross-sectional study was designed to determine the relationship between soy product intake and prevalence of allergic rhinitis in pregnant Japanese women. The study indicated a clear inverse linear trend between intake of dietary *miso* and prevalence of allergic rhinitis (Miyake et al. 2005).

Peanuts are one of the most common foods leading to anaphylactic reactions including fatal and near-fatal food-anaphylactic reactions. Hence, peanut allergy (PNA) has been the target of most research on food allergy therapy. Moreover, PNA is difficult to avoid because of the frequent presence of peanuts in manufactured foods. The prevalence of PNA is increasing in westernized countries (Nowak-Wegrzyn and Sampson 2004, Sampson 2004). Allergen-specific immunotherapy (IT) is currently being re-explored as a treatment option due to the lack of therapeutic modalities. Previously, peanut-specific IT was attempted but was unsuccessful due to significant adverse effects (Oppenheimer et al. 1992). PN allergens are very close to soybean seed storage proteins with respect to amino acid homology (Pons et al. 2004). Hence, it was thought that soy IT could reduce the risk of adverse reactions, while providing some level of desensitization. Further, it may provide a new therapeutic intervention for PNA. Pons et al. (2004) reported that soybean protein IT reduced peanut-allergic responses in the PNA mouse model. Hence, alternative soy-based IT may be useful in the management of PNA.

As PNA has potential life-threatening reactions, animal models of PNA, which closely mimic human PNA, were used to investigate the potential therapies for PNA (Bashir et al. 2004). Zhang et al. (2008) tested the effect of *ImmuBalance* in two different doses on an established murine model of PNA. Furthermore, these authors also tested effects of irradiation sterilized *ImmuBalance* (I-*ImmuBalance*) which contains inactivated microorganisms. PN challenged *ImmuBalance*-treated mice exhibited significantly reduced clinical symptoms as compared with control mice. The effect of I-*ImmuBalance* was comparable to *ImmuBalance*. These results suggest that *ImmuBalance* and perhaps I-*ImmuBalance* may have potential for developing a novel probiotic therapy for PNA and other food allergies.

Japanese cedar pollinosis (JCP) is a common IgE-mediated type I allergic disease which has morbidity of approximately 20% in the Japanese population (Otsuka and Pan 2005). Sneezing, itchy and watery eyes, a runny nose, and a burning sensation in the palate and throat are common symptoms of JCP. JCP causes serious discomfort between January and April of each year which makes it necessary to find an effective prevention for JCP. Otsuka and Pan (2005) examined the effect of *ImmuBalance* on the prevention and treatment of allergic reactions in JCP during the pollen season. The use of *ImmuBalance* results in an interaction of the biological benefits of probiotics, prebiotics, and biogenetics on the host which proved to be more powerful than probiotics and/or prebiotics alone in the prevention and treatment of the allergy. An open-label pilot study on seven individuals with JCP was conducted. Each participant received oral administration of 1.0–2.0 g *ImmuBalance* daily for 3 months. Self-evaluated overall average symptom scores in the peak pollen season showed significant improvement compared with the previous year. Hence, this study suggested effectiveness of dietary *ImmuBalance* in the prevention and treatment of JCP.

AD is a chronic and relapsing skin disease. It is characterized by intense pruritus and the development of inflammatory lesions. AD patients show hyperproduction of IgE due to the strong polarization to Th 2-type responses (Beltrani 2005). Moreover, barrier dysfunction of lesional skin is also observed in AD patients (Leung 2000). Matsuda et al. (2012) studied potential efficacy of *ImmuBalance* for the treatment of AD using a mouse model, NC/Tnd mice for human AD. AD symptoms were found to be reduced by an oral supplementation of *ImmuBalance* in NC/Tnd mice and it was as effective as topical treatment with FK506 ointment. It mainly showed anti-inflammatory effects on production of proinflammatory cytokines in lymphocytes. On the other hand, both high and low fractions of *ImmuBalance* extract suppressed nerve growth factor (NGF)-induced neurite out growth, explaining the antipruritic effect. Finally, it was confirmed that the administration of *ImmuBalance* could be a novel treatment of human AD without serious side effects.

18.4.2 Kefir

The word "*kefir*" derived from the Turkish word "*keif*," symbolizes the "good feeling" one gets after drinking it (Guzel-Seydim et al. 2011). *Kefir* is a fermented milk beverage, slightly acidic with a uniform creamy consistency. In Soviet countries, it has been anecdotally recommended for consumption by healthy people to lower the risk of chronic disease and also to patients for clinical treatment of gastrointestinal and metabolic diseases, ischemic heart disease, and allergy (St-Onge et al. 2002). *Kefir* is also a rich source of vitamins (B_{12} and K2), calcium, folate, and essential amino acids (Otles and Cagindi 2003). It shows antibacterial and antifungal properties as well (Cevikbas et al. 1994).

Fermentation of milk is achieved using *kefir* grains (soft matrix composed of proteins, lipids, a soluble polysaccharide, and a symbiotic community of bacteria *Lactobacillus kefiranofaciens* and yeast *Saccharomyces cerevisiae*), which are recovered after fermentation (Lopitz-Otsoa et al. 2006). Other LAB and yeasts identified in *kefir* grains include *Lactobacillus brevis, Lactobacillus helveticus, Lactobacillus kefir, Leuconostoc mesenteroides, Kluyveromyces lactis, Kluyveromyces marxianus,* and *Pichia fermentans* (Angulo et al. 1993, Lin 1999). Kefiran, an exopolysaccharide produced by *Lb. kefiranofaciens* in *kefir* grains has been suggested to show immunomodulatory effects by suppressing mast cell degranulation and cytokine production, establishing a role in reducing the inflammation associated with allergy. Another clinical study demonstrated that oral feeding of heat-inactivated *Lb. kefiranofaciens* M1 from *kefir* grains significantly inhibited IgE production by modulating the pattern and levels of cytokine production by Th1 and Th2 helper cells in response to ovalbumin (OVA). Further analysis of the immune response using flow cytometry and microarray also revealed upregulation of the expression of *Cd2, Stat4,* and *Ifnr* which skew the Th1/Th2 balance toward Th1 dominance, elevation of the $CD4^+CD25^+$regulatory T (Treg) percentage, and reduction of activated $CD19^+B$ cells. Hence, these findings suggested that *Lb. kefiranofaciens* M1 from *kefir* may have great potential as an antiallergic food and in its utilization in functional food products (Hong et al. 2010).

Soy milk can also be used for the preparation of *kefir* with added benefits. With no cholesterol or lactose and only small quantities of saturated fatty acids, soymilk offers tremendous nutritional health benefits. Studies also support the fact that consumption of fermented soymilk significantly increases the presence of probiotics and improves human intestinal gut microbiome (Cheng et al. 2005). Liu et al. (2006) studied the antiallergenic properties of soymilk *kefir* and its effect on the intestinal bacterial ecosystem of BALB/c mice. It was found that oral consumption of milk *kefir* and soymilk *kefir* for 28 days decreased the serum OVA-specific IgE and IgG1 levels. There was a significant increase in fecal populations of *Bifidobacteria* and *Lactobacillus* along with a significant decrease in the population of *Clostridium perfringens*. This study suggested milk *kefir* and soymilk *kefir* to be promising food systems in combating food allergy.

18.4.3 Red Ginseng

Ginseng (genus *Panax*, family *Araliaceae*)is a perennial plant with fleshy roots, containing ginsenoids as the pharmacologically active compounds (Vogler et al. 1999). Ginsenoids comprise the triterpenoid dammarane structure with variable number of sugar moieties. Red ginseng (RG) is produced by steaming white ginseng at high temperatures (Cho et al. 2006). *Panax ginseng* is harvested when 6 years old, peeled, and heated through steaming at 100°C, and then sun dried. RG is widely used as a traditional herbal medicine in Asian countries as it offers therapeutic properties of restoring normal well-being (Coon and Ernst 2002), enhancing sexual function, and has potent anticancer properties as well as antibiotic properties. RG may contain many biologically active compounds, although the effect of these compounds and their absorption depends upon number, activity, and composition of each individual's intestinal microflora. In the light of this fact, it was suggested that fermentation of RG by treatment with microorganisms and enzymes so as to increase the content of saponin may increase its efficacy (Babayigit et al. 2008, Bae et al. 2009).

Lee et al. (2012) studied the efficacy of RG and fermented red *ginseng* (FRG) on OVA-induced allergic responses in female BALB/c mice. 7-week-old mice were sensitized with 100 μL of OVA solution and 1 week later they were administered 0.1% and 0.3% RG and FRG. The mice sensitized with OVA showed an increased serum concentration of IgG_1, IgE, OVA-IgG_1, and OVA-IgE. In contrast, mice fed with a diet supplemented with RG and FRG showed reduced IgE and IgG_1 levels. OVA-specific IgE and IgG_1 were significantly reduced by 0.1% RG and FRG. There was also a significant suppression of proinflammatory cytokines, IFN-γ, and IL-2. Intestinal barrier-related markers (MMCP-1, IL-4, COX-2, and iNOS mRNA) were also suppressed by RG and FRG leading to reinforcement of the intestinal barrier and reducing the permeability of potential allergens in systemic circulation.

Jung et al. (2011) studied the therapeutic effects of FRG on allergic rhinitis in a double-blind placebo-controlled study. Symptomatic patients with persistent perennial allergic rhinitis were randomly divided into two groups: those receiving FRG tablets (soft capsules—250 mg/capsule) and those receiving a placebo (capsules filled with starch). After 4 weeks of medical treatment, two efficacy variables—total nasal symptom score (TNSS) being the primary variable while rhititis quality of life (RQoL) and skin-prick test being the secondary variables were considered for the study. TNSS scores for the experimental group showed a reduction over time for symptoms such as itching, sneezing, and runny nose while the results for nasal congestion were more encouraging with highly significant reduction compared to the control group, suggesting that FRG shows an early effect on nasal congestion. Also the experimental group showed significant improvement in emotional and activity states after 4 weeks of medication. In the skin-prick test, reduction in size of wheals and flares for histamine and other perennial allergens in experimental groups compared with the control group showed FRG to have an effect not only on histamine but also on other specific allergens.

18.4.4 Milk Products

A long-term consumption of yogurt and other LAB-containing foods have shown alleviation of some of the clinical symptoms of allergy such as atopic rhinitis and nasal allergies and lower IgE levels in serum (Van de Water et al. 1999). Though the mode of alleviation of allergic symptoms is unknown in this case, it is a well-accepted fact that LAB-containing foods are able to promote deviation away from a proallergy phenotype via the mechanism of immunemodulation. The antiallergic effects of LAB have been well reported but very few tablets and powder formulations are available in the market (Peng et al. 2007). The problems associated with these formulations are survivability, loss of efficiency in establishing in the gut, and the psychological illness of patients. These limitations can be overcome by the addition of probiotic LAB in the food, that is, milk products. It also provides nutritional benefits along with health benefits.

18.4.4.1 Fermented Milk

Peng et al. (2007) assessed the antiallergic effect of fermented milk prepared with *Streptococcus thermophilus* MC, *Lactobacillus acidophilus* B, *Lactobacillus bulgaricus* Lb, *Lb. bulgaricus* 448, and *Bifidobacterium longum* B6. Female BALB/c mice were fed fermented milk and immunized intraperitoneally with OVA/complete Freund's adjuvant (CFA). The immune response was observed by evaluating the secretion of cytokines IL-2, IL-4, and IFN-γ and serum antibody IgE. A significant change was not observed in IL-2 spontaneous and OVA-stimulated secretions of splenocytes after supplementation with LAB fermented milk. However, both spontaneous and OVA-stimulated secretions of splenocytes from mice fed LAB fermented milk showed significantly ($P < 0.05$) lower levels of IL-4 (Th2 cytokine) than those from OVA/CFA-immunized mice fed nonfermented milk (Peng et al. 2007). The milk fermented with LAB demonstrated *in vivo* antiallergenic effects on OVA/CFA-immunized mice via increasing the secretion ratio of IFN-γ/IL-4 (Th1/Th2) by splenocytes and decreasing the serum level of OVA-specific IgE.

Kawase et al. (2009) have shown the effect of fermented milk prepared with two probiotic strains on JCP in a double-blind placebo-controlled clinical study. Fermented milk prepared with the *Lactobacillus* GG (LGG) and *Lb. gasseri* TMC0356 (TMC0356) or placebo yogurt was administered for 10 weeks to 40 subjects with a clinical history of JCP f. The mean symptom score for nasal blockage was decreased by consumption of the fermented milk after 9 weeks. The tested strains of LAB-affected cytokine in a strain-dependent manner. The LGG significantly inhibited IL-4 and IL-5 production by peripheral blood mononuclear cells (PBMCs), whereas TMC0356 only suppressed IL-5 production. The fermented milk prepared with LGG and TMC0356 may be beneficial in JCP because of its effect on nasal blockage. The capability of fermented milk to specifically downregulate human Th2 immune response may explain the above results.

18.4.4.2 Yogurt

Dairy products provide a suitable buffering environment and essential nutrients for the growth of LAB. Considering this fact, incorporation of two newly established probiotic strains (*Lb. acidophilus* and *Lactobacillus casei*) in yogurt is more common (Yadav et al. 2005). Jain et al. (2008, 2010) have studied the antiallergic effect of a *dahi* containing probiotic *Lb. acidophilus*, *Lb. casei*, and normal *dahi* culture *Lc. lactis biovar diacetylactis* (named probiotic *dahi*) on OVA-induced allergy in mice. Feeding of probiotic *dahi* completely suppressed the elevation of total and OVA-specific IgE in the serum of OVA-injected mice. Similarly, total and OVA-specific IgE production property of splenocytes was lost in mice fed with probiotic *dahi*. Production of T helper (Th)-1 cell-specific cytokines, that is, IFN-γ and interleukin (IL)-2, increased, while Th2-specific cytokines, that is, IL-4 and IL-6, decreased in the supernatant of cultured splenocytes collected from mice fed with probiotic *dahi*. Moreover, OVA-stimulated lymphocyte proliferation was strongly suppressed by the feeding of probiotic *dahi* in comparison with milk and control *dahi*.

18.4.5 Fermented Fish Oil

Fish oil has been reported as antiallergenic. Fish oil intake alleviates the severity of AD, eczema, and asthma, and downregulates the expression of IL 1, 4, and 13 and IFN-γ in serum (Krauss-Etschmann et al. 2008, Seki et al. 2010). Various omega-3 polyunsaturated fatty acids (n-3 PUFAs) present in fish oil include eicosapentaenoic acid (EPA) and docosahexaenoic acid (DHA) (Seki et al. 2010). EPA is shown to inhibit the production of proinflammatory cytokines (IL-2, IL-12, and IFN-γ), upregulate the expression of anti-inflammatory cytokines (IL-10), and increase the number of Foxp3 and regulatory T cells (Tregs) (Hara et al .2001). DHA helps in reducing the proliferation of effector T cells by increasing mRNA expression of Foxp3, TGF-ß, and IL-10 from Tregs (Yessoufou et al. 2009).

AD is an allergic skin inflammation characterized by pruritus and inflammation, and is regulated partly through the activity of regulatory T cells (Tregs). Differentiation, proliferation, and function of various immune cells including CD4+ T cells are regulated by Tregs. A tremendous capacity of the fermentation process to transform chemical structures to new structures is very common. The beneficial effects of natural fish oil (NFO) have been described in many diseases, but the mechanism of fermented fish oil (FFO) to modulate the immune system and the allergic response is poorly understood. Han et al. (2012) produced FFO and tested its ability to activate CD4, CD25, Foxp3, and Tregs and suppress the allergic inflammatory response. Effectiveness of FFO over NFO was seen by administrating FFO or NFO in drinking water which showed alleviated allergic inflammation in the skin. Immune-suppressive cytokines TGF-β and IL-10 were found to be increased after FFO treatment. Further, increased Foxp3 expression and increased number of CD4, CD25, Foxp3, and Tregs were also found after FFO ingestion. Hence, FFO may be effective in treating the allergic symptoms of AD.

18.4.6 Fermented Dough

Bread has two common allergens, namely gluten and ovomucoid from hen eggs. To overcome the effect of these allergens on the allergy sufferer, it is necessary to find a way to prepare allergen-free bread. The interaction between the allergens in hen eggs (mainly ovomucoid) and gluten also has an effect on the allergy. Toyosaki (2007) determined the effects of peroxides on allergic reactions by closely investigating the relationship between peroxides and proteins. Peroxides are produced from the induction of lipid peroxidation reactions in the process of dough fermentation. The antiallergenic effect of hydroperoxides present in fermented dough on antigen–antibody reaction involving IgE was examined. Crude proteins extracted from the dough including hydroperoxides showed weaker antigen–antibody reactions on allergic tests such as the precipitin ring test with human-specific IgE, and the IgE-binding activity on enzyme-linked immunosorbent assay (ELISA). This inhibitory effect on the antigen–antibody reaction increased with an increased concentration of hydroperoxide. The crude proteins extracted from the dough with hydroperoxides were separated by using affinity chromatography and SDS-PAGE. Each separated protein was examined for the IgE-binding activity on ELISA (Toyosaki 2007). Crude proteins obtained from the dough with hydroperoxide addition during fermentation showed weaker IgE-binding activity on ELISA than proteins of bread made from dough without hydroperoxides. The allergic protein in the dough may be denatured by hydroperoxide which may suppress the antigen–antibody reactions with IgE.

18.4.7 Fermented Preparations from Citrus and Cydonia Fruits

Preparations from lemon, *Citrus medica* L. (citrus) and quince, *Cydonia oblonga* Mill. (Cydonia) are used in pharmaceutical products to treat patients suffering from allergic disorders. Huber et al. (2012) set up an experiment to investigate the immunomodulatory and antiallergenic properties of these preparations. The efficacy was analyzed by their effect on the degranulation capacity from basophilic cells and mediator release from activated human mast cells *in vitro*, including IL-8 and TNF-α secretion. Citrus showed a diminished activity of degranulation of basophilic cells which was comparable to the synthetic drug azelastine. Furthermore, production of IL-8 and TNF-α from human mast cells was found to be inhibited by both citrus and cydonia, which also showed an additive effect at low concentrations. Hence, the data published showed the possibility of use of citrus and cydonia in the treatment of allergic disorders.

18.4.8 Fermented Cabbage

In China, people utilize various ingredients such as *tofu*, mustard, cabbage, and bamboo shoot to produce diverse fermented food products. The manufacturing processes and ingredients give unique flavors to these fermented foods (Li and Hsieh 2004). However, the LAB and other microbes present in these fermented foods are not very well known. Mei et al. (2013) isolated 96 different strains of LAB from various traditional fermented foods in Taiwan. Among these strains, *Lc. lactis* A17 (A17), a strain isolated from fermented cabbage showed significant immunomodulatory potency. The OVA-sensitized BALB/c mice were orally administered live or heat-killed A17. Both live and heat-killed A17 showed modulation in OVA-induced allergic effects. It showed modulation of B-cell response by diminishing IgE production and raising OVA-specific IgG2a production whereas it modulates the T-cell response by increasing IFN- γ production and decreasing IL-4 production.

18.4.9 Potential Antiallergenic Fermented Foods

There are some foods which are prepared by fermentation using LAB making them potentially antiallergenic (Macfarlane and Cummings 1999). Literature on these foods is scant. Hence, investigations and further studies need to be encouraged in this area for exploring their allergy fighting properties. Some representative examples are discussed below.

18.4.9.1 Stinky Tofu

A fermented *tofu* with strong odor is called stinky *tofu*. It is a very popular snack in the Asian region where it is sold at night markets. Traditionally, brine is prepared using fermented milk, vegetable, and meat which take several months for fermentation. Freshly prepared *tofu* is marinated in the brine for a day or two to prepare stinky *tofu*. Though it is commonly used, the LAB indigenous to the fermented brine from which it is made remains poorly understood. Chao et al. (2008) had examined 168 isolates obtained from the original fermented brine (brine A) and two brines in which the hard *tofu* (brine B) and soft *tofu* (brine C) had been soaked. The random amplified polymorphic DNA (RAPD) analysis and 16S rDNA sequencing were used to identify strains. Total 136 representative strains were identified which belong to 7 genera and 32 species: *Enterococcus* (2 species), *Lactobacillus* (14 species), *Lactococcus* (3 species), *Leuconostoc* (6 species), *Pediococcus* (1 species), *Streptococcus* (2 species), and *Weissella* (4 species).

18.4.9.2 Fu-Tsai and Suan-Tsai

The Hakka tribe of Taiwan prepares traditional spontaneously fermented mustard products known as *fu-tsai* and *suan-tsai*. Chao et al. (2009) isolated a variety of LAB strains from five different processing stages of these products and identified them using 16S rRNA gene sequencing. They found 119 representative strains belonging to 5 genera and 18 species, including *Enterococcus* (1 species), *Lactobacillus* (11 species), *Leuconostoc* (3 species), *Pediococcus* (1 species), and *Weissella* (2 species).

18.4.9.3 Tarhana

Tarhana is a traditional fermented product prepared in Turkey using a mixture of spontaneously fermented yogurt and wheat flour. It is made by mixing flour, yogurt or sour milk, and optionally cooked vegetables, salt, and spices. The mixture is fermented, dried, and ground. The lactic acid produced during fermentation gives a characteristic sour taste and good preservative properties. The pH is about 3.4–4.2. The drying step reduces the moisture content to 6%–10% which makes the medium unsuitable to pathogens and spoilage organisms, and preserves the milk proteins (Daglioglu 2000). Sengun et al. (2009) isolated and identified various strains of LAB during the processing of *tarhana* which included *Pediococcus acidilactici* (27%), *Strep. thermophilus* (19%), *Lactobacillus fermentum* (19%), *Ent. faecium* (12%), *Pediococcus pentosaceus* (7%), *Leuconostoc pseudomesenteroides* (5%), *Weissella cibaria* (4%), *Lb. plantarum* (2%), *Lactobacillus delbrueckii* spp. *bulgaricus* (2%), *Leuconostoc citreum* (2%), *Lactobacillus paraplantarum* (1%), and *Lb. casei* (0.5%).

18.4.10 Pu-erh Tea

Tea is one of the most widely consumed beverages in the world. Depending on the method of production, tea can be classified as green tea (unfermented tea), oolong tea (partially fermented tea), black tea (fully fermented tea), and *pu-erh* tea (post fermented tea) (Yamazaki et al. 2012). *Pu-erh* tea is prepared by fermenting green tea leaves with microorganisms such as *Aspergillus*, *Strep. bacillaris*, and *Strep. cinereus* (Jeng et al. 2007, Hou et al. 2010). Yamazaki et al. (2012) investigated the protective action of *pu-erh* tea on an oxazolon-induced mouse type IV allergy. They found that oral administration of 50 mg/kg water extract of *pu-erh* tea showed potent prevention against increase in levels of proinflammatory cytokines specifically IL-12, which is secreted by macrophage-like antigen presenting cells. The effects of "Theabrownin-like fraction" (TBW-ND), the polyphenol complex of pu-erh tea were also studied by oral and percutaneous administration at doses of 18.7 mg/kg and 0.037 mg/ear. A significant decrease in proinflammatory cytokines was observed. It was also found that TBW-ND, the antiallergenic active components are present as complexes consisting of catechins, polysaccharides, and/or proteins.

18.4.11 Fermented Grapes

Polyphenols (flavonoids) have been extensively studied as potent antiallergens. They can alleviate allergic symptoms by modulating the process of allergy formation by directly affecting mast cells and controlling release of inflammatory mediators. Since polyphenols also possess antioxidant capacity they minimize the cellular injury caused by free radicals during allergic responses (Singh et al. 2011). One of the natural foods effective in decreasing effectors of allergy is grape fermented by LAB. Two varieties of black grapes *(Vitis vinifera)*, Negroamaro (Italy) and Koshu (Japan) have been extensively used in studies for their ability to turn down allergic responses. Administration of Koshu-fermented Grape Marc (K-FGM) have shown to reduce the IgE production and eosinophil count in bronchial alveolar lavage fluid in a model of murine asthma. Negroamaro and K-FGM have both shown to suppress human basophil degranulation (Marzulli et al. 2014). Tominaga et al. (2010) investigated the inhibitory effects of lyophilized fine powder of skin and seeds of koshu grapes fermented with *Lb. plantarum* on type 1 allergic response in mice. Oral administration of fermented Grape Marc to BALB/c mice primed with OVA resulted in a significant decrease in the levels of serum IgE compared to the controls. Oral administration of FGM, 30 min prior to OVA challenge significantly suppressed the passive cutaneous anaphylaxis. A clinical study on antiallergenic effect of Koshu grape pomace fermented with *Lb. plantarum* NB strain on rat basophilic leukemia cells showed a significant preventive action on mast cell degranulation (Kondo et al. 2011).

18.5 Conclusions

Food allergy is one of the major concerns worldwide which needs to be addressed for health and nutritive benefits. Use of antiallergenic foods can be a potential approach to solve the allergic response to many foods with their persistent nutritive value. Proteins are known allergens in many food components. Fermentation, specifically by LAB, reduces the immunogenicity of the allergenic protein and also shows immunomodulation. These mechanisms help enhance antiallergenic properties of fermented foods. Fermented foods in all parts of the world based on a wide range of food resources need urgent attention in this respect. Further, the effect of food processing after fermentation on the antiallerginic properties needs to be investigated.

References

Aattouri, N. and D. Lemonnier. 1997. Production of interferon induced by *Streptococcus thermophilus*: Role of CD4+ and CD8+ lymphocytes. *The Journal of Nutritional Biochemistry* 8: 25–31.

Angulo, L., E. Lopez, and C. Lema. 1993. Microflora present in *kefir* grains of the Galician region (northwest of Spain). *Journal of Dairy Research* 60: 263–267.

Babayigit, A., D. Olmez, O. Karaman, H. A. Bagriyanik, O. Yilmaz, B. Kivcak, G. Erbil, and N. Uzuner. 2008. Ginseng ameliorates chronic histopathologic changes in a murine model of asthma. *Allergy and Asthma Proceedings* 29: 493–498.

Babu, K. S., S. H. Arshad, and S. T. Holgate. 2001. Anti-IgE treatment: An update. *Allergy* 56: 1121–1128.

Bae, E. A., H. T. Trinh, H. K. Yoon, and D. H. Kim. 2009. Compound K, a metabolite of ginsenoside Rb1, inhibits passive cutaneous anaphylaxis reaction in mice. *Journal of Ginseng Research* 33: 93–98.

Bashir, M. E., S. Louie, H. N. Shi, and C. Nagler-Anderson. 2004. Toll-like receptor 4 signaling by intestinal microbes influences susceptibility to food allergy. *Journal of Immunology* 172(11): 6978–6987.

Beltrani, V. S. 2005. Suggestions regarding a more appropriate understanding of atopic dermatitis. *Current Opinions in Allergy and Clinical Immunology* 5: 413–418.

Beyer, K. and S. Teuber. 2004. The mechanism of food allergy: What do we know today. *Current Opinion in Allergy and Clinical Immunology* 4: 197–199.

Cevikbas, A., E. Yemni, F. W. Ezzedenn, T. Yardimici, U. Cevikbas, and S. J. Stohs. 1994. Antitumoural, antibacterial and antifungal activities of *kefir* and *kefir* grain. *Phytotherapy Research* 8(2): 78–82.

Chao, S. H., Y. Tomii, K. Watanabe, and Y. C. Tsai. 2008. Diversity of lactic acid bacteria in fermented brines used to make stinky tofu. *International Journal of Food Microbiology* 123(1–2): 134–141.

Chao, S. H., R. J. Wu, K. Watanabe, and Y. C. Tsai. 2009. Diversity of lactic acid bacteria in *suan-tsai* and *fu-tsai*, traditional fermented mustard products of Taiwan. *International Journal of Food Microbiology* 135(3): 203–210.

Cheng, I. C., H. F. Shang, T. F. Lin, T. H. Wang, H. S. Lin, and S. H. Lin. 2005. Effect of fermented soy milk on the intestinal bacterial ecosystem. *World Journal of Gastroenterology* 11: 1225–1227.

Cho, W. C., W. S. Chung, S. K. Lee, A. W. Leung, C. H. Cheng, and K. K. Yue. 2006. Ginsenoside Re of *Panax ginseng* possesses significant antioxidant and antihyperlipidemic efficacies in streptozotocin-induced diabetic rats. *European Journal of Pharmacology* 550 (1–3): 173–179.

Cianferoni, A. and J. M. Spergel. 2009. Food allergy: Review, classification and diagnosis. *Allergology International* 58: 457–466.

Coon, J. T. and E. Ernst. 2002. Review *Panax ginseng*: A systematic review of adverse effects and drug interactions. *Drug Safety* 25(5): 323–344.

Cross, M. L., L. M. Stevenson, and H. S. Gill. 2001. Anti-allergy properties of fermented foods: An important immunoregulatory mechanism of lactic acid bacteria? *International Immunopharmacology* 1: 891–901.

Daglioglu, O. 2000. *Tarhana* as a traditional Turkish fermented cereal food: Its recipe, production and composition. *Nahrung* 44(2): 85–88.

Flohr, C., D. Pascoe, and H. C. Williams. 2005. Atopic dermatitis and the "hygiene hypothesis": Too clean to be true? *British Journal of Dermatology* 152(2): 202–216.

Frias, J., Y. S. Song, C. Martinez-Villaluenga, E. G. De Mejia, and C. Vidal-Valverde. 2008. Immunoreactivity and amino acid content of fermented soybean products. *Journal of Agricultural and Food Chemistry* 56: 99–105.

Guzel-Seydim, Z. B., T. Kok-Tas, A. K. Greene, and A. C. Seydim. 2011. Review: Functional properties of *kefir*. *Critical Reviews in Food Science and Nutrition* 51: 261–268.

Hamelmann, E. and E. W. Gelfand. 1999. Role of IL-5 in the development of allergen-induced airway hyperresponsiveness. *International Archives of Allergy Immunology* 120: 8–16.

Han, S-C., G-J. Kang, Y-J. Ko, H-K. Kang, S-W. Moon, Y-S. Ann, and E-S. Yoo. 2012. Fermented fish oil suppresses T helper 1/2 cell response in a mouse model of atopic dermatitis via generation of CD4 + CD25 + Foxp3 + T cells. *Biomedical Central Immunology* 13: 44–56.

Hara, M., C. I. Kingsley, M. Niimi, S. Read, S. E. Turvey, A. R. Bushell, P. J. Morris, F. Powrie, and K. J. Wood. 2001. IL-10 is required for regulatory T cells to mediate tolerance to alloantigens in vivo. *Journal of Immunology* 166: 3789–3796.

Hong, K-J., C-H. Lee, and S-W. Kim. 2004. *Aspergillus oryzae* GB-107 fermentation improves nutritional quality of food soybean and feed soybean meals. *Journal of Medicinal Food* 7: 430–435.

Hong, W-S., Y-P. Chen, and M-J. Chen. 2010. The antiallergic effect of *Kefir* lactobacilli. *Journal of Food Science* 75(8):244–253.

Hou, C. W., K. C. Jeng, and Y. S. Chen. 2010. Enhancement of fermentation process in pu-erh tea by tea leaf extract. *Journal of Food Science* 75: 44–48.

Huber, R., F. C. Stintzing, D. Briemle, C. Beckmann, U. Meyer, and C. Grundemann. 2012. *In vitro* antiallergic effects of aqueous fermented preparations from citrus and cydonia fruits. *Planta Medica* 78(4): 334–340.

Ishida, Y., I. Bandou, H. Kanzato, and N. Yamamoto. 2003. Decrease in ovalbumin specific IgE of mice serum after oral uptake of lactic acid bacteria. *Bioscience Biotechnology and Biochemistry* 67: 951–957.

Isolauri, E., H. Majamaa, T. Arvola, I. Rantala, E. Virtanen, and H. Arvilommi. 1993. *Lactobacillus casei* strain GG reverses increased intestinal permeability induced by cow milk in suckling rats. *Gastroenterology* 105: 1643–1650.

Jain, S., H. Yadav, and P. R. Sinha. 2008. Stimulation of innate immunity by oral administration of dahi containing probiotic *Lactobacillus casei* in mice. *Journal of Medicinal Food* 11: 652–656.

Jain, S., H. Yadav, P. R. Sinha, S. Kapila, S. Naito, and F. Marotta. 2010. Anti-allergic effects of probiotic *dahi* through modulation of the gut immune system. *Turkish Journal of Gastroenterology* 21(3): 244–250.

Jeng, K. C., C. S. Chen, Y. P. Fang, C. W. Hou, and Y. S. Chen. 2007. Effect of microbial fermentation on content of statin, GABA, and polyphenols in pu-erh tea. *Journal of Agricultural and Food Chemistry* 55: 8787–8792.

Jung, J-W., H-R. Kang, G-E. Ji, M-S. Park, W-J. Song, M-H. Kim, J-W. Kwon et al. 2011. Therapeutic effects of fermented Red ginseng in allergic rhinitis: A randomized, double-blind, placebo-controlled study. *Allergy Asthma and Immunology Research* 3(2): 103–110.

Kanda, T., H. Akiyama, A. Yanagida, M. Tanabe, Y. Goda, M. Toyoda, R. Teshima, and Y. Saito. 1998. Inhibitory effects of apple polyphenol on induced histamine release from RBL-2H3 cells and rat mast cells. *Bioscience, Biotechnology and Biochemistry* 62: 1284–1289.

Kawase, M., F. He, A. Kubota, M. Hiramatsu, H. Saito, T. Ishii, H. Yasueda, and K. Akiyama. 2009. Effect of fermented milk prepared with two probiotic strains on Japanese cedar pollinosis in a double-blind placebo-controlled clinical study. *International Journal of Food Microbiology* 128(3): 429–434.

Kikuchi, T. and T. Yokotsuka. 1972. Studies on the polysaccharides from soy sauce. Part I. Purification and properties of two acidic polysaccharides. *Agricultural and Biological Chemistry* 36: 544–550.

Kitazawa, H., T. Itoh, Y. Tomioka, M. Mizugaki, and T. Yamaguchi. 1996. Induction of IFN-gamma and IL-1 alpha production in macrophages stimulated with phosphopolysaccharide produced by *Lactococcus lactis* sp. *cremoris*. *International Journal of Food Microbiology* 31: 99–106.

Kobayashi, M. 2005. Immunological functions of soy sauce: Hypoallergenicity and antiallergic activity of soy sauce. *Journal of Bioscience and Bioengineering* 100(2): 144–151.

Kobayashi, M., H. Matsushita, K. Yoshida, R. Tsukiyama, T. Sugimura, and K. Yamamoto. 2004. *In vitro* and *in vivo* anti-allergic activity of soy sauce. *International Journal of Molecular Medicine* 14: 879–884.

Kobayashi, M., H. Matsushita, R. Tsukiyama, M. Saito, and T. Sugita. 2005. Shoyu polysaccharides from soy sauce improve quality of life for patients with seasonal allergic rhinitis: A double-blind placebo-controlled clinical study. *International Journal of Molecular Medicine* 15(3): 463–467.

Kondo, K., K. Nakamura, Y. Hamauzu, T. Kawahara, H. Sansawa, M. Suzuki, and H. Yasui. 2011. Inhibitory effect of fermented grape pomace on degranulation in RBL-2H3 cells and an analysis of its active ingredients. *Food Science and Technology Research* 17(3): 241–250.

Krauss-Etschmann, S., D. Hartl, P. Rzehak, J. Heinrich, R. Shadid, M. Del Carmen Ramirez-Tortosa, C. Campoy et al. 2008. Nutraceuticals for healthier life study group: Decreased cord blood IL-4, IL-13, and CCR4 and increased TGF-beta levels after fish oil supplementation of pregnant women. *Journal of Allergy and Clinical Immunology* 121: 464–470.

Lee, E. J., M. J. Song, H. S. Kwon, G. E. Ji, and M. K. Sung. 2012. Oral administration of fermented red ginseng suppressed ovalbumin-induced allergic responses in female BALB/c mice. *Phytomedicine* 19(10): 896–903.

Leung, D. J., Jr. W. R. Shanahan, and H. A. Sampson. 2004. New approaches for the treatment of anaphylaxis. *Novartis Foundation Symposium* 257: 248–260.

Leung, D. Y. 2000. Atopic dermatitis: New insights and opportunities for therapeutic intervention. *Journal of Allergy and Clinical Immunology* 105: 860–876.

Li, J. R. and Y. H. P. Hsieh. 2004. Traditional Chinese food technology and cuisine. *Asia Pacific Journal of Clinical Nutrition* 13(2): 147–155.

Lin, C. W., C. L. Chen, and J. R. Liu. 1999. Identification and characterisation of lactic acid bacteria and yeasts isolated from kefir grains in Taiwan. *Australian Journal of Dairy Technology* 54: 14–18.

Liu, J-R., S-Y. Wang, M-J. Chen, P-Y. Yueh, and C-W. Lin. 2006. The anti-allergenic properties of milk *kefir* and soymilk *kefir* and their beneficial effects on the intestinal microflora. *Journal of the Science of Food and Agriculture* 86: 2527–2533.

Lopitz-Otsoa, F., A. Rementeria, N. Elguezabal, and J. Garaizar. 2006. *Kefir*: A symbiotic yeast-bacteria community with alleged health capabilities. *Iberoamerican Journal of Mycology* 23: 67–74.

Macfarlane, G. T. and J. H. Cummings. 1999. Probiotics and prebiotics: Can regulating the activities of intestinal bacteria benefit health? *British Medical Journal* 318: 999–1003.

Manabe, M., K. Tanaka, T. Goto, and S. Matsura. 1984. Producing capability of kojic acid and aflatoxin by koji mould. *Developments in Food Science* 7: 4–14.

Marzulli, G. A., T. A. Magrone, L. A. Vonghia, M. B. Kaneko, H. B. Takimoto, Y. C. Kumazawa, and J. De. 2014. Immunomodulating and anti-allergic effects of Negroamaro and Koshu *Vitis vinifera* fermented grape marc (FGM). *Current Pharmaceutical Design* 20(6): 864–868.

Matsuda, A., A. Tanaka, W. Pan, N. Okamoto, K. Oida, N. Kingyo, Y. Amagai et al. 2012. Supplementation of the fermented soy product ImmuBalance™ effectively reduces itching behavior of atopic NC/Tnd mice. *Journal of Dermatological Science* 67: 130–139.

Matsuzaki, T., R. Yamazaki, S. Hashimoto, and T. Yokokura. 1998. The effect of oral feeding of *Lactobacillus casei* strain Shirota on immunoglobulin E production in mice. *Journal of Dairy Sciences* 81: 48–53.

Mei, H-C., Y-W. Liu, Y-C. Chiang, S-H. Chao, N-W. Mei, Y-W. Liu, and Y-C. Tsai. 2013. Immunomodulatory activity of *Lactococcus lactis* A17 from Taiwan fermented cabbage in OVA-sensitized BALB/c mice. *Evidence-Based Complementary and Alternative Medicine* 1–11 (not available).

Miyake, Y., S. Sasaki, Y. Ohya, S. Miyamoto, I. Matsunaga, and T. Yoshida. 2005. Soy, isoflavones, and prevalence of allergic rhinitis in Japanese women: The Osaka maternal and child health study. *Journal of Allergy and Clinical Immunology* 115(6): 1176–1183.

Morita, H., F. He, M. Kawase, A. Kubota, M. Hiramatsu, J. Kurisaki, and S. Salminen. 2006. Preliminary human study for possible alteration of serum immunoglobulin E production in perennial allergic rhinitis with fermented milk prepared with *Lactobacillus gasseri* TMC0356. *Microbiology and Immunology* 50: 701–706.

Nowak-Wegrzyn, A. and H. A. Sampson. 2004. Food allergy therapy. *Immunology Allergy Clinics of North America* 24(4): 705–725.

Nowak-Wegrzyn, A. and H. A. Sampson. 2006. Adverse reactions to foods. *Medical Clinics of North America* 90: 97–127.

Ogawa, A., M. Samoto, and K. Takahashi. 2000. Soybean allergens and hypoallergenic soybean products. *Journal of Nutritional Science and Vitaminology* 46(6):271–279.

Ohno, H., S. Tsunemine, Y. Isa, M. Shimakawa, and H. Yamamura. 2005. Oral administration of *Bifidobacterium bifidum* G9–1 suppresses total and antigen specific immunoglobulin E production in mice. *Biological and Pharmaceutical Bulletin* 28: 1462–1466.

Oppenheimer, J. J., H. S. Nelson, S. A. Bock, F. Christensen, and D. Y. Leung. 1992. Treatment of peanut allergy with rush immunotherapy. *Journal of Allergy and Clinical Immunology* 90(2): 256–262.

Ortolani, C. and E. A. Pastorello. 2006. Food allergies and food intolerances. *Best Practice and Research Clinical Gastroenterology* 20(3): 467–483.

Otles, S. and O. Cagindi. 2003. *Kefir*: A probiotic dairy-composition, nutritional and therapeutic aspects. *Pakistan Journal of Nutrition* 2: 54–59.

Otsuka, Y. and W. Pan. 2005. Effects of the novel symbiotic ImmuBalance as a food supplement in relieving clinical symptoms of Japanese cedar pollinosis: A pilot study. *Clinical and Experimental Pharmacology and Physiology* 34: 73–75.

Penas, E., P. Restani, C. Ballabio, G. Prestamo, A. Fiocchi, and R. Gomez. 2005. Assessment of residual immunoreactivity of soybean whey hydrolysates obtained by combined enzymatic proteolysis and high pressure. *European Food Research and Technology* 222: 286–290.

Pene, J., F. Rousset, F. Briere, I. Chretien, J-Y. Bonnefoy, and H. Spits. 1988. IgE production by normal human lymphocytes is induced by interleukin 4 and suppressed by interleukins gamma and alpha and prostaglandin E2. *Proceedings of the National Academy of Sciences* 85: 6880–6885.

Peng, S. J-Y. Lin, and M-Y. Lin. 2007. Antiallergic effect of milk fermented with lactic acid bacteria in a murine animal model. *Journal of Agricultural and Food Chemistry* 55(13): 5092–5096.

Pons, L., U. Ponnappan, R. A. Hall, P. Simpson, G. Cockrell, and C. M. West. 2004. Soy immunotherapy for peanut-allergic mice: Modulation of the peanut-allergic response. *Journal of Allergy and Clinical Immunology* 114(4): 915–921.

Punnonen, J., G. Aversa, B. G. Cocks, and J. E. De Vries. 1994. Role of interleukin-4 and interleukin-13 in synthesis of IgE and expression of CD23 by human B cells. *Allergy* 49: 576–586.

Sampson, H. A. 1999. Food allergy. Part 2: Diagnosis and management. *Journal of Allergy and Clinical Immunology* 103: 981–989.

Sampson, H. A. 2001 Immunological approaches to the treatment of food allergy. *Paediatric Allergy and Immunology* 12(14): 91–96.

Sampson, H. A. 2004. Update on food allergy. *Journal of Allergy and Clinical Immunology* 113(5): 805–819.

Sampson, H. A., L. Mendelson, and J. P. Rosen. 1992. Fatal and near-fatal anaphylactic reactions to food in children and adolescents. *New England Journal of Medicine* 327: 380–384.

Seki, H., T. Sasaki, T. Ueda, and M. Arita. 2010. Resolvins as regulators of the immune system. *Scientific World Journal* 10: 818–831.

Sengun, I. Y., D. S. Nielsen, M. Karapinar, and M. Jakobsen. 2009. Identification of lactic acid bacteria isolated from Tarhana, a traditional Turkish fermented food. *International Journal of Food Microbiology* 135(2): 105–111.

Shekib, L. A. 1994. Nutritional improvement of lentils, chickpea, rice and wheat by natural fermentation. *Plant Foods for Human Nutrition* 46: 201–205.

Sicherer, S. H. and H. A. Sampson. 2009. Food allergy: Recent advances in pathophysiology and treatment. *Annual Review of Medicine* 60: 261–277.

Singh, A., S. Holvoet, and A. Mercenier. 2011. Dietary polyphenols in the prevention and treatment of allergic diseases. *Clinical and Experimental Allergy* 41(10): 1346–1359.

Sinigaglia, F., D. D'Ambrosio, and L. Rogge. 1999. Type I interferons and the Th1/Th2 paradigm. *Developmental and Comparative Immunology* 23: 657–663.

St-Onge, M. P., E. R. Farnworth, T. Savard, D. Chabot, A. Mafu, and P. J. H. Jones. 2002. *Kefir* consumption does not alter plasma lipid levels or cholesterol fractional synthesis rates relative to milk in hyperlipidemic men: A randomized controlled trial. *BMC Complementary and Alternative Medicine* 2: 1–7.

Taylor, S. L. and S. L. Hefle. 2001. Food allergies and other food sensitivities. *Food Technology* 55: 68–83.

Tominaga, T., K. Kawaguchi, M. Kanesaka, H. Kawauchi, E. Jirillo, and Y. Kumazawa. 2010. Suppression of type-I allergic responses by oral administration of grape marc fermented with *Lactobacillus plantarum*. *Immunopharmacology and Immunotoxicology* 32(4): 593–599.

Toyosaki, T. 2007. Anti-allergic effects on addition of hydroperoxide to dough fermentation. *African Journal of Food Science* 1: 51–55.

Valenta, R. 2002. The future of antigen specific immunotherapy of allergy. *Nature Reviews Immunology* 2: 446–453.

Van de Water, J., C. L. Keen, and M. E. Gershwin. 1999. The influence of chronic yogurt consumption on immunity. *Journal of Nutrition* 129: 1492–1495.

Vogler, B. K., M. H. Pittler, and E. Ernst. 1999. The efficacy of ginseng. A systematic review of randomised clinical trials. *European Journal of Clinical Pharmacology* 55: 567–575.

Wheeler, J. G., M. L. Bogle, S. J. Shema, M. A. Shirrell, K. C. Stine, and A. J. Pittler. 1997. Impact of dietary yogurt on immune function. *American Journal of Medical Sciences* 313: 120–123.

Wilson, S., K. Blaschek, and E. Gonzalez de Mejia. 2005. Allergenic proteins in soybean: Processing and reduction of P34 allergenicity. *Nutrition Reviews* 63: 47–58.

Yadav, H., S. Jain, and P. R. Sinha. 2005. Preparation of low fat probiotic. *Journal of Dairying Foods and Home Sci*ences 24: 172–177.

Yamanihi, R., T. Huang, H. Tsuji, N. Bando, and T. Ogawa. 1995. Reduction of the soybean allergenicity by the fermentation with *Bacillus natto*. *Food Science and Technology International* 1: 14–17.

Yamazaki, K., K. Yoshino, C. Yagi, T. Miyase, and M. Sano. 2012. Inhibitory effects of pu-erh tea leaves on mouse type IV allergy. *Food and Nutrition Sciences* 3: 394–400.

Yan, B. M. and E. A. Shaffer. 2009. Primary eosinophilic disorders of the gastrointestinal tract. *Gut* 58: 721–732.

Yessoufou, A., A. Ple, K. Moutairou, A. Hichami, and N. A. Khan. 2009. Docosahexaenoic acid reduces suppressive and migratory functions of CD4 + CD25+ regulatory T-cells. *Journal of Lipid Research* 50: 2377–2388.

Yeung, V. P., R. S. Gieni, D. T. Umetsu, and R. H. De Kruyff. 1998. Heat-killed *Listeria monocytogenes* as an adjuvant converts established murine Th2-dominated immune responses into Th1-dominated responses. *Journal of Immunology* 161: 4146–4152.

Zhang, T., W. Pan, M. Takebe, B. Schofield, H. Sampson, and X-M. Li. 2008. Therapeutic effects of a fermented soy product on peanut hypersensitivity is associated with modulation of Th1 and Th2 responses. *Clinical and Experimental Allergy* 38(11): 1808–1818.

Chapter 19

Antioxidants in Fermented Foods

Santa Ram Joshi and Koel Biswas

Contents

19.1 Introduction

The process of food fermentation is practised by human cultures all over the world. It has become a major component of human survival in places where preserved food has become a necessity. The term "fermentation" comes from a Latin word *fermentum* (to ferment). The definition describes fermentation as the process by which chemical changes in an organic substrate occur as a result of the action of microbial enzymes. Fermentation can also be defined as any process for the making of a product by a mass culture of microorganisms. It is one of the oldest and the most economic forms of food preservation which renders benefits from providing bionutrients and minerals to enhancement of flavor and aroma. Extending the shelf life of foods is one of the major objectives of fermentation, with aspects such as wholesomeness, acceptability, and overall quality. Fermented foods make a major contribution to dietary staples in numerous countries across Africa, Asia, and Latin America and small-scale fermentation technologies contribute substantially to food security and nutrition, particularly in regions that are vulnerable to food shortages (FAO 1998).

Fermentation technologies play an important role in ensuring the food security of millions of people around the world, particularly marginalized and vulnerable groups facing shortage or deficiencies in food supplies. Fermented foods are described as palatable and wholesome and are generally appreciated for several attributes: their pleasant flavors, aromas, textures, and improved cooking and processing properties (Holzapfel and Schillinger 2002). These characteristics in fermented foods are enhanced by virtue of the metabolic activities of the enzymes secreted by microorganisms. Traditional skills have been developed for refining fermentation processes (Hammes 1990). Many fermented products despite their many nutritional advantages are often associated with the stigma of being a "poor man's" food.

19.2 Antioxidants

An antioxidant is a molecule that inhibits the oxidation of other molecules. Oxidation of compounds produces free radicals; in turn these radicals can start a chain reaction. When such a chain reaction occurs in a cell, it causes damage to or the death of the cell. It has been reported that oxygen-free radicals and other reactive oxygen species (ROS) may be formed in the human body and in the food system. Antioxidants terminate the chain reactions by removing the free radical intermediates. Oxidative free radicals are byproducts of the normal reactions within our body. These reactions include the generation of calories, degradation of lipids, the catecholamine response under stress, and inflammatory processes (Ikeda and Long 1990). If the balance between oxidative-free radical production and eradication is maintained, the harmful effects of free radicals in the body are minimized. However, if unwanted free radicals are not eradicated efficiently, oxidative stress occurs. Oxidative stress, caused by reactive oxygen or free radicals, has been shown to be associated with the progression of many lifestyle-related diseases such as atherosclerosis, cirrhosis, arthritis, cancer, heart disease, and depression (McCord 2000, Kovacic and Jacintho 2001, Parola and Robino 2001). In order to protect tissues and organs from oxidative damage, the body possesses both enzymatic and nonenzymatic systems. The main enzymes include superoxide dismutase (SOD), glutathione peroxidase (GSH-Px), and catalase (CAT). These enzymes are front line defenders against oxidative damage. In addition to these enzymes, the nonenzymatic mechanism can also protect the body from damages caused by oxidative stress. One of the most common natural antioxidants is vitamin E. It acts as a peroxyl radical scavenger. Recently, investigators and consumers have been showing interest in seeking natural antioxidant components in the diet, which may help to reduce oxidative damage.

19.2.1 Antioxidants and Health

Antioxidants are believed to play an important role in the body's defense system against oxygen-free radicals and other ROS, which also play a significant pathological role in human diseases (Lin and Yang 2007). Natural antioxidants in plants are related to three major groups: carotenoids, vitamins, and phenolics. Phenolic compounds are plant-derived antioxidants that possess metal chelating capabilities and radical scavenging properties. For example, soybean and its products containing phenolic compounds have been shown to possess antioxidant ability. It has been observed that the intake of antioxidants containing soy food is associated with reduced cardiovascular risk resulting from lower blood pressure, and homocysteine. Dietary intake of soybeans and soybean products also decrease risk of cancer, including breast, colon, and prostate cancers. Many studies reported the protective role of certain components of soybean, especially isoflavone, saponin, vitamin C, tocopherol, and phytate against oxidative stress (Diaz-Batalla et al. 2006, Kumar et al. 2009, 2010). It is emphasized that the intake of food-derived antioxidants in the daily diet may reduce oxidative damage and exerts a corresponding beneficial effect on health. Many other antioxidant components have also been found in soybean foods including fermented soybeans, such as isoflavones, tocopherols, phospholipids, chlorogenic acid isomers, caffeic acid, ferulic acid, peptides, amino acids, and melanoidin.

Owing to the risks of consuming synthetic antioxidants, research studies of natural products containing antioxidant activity have increased, with the aim of replacing synthetic antioxidants or applying associations that reduce their toxic effects (Aungulu et al. 2007, Mendiola et al. 2010). Among the several classes of naturally occurring antioxidant substances, phenolic compounds have drawn particular attention because they inhibit lipid peroxidation (Kristinova et al. 2009) and lipo-oxygenation *in vivo* that is mainly due to the reducing properties of chemical structures that enable neutralization or sequestration of free radicals, as well as the chelation of transition metals, thus avoiding the phase of inhibiting the spread of oxidative processes. Vegetable tissues are good sources of these compounds, often containing simple phenols, phenolic acids (derived from benzoic and cinnamic acid), coumarin, flavonoids, stilbenes, condensed and hydrolyzable tannins, lignins, and lignans (Melo and Guerra 2002, Moon and Shibamoto 2009).

Among the sources of phenolic compounds, rice (*Oryza sativa*) should be highlighted because it is one of the most produced and consumed cereals in the world and plays an important role in the diet–health relationship, and contains distinct phenolic compounds, tocopherols, tocotrienols, and g-oryzanol mainly associated with the pericarp (Iqbal et al. 2005). Another example of a natural source of antioxidants is *Terminalia chebula,* a native plant to India. The dried ripe fruit of *Terminalia chebula* is used in the Indian systems of medicine such as Ayurveda and Siddha. It is a well-known ayurvedic rasayana which possesses adaptogenic properties (Rege et al. 1999). The active principal constituents of *Terminalia chebula* are gallic acid, ellagic acid, tannic acid, ethyl gallate, chebulagic acid, chebulinic acid, corilagin, beta-sitosterol, terchebulin, caffeic acid, mannitol, anthraquinones, ethanedioic acid, terpinene, terpinenol, and so on (Saleem et al. 2002, Kim et al. 2006, Xie et al. 2006).

Since antioxidative peptides can protect the human body from free radicals and slow the progression of many chronic diseases in addition to providing nutritional value, there has been a significant increase in interest in such antioxidants (Rajapakse et al. 2005, GokturkBaydar et al. 2007). Several traditional fermented soybean foods, including *miso, natto, tempe, sufu*, and *douchi*, possess many advantageous properties such as free radical scavenging activity and reducing power and ion-chelating abilities (Santiago et al. 1992, Berghofer et al. 1998, Gibbs et al. 2004). *Miso* has been used as a traditional daily seasoning for several centuries in Japan. It is also used to reduce plasma cholesterol levels (Horii et al. 1990), colonic aberrant crypt foci (Ohara et al. 2002), cerebrovascular disease (Kanazawa et al. 1995), and hypertension (Kanda et al. 1999).

In Indonesia, the fungus used for the preparation of *miso* belongs to a genus other than *Aspergillus* (Sastraatmadja et al. 2002). *Aspergillus* spp. has been used as starter organisms for the preparation of *koji* for thousands of years. They are typically used in the fermentation industry to produce enzymes (Bennett and Klich 1992), organic acids (Raper and Fenell 1965), vitamins (Bennett 1985), soy sauce, *miso*, and *sake* (Hesseltine 1981), and antibiotics (Kozakiewicz 1989). The acceptability, nutritional value, and functionality of the resulting hydrolyzate, such as antioxidant activity, proliferation of both human hybridoma and mouse macrophage cells after 1 h of hydrolysis by *Aspergillus oryzae*, and LAB fermentation have been reported to be improved.

Lactobacillus species are probably the most important bacteria in the food industry. They are widely used as starter cultures and have been reported to play significant roles in the production of fermented food. *Lactobacillus* species are generally recognized as safe (GRAS) and have been reported to have beneficial health properties, as a result of which they are also finding increasing use as probiotics in other health-related applications. An array of beneficial activities such as immunomodulatory, antiallergenic, antimicrobial, antihypertensive, and antitumourigenic effects have been reported (Ishida-Fujii et al. 2007). *Lactobacillus* sp. has also been shown to possess antioxidant activities (Kapila et al. 2006).

19.3 Oxidative Stress

Oxidative stress results when the oxidant/antioxidant ratios tilt in favor of oxidant factors, and it is involved in the aging process and also causes inflammation (Madamanchi et al. 2005). Free radicals attack cellular components leading to oxidation of lipids, proteins, and DNA, thus causing structural and functional changes to these molecules. Oxidation of food constituents is also a key event in food spoilage. This may reduce the nutritional value and safety of food by producing undesirable flavors and toxic substances. The global interest in harnessing the beneficial properties of microbes and their metabolites for human health make it important to explore potential uses of indigenous food grade lactobacilli in the development of functional foods and probiotics. Research has found that *Lactobacillus fermentum* is a superior microbial producer of ferulic acid. Ferulic acid is a naturally found phenolic acid and is a potent antioxidant which is able to neutralize free radicals, such as ROS. ROS have been implicated in DNA damage, cancer, and accelerated cell aging. Recent studies suggest that FA has antitumor activity against breast cancer (Kampa et al. 2003), liver cancer (Lee et al. 2005), and is effective in preventing cancer induced by exposure to various carcinogenic compounds such as benzopyrene (Lesca 1983) and 4-nitroquinoline 1-oxide (Tanaka et al. 1993).

19.4 Naturally Occurring Antioxidants

Naturally occurring antioxidants are found in most plants and animal tissues. The majority of natural antioxidants are phenolic compounds and the most important groups are the tocopherols, flavonoids, and phenolic acids. Antioxidants are substances which significantly inhibit or delay oxidative processes such as lipid peroxidation even at low concentrations. Fermentation involves the transformation of organic substances into simpler compounds such as peptides, amino acids, and other nitrogenous compounds by bacterial or endogenous enzymes. While they are important contributors to the flavor and aroma of fermented products (Mackie et al. 1971, Raksakulthai and Haard 1992), some exhibit an antioxidant capacity (Kitts and Weiler 2003).

Amino acids such as tryptophan and histidine (Houlihan and Ho 1985), glycine and alanine (Hui-Chun et al. 2003) exhibit antioxidative properties. Tyrosine and lysine are generally accepted to be antioxidants (Wang and Gonzalez de Mejia 2005). Amino compounds such as amino acids and peptides can function as primary antioxidants and can also interact with other substances to form Maillard reaction products (MRPs) (Kitts and Weiler 2003). They are nonenzymatic browning reactions that occur in foods. Lysine, as one of the major amino acids in salt-fermented shrimp paste, could have reacted with another substance thus reflecting an increase in activity. Sugar–lysine (Wijewickreme et al. 1999, Jing and Kitts 2004), glucose-glycine (Yoshimura et al. 1997) and sugar-protein (Benjakul et al. 2005) model systems have been shown to exhibit antioxidant activity. In some cases, oxidation reactions show opposite effects on the antioxidant properties of foods. Partially oxidized polyphenols, for instance, exhibit higher antioxidant activity than that of nonoxidized phenols. Thermal processing at elevated temperature, for example, pasteurization, probably influence the transformation of antioxidants into a more active and resistant compound such as MRPs. Antioxidant efficiency of MRPs is influenced by factors such as ratio and type of amino acid compounds and sugar involved, temperature, pH, and water activity (Manzocco et al. 2001).

During the past few decades, significant attention has been paid to dairy and nondairy products containing probiotic bacteria. Today, probiotic microorganisms are available in the market in three different types for direct or indirect human consumption. They include

- Culture concentrate to be added to a food (dried or deep-frozen form) for industrial or home use
- Food products (fermented or nonfermented)
- Dietary supplements (drug products in powder, capsule, or tablet forms)

Consumption of probiotic cells *via* food products are the most popular and widespread way of their intake into the body. Functional foods, designer foods, or medicinal foods are defined as "foods that contain some health-promoting component(s) beyond traditional nutrients." Addition of probiotics is a way in which foods can be changed to become functional (FAO/WHO 2001). Different types of food matrices which have been used as probiotics include various types of cheese, ice cream, milk-based desserts, butter, mayonnaise, powder products or capsules, and fermented foods of vegetable origin (Tamime et al. 2005). In the production of probiotics, an important factor is the food substrate. Besides buffering the bacteria through the stomach, it may contain functional ingredients that interact with the probiotics, altering their activities. Fat content, type of protein, carbohydrates, and pH can affect probiotic growth and survival (Soccol et al. 2010).

Although cholesterol is an important component for body tissues, elevated blood cholesterol is a well-known major risk factor for coronary heart disease (CHD) (Aloglu and Oner 2006). It has been reported that hypercholesterolemia contributes to 45% of heart attacks in Western Europe and 35% of heart attacks in Central and Eastern Europe (Yusuf et al. 2004). CHD is the main cause of death in Canada, the United States, and many other countries around the world (Heart and Stroke Foundation of Canada 2000, American Heart Association 2002). WHO has predicted that by 2030, cardiovascular diseases will remain the leading causes of death, affecting approximately 23.6 million people around the world (WHO 2009). The risk of heart attack is three times higher in those with hypercholesterolemia compared with those who have normal blood lipid profiles (Homayouni et al. 2012). Also, each increase in the serum cholesterol concentration by 1% results in 2%–3% increase in the risk of CHD (Davis et al. 2005, Manson et al. 1992). In healthy adults, about 1 g of cholesterol is synthesized and 0.3 g is consumed per day. The body maintains a relatively constant amount of cholesterol (150–200 mg/dL). This is done mainly through controlling the level of *de novo* synthesis. Dietary intake of cholesterol in part regulates the level of cholesterol synthesis. These cholesterols are then used in the formation of membranes and in the synthesis of the steroid hormones and bile acids (Croft et al. 1988). Bile acid synthesis uses most of this cholesterol.

The cholesterol pool of the liver is used in two important ways. The liver utilizes part of it to produce bile salts, to be stored in the gall bladder as a part of bile, which ends up in the gut. There, the bile salts are involved in the emulsification of fats and in their ingestion and absorption. The rest of the cholesterol is used for other requirements of the body. To do this, the liver combines cholesterol from its pool with triglycerides and covers it with a particular protein so that it can be dissolved in the blood. These are somewhat large molecules, known as very low-density lipoproteins (VLDL). The liver then drains them into the blood. Lipoprotein lipase (LPL) exists in abundance all over the body, especially in the walls of the arteries. This enzyme is involved in removing triglycerides from VLDL cholesterol. In the process, the VLDL shrinks in size and a relatively larger portion of it is made up of what is called intermediate density lipoproteins, or IDL. As the process continues, and more triglycerides are taken away, what is left is a dense molecule referred to as low-density lipoprotein (LDL). This lipoprotein still maintains a large amount of cholesterol. The protein layer allows the tissues to use this cholesterol. It is the LDL receptors on these tissues that make this interaction possible. In tissues such as that of the liver, and the inner layer of the arterial wall, cholesterol is taken away from LDLs. Free radicals in the body are very reactive and oxidative compounds can oxidize LDL cholesterol and help the formation of atherosclerotic plaque in the arteries. Antioxidants in the body can inhibit this process (Jialal 1998). The liver also produces another type of lipoprotein, named high-density lipoprotein (HDL). This is different from VLDL, which is also produced in the liver. It has little triglyceride and cholesterol, and has a particular protein covering. HDL collects the surplus cholesterol that cholesterol metabolizing cells cannot utilize. Lecithin–cholesterol acyl transferase is an enzyme that is responsible for transporting surplus cholesterol back to HDL molecules. Unused cholesterol from arteries, liver, and other tissues are absorbed by HDL cholesterol. There is evidence that even some oxidized LDL can be removed by the LCAT and HDL cholesterol (Hockerstedt et al. 2004). As HDL circulates in the body and collects the cholesterol from tissues, it becomes mature and goes back to the liver. There, it is identified by its lipoprotein covering and is lodged in the liver's cholesterol pool.

Recent approaches and research work done for lowering blood cholesterol levels involve dietary management, behavior modification, regular exercise, and drug therapy (Dunn-Emke et al. 2001). Pharmacological agents available in the markets are used for the treatment of high cholesterol. Although they effectively reduce cholesterol levels, they are expensive and are known to have severe side effects (Bliznakov 2002). Lactic acid bacteria (LAB) with active bile salt hydrolase (BSH) or products containing them are suggested to lower cholesterol levels through interaction with host bile salt metabolism (De Smet et al. 1998). It has been reported by De Smet et al. (1995) that lactobacilli with active BSH have an advantage to survive and colonize the lower small intestine of the host where the enterohepatic cycle takes place and therefore BHS activity may be considered an important colonization factor. Sanders (2000) proposed a mechanism based on the ability of certain probiotic lactobacilli and bifidobacteria to deconjugate bile acids enzymatically, increasing their rates of excretion. Cholesterol being a precursor of bile acids, converts its molecules to bile acids replacing those lost during excretion and this leads to reduction in serum cholesterol. This mechanism could be operated in the control of serum cholesterol levels by conversion of deconjugated bile acids into secondary bile acids by colonic microbes.

Members of the gut microbiota in the large intestine of animals exhibit a variety of enzymatic activities with potential impact on animal health through biotransformation of secondary plant products and xenobiotic compounds (McBain and Macfarlane 1998, Heavey and Rowland 2004, Blaut and Clavel 2007). β-Glucuronidases liberate toxins and mutagens that glucuronate in the liver and excrete into the gut with the bile. This can lead to high local concentrations of carcinogenic compounds within the gut, thus increasing the risk of carcinogenesis (Gill and Rowland 2002). Furthermore, reuptake of the deconjugated compound from the gut and reglucuronidation in the liver leads to an enterohepatic circulation of xenobiotic compounds, which increases their retention time in the body. β-Glucosidases can exert either beneficial or harmful effects, as they form aglycones from a range of different plant glucosides, which might exhibit either toxic/mutagenic or health-promoting effects (Hill 1995, Manach et al. 2004). Some plant glucosides are also subject to deconjugation by host β-glucosidases in the upper gut and may subsequently be glucuronated by the host, making them a substrate for bacterial β-glucuronidases when they reach the colon with the bile (Manach et al. 2004). The resulting aglycones of plant polyphenols may be subjected to further degradation and biotransformation by the gut microbiota (Blaut et al. 2003, Atkinson et al. 2005). Morotomi (1996) reported that *Lactobacillus casei* Shirota strain, a lactic acid bacterium has potential for cancer chemoprevention.

Increased β-glucosidase activity upon soy consumption has been reported in human volunteers (Wiseman et al. 2004). Fecal β-glucuronidase activity increased in rodents after consumption of a high-protein high-fat diet (Eriyamremu et al. 1995) and decreased after consumption of diets high in carbohydrates (Shiau and Chang 1983, Gestel et al. 1994). It has also been reported that cancer patients exhibit higher β-glucuronidase activities than healthy controls (Kim and Jin 2001). Many *in vitro* tests need to be performed while screening for potential probiotic strains (Harzallah and Belhadj 2013). The first step in the selection of a probiotic LAB strain is the determination of its taxonomic classification, which may give an indication of the origin, habitat, and physiology of the strain. All these characteristics have important consequences on the selection of novel strains for probiotic use (Morelli 2007).

Intestinal microbiota is not homogeneous. The number of bacterial cells present in the mammalian gut shows a continuum that goes from 10^1 to 10^3 bacteria per gram of contents in the stomach and duodenum, progressing to 10^4–10^7 bacteria per gram in the jejunum and ileum and culminating in 10^{11}–10^{12} cells per gram in the colon (Sekirov et al. 2010). Additionally, the microbial composition varies between these sites. In addition to the longitudinal heterogeneity displayed by the intestinal microbiota, there is also a great deal of latitudinal variation in the microbiota composition. The microbiota present in the intestinal lumen differs significantly from the microbiota attached and embedded in this mucus layer as well as the microbiota present in the immediate proximity of the epithelium. For instance, *Bacteroides, Bifidobacterium, Streptococcus,* members of Enterobacteriaceae, *Enterococcus, Clostridium, Lactobacillus,* and *Ruminococcus* were all found in feces, whereas only *Clostridium, Lactobacillus,* and *Enterococcus* were detected in the mucus layer and epithelial crypts of the small intestine (Sekirov et al. 2010). β-Glucuronidase, β-glucosidase, and urease activity usually come from these colonic bacteria (Chadwick et al. 1992, Burne and Chen 2000). Urea, which is the end product of nitrogen metabolism, undergoes an enterohepatic circulation, being produced in the liver and then entering the intestinal tract by passive diffusion (Suzuki et al. 1979). Urease has been demonstrated to hydrolyze the substrate urea to form CO_2 and two molecules of NH_3 (Mobley et al. 1995). The NH_3 produced raises the pH of the cytoplasm, thereby buffering the bacteria under acidic environmental conditions. In addition, the NH_3 provides the bacterial cell with an easily assimilated source of nitrogen (Steyert and Kaper 2012).

Improving the viability of probiotic bacteria in different food products (especially fermented products) until the time of consumption has been the subject of hundreds of studies. Viability of probiotic microorganisms, namely, the number of viable and active cells per gram or milliliter of probiotic food products at the moment of consumption is the most critical value of these products which determines their medicinal efficacy (Tamime et al. 2005, Khorbekandi et al. 2011). The addition of L-cysteine, whey protein concentrate, and tryptone improved the viability of *Lactobacillus acidophilus* and bifidobacteria by providing growth factors as these probiotic bacteria lack proteolytic activity (Dave and Shah 1998). Protein derivatives promote probiotic survival due to several reasons namely, their nutritional value for the cells, reducing redox potential of the media as well as increasing buffering capacity of the media (which results in a smaller decrease in pH) (Dave and Shah 1998, Mortazavian et al. 2010). *Lactobacillus* species represent indigenous organisms of the mammalian gastrointestinal (GI) tract and have been used as probiotic agents for the treatment of GI infections and inflammatory bowel disease (IBD) (Madsen 2001, MacFarlane and Cummings 2002). *Lactobacillus* species have been isolated from the intestines of various mammals, including rodents (mice and rats), dogs, cats, ruminants, horses, nonhuman primates, and humans (Savage et al. 1968, Watanabe et al. 1977). These organisms are present in relatively high numbers in the GI tracts of mice and presumably play a beneficial role in healthy animals.

Saturated fatty acids undergo less peroxidation than their unsaturated counterparts. Indeed, supplementation with polyunsaturated as opposed to saturated fatty acids results in a statistically significant increase in lipid peroxidation in the plasma and liver (Song et al. 2000, Song and Miyazawa 2001, Shin 2003). Lactic acid bacteria are promising agents for protecting the liver (Segawa et al. 2008) and very useful as a functional food for maintaining human health (Velayudham et al. 2009). Inhibition of lipid peroxidation is commonly used for analysis of antioxidative activity (Ou et al. 2006). There are reports that have provided evidence of certain LAB possessing antioxidative activity (Kullisaar et al. 2002, Songisepp et al. 2005). Saide and Gilliland (2005) suggested that some lactobacilli strains are a source of dietary antioxidants. It was reported by a study providing new insights into the mechanisms by which LAB with antioxidative properties can help to protect the liver in mammals. Along with the change in dietary patterns to a "Western-style" diet, which contains very little fiber and is deficient in important nutrients, there has been a concurrent increase in the incidence of diseases such as obesity, cardiovascular disease, type 2 diabetes, colon cancer, and constipation (Reddy 1995, Lee and Lee 2000, Lim et al. 2006). Additionally, protective intestinal flora such as LAB are often damaged and reduced as a result of stress and consumption of a Western diet (Bengmark 2000). Intake of fermented foods which reports colonization of probiotic microflora not only can be a source of health-promoting ingredients but also a good source of antioxidants which can terminate or halt the vicious harmful cycle of ROS. There has been a dearth of information on the antioxidant potential of microbes prevalent in fermented foods or food ingredients, but with the benefits reported for fermented foods and associated microbes, there is an urgent need to bioprospect the antioxidant metabolites associated with fermented foods.

19.5 Conclusion

Fermented foods and beverages have occupied an important place in dietary habits and have been a part of the food culture of many communities across the world. The traditional technology behind the development and processing of fermented foods was basically meant for preserving and improving their nutritional value. Fermented foods enhance the flavor and aroma and improve the digestibility of the fermented materials. Texturing and/or biologically active agents' production could be envisaged directly *in situ* of food. Traditionally fermented products have attracted the attention of the food industry because of the involvement of GRAS organisms along with the rheological properties of the products. The health benefits of fermented foods have been an attention gatherer and the beneficial effects of fermented products have been widely reported. The probiotic aspects of fermented foods have focused largely on specific health promoting activities. Among important health protectors and promoters, antioxidant compounds have largely been envisaged as artificial supplements which invariably carry certain risks. Therefore, it is felt that antioxidants from fermented foods can be a potential source for replacing synthetic antioxidants that are available for human use, and thus larger attention is needed to explore and bioprospect antioxidants from fermented foods.

References

Aloglu, H. and Z. Oner. 2006. Assimilation of cholesterol in broth, cream and butter by probiotic bacteria. *European Journal of Lipid Science and Technology* 108(9): 709–713.

Atkinson, C., C.L. Frankenfeld, and J.W. Lampe. 2005. Gut bacterial metabolism of the soy isoflavone daidzein: Exploring the relevance to human health. *Experimental Biology and Medicine* 230: 155–170.

Aungulu, G. 2007. Activity of gaseous phase steam distilled propolis extracts on peroxidation and hydrolysis of rice lipids. *Journal of Food Engineering* 80: 850–858.

Bengmark, S. 2000. Colonic food: Pre- and probiotics. *American Journal of Gastroenterology* 95(Suppl. 1): 5–7.

Benjakul, S., W. Lertittikul, and F. Bauer. 2005. Antioxidant activity of Maillard reaction products from a porcine plasma protein-sugar model system. *Food Chemistry* 93: 189–196.

Bennett J.W. and M.A. Klich. 1992. *Aspergillus: Biology and Industrial Applications*, in J. W. Bennett and M. A. Klich, Eds. 21: 134–137.

Bennett, J.W. 1985. Taxonomy of fungi and biology of the Aspergillus, *Biology of Industrial Microorganisms*, in A. L. Demain and N. A. Solomon, Eds. London: The Benjamin Cummings Publishing Company, Inc., 29: 359–406.

Berghofer, E., B. Grzeskowiad, N. Mundigler, W. B. Sentall, and J. Walcak. 1998. Antioxidant properties of faba bean, soybean and oat tempeh. *International Journal of Food Science and Nutrition* 49: 45–54.

Blaut, M. and T. Clavel. 2007. Metabolic diversity of the intestinal microbiota: Implications for health and disease. *The Journal of Nutrition* 137: 751S–755S.

Blaut, M., L. Schoefer, and A. Braune. 2003. Transformation of flavonoids by intestinal microorganisms. *International Journal for Vitamin and Nutrition Research* 73: 79–87.

Bliznakov, B.G. 2002. Lipid-lowering drugs (statins), cholesterol, coenzyme Q10. The baycol case—A modern Pandoras box. *Biomedice and Pharmacotherapy* 56(1): 56–59.

Burne, R.A. and Y.Y.M. Chen. 2000. Bacterial ureases in infectious diseases. *Microbes and Infection* 2: 533–542.

Chadwick, R.W., S.E. George, and L.D. Claxton. 1992. Role of the gastrointestinal mucosa and microflora in the bioactivation of dietary and environmental mutagens or carcinogens. *Drug Metabolism Reviews* 24: 425–492.

Croft, J.B., J.L. Cresnta, L.S. Webber, S.R. Srinivasan, D.S. Freedman, G.L. Burke, and G.S. Berenson. 1988. Cardiovascular risk in parents of children with extreme lipoprotein cholesterol levels. *Southern Medical Journal* 81(3): 341–353.

Dave, R.I. and N.P. Shah. 1998. Ingredient supplementation effects on viability of probiotic bacteria in yogurt. *Journal of Dairy Science* 81: 2804–2816.

Davis, J., M.J. Iqbal, J. Steinle, J. Oitker, D.A. Higginbotham, R.G. Peterson, and W.J. Banz. 2005. Soy protein influences the development of the metabolic syndrome in male obese ZDFxSHHF rats. *Hormonal Metabolism Research* 37: 316–25.

De Smet. I., L. Van Hoorde, M.V. Woestyne, H. Christiaens, and W. Verstraete. 1995. Significance of bile salt hydrolase activity of lactobacilli. *Journal of Applied Bacteriology* 79: 292–301.

De Smet. I., P. De Boever, and W. Verstraete. 1998. Cholesterol lowering in pigs through enhanced bacterial bile salt hydrolase activity. *British Journal of Nutrition* 79: 185–194.

Diaz-Batalla. L., J.M. Widholm, G.C. Fahey, E. Castano-Tostado, and O. Paredes-Lopez. 2006. Chemical components with health implications in wild and cultivated Mexican common bean seeds (*Phaseolus vulgaris* L.). *Journal of Agricultural and Food Chemistry* 54(6): 2045–2052.

Dunn-Emke, S., G. Weider, and D. Ornish. 2001. Benefits of a low-fat-based diet. *Obesity Research* 9(11): 731.

Eriyamremu, G.E., V.E. Osagie, O.I. Alufa, M.O. Osaghae, and F.A. Oyibu. 1995. Early biochemical events in mice exposed to cycas and fed a Nigerian-like diet. *Annals of Nutrition and Metabolism* 39: 42–51.

FAO. 1998. Fermented fruits and vegetables—A global perspective, FAO Agricultural Services Bulletin No. 134, Rome.

Gestel, G, P. Besancon, and J.M. Rouanet. 1994. Comparative evaluation of the effects of two different forms of dietary fibre (rice bran vs. wheat bran) on rat colonic mucosa and faecal microflora. *Annals of Nutrition and Metabolism* 38: 249–256.

Gibbs, B.F., A. Zougman, R. Masse, and C. Mulligan. 2004. Production and characterization of bioactive peptides from soy hydrolysate and soy-fermented food. *Food Research International* 37: 123–131.

Gill, C.I.R. and I.R. Rowland. 2002. Diet and cancer: Assessing the risk. *British Journal of Nutrition* 88: S73–S87.

GokturkBaydar, N., G. Ozkan, and S. Yasar. 2007. Evaluation of the antiradical and antioxidant potential of grape extracts. *Food Control* 18: 1131–1136.

Hammes, W.P. 1990. Bacterial starter cultures in food production. *Food Biotechnology* 12: 383–397.

Harzallah, D. and H. Belhadj. 2013. Lactic acid bacteria as probiotics: Characteristics, selection criteria and role in immunomodulation of human GI mucosal barrier. *Lactic Acid Bacteria—R & D for Food, Health and Livestock Purposes*, in Dr. J. Marcelino Kongo Ed., ISBN: 978-953-51-0955-6. InTech, DOI: 10.5772/50732.

Heavey, P.M. and I.R. Rowland. 2004. Gastrointestinal cancer. *Best Practice and Research Clinical Gastroenterology* 18: 323–336.

Hesseltine, C.W. 1981. Future of fermented foods. *Process Biochemistry* 16: 2–16.

Hill, M.J. 1995. Carbohydrate metabolism: Role of gut bacteria in human toxicology and pharmacology, in M J Hill Ed. London, UK: Taylor & Francis, 95–104.

Hockerstedt, A., M. Jauhiainen, and M.J. Tikkanen. 2004. Lecithin/cholesterol acyltransferase induces estradiol esterification in high-density lipoprotein, increasing its antioxidant potential. *The Journal of Clinical Endocrinology and Metabolism* 89(10): 5088–5093.

Holzapfel, W.H. and U. Schillinger. 2002. Introduction to pre- and probiotics. *Food Research International* 35: 109–116.

Homayouni, A., L. Payahoo, and A. Azizi. 2012. Effects of probiotics on lipid profile: A review. *American Journal of Food Technology* 7: 251–265.

Horii, M., T. Ide, K. Kawashima, and T. Yamamoto. 1990. Hypo cholesterolemic activity of desalted miso in rats fed an atherogenic diet. *Nippon Shokuhin Kogaku Kaishi* 37:148–153.

Houlihan, C.M. and C. Ho. 1985. Natural antioxidants in flavor chemistry of fats and oils. *American Oil Chemists' Society*, in D. Min, T. H. Smouse Eds., 117–142. American Oil Chemists' Society.

Hui-Chun W., Shiau C., Chen H., and Chiou T. 2003. Antioxidant activities of carnosine, anserine, some free amino acids and their combination. *Journal of Food and Drug Analysis* 11: 48–153.

Ikeda, Y. and D. M. Long. 1990. The molecular basis of brain injury and brain edema the role of oxygen free radicals. *Neurosurgery* 27: 1–11.

Iqbal, S., M.I. Bhanger, and F. Anwar. 2005. Antioxidant properties and components of some commercially available varieties of rice bran in Pakistan. *Food Chemistry* 2: 265–272.

Ishida-Fujii, K., R. Sato, S. Goto, X.P. Yang, S. Hirano, and M. Sato. 2007. Prevention of pathogenic *Escherichia coli* infection in mice and stimulation of macrophage activation in rats by oral administration of probiotic *Lactobacillus casei* 1–5. *Bioscience, Biotechnology and Biochemistry* 71: 866–873.

Jialal, I. 1998. Evolving lipoprotein risk factors: Lipo-protein (a) and oxidized low-density lipoprotein. *Clinical Chemistry* 44: 1827–1832.

Jing, H. and D. Kitts. 2004. Antioxidant activity of sugar-lysine Maillard reaction products in cell free and cell culture systems. *Archives of Biochemistry and Biophysics* 429: 154–163.

Kampa, M., V.I. Alexaki, G. Notas, A.P. Nifli, A. Nistikaki, A. Hatzoglou, E. Bakogeorgou, E. Kouimtzoglou, G. Blekas, and D. Boskou. 2003. Anti proliferative and apoptotic effects of selective phenolic acids on T47D human breast cancer cells: Potential mechanisms of action. *Breast Cancer Research* 6: R63–R74.

Kanazawa, T., T. Osanai, X.S. Zhang, T. Uemura, X.Z. Yin, K. Onoder, Y. Oike, and K. Ohkubo. 1995. Protective effects of soy protein on the peroxidizability of lipoproteins in cerebrovascular disease. *Journal of Nutrition* 125: 639S–646S.

Kanda, A., Y. Hoshiyama, and T. Kawaguchi. 1999. Association of lifestyle parameters with the prevention of hypertension in elderly Japanese men and women: A four-year follow-ip of normotensive subjects. *Asia Pacific Journal of Public Health* 11: 77–81.

Kapila. S., P.R. Vibha, and P.R. Sinha. 2006. Antioxidative and hypocholesterolemic effect of *Lactobacillus casei* ssp. *casei* (biodefensive properties of lactobacilli). *Indian Journal of Medical Science* 60: 361–370.

Khorbekandi, H., A.M. Mortazavian, and S. Iravani. 2011. Technology and stability of probiotic in fermented milks. *Probiotic and Prebiotic Foods: Technology, Stability and Benefits to the Human Health*, in N. Shah, A. G. Cruz, and J. A. F. Faria Eds. New York: Nova Science Publishers, 131–169.

Kim, D.H. and Y.H. Jin. 2001. Intestinal bacterial β-glucuronidase activity of patients with colon cancer. *Archives of Pharmacal Research* 24: 564–567.

Kim, H.G., H.G. Cho, E.Y. Jeong, J.H. Lim, S.H. Lee, and H.S. Lee. 2006. Growth inhibiting activity of active component isolated from *Terminalia chebula* fruits against intestinal bacteria. *Journal of Food Protection* 69(9): 2205–2209.

Kitts D. and K. Weiler. 2003. Bioactive proteins and peptides from food sources: Applications of bioprocesses used in isolation and recovery. *Current Pharmaceutical Design* 9(16): 1309–1323.

Kovacic, P. and J.D. Jacintho. 2001. Mechanisms of carcinogenesis: Focus on oxidative stress and electron transfer. *Current Medicinal Chemistry* 8: 396–773.

Kozakiewicz, Z. 1989. Aspergillus species on stored products. *Mycol. Pap.* 161: 1–187.

Kristinova, V., M. Revilija, S. Ivar, and R. Turid. 2009. Antioxidant activity of phenolic acids in lipid oxidation catalyzed by different prooxidants. *Journal of Agricultural and Food Chemistry* 57: 10377–10385, PMid: 19817371.

Kullisaar, T., M. Zilmer, M. Mikelsaar, T. Vihalemm, H. Annuk, C. Kairane, and A. Kilk. 2002. Two antioxidative lactobacilli strains as promising probiotics. *International Journal of Food Microbiology* 72: 215–224.

Kumar. V., A. Rani, A. Dixit, D. Bhatnagar, and G.S. Chauhan. 2009. Relative changes in tocopherols, isoflavones and antioxidative properties of soybean during different reproductive stages. *Journal of Agricultural and Food Chemistry* 57: 2705–2710.

Kumar, V., A. Rani, A.K. Dixit, D. Pratap, and D. Bhatnagar. 2010. A comparative assessment of total phenolic content, ferric reducing-anti-oxidative power, free radical-scavenging activity, vitamin C and isoflavones content in soybean with varying seed coat colour. *Food Research International* 43: 323–328.

Lee, N.K., C.W. Yun, S.W. Kim, H.I. Chang, C.W. Kang, and H.D. Paik. 2005. Screening of lactobacilli derived from chicken feces and partial characterization of *Lactobacillus acidophilus* A12 as an animal probiotics. *Journal of Microbiology and Biotechnology* 18: 338–342.

Lee, S.M. and W.K. Lee. 2000. Inhibition effects of lactic acid bacteria (LAB) on the azoxymethane-induced colonic preneoplastic lesions. *The Journal of Microbiology* 38: 169–175.

Lesca, P. 1983. Protective effects of ellagic acid and other plant phenols on benzo[a]pyrene-induced neoplasia in mice. *Carcinogenesis* 4: 1651–1653.

Lim, K.S., S.J. You, B.K. An, and C.W. Kang. 2006. Effects of dietary garlic powder and copper cholesterol content characteristics of chicken eggs. *Asian-Australasian Journal of Animal Science* 19: 582–586.

Lin, J-Y. and C-Y. Tang. 2007. Determination of total phenolic and flavonoid contents in selected fruits and vegetables, as well as their stimulatory effects on mouse splenocyte proliferation. *Food Chemistry* 101(1): 140–7.

MacFarlane, G.T. and J.H. Cummings. 2002. Probiotics, infection and immunity. *Current Opinion in Infectious Disease* 15: 501–506.

Mackie, I.M., R. Hardy, and G. Hobbs. 1971. Fermented fish products, FAO, Rome.

Madamanchi, N.R., A. Vendrov, and M.S. Runge. 2005. Oxidative stress and vascular disease, *Arteriosclerosis. Thrombosis and Vascular Biology*. 25: 29–38.

Madsen, K. 2001. The use of probiotics in gastrointestinal disease. *Canadian Journal of Gastroenterology* 15: 817–822.

Manach, C., A. Scalbert, C. Morand, C. Remesy, and L. Jiménez. 2004. Polyphenols: Food sources and bioavailability. *American Journal of Clinical Nutrition* 79: 727–747.

Manson, J.E., H. Tosteson, P.M. Ridker, S. Satterfield, P. Hebert, and G.T. Oconnor. 1992. The primary prevention of myocardial infarction. *The New England Journal of Medicine* 326: 1406–1416.

Manzocco, L., S. Calliaris, D. Mastrocola, M.C. Nicoli, and C. Lerici. 2001. Review of nonenzymatic browning and antioxidant capacity of processed food. *Trends in Food Science Technology* 11: 340–346.

McBain, A.J. and G.T. Macfarlane. 1998. Ecological and physiological studies on large intestinal bacteria in relation to production of hydrolytic and reductive enzymes involved in formation of genotoxic metabolites. *Journal of Medical Microbiology* 47: 407–416.

McCord, J.M. 2000. The evolution of free radicals and oxidative stress. *American Journal of Medicine* 108: 652–659.

Melo, E.A. and N.B. Guerra. 2002. Ação antioxidante de compostos fenólicos atualmente presentes em alimentos. Boletim Sociedade Brasileira de Ciência e Tecnologia-SBCTA 36: 1–11.

Mendiola, J. et al. 2010. Design of natural food antioxidant ingredients through a chemometric approach. *Journal of Agricultural and Food Chemistry* 58: 787–792.

Mobley, H.L., M.D. Island, and R.P. Hausinger. 1995. Molecular biology of microbial ureases. *Microbiological Reviews* 59: 451–480.

Moon, J.K. and T. Shibamoto. 2009. Antioxidant assays for plant and food components. *Journal of Agricultural and Food Chemistry* 57: 1655–1666.

Morelli, L. 2007 *in vitro* assessment of probiotic bacteria: From survival to functionality. *International Dairy Journal* 17: 1278–1283.

Morotomi, M. 1996. Properties of *Lactobacillus casei* shirota strain as probiotics. *Asia Pacific Journal of Clinical Nutrition* 5: 29–30.

Mortazavian, A.M., R. Khosrokhvar, H. Rastegar, and G.R. Mortazaei. 2010. Effects of dry matter standardization order on biochemical and microbiological characteristics of freshly made probiotic Doogh (Iranian fermented milk drink). *Italian Journal of Food Science* 22: 98–102.

Ohara, M., H. Lu, K. Shiraki, Y. Ishimura, T. Uesaka, O. Katoh, and H. Watanabe. 2002. Prevention by long-term fermented miso of induction of colonic aberrant crypt foci by azoxymethane in F344 rats, *Oncology Reports* 9: 69–73.

Ou, C.C., J.L. Ko, and M.Y. Lin. 2006. Antioxidative effects of intracellular extracts of yogurt bacteria on lipid peroxidation and intestine 407 cells. *Journal of Food and Drug Analysis* 14(3): 304–310.

Parola, M., and G. Robino. 2001. Oxidative stress-related molecules and liver fibrosis. *Journal of Hepatology* 35: 297–306.

Rajapakse, N., E. Mendis, W.K. Jung, J.Y. Je, and S.K. Kim. 2005. Purification of a radical scavenging peptide from fermented mussel sauce and its antioxidant properties. *Food Research International* 38: 175–182.

Raksakulthai N. and N. Haard. 1992. Correlation between the concentration of peptides and amino acids and the flavor of fish sauce. *International Food Research Journal* 7: 286–290.

Raper, K.B. and D.I. Fennell. 1965. *The Genus Aspergillus*, Baltimore: Williams and Wilkins, 686.

Reddy, B.S. 1995. Nutritional factors and colon cancer. *Critical Reviews in Food Science and Nutrition* 35: 175–190.

Rege, N.N., U.N. Thatte and S.A. Dahanuka. 1999. Adaptogenic properties of six rasayana herbs used in Ayurvedic medicine. *Phytotherapy Research* 13(4): 275–291.

Saide, J.A. and S.E. Gilliland. 2005. Antioxidative activity of lactobacilli measured by oxygen radical absorbance capacity. *Journal of Dairy Science* 88: 1352–1357.

Saleem, A., M. Husheem, P. Harkonen, and K. Pihlaja. 2002. Inhibition of cancer cell growth by crude extract and the phenolics of *Terminalia chebula* retz fruit. *Journal of Ethnopharmacology* 81(3): 327–336.

Sanders, M.E. 2000. Considerations for use of probiotic bacteria to modulate human health. *The Journal of Nutrition* 130: 384S–390S.

Santiago, L.A., M. Hiramatsu, and A. Mori. 1992. Japanese soybean paste miso scavenges free radicals and inhibits lipid peroxidation. *Journal of Nutritional Science and Vitaminology* 38: 297–304.

Sastraatmadja, D.D., F. Tomita, and T. Kasai. 2002. Production of high-quality oncom, a traditional Indonesian fermented food, by the inoculation with selected mold strains in the form of pure culture and solid inoculum. *J. Graduate School of Agriculture*, Hokkaido University 70: 111–127.

Savage, D.C., R. Dubos, and R. Schaedler. 1968. The gastrointestinal epithelium and its autochthonous bacterial flora. *The Journal of Experimental Medicine* 127: 67–76.

Segawa, S., Y. Wakita, H. Hirata, and J. Watari. 2008. Oral administration of heat-killed *Lactobacillus brevis* SBC8803 ameliorates alcoholic liver disease in ethanol containing diet-fed C57BL/6N mice. *International Journal Food Microbiology* 128: 371–377.

Sekirov, I., S.L. Russell, L.C.M. Antunes, and B.B. Finlay. 2010. Gut microbiota in health and disease. *Physiological Reviews* 90: 859–904.

Shiau, S.Y. and G.W. Chang. 1983. Effects of dietary fiber on fecal mucinase and β-glucuronidase activity in rats. *The Journal of Nutrition* 113: 138–144.

Shin, S.J. 2003. Vitamin E modulates radiation-induced oxidative damage in mice fed a high-lipid diet. *Journal of Biochemistry and Molecular Biology* 36: 190–195.

Soccol, C.R., L.P. de Souza Vandenberghe, M.R. Spier, A.B.P. Medeiros, and C.T. Yamaguishi. 2010. The potential of probiotics: A review. *Food Technology and Biotechnology* 48: 413–434.

Song, J.H. and T. Miyazawa. 2001. Enhanced level of n-3 fatty acid in membrane phospholipids induces lipid peroxidation in rats fed dietary docosahexaenoic acid oil. *Atherosclerosis* 155: 9–18.

Song, J.H., K. Fujimoto, and T. Miyazawa. 2000. Polyunsaturated (n-3) fatty acids susceptible to peroxidation are increased in plasma and tissue lipids of rats fed docosahexaenoic acid-containing oils. *The Journal of Nutrition* 130: 3028–3033.

Songisepp, E., J. Kals, Kullisaar, R. Mandar, P. Hutt, M. Zilmer, and M. Mikelsaar. 2005. Evaluation of the functional efficacy of an antioxidative probiotic in healthy volunteers. *Nutrition Journal* 4: 22.

Steyert, S.R. and J.B. Kaper. 2012. Contribution of urease to colonization by shiga toxin-producing *Escherichia coli*. *Infection and Immunity* 80: 2589–2600.

Suzuki, K., Y. Benno, T. Mitsuoka, S. Takebe, K. Kobashi, and J. Hase. 1979. Urease-producing species of intestinal anaerobes and their activities. *Applied and Environmental Microbiology* 37(3): 379–382.

Tamime, A.Y., M. Saarela, A.K. Sondergaard, V.V. Mistry, and N.P. Shah. 2005. Production and maintenance of viability of probiotic micr-organisms in dairy products. *Probiotic Dairy Products*, in A.Y. Tamime, Ed. Oxford, UK: Blackwell Publishing, 44–51.

Tanaka, T., T. Kojima, T. Kawamori, A. Wang, M. Suzui, K. Okamoto, and H. Mori. 1993. Inhibition of 4-nitroquinoline-1-oxide-induced rat tongue carcinogenesis by the naturally occurring plant phenolics caffeic, ellagic, chlorogenic and ferulic acids. *Carcinogenesis* 14: 1321–1325.

Velayudham, A., A. Dolganiuc, M. Ellis, J. Petrasek, K. Kodys, P. Mandrekar, and G. Szabo. 2009. VSL3 probiotic treatment attenuates fibrosis without changes in steatohepatitis in a diet-induced nonalcoholic steatohepatitis model in mice. *Hepatology* 49: 989–997.

WHO. 2009. Global prevalence of vitamin A deficiency in populations at risk 1995–2005: WHO global database on vitamin A deficiency. Geneva, World Health Organization.

Wang, W. and E. Gonzalez de Mejia. 2005. A new frontier in soy bioactive peptides that may prevent age-related chronic diseases. *Comprehensive Reviews in Food Science and Food Safety* 4: 63–78.

Watanabe, T., M. Morotomi, N. Suegara, Y. Kawai, and M. Mutai. 1977. Distribution of indigenous lactobacilli in the digestive tract of conventional and gnotobiotic rats. *Microbiology and Immunology* 2: 183–191.

Wijewickreme, A.N., Z. Krejpcio, and D. Kitts. 1999. Hydroxyl scavenging activity of glucose, fructose and ribose-lysine model Maillard products. *Journal of Food Science* 64: 457–461.

Wiseman, H., K. Casey, E.A. Bowey, R. Duffy, M. Davies, I.R. Rowland, A.S. Lloyd, A. Murray, R. Thompson, and D.B. Clarke. 2004. Influence of 10 wk of soy consumption on plasma concentrations and excretion of isoflavonoids and on gut microflora metabolism in healthy adults. *American Journal of Clinical Nutrition* 80: 692–699.

Xie, P., S. Chen, Y. Liang, X. Wang, R. Tian, and R. Upton. 2006. Chromatographic fingerprinting analysis—A rational approach for quality assessment of traditional Chinese herbal medicine. *Journal of Chromatography A* 1112(1–2): 171–180.

Yoshimura Y., T. Ijima, T. Watanabe, and H. Nakazawa. 1997. Antioxidative effect of Maillard reaction products using glucose-glycine model system. *Journal of Agriculture Food Chemistry* 45: 4106–4109.

Yusuf S., S. Hawken, S. Ounpuu, T. Dans, A. Avezum, F. Lanas, M. McQueen et al. 2004. INTERHEART study investigators effect of potentially modifiable risk factors associated with myocardial infarction in 52 countries (the INTERHEART study): Case–control study. *The Lancet* 364: 937–952.

Chapter 20

Health Benefits of Nutraceuticals from Novel Fermented Foods

Anil Kumar Anal, Son Chu-Ky, and Samira Sarter

Contents

20.1 Introduction

The history of fermented foods and drinks dates back to more than 4000 years. Wine already existed around 5000 BC, and original forms of soy sauce and fermented milk existed around 3000–2000 BC (Farnworth 2008). Microorganisms seeded in the environment were generally inoculated to use for fermentation and maturation of fermented foods. Regional differences in products, climate, and other environmental factors have developed unique fermented products in various parts of the world. At the same time, regional and racial differences have a greater effect on determining whether some fermented products are considered for consumption or to be discarded. Fermentation is one of the oldest and most economical methods of producing and preserving food (Chavan and Kadam 1989, Billings 1998). In addition, fermentation provides a natural way to reduce the volume of the material to be transported, destroy undesirable components, enhance the nutritive value and appearance of the food, reduce the energy required for cooking, and to make a safer product (Simango 1997).

Food fermentation can be classified into the following types (Soni and Sandhu 1990):

- Lactic acid fermentations mainly carried out by lactic acid bacteria (LAB). For example, fermented cereals, *kimchi,* Sauerkraut, *gundruk,* and so on.
- Alcohol fermentation contributes to the production of ethanol. Yeasts are the predominant organisms, for example, wines, beers, vodka, whiskey, brandy, and bread.
- Acetic acid fermentation produced from the *Acetobacter* species. *Acetobacter* converts alcohol to acetic acid in the presence of oxygen, for example, vinegar.
- Alkaline fermentation takes place during the fermentation of soybeans, fish, and seeds, popularly used as condiment.

The main benefit associated with fermented foods is that it reduces the amount of raw materials, reduces the process of cooking, and improves the quality of protein content, carbohydrate digestibility, and also the availability of micronutrients. This also helps in eliminating toxic materials and antinutritional factors (Sanni 1993, Iwuoha and Eke 1996, Amoa-Awua et al. 1997, Odunfa and Oyewole 1998, Sindhu and Khertapaul 2001). Fermented foods have been traditionally used for preservation and to enhance the shelf life of the products, for example, fermented foods proved to have better nutritional values and better digestibility than unfermented food. Fermentation has another quality of improving the organoleptic quality by enhancing different flavors in different foods (Sarkar and Tamang 1994, Steinkraus 1994). Spoilage and contamination of food is inhibited by the production of organic acid, hydrogen peroxide, antibiotic-like substance, and the lowering of oxidation–reduction potential in the fermented food (Cooke et al. 1987, Mensah et al. 1991, Kingamko et al. 1994, Nout 1994, Lorri and Svanberg 1995, Tanasupawat and Komagata 1995). The microbiology of most fermented food products have not been explored much yet. Mostly these involve a natural process of mixed cultures of fungi, yeasts, and bacteria.

Fermented food products are produced widely using different techniques, raw materials, and microorganisms. There are basically only four types of fermentation process involved in this product development, they are: alcoholic, lactic acid, acetic acid, and alkali fermentation. The preparation of most of the indigenous or traditional fermented foods remains a household art. On the other hand, preparation of soy sauce and many more industrial products are the contributions of biotechnology to the field of fermentation (Bol and de Vos 1997).

20.2 Fermented Cereals

Cereal grains are considered to be one of the best options for abundant supplies of dietary proteins, peptides, amino acids, carbohydrates, oligomers, vitamins, minerals, and fibers (Blandino et al. 2003). The natural processing of cereals leads to a reduced level of carbohydrates as well as some of the non-digestible poly- and oligo-saccharides. Few types of amino acids also get synthesized. Vitamin-B group presence gets improved in the fermented products. The pH of the fermenting media also becomes favorable for enzymatic degradation of phytate; it is present in cereals as a conjugate complex formation with iron, magnesium, and proteins. As a result, a decrease in the quantity of phytate increases the amount of soluble iron, zinc, and calcium by many folds (Khetarpaul and Chauhan 1990, Nout and Motarjemi 1997). The process of fermentation improves the quality of proteins as well as the level of lysine in maize, millet, sorghum, and other cereals (Hamad and Fields 1979). The amount of tryptophan increases during the fermentation of maize or sorghum for the production of *Uji* (McKay and Baldwin 1990). During fermentation of cereals, several volatile complexes are formed as listed in Table 20.1 and contribute to the formation of flavors to the products (Chavan and Kadam 1989).

Common cereal gruels include *ogi* in West Africa, *akasa* or *koko* in Ghana, *uji* in Kenya, *mahewu* or *magou* in South Africa, and *abreh* in Sudan. *Mahewu* is an example of a nonalcoholic sour beverage made from cornmeal, consumed in Africa and some Arabian Gulf countries (Chavan and Kadam 1989). It is a type of food for adults, although it is commonly used to wean children (Shahani et al. 1983). The predominant microorganism in the spontaneous fermentation of African *mahewu* is *Lactococcus lactis* subsp. *lactis* (Steinkraus et al. 1993). *Uji*, a sour cereal gruel is from East Africa. The basic cereal used for uji production is maize, but mixtures of maize and sorghum or millet in the proportion of 4:1 are also used (Mbugua 1984). *Pito* and *burukutu* are brewed concurrently by fermenting malted or germinated single-cereal grains or a mixture of them. *Pito* is a cream-colored liquor while *burukutu* is a brown-colored suspension (Uzogara et al. 1990, Iwuoha and Eke 1996). Rice beers are typically prepared in the Asia-Pacific countries. Those brews include Korean *takju*, Philippine *tapuy*, Indonesian *brem bali*, and Indian *jaanr* (Sankaran

Table 20.1 Compounds Formed During Cereal Fermentation

Organic Acids		*Alcohols*	*Aldehydes and Ketones*	*Carbonyl Compounds*
Butyric	Heptanoic	Ethanol	Acetaldehyde	Furfural
Succinic	Isovaleric	*n*-Propanol	Formaldehyde	Methional
Formic	Propionic	Isobutanol	Isovaleraldehyde	Glyoxal
Valeric	*n*-Butyric	Amyl alcohol	*n*-Valderaldehyde	3-Methyl butanal
Caproic	Isobutyric	Isoamyl alcohol	2-Methyl butanol	2-Methyl butanal
Lactic	Caprylic	2,3-Butanediol	*n*-Hexaldehyde	Hydroxymethyl furfural
Acetic	Isocaproic	β-Phenylethyl alcohol	Acetone	
Capric	Pleargonic		Propionaldehyde	
Pyruvic	Levulinic		Isobutyraldehyde	
Plamitic	Myristic		Methyl ethyl ketone	
Crotonic	Hydrocinnamic		2-Butanone	
Itaconic	Benzylic		Diacetyl	
Lauric			Acetoin	

Source: From Campbell-Platt, G. 1994. Fermented foods: A world perspective. *Food Research International* 27(3), 253–257.

1998, Svanberg and Sandberg 1988). *Sake* is a traditional alcoholic beverage, prepared from rice, consumed particularly in Japan and China (Lotong 1998). *Bouza* is a fermented alcoholic wheat beverage known since the time of the Pharaohs. It is a light yellow, thick, sour drink consumed mainly in Egypt, Turkey, and in some Eastern European countries (Morcos et al. 1973). The biochemical changes of wheat occurring during *bouza* fermentation have been studied by Morcos et al. (1993), who found that the low pH (3.9–4.0) and the high acidity of bouza indicate fermentation by LAB, while the alcohol is due to yeast fermentation. The protein content of bouza ranges from 1.5% to 2.0% and due to the alcoholic fermentation involved in its formation, a significant contribution of vitamin B can be expected.

20.3 Fermented Meat and Fish

20.3.1 Fermented Sausage (Nem Chua)

The storage life of perishable meats can be extended by acid fermentation with added carbohydrates and salts. However, fermentation also brings about new organoleptic properties. The organic acids produced from the added carbohydrates in combination with salt control the extent of acid fermentation and keep the quality of the products. *Nem chua* is a traditional uncooked fermented meat product, which over generations has remained one of the most popular traditional Vietnamese foods. The product formulation and process used in the production of *nem chua* vary considerably between regions (north, middle, and south) of the country. The general *nem chua* formulation and the typical production procedure are shown in Figure 20.1 (Nguyen et al. 2010, Tran et al. 2011, Cao Hoang et al. 2013).

20.3.2 Sour Shrimp (Tom Chua)

Sour shrimps are one of the famous traditional foods of Vietnam, which contain high nutrients and exhibit good taste. In fact, sour shrimps are the products of LAB and protein hydrolysis, made

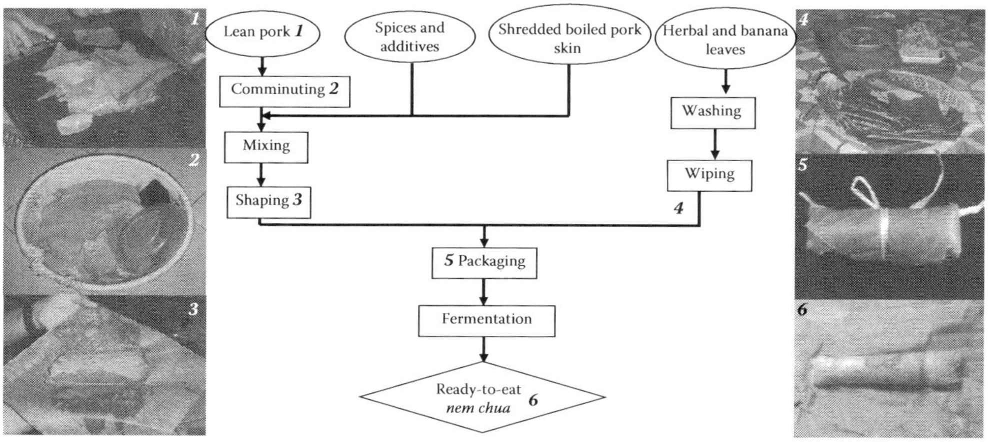

Figure 20.1 General formulation and typical procedure for the production of *nem chua*. Steps with a number in the central scheme are illustrated in the picture with the corresponding number.

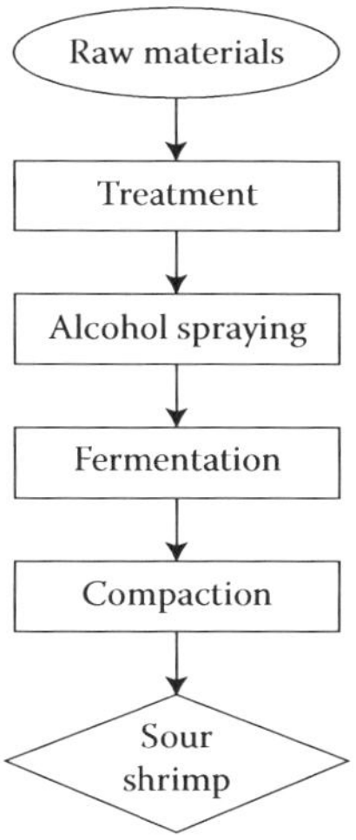

Figure 20.2 Process of production of Hue's sour shrimp (Tom chua).

of shrimps, sticky rice, salt, and spices (Chu 2010) (Figure 20.2). These products are popular in Central and South Vietnam. There is a general formula to make fermented sour shrimps but each area has its own recipe and makes it typical of the region by modulating the recipe and the making process (Cao-Hoang et al. 2013).

20.3.3 Fish Sauce (Nuoc Mam)

Nuoc mam is the most exported Vietnamese fermented product. It is already produced in an industrial way by several traditional or mass-producing firms. The objective of the fermentation is to degrade proteins into amino acids and small peptides. This proteolysis is carried out by enzymes and microorganisms from the fish. In the process, fish are put in a tank with salt in successive layers or in a mixture depending on the size of the fish (mackerel and sardines are popular fishes for this production). Owing to the high content of salt in the fermentation process, the bacteria encountered are mostly halophilic strains with a high proportion belonging to *Bacillus* sp. (Saisithi et al. 1966). In particular, original *Bacillus* strains have been isolated from *nuoc mam* that have been named *Bacillus vietnamensis* sp. nov. (Noguchi et al. 2004). They are able to grow in the presence of up to 15% NaCl at a pH between 6.5 and 10 and with optimal temperatures between 30°C and 40°C. A juice is readily extracted from this preparation. The fermentation process is generally rather uncontrolled, a temperature approaching 37°C is desired but it is in most cases the uncontrolled actual room temperature. Depending on its nitrogen content and organoleptic properties, the juice is reintroduced in the same tank or in a tank containing another fish species to correct its properties. The process lasts about a year in the traditional fermentation way at the end of which, juices are collected to give the various nuoc mam qualities, which are based on the amino acid and the peptide content (Park et al. 2002a). Other parameters have been shown to be important to the final organoleptic properties of the products and particularly volatile fatty acids (Dougan and Howard 1975, Park et al. 2002b). In mass industrial production, *nuoc mam* from different origins (including some homemade products that are collected) are mixed with additives (glutamate and other amino acids, flavoring compounds, etc.) to reach a satisfying organoleptic product (Cao-Hoang et al. 2013).

20.4 Fermented Dairy Products

The primary function of fermenting milk was, originally, to extend its shelf life. With this came numerous advantages, such as an improved taste and enhanced digestibility of milk, as well as the manufacture of a wide variety of products. The traditional methods of fermentation are taking place as a result of the activities of natural flora present in the food or added from the surroundings. Over the period, scientists have tried to isolate and study the characteristics of such desirable organisms. During milk fermentation, certain chemicals are increased (e.g., lactic acid, galactose, free amino acids, flavoring compounds, organic acids, and some antibacterial compounds) whereas the total amount of lactose, proteins, and fats are decreased due to their hydrolysis, producing smaller molecules.

20.5 Fermented Vegetables

Acid-fermented vegetables are important sources of vitamins and minerals. For some of them like *Kimchi*, their positive effect on the physiology of the consumers has been already widely investigated (Lee 1998). *Leuconostoc mesenteroides* has been found to be important in the initiation of fermentation of many vegetables, for example, cabbages, beets, turnips, cauliflower, green beans, sliced green tomatoes, cucumber, olives, and sugarbeet silages (Xiong et al. 2012). In vegetables, *Leuc. mesenteroides* grows rapidly and produces carbon dioxide and acids that quickly lower the pH, thereby inhibiting the development of undesirable microorganisms and the activity of their enzymes as well as preventing unfavorable softening of vegetables (Gardner et al. 2001, Zarour et al. 2012). The carbon dioxide produced replaces air and provides anaerobic conditions that favor the stabilization of ascorbic acid and of the natural colors of the products. *Leuc. mesenteroides* converts glucose to approximately 45% levorotatory D-lactic acid, 25% carbon dioxide, and 25% acetic acid and ethyl alcohol (Bourel et al. 2003, Cao-Hoang et al. 2013). Moreover, fructose is partially reduced to mannitol, which subsequently undergoes secondary fermentation to yield equimolar quantities of lactic acid and acetic acid. The combination of acid and alcohol results in the formation of esters, which impart desirable flavors. Overall, the initial growth of *Leuc. mesenteroides* leads to a modification of the environment that favors the growth of other LAB. Secondary fermentation in these processes, especially by homofermentative *Lactobacillus* species, leads to further reduction of the pH and ultimately to the growth of *Leuc. mesenteroides.*

For the preparation of fermented vegetables (*dua muoi*), fresh cabbage is cut in half or shredded, soaked in approximately 3%–6% brine concentration, and then washed and drained. The minor ingredients are chopped and mixed with shredded radish stuffed between the salted cabbage leaves. *Dua muoi* is then packed in a jar and pressed with a stone in order to submerge them in the juice. *Dua muoi* is fermented for 2–3 days at ambient temperature (Figure 20.3). The dominant species of *Lactobacillus* in the later stages of *kimchi* fermentation vary according to the fermentation temperature; *Lactobacillus plantarum* and *Lactobacillus brevis* dominate fermentations carried out at 20–30°C while *Lactobacillus maltaromicus* and *Lactobacillus bavaricus* dominate at 5–7°C. *Lb. plantarum* is homofermentative and is the highest acid-producing species of this group, yielding three or four times higher DL-lactic acid content than *Leuconostoc* species. Low temperature is preferred for *kimchi* fermentation to prevent the production of high amounts of lactic acid and over ripening as well as to extend the period of optimum taste.

Fermented mustard leaves are a popular traditional food of Vietnam. This product is normally manufactured by spontaneous fermentation in a period of time from few days to 1 week at a small

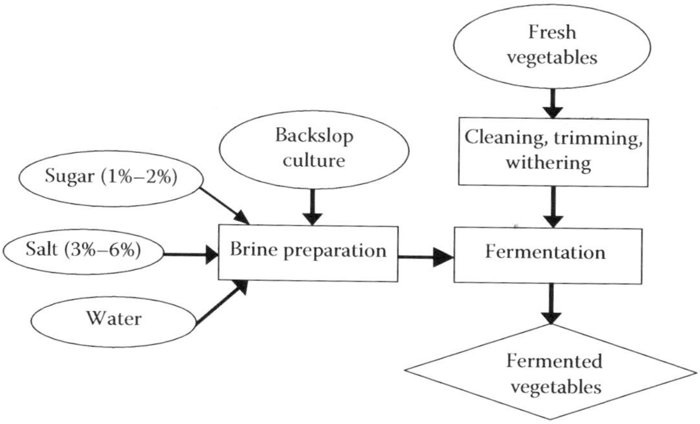

Figure 20.3 The processing procedures of Vietnamese fermented vegetables (*dua muoi*).

scale, and therefore, could be easily contaminated. A microbiological survey on 32 samples of fermented mustard leaves available in the markets in Hanoi during the period between November 2008 and May 2009 was conducted by Hanoi University of Science and Technology (project report "Technological solutions to reduce food poisoning microorganisms in fermented vegetables," Ministry of Agriculture and Rural Development, 2008–2009). Preliminary result showed that dominant microorganisms in fermented mustard were LAB at the level of 8–10 log CFU/mL. However, more than 70% of test samples did not meet the Vietnamese regulation (Regulation by Ministry of Health 46/2007/QĐ-BYT) on microorganisms (90% on coliforms, 70% on *Escherichia coli*, 90% on yeast and mold). There is a concern about coliforms and *E. coli* contamination due to the common practice of using animal manure in vegetable farming.

20.6 Probiotics for Fermentation

Probiotics and prebiotics provide alternate sources for the management of different intestinal disorders. It was demonstrated that the amount of bacterial count in the fecal matter in children is more than the adults with high amounts of *Lactobacillus* and *Bifidobacterium*. Disorders such as gastroenteritis is able to imbalance the biochemical environment of the gut, but the intake of probiotic functional food can stabilize the colonic microflora and can also help in relieving the adverse effect of antibiotics. LAB belong to a group of Gram-positive facultative anaerobic bacteria that synthesize lactic acid as their main product of fermentation into the culture medium. LAB were among the first organisms to be used in food development. Today LAB play crucial roles in the manufacturing of fermented milk products, vegetables, and meat, as well as in the processing of other products such as wine. To understand and especially to manipulate the roles of these LAB in these fermentation processes, LAB have been studied extensively and are now among the best characterized microorganisms with respect to their genetics, physiology, and applications (Table 20.2). The relative simplicity of LAB make them excellent candidates for complete analysis of the metabolic pathways in the near future. Currently, the genomes of several LAB are being sequenced and the first completely sequenced genome of the LAB *L. lactis* IL1403 has recently been presented (Bolotin et al. 1999).

Some works deal with gut bacteria that can be good candidates for probiotic formulation as they are already able to colonize the intestinal tract and exhibit several important properties

Table 20.2 The Contributions of Probiotics

Disease Type	*Contribution by the Probiotics*	*Reference*
Intestinal flora	Inhibits the growth of pathogenic species like *Shigella dysenteriae, Salmonella typhosa and E. coli* and this results in the less occurrence of diarrhea and vomiting	Asahara et al. (2001)
Lactose intolerance	Lactose supplement could help in the digestion of lactose by helping in its fermentation.	Jiang and Savaiano (1997)
Immuno-modulatory effects of probiotics	Administration of probiotics have proven to show the activity on Peyers's patches, NK cell activity, enhancement of IgA production in intestine, development of GALT (gut-associated lymphoid tissue).	Palma et al. (2006), Hosono et al. (2003), Hoentjen et al. (2005), Nakamura et al. (2004), Pierre et al. (1997)
Preventing cancer	Recent research showed that butyric acid production by the fermentation of probiotics plays a lead role in cancer prevention. This acid helps in the chemopreventive efficacy in carcinogenesis, and also against colon cancer by the promotion of differentiation of cell. Another breakthrough is the propionate, having anti-inflammatory effect on colon cancer cells. In another research probiotics showed the inhibition on colon tumor-forming azoxymethane by the probiotics in association with probiotics (inulin).	Femia et al. (2002), Munjal et al. (2009)
Lipid metabolism	Probiotics have been proven to show a positive effect on the hepatic lipid metabolism. Experiment on rats has shown a decrease in the level of cholesterol and triglycerides by 15% and 50%, respectively. The reason behind this is the suppression activity of the lipogenic enzyme activity.	Delzenne et al. (2002), Delzenne and Kok (2001), Williams and Jackson (2002)
Autism spectrum disorders	A potential probiotic *Lb. fermentum* HA6 strain, isolated from fermented vegetables, was identified and was found to have antifungal activity against eight among the 10 tested food originated fungi. This strain demonstrated inhibitory ability toward proliferation of four types of human cancer cell *in vitro*. This strain was also reported to have PepX (PepX, EC 3.4.14.5) activity to digest exorphins, products of incomplete digestion of food proteins, which may lead to accumulation of opioid peptides in brain and resulting in neurological disorders, for example, autism spectrum disorders. Abnormal peptide content has been described in the urine of most autistic patients. Exorphin opioids	Chu-Ky et al. (2014)

Continued

Table 20.2 (Continued) The Contributions of Probiotics

Disease Type	*Contribution by the Probiotics*	*Reference*
	(e.g., casomorphins, gluteomorphins, and gliadomorphins) derived from casein and gluten were found to cross the blood–brain barrier and cause social indifference symptoms. It was suggested that autism was based in genetic errors of peptide digestion, possibly of enzyme dipeptidylpeptidase IV (DPP IV or pepX, EC 3.4.14.5), and autistic symptoms could be explained by stimulant activity of exorphin toward the brain. Although conflicting reports exist, addition of ingestible genomeceutical compounds, which increase the user's expression of DPP IV or like substances, or supplementing with probiotics to improve autism spectrum disorders has been proposed.	

resulting in good probiotic qualities such as the ability to favor growth and weight gain in chicken (Pham and Le 2001, 2004a,b, Pham et al. 2001, 2003). Species from LAB as *Lactobacillus delbueckii* subsp. *bulgaricus, Lactobacillus acidophilus, Lactobacillus casei, Lactobacillus paracasei, Lb. plantarum, Lactobacillus rhamnosus, Enterococcus faecium* and recently from *Bifidobacterium longum, Bifidobacterium bifidum, Bifidobacterium lactis, and Bifidobacterium infantis* are selected for probiotic formulations. By using the adequate tests, it is also possible to isolate very interesting strains from fermented food and this is becoming an interesting target for selection. For instance, LAB were isolated from Vietnamese natural fermented foods and then tested for survival in simulated gastric juice at acidic pH 2.0 and simulated small intestinal juices with 0.3% bile salts at pH 8.0. Tolerant strains were observed morphologically and were identified using their carbohydrate fermentation patterns. The identification of LAB strains was confirmed by molecular methods using partial 16s rDNA sequence, genus–specific, and species-specific polymerase chain reaction (PCR) assays. The identified strains were tested for adhesiveness onto human epithelial cell lines Caco-2, and then were investigated for their health benefits. A potential probiotic strain was identified as *Lactobacillus fermentum* HA6 and was found to have antifungal activity against eight among the 10 tested food-borne fungi. This strain also demonstrated inhibitory ability toward proliferation of four types of human cancer cells *in vitro* (Ho and Adams 2006). Studies on *Lb. fermentum* HA6 demonstrated exorphin digestion activity of the test bacterium both in the form of enzyme crude extract as well as in whole cell after exposure to gastrointestinal condition (Ho et al. 2011a, Chu-Ky et al. 2014). The finding suggested that *Lb. fermentum* HA6 could be used to improve the symptoms of diseases related to exorphins. Later on, the strain of interest was investigated for its ability to be incorporated into food matrices, such as litchi concentrate and tomato juice (Ho et al. 2011b) (Cao-Hoang et al. 2013, Chu-Ky et al. 2014). The major benefits associated with probiotics on human health are in maintaining proper colon function and in improving metabolism. They are also responsible for enhancing the expression of short-chain fatty acids, the increase in fecal weight, the decrement in pH of the colon, reduced release of nitrogenous material from the body, and reductive enzymes (Bournet et al. 2002, Forchielli and Walker 2005, Qiang et al. 2009).

The extensive knowledge gained of LAB has opened new possibilities for their application (Table 20.3). Tailor-made LABs with desired physiological traits can be constructed and can be

Table 20.3 Health Benefits of Nutraceuticals from Fermented Foods: Case Studies

Work Done	*Benefit of Nutraceuticals*	*Reference*
Case Study 1		
Enhanced antioxidant activity of the fermented food by the addition of ginger to the culture of *Monascus* sp.	Nutraceutical with greater anti-atherosclerotic Value.	Kuo et al. (2009).
Case Study 2		
The study demonstrated considerable variation in the phenolic profiles of Sri Lankan tea. Total catechins, total flavonols, and total aflavins were higher in fermented leaves compared with the unfermented tea leaves.	Tea contains several flavonoid compounds that are responsible for its distinctive taste and color and for its purported beneficial health effects.	Jayasekera et al. (2014)
Case Study 3		
It is recognized that milk fermentation with LAB can generate a large number of peptides including some with potentially bioactive properties. Milk fermented with different strains of *Enterococcus faecalis* contained peptides with ACEI and antihypertensive activity.	Identified two peptides, corresponding to β-casein *f* (133–138) and β-casein *f* (58–76). They exhibit inhibitory activity for angiotensin-converting enzyme (ACEI). These peptides have antihypertensive activity, when given orally to rats.	Quiros et al. (2007)
Case Study 4		
Development of fermented sausage after the addition of vegetable extract, cocoa extract, and grape seed extract. There was an elevation of phenolic contents. After the completion of aging process, catechin and epicatechin were at 54%–61%, gallic acid and galloylated flavan-3-ols at 59%–91%, oligomeric flavan-3-ols at 72%–95%, and glycosylated flavonols at 56%–88% (in cocoa treatment) and 82%–94% (in GSE treatment) of the contents that were added to the meat batter.	It was a good fermented meat product with balanced quantities of phenolic and other bioactive compounds. All phenolic compound levels did not decrease further significantly after aging until the end of shelf life.	Ribas-Agustí et al. (2014)

Case Study 5		
Study was conducted on the positive effect of fermented papaya preparation (FPP) on type-2 diabetes. The evaluation was done by studying its effect on the human antioxidant status and erythrocyte integrity on a multi-ethnic pre-diabetic population. Fermented papaya exhibited effective *in-vitro* free radical scavenging activities thought to be attributed to residual phenolic or flavonoid compounds.	The experiment suggested that a dose of 6 g FPP/day for a period of 14 weeks was observed to notably reduce the rate of hemolysis and accumulation of protein carbonyls in the blood plasma of prediabetic patients. FPP if consumed on a daily basis strengthen antioxidant defense system *in vivo* was clearly demonstrated by the marked increase of total antioxidant status in the FPP-supplemented prediabetic patients.	Somanah et al. (2014)
Case Study 6		
Adlay angkak a new developed product from an adlay substrate fermented by *Monascus* fungus can be used both as a natural colorant and as a dietary supplement. However, not only useful secondary metabolites such as mevinolin and pigments are produced.	Bioactive component obtained from e fermentation is the blood-reducing cholesterol substance called mevinolin ($C_{24}H_{36}O_5$), a substance that prohibits the creation of cholesterol by blocking a key enzyme, HMG-CoA reductase (activates cholesterol synthesis). However, not only useful secondary metabolites such as mevinolin and pigments are produced, the fungi also produce toxin substance called citrinin.	Pattanagul et al. (2008)
Case Study 7		
Fruit juices of Xisha Noni (*Morinda citrifolia* L.) were studied on the basis of post-fermentation. There was an increase in the amount of phenolic compound having the antioxidant activity and several compounds of fermented noni fruit juice.	Study verified that the possible antioxidative mechanism of fermented noni fruit juice was partially due to the scavenging ability of a group of phenolic compounds (such as asisoscopoletin, aesculetin, and quercetin). Quercetin, one of the most abundant flavonoids in human diet, has been popular for its various bioactivities, such as antiulcer, antiallergic, antiviral, immunomodulating activities, and inhibition of lipid peroxidation. Isoscopoletin, another phenolic compound due to its high scavenging activity has the ability to prevent oxidation-related diseases.	Chang-hong et al. (2007)

Continued

Table 20.3 (Continued) Health Benefits of Nutraceuticals from Fermented Foods: Case Studies

Work Done	*Benefit of Nutraceuticals*	*Reference*
Case Study 8		
Bioactivity compound generated due to the fermentation of soybean to form *tempe*, the traditional food from Indonesia. Soybean *tempe* extracts powerfully repressed the adhesion of entero-toxigenic *E. coli* (ETEC) strains tested. All *tempe* made from other leguminous seeds were as bioactive as soybean *tempe*.	The bioactivity of the *tempe* is due to its inhibition of the adhesion of (ETEC) to intestinal cells.	Roubos-van den Hil (2010)
Case Study 9		
Salt-shrimp fermentation in the Philippines has added beneficial information to this research. There was noticeable increase in the oxidation scavenging activity and bioactive components after the shrimp was kept for prolonged fermentation. The fermentation period of 90 days showed a dramatic increase in free amino acids.	Amino compounds such as free amino acids and peptides function as a primary antioxidant. The major free amino acids in shrimp paste are taurine, glycine, alanine, leucine, lysine, and arginine, and most of them increased dramatically during fermentation. These free amino acids are interrelating with other substances to form compounds exhibiting antioxidant activity such as Maillard reaction products (MRPs). MRPs formed in food have been reported to exhibit high antioxidant activity.	Peralta et al. (2008)
Case Study 10		
Fermentation of rice is done by traditional method in Thailand. The study was conducted to evaluate the bioactive components of the Thai rice (*Oryza sativa* L. var. *indica*) fermentation, including white plain, purple plain, brown plain, white glutinous, and purple glutinous rice were fermented with *lookpang* (a mixed culture of yeasts and molds).	The sap sample of the fermentation of purple plain rice showed the highest free radical scavenging (the sample concentrations that scavenged 50% of the DPPH radicals, SC_{50} at 14.51 ± 2.21 mg/mL), tyrosinase inhibition (the sample concentrations that inhibited 50% of tyrosinase activity, IC_{50} at 15.05 ± 2.92 mg/mL) and MMP-2 inhibition activities (62.22 ± 3.78%).	Manosroi et al. (2011)

	Tyrosinase is the main enzyme that catalyzes melanin synthesis. MMPs are the matrix metalloproteinases, enzymes to degrade the collagen matrix plus arthritis, inflammations, heart-related diseases, cancer, and skin aging. Many MMPinhibitors are basically vitamin C and vitamin E.	
Case Study 11		
Fermentation of pork sausage (*Nham*) was found with high amounts of GABA in this study. The enhancement of these bioactive compounds was achieved by the addition of 0.5% monosodium glutamate (MSG) together with inoculums (*Pediococcus pentosaceus* HN8 and *Lactobacillus namurensis* NH2, ratio 1:1) with a size of roughly 6 log CFU/g in this experiment, a unique *nahm* was formulated containing a high amount of GABA but low in fat, carbohydrate, and energy.	GABA is a nonprotein amino acid that acts as the major inhibitory neurotransmitter in the sympathetic nervous system and also plays an important role in cardiovascular function. Other reports on GABA show its health benefits as a food additive such as reducing hypertension, its diuretic effect, inhibiting the proliferation of cancer cells, and preventing diabetes. Most GABA-containing functional foods have been reported in fermented beverages, for example, fermented seaweed beverage, raspberry juice, and dairy products.	Ratanaburee et al. (2013)
Case Study 12		
Herbs are known as rich sources of bioactive compounds entering in the preparation of traditional beverages (antioxidant, anti-inflammatory, antimicrobial). Traditional dates juice (*Phoenix dactylifera*), Tassabount in Morocco, is a preparation using medicinal and aromatic plants macerate which is fermented over 3–5 days. A variety of plants are used including more than 20 species (basil, clove, thyme, lemon, iris, myrthe, oregano, nutmeg, rosemary, mandrak). The fermentation process has the potential to produce new beneficial compounds, resulting in the increase of biological properties of traditional preparations.	This aromatic extract has been reported to contain bioactive compounds such as carvacrol, thymol, and phenolic compounds providing antimicrobial properties (Cowan 1999) and improving the safety status and shelf life of the traditional juice.	Fernandez-Panchon et al. (2008), Harbourne et al. (2013), Harrak et al. (2012).

Continued

Table 20.3 (Continued) Health Benefits of Nutraceuticals from Fermented Foods: Case Studies

Work Done	*Benefit of Nutraceuticals*	*Reference*
Case Study 13		
The viability of the probiotic bacterium *Lb. fermentum* HA6 isolated from naturally fermented vegetables in Vietnam was improved by growing the bacterium into a mild acid condition (pH4.0). Viability and probiotic functionality (PepX) activity of the acid-adapted bacterium exposed to simulated gastrointestinal conditions were investigated. The performance of acid-adapted bacteria in simulated gastric juice, specific PepX, and simulated small intestinal fluid were better compared with those of the control bacterium.	Acid adaptation has a key role in acquiring cross-protection mechanism, which in this study resulted in higher survival of *Lb. fermentum* HA6 after simulated gastrointestinal stresses. The strategy of acid adaptation could be valuable for the production of robust probiotics.	Chu-Ky. et al. (2014)
Case Study 14		
In Hunan Province of China, *Fuzhuan* tea *Camellia sinensis* L. is traditionally prepared by fungal fermentation using *Eurotium cristatum*. The *fuzhuan* tea extracts (TEs) were compared with nonfermented green tea extracts using ultraperformance liquid chromatography/time of flight-mass spectrometry (UPLC-ToF-MS). The data from this metabolomic analysis revealed significant increase in the amount of fatty acid amides in the aqueous fermented *fuzhuan* TE. This fermented *Fuzhuan* tea was also found to be biologically active against the growth of Gram-negative *Staphylococcus sonnei*, as well as Gram-positive *Staphlococcus aureus*.	Stimulation of pancreatic amylase and protease *in vitro*, which suggests digestive and intestinal health benefits. The growth of food-borne pathogens *Bacillus cereus*, *Bacillus subtilis*, *Clostridium perfringens*, *Clostridium sporogenes* were inhibited.	Keller et al. (2013)

Case Study 15		
In this study, the potential of two-step fermentation and its synergistic effect to preserve tea polyphenols in functional soy-tea beverage was examined. *Streptococcus thermophilus, Lactobacillus delbrueckii* ssp. *bulgaricus* and *Bif. longum* were cultured in soy milk supplemented with TE to produce fermented soy milk tea (FST). Based on experimental results obtained from this two-step fermentation, there was increase in total antioxidant content, antiradical activity, and stability of tea polyphenols.	This functional beverage containing tea polyphenols, soy isoflavones, and functional bacteria can have potential health benefits.	Zhao and Shah (2014)
Case Study 16		
ImmuBalance is one of the Japanese fermentation products (Nichimo Co. Ltd., Tokyo, Japan) made by fermenting defatted soybeans with *Aspergillus oryzae* and LAB *(Pediococcus paevulus* and *E. faecium).*	ImmuBalance has exhibited suppressive properties on skin disorders, like atopic dermatitis (AD) by downregulation of the itch sensation.	Matsuda et al. (2012)

applied to optimize the food-manufacturing processes or to manipulate the organoleptic properties (i.e., the overall flavor and texture) of the products. Figure 20.4 shows the recent study of probiotic mechanism on health enhancement.

Lb. plantarum is a nonpathogenic Gram-positive bacterium found in the human gut. Besides, *Lactobacillus* is a facultative anaerobic bacterium because it can grow both in the presence and absence of oxygen. In the case of presence of oxygen, this probiotic will use the oxygen content to increase the biomass. Nevertheless, in the absence of oxygen, *Lb. plantarum* will convert sugar into lactic acid and alcohol. Moreover, the lactic acid produced is a combination of *D*- and *L*-isomers. Moreover, because of being able to produce lactic acid, approximately 50 species of *Lb. plantarum* have been applied popularly in traditional fermentation food technology such as the production of fermented products from meat, vegetable, and dairy. Furthermore, improving the conversion, flavor, and texture characteristics of the fermented food are considered as main reasons for this probiotic strain to use in industrial food technology. Besides, the safety of *Lb. plantarum* is confirmed by history of its use in sauerkraut and olive preparation. The environmental conditions in stomach and bile are recognized as an extreme condition with microorganism. However, the survival of *Lb. plantarum* is commended higher than *Lc. lactic* and *Lc. fermentum* which are 7 ± 2%, 1 ± 0.8%, and 0.5 ± 0.5%, respectively. Moreover, the colonization capacity of Lactobacillus plantarum is

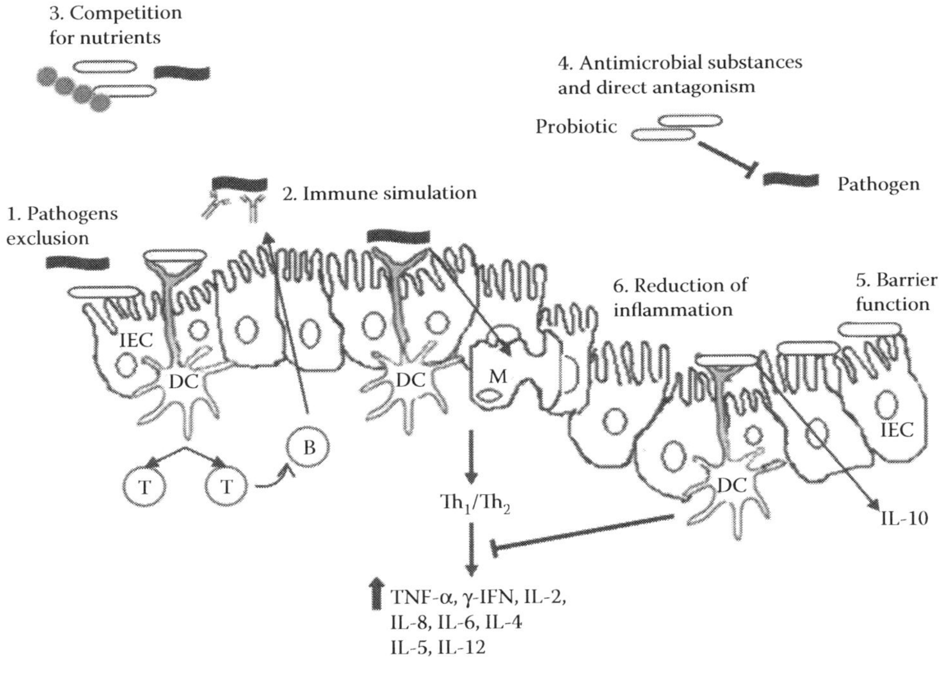

Figure 20.4 Some probiotic mechanisms whereby induce several beneficial host responses. Most effects consist of: (1) exclusion and competing with pathogen to epithelial cells adhesion, (2) innate immune stimulation, (3) competition for nutrients and prebiotic products, (4) production of antimicrobial substances and thereby pathogen antagonism, (5) protection of intestinal barrier integrity, and (6) regulation of anti-inflammatory cytokine and inhibition of proinflammatory cytokine production. IEC: intestinal epithelium cells, DC: dendritic cell; IL: interleukin; M: intestinal M cell. (From Saad et al. 2013. *LWT-Food Science and Technology* 50, 1–16.)

higher than *Lactobacillus reuti, Lactobacillus gasseri, Lb. acidophilus, Lb. casei, and Lactobacillus agilis* (Maaike et al. 2006).

Many studies focus on the survival of probiotics after passing through stomach and bile. Research of characterization and probiotic potential of *Lb. plantarum* is one of the studies to ensure the probiotic properties Ninety-eight *Lactobacillus* strains were isolated from Italian and Argentinean cheese to check the probiotic potential (Miriam Zago 2011). In the case of *in-vitro* resistance to lysozyme condition, 50 strains of *Lb. plantarum* could be found in a lysozyme resistance experiment at 68% survival. Moreover, the survival ability of this probiotic in bile condition was recognized higher than the lysozyme condition, 95% survival of *Lb. plantarum* 804, 805, and 994 strains; 95.98% *Lb. plantarum* 790 strains. In simulated gastric juice, only 9 strains can survive at pH 2 during 90 min, which was 10^6 CFU/mL.

To improve the stability of *Lb. plantarum* in an extreme environment such as stomach and bile, microencapsulation technique is applied. In this experiment, *Lb. plantarum* was covered twice by pectin, sodium alginate, and another pectin, sodium alginate. In the simulated gastrointestinal medium and the simulated gastric medium, the survival of this probiotic between free cells and encapsulated cells was similar. Nevertheless, the living cell of the encapsulated *Lb. plantarum* cell was higher than the free cell under refrigerated condition. Moreover, the combination of 4% pectin, 3% sodium alginate coated with chitosan, and a mixture of 2% (w/v) sodium alginate, and 2% (w/v) pectin was recognized as the best method used to survive the viability of the encapsulated cell. Furthermore, the loss of living cell in yogurt was 0.55 log cycles during 38 days of storage (Brinques and Ayub 2011).

Viability and probiotic functionality (X-prolyl dipeptidyl aminopeptidase [PepX] activity) of the acid-adapted bacterium exposed to simulated gastrointestinal conditions were investigated. After 180 min in the simulated gastric juice (0.3 g/L pepsin, pH 2.0), the viability of acid-adapted *Lb. fermentum* HA6 (11.5%) was higher than that of control *L. fermentum* HA6 (2.2%). Specific PepX activity of acid-adapted cells (24.5 U/mg) was higher than that of control cells (17.8 U/mg). After 180 min exposure to the simulated small intestinal medium (0.3 g/L bile salts, 0.1 g/L pancreatin, pH 8.0), the viability of acid-adapted *Lb. fermentum* HA6 (13.5%) was two-fold as high as that of control *Lb. fermentum* HA6 (8.0%). Our results suggested that acid adaptation has a key role in acquiring the cross-protection mechanism, which in this study resulted in higher survival of *Lb. fermenturm* HA6 after simulated gastrointestinal stresses. The strategy of acid adaptation could be valuable for the production of robust probiotics (Chu-Ky et al. 2014).

20.6.1 Probiotic-Based Dairy Food and Beverage

Owing to the many advantages of *Lb. plantarum*, this probiotic strain was applied popularly in both dairy food and nondairy food. According to Gülden Bas yiğit Kilic et al. (2009), Turkey Beyar cheese material was available to add by *Lb. plantarum*. Turkey Beyar cheese is a traditional fermented food having both nutritional and economic value. Moreover, this special cheese was produced from the milk of sheep and cow without heat treatment. According to the recorded result of this research, probiotic can be available during the 4-month storage of the cheese product. Furthermore, population of this probiotic was 10^8 CFU/g in MRS and M17 medium. Nevertheless, the living probiotic cells decrease after 120 days of storage, which was 10^5 CFU/g. However, sensory value was considered as an important factor when adding probiotics to cheese because an increase in the content of acetic acid and a decrease in diacetyl content of cheese after 120 days of storage reduce the flavor of the product.

Kefir is a traditional milk product, a combination of LAB and yeast. Special taste and aroma was found in kefir product, a combination of lactic acid and alcohol. Moreover, fresh milk was usually fermented by kefir grain, insoluble in water and containing the group of microorganism. Moreover, *Lactobacillus* species are considered as the majority of bacteria in kefir. Therefore, kefir product was recognized as having antimicrobial activity because kefir grain will produce lactic acid, volatile acids, hydrogen peroxide, carbon dioxide, diacetyl, and acetaldehyde. Moreover, *Lb. plantarum* ST8KF was seen as one of the LAB in kefir grain. The activity of *Lb. plantarum* in kefir was stable with α-amylase while this bacteria was destroyed during treatment with proteinase K and pronase. Moreover, *Lb. plantarum* was stable at pH from 2 to 10 at 30°C (Powell et al. 2007).

20.6.2 Probiotic-Based Nondairy Food and Beverage

Besides cheese, *Lb. plantarum* was also applied in nondairy foods, among them, instant Chinese noodle was considered as material to carry out this experiment. To improve the texture of the noodle, strong wheat and Kansvi, a mixture of alkaline salt such as potassium carbonate, sodium carbonate, were used in noodle processing. However, application of lactic acid by *Lb. plantarum* can replace the chemical Kansvi increasing elasticity and color. Therefore, 46 LAB strains were cultured in strong wheat material to improve the quality of instant Chinese noodles. However, only night strains can grow at a higher population at a pH of less than 5.5 after 24 h fermentation. Among the night probiotic strains, *Lb. plantarum* NRIC 0380 isolated from Thai pickle was recognized as the most suitable strains because 9.79 g/kg of acid lactic and 0.99 g/kg of acetic acid were produced after 24 h of fermentation. However, there were many disadvantages when applying *Lb. plantarum* to noodle such as the available cell reduced from 6.8 10^8 to 1.7 10^8 CFU/g after storage, pH in the material decreased dramatically and the color of the noodle changed from yellow to white. However, using this probiotic improved the texture and increased the nutritional properties of the Chinese noodle such as amino acids and vitamins (Sawatari et al. 2011).

Many studies have focused on research of the survival capacity of *Lb. plantarum* in cereal and fruit materials such as oat flour, malt, barley, and cabbage juice. Moreover, cereal and fruit were considered as materials having valuable health benefits and containing many nutrients and such as bioactive compounds and so on. Therefore, in the experiment, *Lb. plantarum* was found at the highest maximum biomass production in white flour. Similar to white flour, probiotic bacteria reached the stationary phase only at 6 h of fermentation in malt, barley, and a mixture of malt and barley cultured 1% *Lb. plantarum*. Moreover, a large amount of amino acid was found in malt after fermentation with this strain (Rathore 2011). Furthermore, fruit and vegetable are considered rich sources of functional components such as minerals, vitamins, dietary fibers, and antioxidants. Cabbage also contains a large amount of minerals, vitamin C, dietary fibers, and phytochemicals. Therefore, this material was also applied as material to culture *Lb. plantarum*. According to the result of this research, probiotics can grow in cabbage rapidly after 48 h of fermentation at 30°C which was 10^{10} CFU/g. The large population of *Lb. plantarum* was found after 4 weeks of storage, which was 4.1 10^7 CFU/g. Nevertheless, the survival of this probiotic is based on many factors such as oxygen, oxygen permeation, fermentation time, and storage time (Kyung et al. 2006).

20.7 Nutraceuticals from Fermented Foods and Beverages

Nutraceuticals are diet supplements that deliver a concentrated form of a presumed bioactive agent from a food, presented in a nonfood matrix, and used with the purpose of enhancing health in dosages that exceed those that could be obtained from normal foods (Zeisel 1999). Nutraceuticals are sold in presentations similar to drugs: pills, extracts, tablets, and so on. The Food and drug administration (FDA) regulates dietary supplements under a different set of regulations than those covering conventional foods and drug products. However, no specific regulation exists in Europe to control nutraceuticals. The boundary between nutraceuticals and functional foods is not always clear. For example, when a phytochemical or phytochemical extract is included in a food formulation, that is, 300 mg of extract dissolved in 1 L of juice, a new potential functional food can be formulated. The same amount of phytochemical or phytochemical extract included in a capsule will constitute new nutraceuticals (Espín et al. 2007).

20.8 Conclusions

Fermented foods are of great significance because they provide and preserve vast quantities of nutritious foods in a wide diversity of flavors, aromas, and textures, which enrich the human diet. Fermented foods have been with us since man's first existence on the earth. These products will remain important in the future as they are the source of alcoholic foods/beverages, vinegar, pickled vegetables, sausages, cheeses, yogurts, vegetable protein amino acid/peptide sauces, and pastes with meat-like flavors, leavened and sourdough breads. The release of organic acids such as hydrogen peroxide, ethanol, and diacetyl not only contribute to the antimicrobial activity in starter cultures, rather other LAB metabolites also contribute to it. Bacteriocin is among such metabolites, as LAB strains are GRAS for usage in food production, therefore the detection and identification of bacteriocins have got much importance for its "natural" preservation quality. Lactic acid fermentation of vegetables, cereals, and marine products is a valuable technique, for ensuring the suppression of unwanted, hazardous growth of microorganisms in regions, where proper hygienic condition is away from reasonable reach. Fermentation has been proving itself since history as the best method to maintain hygienic conditions, and also an alternate for those recons in world to maintain food in poor and underdeveloped countries. This can be achieved just by providing them proper knowledge and adequate training to maximize the available resource in a proper way. The knowledge of traditional fermentation can be shared for the better application of fermented foods and for improvement of nutraceuticals. More research on fermented foods is needed, and mechanisms to exchange knowledge between these regions should be established in order to stimulate regional research and expand the benefits of new findings.

References

Amoa-Awua, W.K., Frisvad, J. C., Sefa-Dedeh, S., and Jakobsen, M. 1997. The contribution of moulds and yeasts to the fermentation of "agbelima" cassava dough. *Journal of Applied Microbiology* 83: 288–296.

Asahara, T., Nomoto, K., Shimizu, K., Watanuki, M., and Tanaka, R. 2001. Increased resistance of mice to Salmonella entericaserovar Typhimurium infection by synbiotic administration of Bifidobacteria and transgalactosylated oligosac-charides. *Journal of Applied Microbiology* 91: 985–996.

Billings, T. 1998. On fermented foods. Also available online at http://www.livingfoods.com

Blandino, A., Al-Aseeri, M. E., Pandiella, S. S., Cantero, D., and Webb, C. 2003. Cereal-based fermented foods and beverages. *Food Research International* 36(6): 527–543.

Bol, J., and de Vos, W. M. 1997. Fermented foods: An overview. In: J. Green (Ed.), *Biotechnological Innovations in Food Processing*. Oxford: Butterworth-Heinemann.

Bolotin, A., Mauger, S., Malarme, K., Ehrlich, S. D., and Sorokin, A. 1999. Low-redundancy sequencing of the entire Lactococcus lactis IL1403 genome. In: *Lactic Acid Bacteria: Genetics, Metabolism and Applications*. Netherlands: Springer, pp. 27–76.

Bourel, G., Henini, S., Divies, C., and Garmyn, D. 2003. The response of Leuconostoc mesenteroides to low external oxidoreduction potential generated by hydrogen gas. *Journal of Applied Microbiology* 94(2): 280–288.

Bournet, F. R., Brouns, F., Tashiro, Y., and Duvillier, V. 2002. Nutritional aspects of short-chain fructooligosaccharides: Natural occurrence, chemistry, physiology, and health implications. *Digestive and Liver Disease* 34: S111e–S120.

Brinques, G. B., and Ayub, M. A. Z. 2011. Effect of microencapsulation on survival of Lac. plantarum in simulated gastrointestinal conditions, refrigeration, and yogurt. *Journal of food engineering* 103(2): 123–128.

Campbell-Platt, G. 1994. Fermented foods: A world perspective. *Food Research International* 27(3): 253–257.

Cao-Hoang, L., Chu-Ky, S., Ho, P.-H., Husson, F., Le, T.-B., Le-Thanh, M. et al. 2013. Tropical traditional fermented food, a field full of promise. Examples from the Tropical Bioresources and Biotechnology programme and other related French-Vietnamese programmes on fermented food. *International Journal of Food Science and Technology* 48: 1115–1126.

Chang-hong, L. I. U., Ya-rong, X. U. E., Yong-hang, Y. E., Feng-feng, Y. U. A. N., Jun-yan, L. I. U., and Jing-lei, S. H. U. A. N. G. 2007. Extraction and Characterization of antioxidant compositions from fermented fruit juice of Morinda citrifolia(Noni). *Agricultural Sciences in China* 6(12): 1494–1501.

Chavan, J. K., and Kadam, S. S. 1989. Critical reviews in food science and nutrition. *Food Science* 28: 348–400.

Chu, D. 2010. Role of Lactic Acid Bacteria in the Fermented Shrimp (Tom chua) Making Process. Hanoi: Hanoi University of Agriculture.

Chu-Ky, S., Bui, T. K., Nguyen, T. L., and Ho, P. H. 2014. Acid adaptation to improve viability and X-prolyl dipeptidyl aminopeptidase activity of the probiotic bacterium Lactobacillus fermentum HA6 exposed to simulated gastrointestinal tract conditions. *International Journal of Food Science and Technology* 49(2): 565–570.

Cooke, R. D., Twiddy, D. R., and Reilly, P. J. A. 1987. Lactic acid fermentation as a low cost means of food preservation in tropical countries. *FEMS Microbiological Reviews* 46: 369–379.

Cowan, M. M. 1999. Plant products as antimicrobial agents. *Clinical Microbiology Reviews* 12: 564–582.

Delzenne, N. M., and Kok, N. 2001. Effects of fructan-type prebiotics on lipid metabolism. *American Journal of Clinical Nutrition* 73: 456–458.

Delzenne, N. M., Daubioul, C., Neyrinck, A., Lasa, M., and Taper, H. S. 2002. Inulin and oligofructose modulate lipid metabolism in animals: Review of biochemical events and future prospects. *British Journal of Nutrition* 87(S2): S255–S259.

Dougan, J., and Howard, G. E. 1975. Some flavouring constituents of fermented fish sauces. *Journal of the Science of Food and Agriculture* 26(7): 887–894.

Espin, J. C., Garcia-Conesa, M. T., and Tomas-Barberan, F. A. 2007. Nutraceuticals: Facts and fictio. *Phytochemistry* 68: 2986–3008.

Farnworth, E. R. T. (Ed.). 2008. *Handbook of Fermented Functional Foods*. CRC press Taylor & Francis Group, Boca Raton.

Femia, A. P., Luceri, C., Dolara, P., Giannini, A., Biggeri, A., Salvadori, M., and Caderni, G. 2002. Antitumorigenic activity of the prebiotic inulin enriched with oligofructose in combination with the probiotics Lactobacillus rhamnosusand Bifidobacterium lactis on azoxymethane-induced colon carcinogenesis in rats. *Carcinogenesis* 23(11): 1953–1960.

Fernandez-Panchon, M. S., Villano, D., Troncoso, A. M., and Garcia-Parrilla, M. C. 2008. Antioxidant activity of phenolic compounds: From in vitro results to in vivo evidence. *Critical Reviews in Food Science and Nutrition* 48(7): 649–671.

Forchielli, M. L., and Walker, W. A. 2005. The role of gut-associated lymphoid tissues and mucosal defence. *British Journal of Nutrition* 93(Suppl. 1): 41–48.

Gardner, C. D., Newell, K. A., Cherin, R., and Haskell, W. L. 2001. The effect of soy protein with or without isoflavone relative to milk protein on plasma lipids in hypercholesterolemic postmenopausal women. *The American Journal of Clinical Nutrition* 73(4): 728–735.

Hamad, A. M., and Fields, M. L. 1979. Evaluation of protein quality and available lysine of germinated and ungerminated cereals. *Journal of Food Science* 44: 456–459.

Harbourne, N., Marete, E., Jacquier, J. C., and O'Riordan, D. 2013. Stability of phytochemicals as sources of anti-inflammatory nutraceuticals in beverages: A review. *Food Research International* 50: 480–486.

Harlander, S. 1992. Food biotechnology. In: J. Lederberg (Ed.), *Encyclopaedia of Microbiology.* New York: Academic Press.

Harrak, H., Lebrun, M., Alaoui, M. M. I., Sarter, S., and Hamouda, A. 2012. Physico-chemical, biochemical and microbiological phenomena of the medicinal and aromatic plants extract used in the preparation of Tassabount date juice in Morocco. In: J. K. Mworia (Ed.), *Botany.* Croatie: InTech.

Ho, P.-H., and Adams, M. 2006. Selection and identification of a novel probiotic strain of Lactobacillus fermentum isolated from Vietnamese fermented food. In: N. Le-Van and A. To-Kim (Eds.), *20th Scientific Conference.* Hanoi: Hanoi University of Technology.

Ho, P.-H., Adams, M. C., Rothkirch, T. B., Dunstan, R. H., and Roberts, T. K. 2011a. Opioid peptide digestion by newly isolated potential probiotic bacteria from foods. *Journal of Science and Technology* 49: 161–168.

Ho, P. H., Tien, L. H., and Chi, L. T. L. 2011b. Incorporation of probiotic Lactobacillus fermentum HA6 into food products: An exploratory study. *Journal of Science and Technology* 82A: 27–31.

Hoentjen, F., Welling, G. W., Harmsen, H. J., Zhang, X., Snart, J., Tannock, G. W. et al. 2005. Reduction of colitis by prebiotics in HLA-B27 transgenic rats is associated with microflora changes and immunomodulation. *Inflammatory Bowel Disease* 11: 977–985.

Hosono, A., Ozawa, A., Kato, R., Ohnishi, Y., Nakanishi, Y., Kimura, T., and Nakamura, R. 2003. Dietary fructooligosaccharides induce immunoregulation of intestinal IgA secretion by murine Peyer's patch cells. *Bioscience, Biotechnology, and Biochemistry* 67(4): 758–764.

Iwuoha, C. I., and Eke, O. S. 1996. Nigerian indigenous fermented foods: Their traditional process operation, inherent problems, improvements and current status. *Food Research International* 29: 527–540.

Jayasekera, S., Kaur, L., Molan, A. L., Garg, M. L., and Moughan, P. J. 2014. Effects of season and plantation on phenolic content of unfermented and fermented Sri Lankan tea. *Food Chemistry* 152: 546–551.

Jiang, T., and Savaiano, D. A. 1997. Modification of colonic fermentation by bifidobacteria and pH in vitro (impact on lactose metabolism, short-chain fatty acid, and lactate production). *Digestive Diseases and Sciences* 42(11): 2370–2377.

Keller A. C., Weir T. L., Broeckling C. D., and Ryan E. P. 2013. Antibacterial activity and phytochemical profile of fermented Camellia sinensis (fuzhuan tea). *Food Research International* 53: 945–949.

Khetarpaul, N., and Chauhan, B. M. 1990. Effect of fermentation by pure cultures of yeasts and lactobacilli on the available carbohydrate content of pearl millet. *Tropical Science* 31: 131–139.

Kılıc, G. B., Kuleaşan, H., Eralp, İ., and Karahan, A. G. 2009. Manufacture of Turkish Beyaz cheese added with probiotic strains. *LWT-Food Science and Technology* 42(5): 1003–1008.

Kingamko, R., Sjogren, E., Svanberg, U., and Kaijser, B. 1994. pH and acidity in lactic-fermenting cereal gruels: Effects of variability of enteropathogenic microorganisms. *World Journal of Microbiology and Biotechnology* 10: 664–669.

Kuo, C. F., Hou, M. H., Wang, T. S., Chyau, C. C., and Chen, Y. T. 2009. Enhanced antioxidant activity of Monascus pilosusfermented products by addition of ginger to the medium. *Food Chemistry* 116(4): 915–922.

Kuo, C. F., Hou, M. H., Wang, T. S., Chyau, C. C., and Chen, Y. T. 2009. Enhanced antioxidant activity of *Monascus pilosus* fermented products by addition of ginger to the medium. *Food Chemistry* 116(4): 915–922.

Kyung, Y. Y., Woodams, E. E., and Hang, Y. D. 2006. Production of probiotic cabbage juice by lactic acid bacteria. *Bioresource Technology* 97: 1427–1430.

Lee, C.-H. 1998. Lactic acid fermented foods and their benefits in Asia. *Food Control* 8: 259–269.

Lorri, W., and Svanberg, U. 1995. An overview of the use of fermented foods for child feeding in Tanzania. *Ecology of Food and Nutrition* 34(1): 65–81.

Lotong, N. K. 1998. In J. B. Wood (Ed.), *Microbiology of Fermented Foods.* London: Blackie Academic and Professional, pp. 658–695.

Maaike, C. de Vries, Elaine, E. V., Kleerebezem, M., and de Vosa, W. M. 2006, Lactobacillus plantarum—Survival, functional and potential probiotic properties in the human intestinal tract. *International Dairy Journal* 16: 1018–1028.

Manosroi, A., Ruksiriwanich, W., Kietthanakorn, B. O., Manosroi, W., and Manosroi, J. 2011. Relationship between biological activities and bioactive compounds in the fermented rice sap. *Food Research International* 44(9): 2757–2765.

Matsuda, A., Tanaka, A., Pan, W., Okamoto, N., Oida, K., Kingyo, N., and Matsuda, H. 2012. Supplementation of the fermented soy product ImmuBalance™ effectively reduces itching behavior of atopic NC/Tnd mice. *Journal of Dermatological Science* 67(2): 130–139.

Mbugua, S. K. 1984. Isolation and characterization of lactic acid bacteria during the traditional fermentation of uji. *East African Agricultural and Forestry Journal* 50: 36–43.

McKay, L. L. and Baldwin, K. A. 1990. Applications for biotechnology: Present and future improvements in lactic acid bacteria. *FEMS Microbiology Reviews* 87: 3–14.

Mensah, P., Tomkins, A. M., Brasar, B. S., and Harrison, T. J. 1991. Antimicrobial effect of fermented Ghanaian maize dough. *Journal of Applied Bacteriology* 70: 203–210.

Miriam Z., Maria E. F., Domenico C., Patricia B., Viviana S., Gabriel V. et al. 2011. Characterization and probiotic potential of Lactobacillus plantarum strains isolated from cheeses. *Food Microbiology* 28: 1033–1040.

Morcos, S. R., Hegazi, S. M., and Ell-Damhoughy, S. I. T. 1973. Fermented foods in common use in Egypt. II. The chemical composition of Bouza and its ingredients. *Journal of Science Food and Agriculture* 24: 1151–1561.

Morcos, S. R., Hegazi, S. M., and Ell-Damhougy, S. I. T. 1993. Egyptian bouza. In: K. H. Steinkraus (Ed.), *Handbook of Indigenous Fermented Foods*. New York: Marcel Dekker, pp. 421–425.

Munjal, U., Glei, M., Pool-Zobel, B. L., and Scharlau, D. 2009. Fermentation products of inulin-type fructans reduce proliferation and induce apoptosis in human colon tumour cells of different stages of carcinogenesis. *British Journal of Nutrition* 27: 1–9.

Nakamura, Y., Nosaka, S., Suzuki, M., Nagafuchi, S., Takahashi, T., Yajima, T., and Moro, I. 2004. Dietary fructooligosaccharides up-regulate immunoglobulin A response and polymeric immunoglobulin receptor expression in intestines of infant mice. *Clinical and Experimental Immunology* 137(1): 52–58.

Nguyen, H. T., Elegado, F. B., Librojo-Basilio, N. T., Mabesa, R. C., and Dizon, E. I. 2010. Isolation and characterisation of selected lactic acid bacteria for improved processing of Nem chua, a traditional fermented meat from Vietnam. *Beneficial Microbes* 1(1): 67–74.

Noguchi, H., Uchino, M., Shida, O., Takano, K., Nakamura, L. K., and Komagata, K. 2004. Bacillus vietnamensis sp. nov., a moderately halotolerant, aerobic, endospore-forming bacterium isolated from Vietnamese fish sauce. *International Journal of Systematic and Evolutionary Microbiology* 54(6): 2117–2120.

Nout, M. J. R. 1994. Fermented foods and food safety. *Food Research International* 27(3): 291–298.

Nout, M. J. R., and Motarjemi, Y. 1997. Assessment of fermentation as a household technology for improving food safety: A joint FAO/WHO workshop. *Food Control* 8: 221–226.

Odunfa, S. A., and Oyewole, O. B. 1998. African fermented foods. In: J. B. Woods (Ed.), *Microbiology of Fermented Foods*. London: Blackie Academic and Professional.

Palma, A. S., Feizi, T., Zhang, Y., Stoll, M. S., Lawson, A. M., Diaz-Rodriguez, E. et al. 2006. Ligands for the beta-glucan receptor, Dectin-1, assigned using "designer" microarrays of oligosaccharide probes (neoglycolipids) generated from glucan polysaccharides. *Journal of Biological Chemistry* 281: 5771–5779.

Park, J. N., Ishida, K., Watanabe, T., Endoh, K. I., Watanabe, K., Murakami, M., and Abe, H. 2002b. Taste effects of oligopeptides in a Vietnamese fish sauce. *Fisheries Science* 68(4): 921–928.

Park, J. N., Watanabe, T., Endoh, K. I., Watanabe, K., and Abe, H. 2002a. Taste-active components in a Vietnamese fish sauce. *Fisheries Science* 68(4): 913–920.

Pattanagul, P., Pinthong, R., Phianmongkhol, A., and Tharatha, S. 2008. Mevinolin, citrinin and pigments of adlay *angkak* fermented by *Monascus* sp. *International Journal of food Microbiology* 126(1): 20–23.

Peralta, E. M., Hatate, H., Kawabe, D., Kuwahara, R., Wakamatsu, S., Yuki, T. et al. 2008. Improving antioxidant activity and nutritional components of Philippine salt-fermented shrimp paste through prolonged fermentation. *Food Chemistry* 111(1): 72–77.

Pham, T. N. L., and Le, T. B. 2001. Improvement of weight gain in growing broiler chicken by administration of probiotic Lactobacillus strains. *Advance in Natural Science* 2: 69–76.

Pham, T. N. L., and Le, T. B. 2004a. 16 Ribosomal DNA terminal restriction fragment pattern analysis of jejunal and cecal microbiota of young chick fed two probiotic *Lactobacillus* strains. *Advance in Natural Science* 5: 297–311.

Pham, T. N. L., and Le, T. B. 2004b. Effect of two probiotic Lactobacillus strains on the jejunal and cecal microbiota and growth performance of Young broiler chick. *Advance in Natural Science* 5: 78–84.

Pham, T. N. L., Le, T. B., and Yoshimi, B. 2001. Effect of probiotic Lactobacillus strains on Lactobacillus flora in intestine of broiler chicken. *Advance in Natural Science* 3: 71–79.

Pham, T. N. L., Le, T. B., and Yoshimi, B. 2003. Impact of two probiotic Lactobacillus strains on fecal lactobacilli and weight gains in chicken. *Journal of General and Applied Microbiology* 49: 29–39.

Pierre, F., Perrin, P., Champ, M., Bornet, F., Meflah, K., and Menanteau, J. 1997. Shortchain fructo-oligosaccharides reduce the occurrence of colon tumors and develop gut-associated lymphoid tissue in Min mice. *Cancer Research* 57: 225–228.

Powell, J. E., Witthuhn, R. C., Todorov, S. D., and Dicks, L. M. T. 2007. Characterization of bacteriocin ST8KF produced by a kefir isolate *Lactobacillus plantarum* ST8KF. *International Dairy Journal* 17: 190–198.

Qiang, X., YongLie, C., and QianBing, W. 2009. Health benefit application of functional oligosaccharides. *Carbohydrate Polymers* 77(3): 435–441.

Quiros, A., Ramos, M., Muguerza, B., Delgado, M. A., Miguel, M., Aleixandre, A. et al. 2007. Identification of novel antihypertensive peptides in milk fermented with *Enterococcus faecalis*. *International Dairy Journal* 17(1): 33–41.

Ratanaburee, A., Kantachote, D., Charernjiratrakul, W., and Sukhoom, A. 2013. Selection of γ-aminobutyric acid-producing lactic acid bacteria and their potential as probiotics for use as starter cultures in Thai fermented sausages (Nham). *International Journal of Food Science and Technology* 48(7): 1371–1382.

Ribas-Agustí, A., Gratacós-Cubarsí, M., Sárraga, C., Guàrdia, M. D., García-Regueiro, J. A., and Castellari, M. 2014. Stability of phenolic compounds in dry fermented sausages added with cocoa and grape seed extracts. *LWT—Food Science and Technology*, 57(1): 329–336.

Roubos-van den Hil, P. J., Nout, M. J., van der Meulen, J., and Gruppen, H. 2010. Bioactivity of tempe by inhibiting adhesion of ETEC to intestinal cells, as influenced by fermentation substrates and starter pure cultures. *Food Microbiology* 27(5): 638–644.

Saad, N., Delattre, C., Urdaci, M., Schmitter, J. M., and Bressollier, P. 2013. An overview of the last advances in probiotic and prebiotic field. *LWT–Food Science and Technology* 50: 1–16.

Saisithi, P., Kasemsarn, R. O., Liston, J., and Dollar, A. M. 1966. Microbiology and chemistry of fermented fish. *Journal of Food Science* 31(1): 105–110.

Sankaran, R. 1998. Fermented food of the Indian subcontinent. In: J. B. Wood (Ed.), *Microbiology of Fermented foods*. London: Blackie Academic and Professional, pp. 753–789.

Sanni, A. I. 1993. The need for process optimization of African fermented foods and beverages. *International Journal of Food Microbiology* 18(2): 85–95.

Sarkar, P. K., and Tamang, J. P. 1994. The influence of process variables and inoculum composition on the sensory quality of kinema. *Food Microbiology* 11: 317–325.

Sawatari, Y., Sugiyama, H., Suzuki, Y., Hanaoka, A., Saito, K., Yamauchi, H., and Yokota, A. 2011. Development of fermented instant Chinese noodle using *Lactobacillus plantarum*. *Food Microbiology* 22(6): 539–546.

Shahani, K. M., Friend, B. A., and Bailey, B. J. 1983. Antitumor activity of fermented colostrums and milk. *Journal of Food Proteins* 46: 385–386.

Simango, C. 1997. Potential use of traditional fermented foods for weaning in Zimbabwe. *Social Science & Medicine* 44(7): 1065–1068.

Sindhu, S. C., and Khertapaul, N. 2001. Probiotic fermentation of indigenous food mixture: Effect on antinutrients and digestibility of starch and protein. *Journal of Food Composition and Analysis* 14: 601–609.

Somanah, J., Bourdon, E., Rondeau, P., Bahorun, T., and Aruoma, O. I. 2014. Relationship between fermented papaya preparation supplementation, erythrocyte integrity and antioxidant status in pre-diabetics. *Food and Chemical Toxicology* 65: 12–17.

Soni, S. K., and Sandhu, D. K. 1990. Indian fermented foods: Micro- biological and biochemical aspects. *Indian Journal of Microbiology* 30: 135–157.

Steinkraus, K. H. 1994. Nutritional significance of fermented foods. *Food Research International* 21: 259–267.

Steinkraus, K. H., Ayres, R., Olek, A., and Farr, D. 1993. Biochemistry of Saccharomyces. In: K. H. Steinkraus (Ed.), *Handbook of Indigenous Fermented Foods*. Marcel Dekker, New York, pp. 517–519.

Suskovic, J., Kos, B., Matosic, S., and Maric, V. 1997. Probiotic properties of Lactobacillus plantarum L4. *Food Technology and Biotechnology* 35: 107–112.

Svanberg, U. and Sandberg, A. S. 1988. Improved iron availability in weaning foods through the use of germination and fermentation. pp. 366–373.

Tanasupawat, S., and Komagata, K. 1995. Lactic acid bacteria in fermented foods in Thailand. *World Journal of Microbiology and Biotechnology* 11: 253–256.

Tran, K., May, B. K., Smooker, P. M., Van, T. T., and Coloe, P. J. 2011. Distribution and genetic diversity of lactic acid bacteria from traditional fermented sausage. *Food Research International* 44(1): 338–344.

Uzogara, S. G., Agu, L. N., and Uzogara, E. O. 1990. A review of traditional fermented foods, condiments and beverages in Nigeria: Their benefits and possible problems. *Ecology of Food and Nutrition* 24(4): 267–288.

Williams, C. M., and Jackson, K. G. 2002. Inulin and oligofructose: Effects on lipid metabolism from human studies. *British Journal Nutrition* 87: 261–264.

Xiong, T., Guan, Q., Song, S., Hao, M., and Xie, M. 2012. Dynamic changes of lactic acid bacteria flora during Chinese sauerkraut fermentation. *Food Control* 26(1): 178–181.

Zarour, K., Benmechernene, Z., Hadadji, M., M.-B., B., Henni, D. J., and Kihal, M. 2012. Bioprospecting of Leuconostoc mesenteroides strains isolated from Algerian raw camel and goat milk for technological properties useful as adjunct starters. *African Journal of Microbiology Research* 6: 3192–3201.

Zeisel, S. H. 1999. Regulation of nutraceuticals. *Science* 285: 1853–1855.

Zhao, D., and Shah, N. P. 2014. Antiradical and tea polyphenol-stabilizing ability of functional fermented soymilk–tea beverage. *Food Chemistry* 158: 262–269.

Chapter 21

From Gut Microbiota to Probiotics: Evolution of the Science

Neerja Hajela, G. Balakrish Nair, and Sarath Gopalan

Contents

21.1 Introduction

A visit to any supermarket these days immediately draws one's attention to the variety of probiotic supplemented dairy products displayed on the shelves. A quick search on Google using the term "probiotic" as the key search word will reveal a mind-boggling number of hits. According to the latest report titled "Dairy Industry in India: 2013–2019," the Indian probiotics market is expected to experience exponential growth at a compound annual growth rate of 25% during 2014–2019. Among others, this spurred interest in probiotics is catalyzed by a large population of youth, an increasing consumer interest in health and wellness, a rising prevalence of stress-related and lifestyle diseases, and urbanization (IMARC Group).

In many ways, probiotics is riding the crest of another unfolding area of research on the human microbiome, particularly the role of the gut microbiota. In fact, probiotics may be operationally defined as a mirror of the beneficial effects of the gut microbiota (Shanahan et al. 2012). Another reason that is driving the interest in probiotics is the voluminous research emanating from the study of the human microbiome particularly the gut microbiome in the last two decades or so. Such research leads to the vital role the gut microbiome plays in maintaining health and preventing disease in ways similar to which probiotics or beneficial bacteria do in the gut. The important strides made in understanding the role of the gut microbiome in health and disease leads to the concept of personalized microbiomes where treatment for chronic medical conditions such as diarrhea and obesity can be effected by genome-informed microbial selection (Sharon and Banfield 2013).

Clearly, probiotics have caught the imagination and attention of both academics and commerce. This chapter will focus on the latest firm evidence-based information that is now being generated on the usefulness of probiotics in acute, chronic, systemic, and localized diseases with particular emphasis on diarrheal diseases.

21.2 History of Probiotics

In 1907, the Russian Nobel laureate Elie Metchnikoff, fascinated by the unusual longevity of Bulgarian farmers who consumed lactic acid bacteria by way of traditionally fermented milk products, suggested that the ingestion of microbes could benefit human health. Although Dr. Metchnikoff's recommended strain for the purpose proved largely ineffective, the concept was carried forward with moderate success until the war on bugs began because of the advent of sulfa drugs and antibiotics (Scott 2012). However, soon after their rampant use and the realization of the hazardous effects of antibiotic therapy, researchers turned yet again to ecological notions and the soil was fertile for the advent of probiotics. By the 1980s the term had stabilized both in medical and veterinary literature. The mid-1990s witnessed a surge of research in the area of probiotics, the definition of probiotics emerged in 2001 and the years that followed saw tremendous progress in the science.

Almost parallel was a reawakening of interest in the study of the gut microbiota when Alfred Nissle demonstrated that transferring members of the human gut microbiota to healthy typhoid carriers resulted in *Salmonella* being cleansed from the system (Nissle 1916). This, for the first time pointed to the importance of the gut microbes in prevention of infection. What followed was the advent of culture independent, high-throughput sequencing technologies, and success of the two most ambitious projects—Human Microbiome project (Turnbaugh et al. 2007) and the European MetaHit project (Metahit 2009, Qin et al. 2010)—that provided fascinating insights into the highly complex microbial ecosystem harbored by the human body. By 2001, the term microbiome (refers to the collective genome of our microbial inhabitants) had entered literature and what emerged was the significant role of the gut microbiota in promoting and maintaining health.

21.3 What are the Findings?

New insights from this rapidly developing field of research have revealed that the microbes we harbor outnumber the number of human cells by a factor of 10. Largest consortiums of these organisms are present in the gut and are called gut microbiota, which comprises nearly 10^{14} microorganisms and as many as 1000 species. This virtual organ system aids host nutrition and maintains homeostasis and even more importantly, with 70% of the immune cells being located in the gut, the enteric microbiota interacts with the immune system providing signals for promoting the maturation of immune cells and the normal development of immune functions (Chow et al. 2010).

The critical role of the gut microbiota in maintaining health comes from findings in germ-free animals that have reduced secretory IgA, defects in development of gut-associated lymphoid tissues and smaller Peyer's patches and mesenteric lymph nodes as compared to their conventional counterparts. IgA induced in response to colonization by specific commensal bacteria plays a fundamental role in mucosal immunity and in the protection of mucosal surfaces that contribute to host microbe mutualism. Normal nutrition, growth, and development are therefore severely compromised and the animal is far more susceptible to infection as compared with conventional animals (Clemente et al. 2012).

21.4 Dysbiosis

The composition of the intestinal microbiota of the otherwise stable gut microbiota fluctuates over time with intercurrent infections, treatment with oral antibiotics, stress, and aging. An alteration in the balance resulting in dysbiosis of the gut microbiota is being identified as a cause for clinical disease expression. A recent study in twins revealed that a reduced abundance of the commensal bacterium *Fecalibacterium prauznitzi* and an increased abundance of *Escherichia coli* species were associated with ileal Crohn's disease phenotype. Decreased diversity in infancy seems to be associated with an increased risk of atopic diseases later in childhood (Vael and Desager 2009). Decreased diversity of the gut microbiome is also a recurring theme in a variety of conditions that are potentially related to dysbiosis including chronic Inflammatory Bowel Disease (IBD) (Tannock 2008), chronic diarrhea, and necrotizing enterocolitis (NEC) (Swidsinski et al. 2008).

A new epoch is emerging with these findings in basic research and it is becoming clear that certain pathologies, which are associated with an altered microbiome are connected to disease and infection (Shanahan 2012).

21.5 From Microbiota to Probiotics

Because the microbiota represents a health asset with some of the microbial constituents becoming a liability, the rationale for using dietary interventions is to enhance the microbial assets and offset the liabilities. With scientific and clinical evidences having progressed rapidly for the possible role of probiotics in favorably modulating the gut microbiota and thereby manipulating its plasticity, there is both academic and clinical excitement in its utility for the improvement of health and prevention of disease (Simren and Dore 2012).

Probiotics are defined as live microorganisms which when administered in adequate amounts confer a health benefit to the host (FAO/WHO 2001). Operationally a probiotic may be defined as a of the beneficial effects of the gut microbiota and therefore probiotic therapy is in essence an attempt to harness the beneficial effects of the commensal microbiota for the host (Shanahan 2010).

21.6 Probiotic Selection

To exert their effect on the intestinal microbiota, it is generally accepted that a probiotic strain unless protected by a capsule should be intrinsically resistant to low pH, bile, and pancreatic enzymes and thus be able to survive transit through the gastrointestinal (GI) tract in numbers adequate enough to elicit a beneficial effect (Sorokulova 2008).

Just as all pills or tablets are not the same, all bacteria are not the same and all probiotics are not the same (Shanahan et al. 2012). Probiotics are defined by their genus, species, and strain and clubbing all probiotic bacteria of one genera and species together is a folly, some have no probiotic effect and those that do differ profoundly in their genotype and phenotype. Therefore, the effect of one probiotic strain cannot be extrapolated to another even if it belongs to the same genus and species. It is therefore important that each probiotic strain is supported by its own dossier of scientific evidence with relevant studies conducted using similar intervention levels as those recommended for daily consumption (Thomas and Versalovic 2010). The merit of employing a single organism versus a combination of probiotic strains also remains a point of ongoing contention even among experts in the field.

21.7 Probiotic Organisms

Many different species of bacteria as well as yeasts have been used as probiotics. The most common are Bifidobacteria and Lactobacilli; the latter are lactic acid bacteria that have been used for centuries in fermented foods. Currently, the yeast *Saccharomyces boulardii* and bacteria that comply with the current definition of probiotics including species of *Lactobacillus, Streptococcus, Entercoccus, Bifidobacterium, Propioniibacterium, Bacillus,* and *Escherichia coli* are being used as probiotics. Strictly speaking, the term probiotic is reserved for live microbes that have been shown to demonstrate a health benefit in controlled human studies.

21.8 Safety

Traditionally, lactic acid bacteria have been associated with food fermentation and are generally considered safe for oral consumption as a part of foods and supplements for the generally healthy population and at levels traditionally used. On the basis of the prevalence of *Lactobacilli* in fermented foods, as normal colonizers of the human body and given the low level of infection attributed to them, the safety of these microbes has been reviewed and their pathogenic potential is deemed to be quite low. However, some studies have highlighted that probiotics may be ill advised in specific patient populations, for example, where bacteremia, sepsis, and meningitis have been described on rare occasions in children and adults. It also remains to be determined whether patients with severe immune deficiencies could pose too great a risk for the development of serious complications (Gareau et al. 2010).

21.9 Quantities

There is no general minimal level for the probiotic count, the viable count is strain specific (Thomas and Versalovic 2010) and probably depends on the type of benefit sought by the administration of the probiotic. For example, *Bifidobacterium infantis* 35624 was effective in alleviating symptoms of irritable bowel syndrome (IBS) at 100 million CFU/day, whereas studies with VSL#3 have used sachets with 300–450 billion CFU/day (Guarner et al. 2012). It should also be noted that probiotics are transient colonizers, and therefore should be taken on a regular basis. They are only detected for limited periods of time after the end of consumption period.

21.10 Probiotic Mechanisms

Illuminating work during the past decade has highlighted that probiotic bacteria can exert their beneficial effect on the host through various mechanisms which range from their ability to antagonize pathogenic bacteria by reducing luminal pH, inhibiting bacterial adherence and translocation, or producing antibacterial substances such as bacteriocins and defensins. In addition, probiotics can influence mucosal cell–cell interactions and cellular stability by enhancement of intestinal barrier function and exerting their effects on numerous cell types involved in innate and adaptive immune responses such as epithelial cells, dendritic cells, monocytes/macrophages, B cells, T cells, and NK cells. Metabonomic studies have shown that probiotics can modulate the gut microbiome and the metabolism of short-chain fatty acids (SCFAs), amino acids, bile acids, and plasma lipoproteins demonstrating the diversity of symbiotic co-metabolic connections between the gut microbial content and the host (Gareau et al. 2010).

21.11 Clinical Evidence

Given that the intestinal tract is the largest reservoir of microbes in the human body, it is not surprising that the use of probiotic organisms in diseases has been investigated extensively in intestinal disorders. In general, the strongest clinical evidence for probiotics is related to their use in improving gut health and stimulating immune function.

21.11.1 Infectious Diarrhea

While research using probiotics has extended to a vast array of diseases, the most investigated field continues to remain infectious diarrhea and compelling evidence comes from randomized placebo-controlled trials (RCTs). The evidence from studies on viral diarrhea is however more convincing than from bacterial or parasitic infections. The rationale for using probiotics in acute infectious diarrhea is based on the assumption that they act against intestinal pathogens, synthesize antimicrobial substances, and competitively inhibit adhesion of pathogens.

A Cochrane review that included 63 randomized and quasi-randomized controlled trials that included 8014 participants concluded that probiotics reduced the duration of diarrhea although the size of the effect varied considerably between studies (Allen et al. 2010). Two RCTs evaluated probiotics for children with persistent diarrhea and reported dramatic reduction in diarrhea duration—4.8 and 3.9 days in Argentina (Gaon et al. 2003) and India (Basu et al. 2007), respectively. Two trials evaluated probiotics for diarrhea prevention, where children in Peru had 13% fewer diarrheal episodes after 15 months of receiving *Lactobacillus rhamnosus* GG (Oberhelman et al. 1999) whereas diarrhea frequency was reduced by 14% among children in India who received daily doses of *Lactobacillus casei* Shirota (LcS) for 12 weeks with a 12-week follow-up period (Sur et al. 2011).

The use of probiotics for acute infectious diarrhea in children is an accepted therapy in Europe. The European Society for Pediatric Gastroenterology, Hepatology and Nutrition and the European Society of Pediatric Infectious Diseases Expert Working group have stated that selected probiotics with proven clinical efficacy and in appropriate dosages according to the strain and population, may be used as an adjunct to conventional therapy for the management of acute gastroenteritis in children being given rehydration therapy (Guarino et al. 2008).

21.11.2 Antibiotic-Associated Diarrhea

The incidence of antibiotic-associated diarrhea (AAD) ranges between 1% and 44% and symptoms vary from mild episodes that resolve when antibiotics are stopped to serious complications. Risk is increased with extremes of age, comorbidity, and use of oral broad-spectrum antibiotics. Potentially probiotics maintain or restore gut microecology during or after antibiotic treatment through receptor competition, competition for nutrients, inhibition of epithelial and mucosal adherence of pathogens, stimulation of immunity or production of antimicrobial substances (Butler et al. 2012).

A meta-analysis of 34 masked, randomized, placebo-controlled trials, of which only one was community based from a developing country, revealed that probiotics significantly reduced the incidence of AAD by 52% (95% CI 35%–65%) (Sazawal et al. 2006). A very recent meta-analysis that included 82 RCTs revealed that the pooled relative risk in meta-analysis of 63 RCTs which included 11,811 participants indicated a statistically significant association of probiotic administration with reduction in AAD (RR −0.58, 95% CI 0.50–0.68; $p < 0.001$). The majority of trials used *Lactobacillus*-based interventions alone or in combination with other genera but the strains were poorly documented. Therefore, additional research is needed to determine which probiotics are associated with the greatest efficacy and the antibiotic against which the probiotic would be efficacious (Hempel et al. 2012). A recent study indicates that *L casei* strain Shirota (LcS) was useful in reducing the incidence of AAD in hospitalized spinal cord injury patients (Wong et al. 2014).

21.11.3 **Clostridium difficile** *Diarrhea*

More recently, the role of probiotics has extended to the prevention of *Clostridium difficile* diarrhea, which is responsible for around 10%–20% of all cases of AAD (Bartlett 2002). While the organism can remain latent in many patients, those receiving antibiotics have an increased risk of developing diarrhea and pseudomembranous colitis (Gerding et al. 1986). The three risk factors include antibiotic use, increasing age, and hospitalization. A recent meta-analysis showed that administration of probiotics led to a statistically significant relative risk reduction of *Clostridium difficile*-associated diarrhea (CDAD) by 71% (Avadhani and Miley 2011).

A systematic review and meta-analysis of 20 trials that included 3818 participants concluded that probiotics reduced the incidence of CDAD by 66% (pooled RR, 0.34, 95% CI 0.24–0.49). In a population with 5% incidence of antibiotic-associated CDAD (median control group risk), probiotic prophylaxis would prevent 33 episodes (95% CI 25–38 episodes) per 1000 persons. Of probiotic-treated patients, 9.3% experienced adverse events, compared with 12.6% of control patients (Johnston et al. 2012).

21.11.4 Constipation

Constipation is a common condition affecting children and adults. Differences in the intestinal microbiota between constipated and healthy children have been observed. In constipated children, the number of Bifidobacteria was lower than the number of nonpathogenic *E. coli*, Bacteroides, and the total number of organisms. It has also been reported that constipation predominant IBS patients showed increased amounts of *Veillonella* species (Van den Berg et al. 2006). The effect of probiotics on various forms of constipation has been explored only in a few studies and that too without controls. Constipation nevertheless has a significant impact on the quality of life and the beneficial effects of probiotics in the treatment of constipation appear promising. A recent meta-analysis of 5 RCTs with a total of 377 subjects of which 266 were adults and 111 were children concluded that *Bifidobacterium lactis* DN-173010, *L casei* Shirota and *E. coli* Nissle 1917 had a favorable effect on defecation frequency and stool consistency in adults and *Lb. caseirhamnosus* Lcr35 had a positive impact on children (Chmielewska and Szajewska 2010).

The role of LcS in the improvement of symptoms of constipation has further been underpinned in two randomized controlled trials which showed that regular consumption of LcS improved both the defecation frequency and stool consistency after 2 weeks of intervention of the probiotic. The beneficial effects on constipation may be explained due to various mechanisms including changes in the composition of the intestinal flora, changes in metabolites of bacterial fermentation resulting in enhanced motility, and shortening of intestinal transit time (Koebnick et al. 2003, Krammer et al. 2011).

21.11.5 Irritable Bowel Syndrome

Irritable bowel syndrome (IBS) is the most common GI disorder thought to affect at least 15% of the population. It is a heterogeneous condition often diagnosed by exclusion of other underlying diseases including IBD. Disease risk factors include those that disturb the gut microbiota such as antibiotics, gastrointestinal surgery, and infection. Differences in the gut microbiota are evident in IBS sufferers and controls, with the former demonstrating significantly lower concentrations of Bifidobacteria and Lactobacilli and higher concentrations of Streptococci, *E. coli*, and *Clostridia*. Such observations have encouraged investigations of the potential role of probiotics in this disorder. A wide range of strains and dosages have been studied with *Lactobacilli, Bifidobacteria,* and *Streptococcus* being the most widely researched (Barrett et al. 2008).

A meta-analysis (McFarland and Dublin 2008) reviewed 20 IBS trials and reported that probiotic use was associated with improvement of IBS symptoms compared to controls, particularly for less abdominal pain; however, more data are needed. A review of 19 randomized controlled clinical trials (Moayyedi et al. 2010) that included 1650 patients with IBS concluded that probiotics were better than placebo [relative risk of IBS not improving 0.71 (95% CI 0.57–0.88) with a number needed to treat 4 (95% CI 3.0–12.5)]. In another review of 42 RCTs (Clarke et al. 2012) for the effect of probiotic bacteria on IBS symptoms, 34 trials reported benefit in at least one of the endpoints studied.

In yet another 16 strictly selected RCTs (Brenner et al. 2009), it was found that 11 studies were inadequately blinded, of too short duration, of too small sample size, and/or lacked intention-to-treat analysis. It was concluded that only two of the studies showed significant improvement in abdominal pain/discomfort, bloating/distension, and/or bowel movements as compared with placebo (O'Mohanny et al. 2005, Whorwell et al. 2006). Several mechanisms of activity may be involved including a change in the intestinal microbiota resulting in lower numbers of potentially harmful bacteria and less gas production, increased SCFAs and fecal microbiota mass, and better bile acid metabolism (Moayyedi et al. 2010).

In the above studies, various Lactobacilli species when taken either alone or coadministered with bifidobacteria resulted in an improvement in symptoms in patients with IBS (Moayyedi et al. 2010). However, given the heterogeneity of IBS, research that focuses on the use of probiotics for specific IBS subgroups for specific IBS-related symptoms is probably the best way forward.

21.11.6 Inflammatory Bowel Disorder

Although no single enteric pathogen is associated with the development of the disease, changes in the gut microbiota have been associated with IBD. Adherent-invasive E. coli (AIEC) strains isolated from Crohn's disease have the ability to bind to and invade intestinal epithelial cells (Gareau et al. 2010). The intestinal microbiota in patients with IBD seems to drive an overactive immune response which leads to disease expression and concurrent morbidity. The potential for probiotics to modulate the microbiota, provide beneficial immunomodulatory effectors, and restore epithelial barrier defects suggests that a probiotic strategy might prove a viable future treatment option for patients with IBD (Gareau et al. 2010). Benefit has been reported in some, but not all human trials. Investigations have focused mostly on remission maintenance rather than treatment of active disease, with evidence strongest for pouchitis > ulcerative colitis > Crohn's disease.

Early success with VSL#3 was reported to significantly reduce pouchitis recurrence (Gionchetti et al. 2003). For ulcerative colitis, benefits have been described for a combination of *Lactobacillus*, *Bifidobacterium*, and *Streptococcus* probiotic species or for *E. coli* Nissle in inducing and maintaining remission of disease activity in mild-to-moderately severe ulcerative colitis (UC). Treatment with *E. coli* Nissle 1917 alone has been reported to be as effective as mesalazine in maintaining UC remission (Kruis et al. 2004, Sanders et al. 2013). Combined probiotic treatment has also been shown to help with diverticulitis. Studies of probiotics in Crohn's disease have been disappointing with the Cochrane Systematic Review concluding that there is no evidence to suggest that probiotics are beneficial for the maintenance of remission in Crohn's disease (Butterworth et al. 2008).

21.11.7 Eradication of Helicobacter pylori

This pathogen is associated with chronic gastritis, peptic ulcer, and gastric cancer. Animal studies have shown some benefit with *Lactobacilli* probiotic because lactic acid is more inhibitory to pathogens than acetic or hydrochloric acid (Midolo et al. 1995). A recent meta-analysis of 14 randomized trials suggests that supplementation of anti-*H. pylori* antibiotic regimens with certain probiotics may also be effective in increasing eradication rates and may be considered helpful for patients with eradication failure (Guarner et al. 2012). There is currently insufficient evidence to support the concept that a probiotic alone without concomitant antibiotic therapy would be effective. They may be helpful as adjuvant therapy with antibiotics for the eradication of *H. pylori* infection (Sykora et al. 2005).

21.11.8 Necrotizing Enterocolitis

Necrotizing enterocolitis (NEC) is a major cause of morbidity and mortality in premature infants; the etiology of the disease has yet not been fully clarified. The rationale for probiotic supplementation in preterms is based on the fact that they have a restricted number of species with typically only three bacterial species found at 10 days of age which include enterobacteria such as *E. coli* and *Klebsiella* species, Enterococci, that is, *Enterococcus fecalis* and Staphylocococci such as *Staphylococcus aureus, Staphylococcus hemolyticus*, and *Staphylococcus epidermidis* (Gewolb et al. 1999). All these facultative anaerobes persist at high levels in the fecal flora of preterm infants which is a key feature of intestinal microbiota in preterm infants compared with healthy counterparts. Moreover, the immature intestine of preterm infants is especially prone to inflammation and loss of epithelial integrity. Since probiotics have the potential to interfere with this progression, they have been tested clinically for NEC (Sanders et al. 2013).

A systematic review reported in 2007 identified 7 RCTs and found that most of the investigated probiotics might reduce the risk of NEC in preterm neonates with <33 weeks of gestation. Risk of sepsis did not differ significantly among groups (Deshpande et al. 2007). Similarly, the Cochrane review published in 2008 found that enteral supplementation of certain probiotics reduced the risk of severe NEC and mortality in preterm infants born <1500 g (Alfaleh and Bassler 2008). It has also been suggested that enteral administration of probiotics to preterm newborn could prevent infections and NEC and reduce the use of antibiotics (Caplan and Jilling 2000). Although the American Academy of Pediatrics recognizes that there is evidence that probiotics prevent NEC in very low birth weight infants they call for more studies to clarify the effective dose and strain of probiotic before issuing a clinical recommendation. The efficacy and safety of probiotic supplementation in premature infants <1000 g needs to be well defined (Wolvers et al. 2010).

21.11.9 Hepatic Encephalopathy

Recent studies suggest that the composition of the gut microbiome is linked with cognition in patients with liver disease (Davila et al. 2013). An increase in Veillonellaceae was found in cirrhotics with hepatic encephalopathy compared with those without encephalopathy (Bajaj et al. 2013). Minimal hepatic encephalopathy was reversed in 50% of patients treated with a symbiotic preparation (4 probiotic strains and 4 fermentable fibers, including inulin and resistant starch) for 30 days (Shukla et al. 2011). However, there is insufficient data for the regular use of probiotics in hepatic encephalopathy.

21.11.10 Prevention of Cancer

The possible involvement of intestinal microbiota in colonic carcinogenesis comes from the fact that proteolytic Clostridia and Bacteroides have higher levels of carcinogenic enzymes compared to Lactobacilli and Bifidobacteria, and certain intestinal species produce harmful metabolites (Commane et al. 2005). Many probiotic mechanisms of activity are relevant to cancer, prompting studies which have generally used biomarkers to evaluate benefit. An EU funded SYNCAN study tested the effect of oligofructose plus two probiotic strains in patients at risk of developing colonic cancer (Van Loo et al. 2005). The results of the study suggest that a symbiotic preparation can decrease the expression of biomarkers for colorectal cancer.

In a large intervention trial on 398 subjects who had at least two colorectal tumors removed and were given wheat bran, LcS and wheat bran or LcS alone it was observed that the probiotic alone was associated with a significant reduction of the rate of progression of new tumors, but did not reduce their incidence (Ishikawa et al. 2005). In a case-controlled study (Ohashi et al. 2002), a group of 180 bladder cancer cases were compared with 445 population matched controls in relation to the consumption of LcS over the past 10–15 years. The authors concluded a negative correlation. This was supported by a 1-year placebo-controlled intervention trial with 58 patients who had previously had surgery for superficial bladder cancer. Intake of LcS was associated with a significantly reduced recurrence rate (Aso et al. 1992). Similar results were found in larger studies with 125 and 207 patients (Aso et al. 1995, Naito et al. 2008). A recent population-based case-controlled study of 306 cases with breast cancer and 662 control aged 40–55 years concluded that regular consumption of beverages containing *L casei* strain Shirota (BLS) and isoflavones since adolescence were inversely associated with the incidence of breast cancer in Japanese women (Toi et al. 2013).

21.11.11 Allergy and Atopic Diseases in Children

The so-called hygiene hypothesis (Strachan 1989) has suggested that a decreased microbial diversity in infancy seems to be associated with an increased risk of atopic disease later in childhood. This is mostly due to smaller families, better household amenities, and higher standards of personal cleanliness, which result in an imbalanced Th1:Th2 immune response (Guarner 2007). It has been suggested that in countries where there is an increasing trend for cesarean section, the resultant early adverse effects on biodiversity of the infant's intestinal bacteria can be linked to an increasing incidence of common childhood diseases like asthma. More recently, it has been shown that babies delivered by cesarean section may be at an increased risk of developing obesity in early childhood.

L rhamnosus GG was administered to pregnant women 1 month before delivery and to the babies for 6 months after birth (Kalliomaki et al. 2001). Incidence of atopic eczema during the first 4 years was reduced to 50% in the probiotic group compared to those on placebo (Kalliomaki et al. 2003). Even 7 years later, the children's risk of developing eczema was significantly lower although the difference was less (Kalliomaki et al. 2007). Several studies have shown a persistent and significantly reduced rate of atopic dermatitis for up to 7 years following probiotic consumption (Folster-Holst 2010, Shane et al. 2010). However, no effect on the expression of asthma later in childhood has been observed. Rhinitis studies have also given mixed results.

Unfortunately, the enormous heterogeneity of studies, strains, duration of therapy, and doses used does not allow the drawing of a univocal interpretation.

21.11.12 Respiratory Infections

Recent studies have provided positive results on the effects of probiotics on the respiratory system, especially with regard to prevention, and to reducing the severity of respiratory infections due to an increase in the IgA-secreting cells in the bronchial mucosa (Aureli et al. 2011). Positive effects were found in regular smokers usually affected by reduced NK cell activity (Morimoto et al. 2005).

21.11.13 Obesity and Diabetes

Recent insights have suggested that microbiota play a crucial role in the pathogenesis of metabolic syndrome resulting in a paradigm shift in our approach to battle the obesity and diabetes syndrome (Parekh et al. 2014). Both these conditions are associated with divergent changes in the gut microbiota. The gut microbiome in obese rodents and humans has shown an overall decrease in microbial diversity with an increase in the phylum Firmicutes and a decrease in phylum Bacteroidetes (Hildebrandt et al. 2009). Two recent studies (Ma et al. 2008, Kadooka et al. 2010) have revealed that probiotics may have a beneficial influence on metabolic disorders by lowering effects on abdominal adiposity, body weight, and other measures. It has been suggested that an altered intestinal microbiota leads to an increased intestinal permeability and mucosal immune response contributing to the development of diabetes. Evidence available from experimental studies and clinical trials point to the fact that modulation of intestinal microbiota by probiotics may be effective toward prevention and management of type 1 and type 2 diabetes (Gomes et al. 2014).

21.12 Microbiota–Gut–Brain Axis

Dysbiosis of the enteric milieu is marked by an increase in anxiety, depressive behavior, and memory impairment along with decreased concentration of key neurotrophic factors involved in plasticity like the brain-derived neurotrophic factor (BDNF) (Neufeld et al. 2011). Recent findings have revealed that the vagus nerve is an important mediator of microbiota–gut–brain interaction and may depend on the bacterial strain used. The exact modalities of how the vagus nerve interacts with the microbiota to induce such effects remains unclear (Bercik et al. 2011a). It has been observed albeit in relatively small cohorts that autistic spectrum disorders may be associated with an alteration in microbiota composition and metabolism (Critchfield et al. 2011, Mulle et al. 2013). Preclinical data support the concept that probiotics affect enteric nervous system and brain signaling; and the beneficial effects of probiotics on visceral nociceptive reflexes in rodents have also been described. However, larger clinical trials need to be conducted to point to the benefit of probiotics in preventing neurological disorders.

21.13 What to Expect?

It is important to remember that probiotics are not drugs; they are not alternatives or substitutes for conventional therapy. They are in fact supplements and like many naturally occurring agents modest benefits should be expected when used as adjuncts with conventional therapy. The challenge in nutritional science is not to tackle disease with a pharmaceutical approach but rather to maintain health and thereby reduce the risk of disease. Instead of testing clinical end points of reduction in disease, it is the markers of risk of disease that need to be checked and validated in nutritional intervention studies.

21.14 A Glimpse into the Future

With the microbiota of a number of diseases being currently examined to identify potential co-relations, the promise of microbiome research relies largely on the future of probiotics. Probiotic research aims to find single interventions with beneficial effects on multiple health conditions by impacting the plasticity of the gut microbiota. More research, bigger and better clinical trials, and enhanced understanding of the host microbe in health and disease will pave the way for probiotic progress. Although, the Indian market is still nascent in capturing the understanding and need for the category, the increasing scientific credibility and the new emerging holistic concept of health that focuses on promoting good health rather than focusing on the manifestations of ill health will see the probiotic category advance as an important functional food for promoting and maintaining good health.

References

Alfaleh, K. and Bassler, D. 2008. Probiotics for prevention of necrotizing enterocolitis in preterm infants. *Cochrane Database Syst Rev* 23(1): CD005496. doi: 10:1002/14651858.CD005496.

Allen, S.J., Martinez, E.G., Gregori, G.V., and Dans, L.F. 2010. Probiotics for treating infectious diarrhoea. *Cochrane Database of Syst Rev* 10: CD003048.

Aso, Y. and Akazan, H. 1992. Prophylactic effect of a *Lactobacillus casei* preparation on the recurrence of superficial bladder cancer. *Urol Int* 49: 125–129.

Aso, Y., Akaza, H., Kotake, T. et al. 1995. Preventive effect of a *Lactobacillus casei* preparation on the recurrence of superficial bladder cancer in a double blind trial. *Eur Urol* 27: 104–109.

Aureli, P., Capurso, L., Castellazzi, A.M. et al. 2011. Probiotics and health: An evidence-based review. *Pharmacological Research* 63: 366–376.

Avadhani, A. and Miley, H. 2011. Probiotics for prevention of antibiotic-associated diarrhea and *Clostridium difficile*-associated disease in hospitalized adults—A meta-analysis. *J Am Acad Nurse Pract* 23: 269–274.

Bajaj, J.S., Heuman, D.M., Sanyal, A.J. et al. 2013. Modulation of the metabiome by rifaximin in patients with cirrhosis and minimal hepatic encephalopathy. *PLoS ONE* 8: e60042.

Barrett, J.S., Canale, K.E.K., Gearry, R.B. et al. 2008. Probiotic effects on intestinal fermentation patterns in patients with irritable bowel syndrome. *World J Gastroenterol* 14(32): 5020–5024.

Bartlett, J.G. 2002. Clinical practice: Antibiotic associated diarrhea. *N Engl J Med* 346: 334–339.

Basu, S., Chatterjee, M., Ganguly, S. et al. 2007. Effect of *Lactobacillus rhamnosus* GG in persistent diarrhoea in Indian children: A randomized controlled trial. *J Clin Gastroenterol* 41: 756–760.

Bercik, P., Denou, E., Collins, J. et al. 2011a. The intestinal microbiota affect central levels of brain-derived neurotropic factor and behaviour in mice. *Gastroenterology* 141: 599–609.

Brenner, D.M., Moeller, M.J., Chey, W.D. et al. 2009. The utility of probiotics in the treatment of irritable bowel syndrome: A systematic review. *Am J Gastroenterol* [Review] 104: 1033–1049.

Butler, C.C., Duncan, D., and Hood, K. 2012. Does taking probiotics routinely with antibiotics prevent antibiotic associated diarrhea? *BMJ* 344: e682.

Butterworth, A.D., Thomas, A.G. Akobeng, A.K. 2008. Probiotics for induction of remission in Crohn's disease (Review). *Cochrane Database Syst.* Rev 3: CD006634.

Caplan, M.S. and Jilling, T. 2000. Neonatal necrotizing enterocolitis: Possible role of probiotic supplementation. *J Pediatr Gastroenterol Nutr* 30: Suppl 2: S18–S22.

Chmielewska, A. and Szajewska, H. 2010. Systematic review of randomised controlled trials: Probiotics for functional constipation. *World J Gastroenterol* 16(1): 69–75.

Chow, J., Lee, S.M., Shen, Y., Khosravi, A., and Mazmanian, S.K. 2010. Host-bacterial symbiosis in health and disease. *Adv Immunol* 107: 243–274.

Clarke, G., Cryan, J.F., Dinan, T.G. et al. 2012. Review article: Probiotics for the treatment of irritable bowel syndrome—focus on lactic acid bacteria. *Aliment Pharmacol Ther*[Research Support, Non-U.S. Gov't Review] 35: 403–413.

Clemente, J.C., Ursell, L.K., Parfrey, L.W., and Knight, R. 2012. The impact of the gut microbiota on human health: An integrative view. *Cell* 148: 1258–1270.

Commane, D.1., Hughes, R., Shortt, C., and Rowland, I. 2005. The potential mechanisms involved in the anti-carcinogenic action of probiotics. *Mutant Res* 11: 591(1–2): 276–289.

Critchfield, J.W., van Hemert, S., Ash, M., Mulder, L., and Ashwood, P. 2011. The potential role of probiotics in the management of childhood autism spectrum disorders. *Gastroenterol Res Pract* 2011: 161358.

Davila, A.M., Blachier, F., Gotteland, M. et al. 2013. Re-print of "Intestinal luminal nitrogen metabolism: Role of the gut microbiota and consequences for the host." *Pharmacol Res* 69:114–126.

Deshpande, G., Rao, S., and Patole, S. 2007. Probiotics for prevention of necrotizing enterocolitis in preterm neonates with very low birthweight: A systematic review of randomised controlled trials. *Lancet* 369: 1614–1620.

FAO/WHO. Health and nutritional properties of probiotics in food including powder milk with live lactic acid bacteria. 2001. Available at: http://www.who.int/foodsafety/publications/fs_management/en/probiotics.pdf. Accessed June 4, 2012.

Folster-Holst, R. 2010. Probiotics in the treatment and prevention of atopic dermatitis. *Ann Nutr Metab* 57: 16–19.

Gaon, D., Garcia, H., Winter, L. et al. 2003. Effect of *Lactobacillus* strains and *Saccharomyces boulardii* on persistent diarrhoea in children. *Medicina (B Aires)* 63: 293–298.

Gareau, M.G., Sherman, P.M., and Walker, W.A. 2010. Probiotics and the gut microbiota in intestinal health and disease. *Nat Rev Gastroenterol Hepatol* 7(9): 503–514.

Gerding, D.N., Olson, M.M., Peterson, L.R. et al. 1986.*Clostridium difficile*-associated diarrhea and colitis in adults. A prospective case-controlled epidemiologic study. *Arch Intern Med* 146: 95–100.

Gewolb, I.H., Schwalbe, R.S., Taciak, V.L., Harrison, T.S., and Panigrahi, P. 1999. Stool microflora in extremely low birthweight infants. *Arch Dis Child Fetal Neonatal Ed* 80: F167–F173.

Gionchetti, P., Rizzello, F., Helwig, U., Venturi, A., Lammers, K.M., Brigidi, P., Vitali, B., Poggioli, G., Miglioli, M., and Campieri, M. 2003. Prophylaxis of pouchitis onset with probiotic therapy: A double-blind, placebo-controlled trial. *Gastroenterology* 124(5): 1202–1209.

Gomes, A.C., Bueno, A.A. et al. 2014. Gut microbiota, Probiotics and diabetes. *Nutr J* 13(1): 60.

Guarino, A., Albano, F., Ashkenazi, S., Gendrel, D., Hoekstra, J.H., Shamir, R., and Szajewska, H. 2008. European Society for Paediatric Gastroenterology, Hepatology and Nutrition/European Society for Paediatric Infectious Diseases evidence-based guidelines for the management of acute gastroenteritis in children in Europe: Executive summary. *J Pediatr Gastroenterol Nutr* 46: 619–621.

Guarner, F. 2007. Hygiene, microbial diversity and immune regulation. *Curr Opin Gastroenterol* 23(6): 667–672.

Guarner, F., Khan, A.G., Garisch, J. et al. 2012. World gastroenterology organisation global guidelines: Probiotics and prebiotics October 2011. *J Clin Gastroenterol* 46(6): 468–481.

Hempel, S., Newberry, S.J., Maher, A.R. et al. 2012. Probiotics for the prevention and treatment of antibiotic-associated diarrhea. *JAMA* 307(18): 1959–1969.

Hildebrandt, M.A., Hoffmann, C., Sherrill-Mix, S.A. et al. 2009. High-fat diet determines the composition of the murine gut microbiome independently of obesity. *Gastroenterology* 137(5): e1–e2. doi:10.1053/j.gastro.2009.08.042.

IMARC Group. Dairy Industry in India: 2013–2019. http://www.digitaljournal.com/pr/1829000

Ishikawa, H., Akedo, I., Otani, T. et al. 2005. Randomized trial of dietary fiber and *Lactobacillus casei* administration for prevention of colorectal tumors. *Int J Cancer* 116: 762–767.

Johnston, B.C., Ma, S.S., Goldenberg, J.Z. et al. 2012. Probiotics for the prevention of *Clostridium difficile*-associated diarrhea: A systematic review and meta-analysis. *Ann Intern Med* 157(12): 878–888.

Kadooka, Y. et al. 2010. Regulation of abdominal adiposity by probiotics (*Lactobacillus gasseri* SBT2055) in adults with obese tendencies in a randomized controlled trial. *Eur J Clin Nutr* 64(6): 636–643.

Kalliomaki, M., Salminen, S., Arvilommi, H., Kero, P., Koskinen, P., and Isolauri, E. 2001. Probiotics in primary prevention of atopic disease: A randomised placebo controlled trial. *Lancet* 357: 1076–1079.

Kalliomaki, M., Salminen, S., Poussa, T. et al. 2003. Probiotics and prevention of atopic disease: 4-year follow-up of a randomised placebo-controlled trial. *Lancet* 361: 1869–1871.

Kalliomaki, M., Salminen, S., Poussa, T., and Isolauri, E. 2007. Probiotics during the first 7 years of life: A cumulative risk reduction of eczema in a randomized, placebo controlled trial. *J Allergy Clin Immunol* 119: 1019–1021.

Koebnick, C., Wagner, I., Leitsmann, P., Stern, U., and Zunfit, H.J.F. 2003. Probiotic beverage containing *Lactobacillus casei* Shirota improves gastrointestinal symptoms in patients with chronic constipation. *Can J Gastroenterol* 17(11): 655–659.

Krammer, H.J. et al. 2011. Effect of *Lactobacillus casei* Shirota on colonic transit time in patients with chronic constipation. *Coloproctology* 33: 109–113.

Kruis, W., Fric, P., Pokrotnieks, J. et al. 2004. Maintaining remission ofulcerative colitis with the probiotic *Escherichia coli* Nissle 1917 is as effective as with standard mesalazine. *Gut* 53(11): 1617–1623.

Ma, X, Hua, J., Li, Z. 2008. Probiotics improve high fat diet-induced hepatic steatosis and insulin resistance by increasing hepatic NKT cells. *J Hepatol* 49(5): 821–830.

McFarland, L.V. and Dublin, S. 2008. Meta-analysis of probiotics for the treatment of irritable bowel syndrome. *World J Gastroenterol* 14(17): 2650–2661.

Metahit. Metagnomics of the human intestinal tract; 2009. http://www.metahit.eu/fileadmin/Content/Management_Files/Periodic_Report/First_periodic_MetaHIT_report_extended_summarypdf.

Midolo, P.D., Lambert, J.R., Hull, R., Luo, F., and Grayson, M.L. 1995. *In vitro* inhibition of *Helicobacter pylori* NCTC 11637 by organic acids and lactic acid bacteria. *J Appl Bacteriol* 79(4): 475–479.

Moayyedi, P., Ford, A.C., Talley, N.J. et al. 2010. The efficacy of probiotics in the treatment of irritable bowel syndrome: A systematic review. *Gut* 59: 325–332.

Morimoto, K., Takeshita, K., Nanno, M., Tokudome, S., and Nakayama, K. 2005. Modulation of natural killer cell activity by supplementation of fermented milk containing *Lactobacillus casei* in habitual smokers. *Prev Med* 40: 589–594.

Mulle, J.G., Sharp, W.G., and Cubells, J.F. 2013. The gut microbiome: A new frontier in autism research. *Curr Psychiatry Rep* 15: 337.

Naito, S., Koga, H., Yamaguchi, A. et al. 2008. Prevention of Recurrence with Epirubicin and *Lactobacillus casei* after transurethral resection of bladder cancer. *J Urol* 179: 485–490.

Neufeld, K.M., Kang, N., Bienenstock, J., and Foster, J.A. 2011. Reduced anxiety-like behavior and central neurochemical change in germ-free mice. *Neurogastroenterol Motil* 23: 255–264.

Nissle, S. 1916.Ueber die Grundlageneinerneuenursaechlichen Bekaempfungderpathologischen Darmflora. *Dtsch Med Wochenschr* 42: 1181–1184.

Oberhelman, R.A., Gilman, R.H., Sheen, P. et al. 1999. A placebo-controlled trial of *Lactobacillus* GG to prevent diarrhoea in undernourished Peruvian children. *J Pediatr* 134: 15–20.

Ohashi, Y., Nakai, S., Tsukamoto, T. et al. 2002. Habitual intake of lactic acid bacteria and risk reduction of bladder cancer. *UrolInt* 68: 273–280.

O'Mohanny, L., McCarthy, J., Kelly, P. et al. 2005. *Lactobacillus* and *Bifidobacterium* in irritable bowel syndrome: Symptom responses and relationship to cytokine profiles. *Gastroenterology* [Clinical Trial Randomised Controlled Trial Research Support, Non-U.S. Gov't] 128: 541–551.

Parekh, P.J., Arusi, E., Vinik, A.I., and Johnson, D.A. 2014. The role and influence of gut microbiota in pathogenesis and management of obesity and metabolic syndrome. *Front Endocrinol* (Lausanne) 5: 47.

Qin, J., Li, R., Raes, J. et al. 2010. MetaHIT Consortium. A human gut microbial gene catalogue established by metagenomic sequencing. *Nature* 464: 59–65.

Sanders, M.E., Guarner, F., Guerrant, R. et al. 2013. An update on the use and investigation of Probiotics in health and disease. *Gut* 62: 787–796.

Sazawal, S., Hiremath, G., Dhingra, U., Malik, P., Deb, S., and Black, R.E. 2006. Efficacy of probiotics in prevention of acute diarrhea: A meta-analysis of masked, randomised, placebo-controlled trials. *Lancet Infect Dis* 6: 374–382.

Scott, H. P. 2012. Metchnikoff and the microbiome. *Lancet* 380(9856): 1810–1811.

Shanahan, F. 2010. Probiotics in perspective. *Gastroenterology* 139: 1808–1812.

Shanahan, F. 2012. The gut microbiota—A clinical perspective on lessons learned. *Nat Rev Gastroenterol Hepatol* 9: 609–614.

Shanahan, F., Dinan, T.G., Ross, P., and Hill, C. 2012. Probiotics in transition. *Clin Gastroenterol Hepatol* 10: 1220–1224.

Shane, A.L., Cabana, M.D., Vidry, S. et al. 2010. Guide to designing, conducting, publishing and communicating results of clinical studies involving probiotic applications in human participants. *Gut Microbes* 1: 243–253.

Sharon, I. and Banfield, J.F. 2013. Microbiology. Genomes from metagenomics. *Science* 342(6162): 1057–1058.
Shukla, S., Shukla, A., Mehboob, S., and Guha, S. 2011. Meta-analysis: The effects of gut flora modulation using prebiotics, probiotics and synbiotics on minimal hepatic encephalopathy. *Aliment Pharmacol Ther* 33: 662–671.
Simren, M. and Dore, J. 2012. Gut microbiota for health—current insights and understanding. *Eur Gastroenterol Hepatol Rev* 8(2): 77–81.
Sorokulova, I. 2008. Preclinical testing in the development of probiotics: A regulatory perspective with *Bacillus* strains as an example. *Clin Infect Dis* 46(Suppl. 2): S92–S95.
Strachan, D.P. 1989. Hay fever, hygiene and household size. *BMJ* 299(6710): 1259–1260.
Sur, D., Manna, B., Niyogi, S.K. et al. 2011. Role of probiotic in preventing acute diarrhoea in children: A community-based, randomized, double-blind placebo-controlled field trial in an urban slum. *Epidemiol Infect* [Randomized Controlled Trial Research Support, Non-U.S. Gov't] 139: 919–926.
Swidsinski, A., Loening-Baucke, V., Verstraelen, H., Osowska, S., and Doerffel, Y. 2008. Biostructure of fecal microbiota in healthy subjects and patients with chronic idiopathic diarrhea. *Gastroenterology* 135: 568–579.
Sykora, J., Valeckova, K., Amlerova, J. et al. 2005. Effects of a specially designed fermented milk product containing probiotic *Lactobacillus casei* DN-114 001 and the eradication of *H. pylori* in children: A prospective randomized double-blind study. *J Clin Gastroenterol* 39: 692–698.
Tannock, G.W. 2008. Molecular analysis of the intestinal microflora in IBD. *Mucosal Immunol* 1(Suppl 1): S15–S18.
Thomas, C.M. and Versalovic, J. 2010. Probiotics-host communication: Modulation of signalling pathways in the intestine. *Gut Microbes* 1: 1–16.
Toi, M., Hirota, S., Tomotaki, Ai. et al. 2013. Probiotic beverage with soy isoflavone consumption for breast cancer prevention: A case–control study. *Curr Nutr Food Sci* 9: 194–200.
Turnbaugh, P.J., Ley, R.E., Hamady, M., Fraser-Liggett, C.M., Knight. R., and Gordon, J.I. 2007. The human microbiome project. *Nature* 449: 804–810.
Vael, C. and Desager, K. 2009. The importance of the development of the intestinal microbiota in infancy. *Curr Opin Pediatr* 21: 794–800.
Van den Berg, M.M., Benninga, M.A., and Di Lorenzo, C. 2006. Epidemiology of childhood constipation: A systematic review. *Am J Gastroenterol* 101: 2401–2409.
Van Loo, J., Clune, Y., Bennett, M., and Collins, J.K. 2005. The SYNCAN project: Goals, set-up, first results and settings of the human intervention study. *Br J Nutr* 93(Suppl 1): S91–S98.
Whorwell, P.J., Altringer, L., Morel, J. et al. 2006. Efficacy of an encapsulated probiotic *Bifidobacterium infantis* 35624 in women with irritable bowel syndrome. *Am J Gastroenterol* [multicenter Study Randomized Controlled Trial Research Support, Non-U.S. Gov't] 101: 1581–1590.
Wolvers, D., Antoine, J.M., Myllyluoma, E. et al. 2010. Guidance for substantiating the evidence for beneficial effects of probiotics: Prevention and management of infections by probiotics. *J Nutr* 140: 698S–712S.
Wong, S., Jamous, A. et al. 2014. A *Lactobacillus casei* Shirota probiotic drink reduces antibiotic-associated diarrhoea in patients with spinal cord injuries: A randomised control trial. *Br J Nutr* 111(4): 672–678.

Index

D

E

F

I

M

N

O

Q

R

S

T

U

V